SECOND EDITION

FORENSIC NURSING

A Handbook for Practice

Edited by

Rita M. Hammer, PhD, RN, BC
Professor of Nursing, Retired
New Smyrna Beach, Florida

Barbara Moynihan, PhD, APRN, BC, AFN
Professor of Nursing
Quinnipiac University
Hamden, Connecticut

Elaine M. Pagliaro, JD, MS
Forensic Scientist
Henry C. Lee Institute of Forensic Science
University of New Haven
West Haven, Connecticut

JONES & BARTLETT
LEARNING

D1716554

World Headquarters
Jones & Bartlett Learning
5 Wall Street
Burlington, MA 01803
978-443-5000
info@jblearning.com
www.jblearning.com

Jones & Bartlett Learning books and products are available through most bookstores and online book-sellers. To contact Jones & Bartlett Learning directly, call 800-832-0034, fax 978-443-8000, or visit our website, www.jblearning.com.

Substantial discounts on bulk quantities of Jones & Bartlett Learning publications are available to corporations, professional associations, and other qualified organizations. For details and specific discount information, contact the special sales department at Jones & Bartlett Learning via the above contact information or send an email to specialsales@jblearning.com.

The authors, editors, and publisher have made every effort to provide accurate information. However, they are not responsible for errors, omissions, or for any outcomes related to the use of the contents of this book and take no responsibility for the use of the products and procedures described. Treatments and side effects described in this book may not be applicable to all people; likewise, some people may require a dose or experience a side effect that is not described herein. Drugs and medical devices are discussed that may have limited availability controlled by the Food and Drug Administration (FDA) for use only in a research study or clinical trial. Research, clinical practice, and government regulations often change the accepted standard in this field. When consideration is being given to use of any drug in the clinical setting, the health care provider or reader is responsible for determining FDA status of the drug, reading the package insert, and reviewing prescribing information for the most up-to-date recommendations on dose, precautions, and contraindications, and determining the appropriate usage for the product. This is especially important in the case of drugs that are new or seldom used.

Production Credits
Publisher: Kevin Sullivan
Acquisitions Editor: Amanda Harvey
Editorial Assistant: Sara Bempkins
Associate Production Editor: Sara Fowles
Associate Marketing Manager: Katie Hennessy
V.P., Manufacturing and Inventory Control: Therese Connell
Composition: Paw Print Media
Cover Design: Kristin E. Parker
Cover Image: © Cammeraydave/Dreamstime.com
Printing and Binding: Malloy, Inc.
Cover Printing: Malloy, Inc.

Some images in this book feature models. These models do not necessarily endorse, represent, or participate in the activities represented in the images.

Library of Congress Cataloging-in-Publication Data
Forensic nursing: a handbook for practice/[edited by] Rita M. Hammer, Barbara Moynihan, Elaine M. Pagliaro. — 2nd ed.
p. ; cm.
Includes bibliographical references and index.
ISBN 978-0-7637-9200-8 (pbk.)
I. Hammer, Rita M. II. Moynihan, Barbara. III. Pagliaro, Elaine M.
[DNLM: 1. Forensic Nursing. 2. Mandatory Reporting. WY 170]
LC classification not assigned
614'.1—dc23
                            2011031935

6048

Printed in the United States of America
23 22 21   10 9 8 7 6 5 4

Contents

PART I: FOUNDATIONS

PART II: POPULATIONS

PART III: PRACTICAL ASPECTS OF FORENSIC NURSING

PART IV: SPECIALIZED FORENSIC NURSING ROLES

PART V: CONCEPTS FOR THE 21ST CENTURY

Foreword

In 1994, I authored federal legislation for the Violence Against Women Act that provided 1.6 billion dollars over 5 years to state and local authorities and victim service providers for the investigation, prosecution, treatment, and prevention of domestic violence, sexual assault, and stalking. This Act was reauthorized in 2000 and in 2005 providing an additional $3.33 and $3.935 billion, respectively, for each 5-year period. I also overhauled our nation's federal criminal laws to better prosecute these crimes. Significantly, the Violence Against Women Act mandated the Attorney General to evaluate and recommend standards for training and practice for licensed health care professionals performing sexual assault forensic exams.

In the course of drafting the Violence Against Women Act, I became aware of the critical work sexual assault forensic nurses do in our country's hospitals. I learned that these nurses are particularly sensitive to the trauma of sexual assault and try to ensure that the patient is not revictimized after reporting the crime. When forensic nurses are involved in the treatment of a sexual assault victim, there is typically better collaboration with law enforcement, higher reporting rates, better documentation of the crime, accurate forensic evidence collection, and more successful prosecutions of the assailants. Forensic nurses play an integral role in bridging the gap between law and medicine. They should be in each and every emergency room.

Ten years ago, DNA analysis cost thousands of dollars and took months to get results. Today, it can be done for $40 in a matter of days and technologies currently being tested will reduce that time period to hours. Ten years ago, it took a bottle cap of blood for forensic scientists to do the tests. Now, testing can be done with a sample the size of a pinhead. Today, DNA testing is 99.9 percent accurate. The changes in DNA technology are remarkable and mark a sea of change in how forensic science can help us fight crime, particularly sexual assault crimes. But DNA matching is only effective if the evidence is collected and maintained appropriately. It is clear that if we are going to capitalize on the power of DNA, forensic nurses must be key players. Arming our forensic nurses with resources and tools will help us bring to justice thousands of criminals who are only one DNA test away from conviction.

The examples of what can be done are clear. In 2003, Alabama authorities charged a man in the rape of an 85-year-old woman almost 10 years after the assault because he was linked to the case by a DNA sample he was compelled to submit while in prison on unrelated charges. In Colorado, prosecutors brought to trial a case against a man accused of at least 14 rapes and sexual assaults. Due to the national DNA database, prosecutors were able to trace the defendant to rapes and assaults that occurred in Colorado, California, Arizona, Nevada, and Oklahoma between 1999 and 2002.

Undoubtedly, DNA matching by comparing evidence gathered at the crime scene with offender samples entered on the national DNA database has proven to be the deciding factor in solving stranger sexual assault cases—it has revolutionized the criminal justice system and brought closure and justice for victims. Federal, state, and local lawmakers have begun to focus attention on DNA evidence and ensure that our professionals, including forensic nurses, have adequate tools to harness the power of DNA.

In 2003 Congress passed new federal legislation (the Advancing Justice through DNA Technology Act of 2003), passed legislation such as the DNA Analysis Backlog Elimination Act and held several hearings that focused on DNA and sexual assault crimes and oversight of the forensic sciences. In 2004, The Administration also launched a DNA initiative, calling for, among its many goals, the use of DNA to clear suspects and to exonerate persons mistakenly accused of or convicted of crimes.

Forensic nurses are foot soldiers in the response to and treatment of violence against women. Therefore, I am pleased that this textbook will help educate and prepare tomorrow's forensic nurses. Recognizing the complexity of forensic nursing, this textbook covers a wide variety of issues, such as forensic photography, offender profiling, and court testimony. It also devotes an entire chapter to disaster management, human trafficking, and crimes committed against the elderly.

Forensic Nursing: A Handbook for Practice, Second Edition brings together in one volume many of the field's most accomplished experts. I am certain that this textbook will serve as an invaluable resource for the entire forensic examiner community and help shape a new generation of forensic nurses.

Joseph R. Biden, Jr.
Vice President
United States

Preface

Forensic nursing is an area of clinical expertise that has evolved into a significant independent nursing specialty. Its development reflects a response designed to fulfill a societal need: The growing public health problem of societal violence. A few enthusiastic and dedicated individuals with a vision recognized not only the need for forensic nurses and forensic nursing, but also the fact that nurses have been practicing in forensic roles for many years. This role was informally recognized among nurses themselves, but never formally acknowledged. A pioneer among those visionary nurses was Virginia Lynch, the founding president of the International Association of Forensic Nurses and a contributing author of this text. The growing public health problem of societal violence remains with us and seeks to involve forensic nurses locally, nationally, and internationally. This handbook was developed in recognition of the need for a resource that could enhance the ability of the forensic nurse to function effectively in this demanding evolving role. Thus, it is a book intended for use by both practicing forensic nurses as well as those just beginning the study of forensic nursing and a resource for other healthcare professionals involved in forensic medical issues.

Current global conditions have our attention riveted on violence as an international concern. Although war and acts of terrorism are indeed a real and omnipresent threat, no less demanding of our attention is the issue of violence within our own borders. Until recently, the death and disability caused by violence was viewed as a social problem that came under the purview of the criminal justice system. Recognizing violence as a public health problem mandates that successful interventions must encompass a collaborative effort among healthcare professionals, scientists, and professionals within the criminal justice system. A coalition of these professionals gives rise to the hope that strategies will be created and tested that address the problem of violence from the standpoint of both prevention and intervention. To develop interventions to prevent violent behavior and to protect at risk populations, professionals are needed who understand the dynamics of both victimization and criminal behavior. Forensic nurses are uniquely positioned to fulfill this role and to form the necessary collaborative relationships and coalition of resources that need to exist among the healthcare system, forensic science, and the criminal justice system.

These disciplines have come together with the common goal of meeting the needs of individuals and groups who have been affected by violence. In addition, there are forensic situations that are not associated with interpersonal violence, such as natural disaster, organ procurement, Internet safety, and others. Holistic forensic nursing practice recognizes the uniqueness of each situation and draws upon the expertise of the nurse in all three purviews—nursing, science, and the law.

This handbook is organized around what the authors consider to be significant concepts that support forensic nursing practice, as well as what they consider to be challenges to that practice in the 21st century. Basic foundations of forensic nursing are explored, as are some significant roles of the forensic nurse and the skills required to meet the challenges of those roles. In this handbook, individuals with diverse expertise have been brought together to share their knowledge, experience, and insights. The editors hope that the reader will benefit from the broad scope of content and the depth of knowledge presented by these experts, who are highly renowned in their respective fields.

Since the publication of the first edition of our book we have seen an expansion of the scope and practice of forensic nursing that warrants expansion of original content or inclusion of topics not previously covered. The organization of the book has been altered somewhat to reflect this expansion while still providing a logical flow of subject areas. The extraordinary expansion of Internet technology with its accompanying potential problems for adults as well as children dictated a need for expanded content in this area. New developments in the field of biological evidence and DNA analysis have been explicated in this edition. Changing statistical information relative to violence and violent crime necessitated an overhaul of the chapter dealing with this issue. Major changes in the system of homeland security and the response to disaster management are reflected in the revision of this chapter. Two areas of interest not previously included have been added, human trafficking and crimes against the elderly. A new feature designed to enhance the reader's ability to envision the clinical and practical aspects of the forensic problem is the addition of case studies in each chapter. To accommodate the additional information necessary to make this second edition current and authoritative without becoming unwieldy, it was necessary to remove some information and consolidate or incorporate selected information into other chapters. We chose which content to remove based not on our belief that it was not important but with the knowledge that the edited content could be found elsewhere, which we have indicated within the book. Thus the reader will note the absence of the chapters specific to arson, media relations, and nursing leadership. The visual and physical presentation of this second edition reflects our desire to provide a more convenient resource as well as a more engaging one. We hope that we have succeeded in accomplishing our desire to provide a new and exciting edition of this book devoted to such an important and relevant topic as forensic nursing practice in the 21st century both nationally and globally.

Acknowledgments

Many people generously gave their time to provide insight and assistance during the writing of this book. Among those who deserve particular thanks are Eva Amenta, a Pennsylvania State University graduate student who assisted with editing, and the editorial and production staffs of Jones & Bartlett Learning. In addition, we would like to thank the contributing authors for their time, expertise, and dedication to this project.

We would also like to thank our students, co-workers, and other professional colleagues, especially those at the Henry C. Lee Institute of Forensic Science at the University of New Haven and the Connecticut Department of Public Safety Division of Scientific Services, who provided ideas, comments, and encouragement throughout this endeavor.

Finally, a special thank you is extended to our families and friends for their patience, understanding, and support throughout the entire project.

Contributors

Frederick Berrien, MD
St. Francis Medical Center
Hartford, Connecticut

Edwin "Ted" Brandhurst, PhD, CCFC
Therapist
Center for the Treatment of Problem
    Sexual Behavior
Middletown, Connecticut

Nancy B. Cabelus, DNP, MSN, RN, FAAFS
Forensic Nurse Consultant
Belleair, Florida

Jacquelyn C. Campbell, PhD, RN, FAAN
Associate Dean
Johns Hopkins University School of
    Nursing
Baltimore, Maryland

Bonnie R. Bentley Cewe, JD
Office of the State's Attorney
Danielson, Connecticut

Paul T. Clements, PhD, APRN-BC, DF-IAFN
Associate Clinical Professor
Drexel University
Philadelphia, Pennsylvania

David A. D'Amora, MS, LPC, CFC
Director–CQI-TCI
Center for the Treatment of Problem
    Sexual Behavior
Middletown, Connecticut

Linda C. Degutis, DrPH, MSN
Director, Connecticut Partnership for Public
    Health Workforce Development
Director of the National Center for Injury
    Prevention and Control
Centers for Disease Control and Prevention
Atlanta, Georgia

Joseph T. DeRanieri, PhD, RN, CAN, BCECR
CFO, COPE Consultants, LLC, Trauma
    Response Specialist
Assistant Professor
Thomas Jefferson University
Philadelphia, Pennsylvania

David Duff, MPA
Public Policy Consultant
Owner, SPR Consulting
Fargo, North Dakota

Monique Mattei Ferraro, JD
Associate Professor
Post University
Waterbury, Connecticut

Mary M. Galvin, JD
Senior Counsel Claim Legal Group
The Travelers Indemnity Companies
Hartford, Connecticut

Mario Thomas Gaboury, JD, PhD
Acting Dean and Professor of
    Criminal Justice
Henry C. Lee College of Criminal Justice
    and Forensic Sciences
Haven, Connecticut

Rita M. Hammer, PhD, RN, BC
Professor of Nursing, Retired
New Smyrna Beach, Florida

Tracey Creegan Hammer, JD
Attorney at Law
Westport, Connecticut

Shadonna L. Hawkins, BSN, RN
Johns Hopkins University School of
    Nursing
Baltimore, Maryland

Anita G. Hufft, PhD, RN
Dean of College of Nursing
Valdosta State University
Valdosta, Georgia

Arlene Kent-Wilkinson, PhD, RNN
Associate Professor of Nursing
University of Saskatchewan
Saskatoon, Saskatchewan, Canada

Anne Klein, APR, Fellow PRSA
President
Anne Klein & Associates
Marlton, New Jersey

Carll Ladd, PhD
Forensic Scientist 3
CT Forensic Science Laboratory
Meriden, Connecticut

Patricia LaMonica, MSN, SANE
Director
Emergency Department
St. Francis Hospital and Medical Center
Hartford, Connecticut

Henry C. Lee, PhD
Chaired Professor of Forensic Science
University of New Haven
Chief Emeritus
CT Forensic Science Laboratory
Meriden, Connecticut

Nathan Light, PhD
Senior Researcher
Max Planck Institute for Social
   Anthropology/Advokatenweg
Halle, Germany

Virginia A. Lynch, MS, RN
Director of Forensic Health Science
University of Colorado
Colorado Springs, Colorado

Jennifer L. Makely, BSN, RN
Johns Hopkins University School of
   Nursing
Baltimore, Maryland

Edward T. McDonough, MD
Assistant Chief Medical Examiner
State of Delaware
Dover, Delaware

Barbara Moynihan, PhD, APRN, BC, AFN
Professor of Nursing
Quinnipiac University
Hamden, Connecticut

Michael E. Moynihan, MSW
President and CEO
United Way of Camden County
Camden, New Jersey

Catherine R. Nash, MSN, RN
Johns Hopkins University School of
   Nursing
Baltimore, Maryland

Douglas Olsen, PhD, RN
Yale School of Nursing
New Haven, Connecticut

Elaine M. Pagliaro, MS, JD
Forensic Scientist
Henry C. Lee Institute of Forensic Science
University of New Haven
West Haven, Connecticut

Paul Penders, CFPEI
CT Forensic Science Laboratory
Meriden, Connecticut

Edwin F. Renaud, LCSW, PhD
Clinical Director of Outpatient Behavioral
   Health Services
The Connection, Inc.
Middletown, Connecticut

Daniel J. Sheridan, PhD, RN, FAAN
Associate Professor
Johns Hopkins University School of
   Nursing
Baltimore, Maryland

Deborah Smith, RN, BSN, CEN
Manager, Clinical Services
Yale New Haven Center for Emergency
    Preparedness and Disaster Response
New Haven, Connecticut

Katherine Spangler, MS, RN
Forensic Nurse Consultant
Jupiter, Florida

Tracy A. Swan, MPA, MCJ
Rutgers University
Camden, New Jersey

Randall Wallace, PsyD
Licensed Psychologist
Juvenile Coordinator, CTPSB
Middletown, Connecticut

Kenneth B. Zercie, MS
Director
CT Forensic Science Laboratory
Meriden, Connecticut

CHAPTER ONE

Forensic Nursing Science

Virginia A. Lynch

This chapter defines the evolving field of forensic nursing, introduces an innovative framework for the provision of forensic health care, and identifies the opportunities and challenges inherent in the development of forensic nursing practice.

 ## CHAPTER FOCUS

» History and Development
» Forensic Nursing Defined
» Advent of Forensic Nursing
» A Framework to Guide Forensic Nursing Practice

» Roles and Responsibilities of Forensic Nurses
» Present and Future Trends

KEY TERMS

» clinical forensic practice
» forensic case management
» forensic health care
» forensic nursing
» forensic patient/client

» International Association of Forensic Nurses
» multidisciplinary team approach

Introduction

Forensic nursing is an innovative and evolving nursing specialty that seeks to address healthcare issues that have a medicolegal component. Although forensic nursing has been practiced informally by nurses in various sectors for many years, it has only recently been recognized formally in response to an increasing level of sophistication in identifying its unique body of knowledge.

Crime and violence bring together two of the most powerful systems that impact the daily lives of citizens throughout the world: health and justice. Violent crime and its associated trauma are issues that concern physicians, nurses, attorneys, judges, sociologists, psychologists, social workers, forensic and political scientists, advocates, and activists, as well as criminal justice agencies. No one from any of these disciplines can continue to work in isolation. Effective **forensic case management** has been hampered by lack of sufficient policy and legislation to ensure protection of patients' legal, civil, and human rights. Reducing and preventing human violence requires a multidisciplinary, multidirectional approach.

This new nursing specialty is evolving in response to the healthcare issues presented by criminal violence. This chapter will introduce an innovative framework for forensic health care and for the nurse's role in processing victims, perpetrators, and families through the health and justice systems. In partnership with the forensic medical sciences and the criminal justice system, the emerging discipline of forensic nursing science is assuming responsibility for those affected by human violence and liability-related accidents.

The forensic nurse examiner as clinical investigator represents one member of an alliance of healthcare providers, law enforcement officials, and forensic scientists joined in a holistic approach to the study and intervention of physical, psychological, and sexual violence. While the role of a forensic nurse specialist augments and enhances traditional nursing with exciting and intellectually stimulating responsibilities, it also brings with it a new identity, new language, new terms, and new definitions. It expands the traditional concept of holistic practice—*body, mind, spirit*—to include *the law* (Lynch, 2006).

It is important to emphasize that the forensic nurse does not serve as a criminal investigator; this function remains outside the boundaries of nursing practice. Forensic nurses do not compete with, replace, or supplant other practitioners—rather, they fill voids by performing select forensic tasks in cooperation with other health and justice professionals. Forensic nursing brings to forensic medicine a perspective that historically has been absent, providing the practice with a uniquely qualified clinician who blends biomedical knowledge with an understanding of the basic principles of law and human behavior.

The conceptual framework for the forensic nursing specialty has evolved from society's need to reduce and prevent interpersonal violence and criminal behavior. Benefits derived from clinical forensic intervention, collection, and preservation of forensic evidence, effective sexual assault examinations, identification and reporting of abuse, investigation of suspicious deaths, court-ordered mental health evaluations, and expert testimony by forensically skilled experts in nursing are clearly recognized. These forensic services have been historically absent or insufficient as a result of the failure to integrate the practice of clinical forensic medicine or the principles of forensic pathology into traditional clinical medicine and nursing curricula.

Background Perspectives

Daily, nurses are faced with the extremes of human behavior—child abuse, domestic violence, crimes against the elderly, catastrophic accidents, self-inflicted injuries, blatant neglect, and maltreatment. These incidents must be reported to a law enforcement agency and investigated. Special skills are also required of nurses who provide treatment to or court-ordered assessments of patients in legal custody. As trends in crime and violence change, new legislation is implemented as a means of antiviolence strategies; new resources are required in order to meet the needs of a society at war against crime. Nurses have been challenged to conjoin patient care with the legal system in order to augment resources available to patients with liability-related injuries, mentally disordered offenders, crime victims, and suspects or offenders in police custody.

Forensic nursing represents a new perspective on the holistic approach to legal issues surrounding patient care in clinical or community-based settings. The application of forensic science to contemporary nursing practice allows practitioners a wider role in the clinical investigation of crime and the legal process that contributes to public health and safety (Lynch, 1995). It is not surprising that there is strong support for nurse specialists who possess the combination of knowledge and skills required to go beyond the traditional treatment of forensic patients to fulfill today's requirements for forensic expertise in health care.

Because many forensic patients first present to the emergency department, trauma care providers must be aware of the indicators of liability-related injuries, abuse of children and the elderly, sexual assault, interpersonal violence, and unnatural deaths. Other forensic patients will present in different departments of the hospital, private or public clinics, law offices, jails, penal institutions, psychiatric hospitals, disaster sites, and the morgue or mortuary.

All trauma is classified as a forensic situation until proven otherwise. Injuries presented in a hospital emergency department require a clinical and criminal investigation in order to confirm or rule out use of force and criminal intent. Failure to meet forensic requirements in the clinical setting can compromise the investigation. A nurse's ignorance of forensic issues could leave unanswered questions related to trauma that later may be of relevance in a court of law.

Despite the urgency presented by many cases within the emergency department, as part of the multidisciplinary team attending the victim(s), it is the nurse's responsibility to collect and preserve all forensic evidence. Staff members in these situations are recognizing the need to develop evidence-based procedures for forensic evidence collection within the emergency department (Eisert et al., 2010).

Forensic Nursing Defined

Forensic nursing is defined as the application of the nursing process to public or legal proceedings, and the application of **forensic health care** in the scientific investigation of trauma and/or death related to abuse, violence, criminal activity, liability, and accidents (Lynch, 2004). In order to understand the concept of a forensic nurse specialist, we must first accurately define the term *forensic*. Healthcare and justice professionals in the United States often misinterpret and misuse this term. According to *Taber's Cyclopedic Medical Dictionary* (2009), forensic means "pertaining to the law," specifically, that which is related to public debate (Latin: *forensis*; a forum) in a court of law, implying the debate between the prosecution and defense to determine the innocence or guilt of the accused. The forensic nurse provides direct services to individual clients, consultation services to nursing, medical and law-related agencies, as well as providing expert court testimony in areas dealing with questioned death investigative processes, adequacy of services delivery and specialized diagnoses of specific conditions as related to nursing" (Lynch, 1991b, p. 1). This description was derived from original research at the University of Texas in Arlington, which was published in 1990. Since that time, this description has remained the standard, while at the same time expanding and evolving into broader definitions and emerging subspecialties. A theoretical framework evolved from the 1990 study and continues to evolve as the practice of forensic nursing expands to address society's needs for forensic intervention in health care. The consequences of criminal and interpersonal violence have been recognized as a primary healthcare and human rights concern. As a public service profession, nursing has a responsibility to maintain standards of practice in forensic-related cases. Because of the legal issues involved in caring for victims of human violence, the risk of using forensically unskilled personnel to provide healthcare intervention has become antiquated. Today, enlightened healthcare institutions, death investigation systems, government agencies, and institutes of higher learning have recognized the benefits of the forensic nurse.

A forensic nurse has advanced knowledge in forensic evidence collection and preservation, treatment protocols for victims of sexual assault, domestic violence, child and elder abuse, human trafficking, legal proceedings, legal expert court testimony, death investigation, forensic psychiatric nursing, and correctional nursing. Forensic nursing focuses on those areas where medicine, nursing, and individuals impacted by violence interface with the law.

Thus the potential venues for clinical practice within the field are many and varied. The forensic nurse practices in a collaborative manner with various members within the field of forensic science.

Forensic Science Defined

Forensic science is defined as the application of science to the just resolution of legal issues (American Academy of Forensic Sciences, 2010). The American Academy of Forensic Sciences remains the oldest and most prestigious organization of forensic specialists worldwide. "The objectives of the Academy are to promote integrity, competency, education, foster research, improve practice, and encourage collaboration in the forensic sciences" (American Academy of Forensic Sciences, 2010). The academy, established in 1948, was the first formal association to recognize forensic nursing as a scientific discipline and give credence to this new specialty (Lynch, 1991b). Forensic medicine, one of many specialties within the forensic sciences, applies the standards and principles of medical practice to questions of law. This specialty includes both forensic pathology and clinical forensic medicine.

Other specialties within the boundaries of the forensic sciences include psychiatry and behavioral science, anthropology, odontology, criminalistics, questioned document examination, radiology, biology, jurisprudence, engineering, toxicology, and others. The newest specialties in forensic science comprise unique, emerging areas of expertise, specialties represented by professionals who practice in such innovative areas as forensic accounting, voice analysis, forensic wildlife, and forensic botany; however, these growing specialties will remain uncategorized until a sufficient number of experienced experts in each group are identified. The original application for recognition as a scientific discipline within the American Academy of Forensic Sciences described forensic nursing as "the application of the forensic aspects of health care combined with the bio/psycho/social/spiritual education of the registered nurse in the scientific investigation and treatment of trauma and/or death" (Lynch, 1990).

History and Development

The concept of forensic nursing emerged from the practice of clinical forensic medicine. A subspecialty of forensic medicine defined as the application of forensic medical knowledge and techniques to living patients has existed in Europe and Great Britain as well as Asia, South America, Australia, Africa, and many other countries for more than 2 centuries (McLay, 1990). Medical professionals in this field go by various titles but most often are referred to as police surgeons, forensic medical officers, and most recently, forensic medical examiners. The role of the police surgeon or forensic medical examiner in the United Kingdom served as the conceptual model for the development of the clinical forensic nurse.

Clinical forensic medicine is defined as a medical specialty that applies the principles and practices of clinical medicine to the elucidation of questions in judicial proceedings for the protection of the individual's legal rights prior to death (Eckert et al., 1986). Historically, this healthcare role had been viewed worldwide as a medical specialty and had been restricted to physicians alone. Until recently, practitioners of clinical medicine and nursing in the United States have largely ignored forensic issues in the care of the living patient (Smock, 1998, 2004). Medical examiners or coroners, or combined coroner–medical examiner systems (which are responsible for the investigation of unnatural and suspicious deaths), traditionally have not been assigned the responsibility of dealing with living forensic patients. Yet forensic pathologists strongly believe that if vital legal questions are not addressed during the care of the living patient, justice will suffer, criminals will go free, and innocent persons could be convicted of crimes they did not commit. The practice of clinical forensic medicine is often either unrecognized as such or is consciously or subconsciously evaded by practicing clinical physicians. If clinical physicians and forensic pathologists do not consider themselves responsible for the forensic issues surrounding living patients, who does?

By the 1980s, U.S. physicians and forensic pathologists were beginning to recognize the inadequacies of the medicolegal structure and the need to establish a more effective partnership between the health and justice systems. The first article to appear in American emergency medicine literature regarding clinical forensic medicine was published in the *Emergency Medicine Clinics of North America* (Smialek, 1983). Smialek stated that "medical care of the critically ill in the emergency department has a significant impact on the practice of forensic medicine. Many victims of homicide or accidents receive some degree of medical or surgical treatment prior to expiration" (p. 699). Smialek recognized that the evidence necessary to accurately reconstruct the event, prove guilt, or establish innocence was disappearing or being destroyed, either by commission or omission, during trauma treatment. That same year, the *American Journal of Nursing* published the article, "Preserving Evidence in the Emergency Department," by Roger Mittleman, a forensic pathologist, Hollace Goldberg, an emergency nurse, and David Waksman, a state attorney in Florida (Mittleman, Goldberg, & Waksman, 1983). This article emphasized the importance of recognizing and preserving the evidence found on patients presenting to the emergency department—to avoid unnecessary negative consequences for both individuals and the system.

In 1988, Dr. C. Everett Koop, then U.S. surgeon general, criticized our social and legal systems' responses to forensic victims as late and inadequate. He also pointed out that the resources available to help law enforcement and the courts—resources from community and social service organizations—should include those of medicine and health care. Koop stated that it is the responsibility of healthcare professionals—doctors, nurses, physician assistants, paramedics, emergency medical technicians, hospital administrators, and other executives with the power to influence change—to maintain a high index of suspicion in the protection of the victim's rights (Koop, 1988).

As medical professionals began to weigh risk and liability issues involved in the medicolegal management of forensic patients they were required by law to treat, a concerted effort by Dr. William Smock and Dr. George Nichols II of the University of Louisville, Kentucky, established the first clinical forensic medicine program in 1993 (Smock, Nichols, & Fuller, 1993).

With the exception of some academic emergency medical centers and progressive medical examiner/coroner programs, clinical forensic medicine has not enjoyed the same success as forensic nursing (Smock, from Lynch, 2006). In 2000, the American College of Emergency Physicians still had no position or statement regarding the role of clinical forensic physicians (police surgeons) in emergency departments in America. The college's only training guidelines related to the collection of evidence are those for recognizing, assessing, and intervening in case of child abuse. On the other hand, the American College of Emergency Physicians has recognized the benefits of sexual assault nurse examiners and strongly supports their presence in the emergency department (American College of Emergency Physicians, 2000). In spite of some initial resistance from the medical and legal communities, forensic nursing has become the moving force in clinical forensic practice in the United States and Canada. In countries where clinical forensic medicine is already established, current restructuring of forensic services will no doubt result in a greater emphasis on forensic nursing science.

Clinical Forensic Practice

The combined energies of medicine, nursing, and the law have developed into a mutually beneficial, collaborative practice in which knowledge and responsibility are shared in order to reach common goals. The evolution of forensic nursing science has revolutionized the medicolegal management of forensic patients and has reduced the risk of liability due to violation of patients' legal rights for clinical and community facilities in the United States.

Clinical forensic practice is now defined as the application of medical and nursing sciences to the care of living victims of crime or liability-related accidents, as opposed to forensic pathology, which focuses upon the deceased. Clinical forensic practice also applies the principles and philosophies of forensic science to the investigation of trauma in living patients, with the aim of the just resolution of legal issues. Forensic scientists and police have long recognized that there are intervals between the forensic patient's trauma, emergency care, admission to the clinical setting, and initiation of the investigation. During these periods of time, a series of events occur that may compromise the recovery, preservation, and security of forensically significant trace and physical evidence. Biological evidence, which is highly perishable and fragile, is often the most essential evidence that links the perpetrator to the victim or the crime scene. When the clinical staff handling the case lacks forensic education and skills, the loss and destruction of such evidence is predictable.

Advent of Forensic Nursing

As a medicolegal death investigator member of the American Academy of Forensic Sciences and the National Association of Medical Examiners, Lynch recognized the value of forensic education and forensic roles for nurses and proposed the development of a forensic nursing specialty in 1986. The concept became a reality when the University of Texas at Arlington School of Nursing's department of graduate studies accepted the proposed curriculum and implemented the first master's degree for forensic clinical nurse specialists. Although the original proposal focused on preparing the forensic nurse to assist forensic pathologists in death investigations, Lynch rapidly expanded this focus to include the practice of clinical forensic nursing. The first articles on the subject of forensic nursing were incorporated into the introduction of clinical forensic medicine presented at the 1988 annual meeting of the American Academy of Forensic Sciences. These articles, influenced by Lynch's association with the forensic pathologists in the National Association of Medical Examiners, combined with the mandate from Dr. Koop, became the impetus to define forensic nursing as a scientific discipline.

Lynch identified all areas of nursing in which nurses were providing a *nursing* service within a forensic environment to forensic patients, or were providing a *forensic* service within a healthcare environment to forensic patients. At that time, these nurses had no specialty practice recognition, yet they were highly aware that they were filling a unique role. Their jobs included providing death scene investigations, sexual assault examinations, psychiatric evaluations, and treatment of offenders. There were nurses practicing in various venues including law offices, penal institutions, and other areas where they interfaced with the law.

The initial intent of the forensic nursing curriculum was to combine instruction in nursing science, forensic science, and the law, expanding existing nursing education to address critical healthcare and legal issues surrounding patient care. Traditional nursing education was conspicuously lacking in forensic knowledge and skills, yet nurses were expected daily to provide forensic services. By 1995, however, forensic nursing had been recognized as one of the four major areas for nursing development in the 21st century (Marullo, 1995). That same year the International Association of Forensic Nurses (IAFN) was formed by a group of sexual assault nurses whose original intent was to form an organization to meet their specific needs in this narrow field of practice. The specialty was formally recognized by the American Academy of Forensic Sciences in 1991 and by the American Nurses Association (ANA) in 1995. In 1997 the Scope and Standards of Forensic Nursing Practice was developed and published through the joint efforts of the IAFN and the ANA. The framework for the specialty was poised to meet legal requirements and to ensure that the Joint Commission on Accreditation for Healthcare Organizations guidelines were fulfilled with reasonable certainty (JCAHO, 1995).

An Integrated Practice Model

As a graduate student at the University of Texas at Arlington, Lynch finalized research, titled "Clinical Forensic Nursing: A Descriptive Study in Role Development" (Lynch, 1990). The purpose of this descriptive study was to identify forensic role behaviors and to clarify role expectations of the emergency department nurses working with trauma victims. It further sought to identify and examine the differences between the frequency and perceived importance of selected forensic role behaviors performed by emergency department nurses. This study promoted the need for a **multidisciplinary team** approach to the identification of forensic trauma and the recovery and preservation of evidence. Research results defined the appropriate application of selected forensic concepts to professional nursing practice and education and described the potential for a forensic clinical nurse specialist. Since that time, replications of this study have assessed trauma centers and first responders, as opposed to emergency departments, further validating the significance of forensic health care.

Progressive trauma centers that include forensic nurses assign a high value to the services provided. The American College of Surgeons encourages establishment of comprehensive systems to assure that standards of trauma care are being met in the form of trauma centers that provide state-of-the-art care to patients with life-threatening injuries (American College of Surgeons, 1999). While recognizing the overwhelming importance of the physiological need of the patient, the clinician must also acknowledge the patient's psychological trauma and the priority of legal requirements (Rooms, 2004). The application of forensic science to contemporary nursing practice reveals a wider role for the nurse in the clinical investigation of crime and the legal process that contributes to public health and safety (Lynch, 1995).

The integrated practice model for forensic nursing science incorporates a synthesis of shared theory from a variety of disciplines, including social science, nursing science, and forensic science. It presents a global perspective on the interrelated disciplines and knowledge bases that affect forensic nursing practice and social justice. An integrated practice model is especially relevant to the applied health sciences.

Theoretical Foundations

Forensic nursing derives its theoretical foundations from several mainstream nursing theories, which are integrated with theories from sociology and philosophy. Like every nursing specialty, forensic nursing offers specific strategies and considerations for addressing the biological, psychological, social, and spiritual dimensions of patient care—with the important addition of the legal dimension. The connection that brings the philosophies of nursing science together with the law defines forensic nursing's body of knowledge (Lynch, 2006).

Forensic nursing theory incorporates the various human dimensions pertinent to all nursing theories of care, yet projects beyond the biological, psychological, social, spiritual and cultural aspects to incorporate the dimension of law. Forensic nursing is holistic in nature, addressing these concepts individually and collectively, and has been recognized by the professional bodies of nursing that direct the development of nursing education, research, and practice (Lynch, 2006).

Truth as a Central Paradigm

The forensic nursing practice model integrates sociology (sociopolitical impact), criminology (crime, violence, criminal justice, social sanctions, and human rights), clinical and criminal investigation (forensic science), and education (nursing and medicolegal knowledge, education of staff and **forensic patient/clients**). The cyclic nature of the model speaks to continuance, perpetuation, and balance. The scales of justice are balanced when justice is served to those who have been victimized, to those accused of a crime, and to society as a whole. Justice is served when truth is identified, verified, and demonstrated. Thus, the forensic nurse becomes an advocate for justice and an advocate for truth. Truth and justice perpetuate holistic health in its biological, psychological, sociological, spiritual, and cultural dimensions (Lynch, 2006).

The dynamics of the interlocking circles are omnidirectional (see **Figure 1-1**). The outer circle, framing and encompassing these components, is symbolic of the environment—society, education, and other social systems. At the center of the internal triangle, the symbol of forensic nursing is displayed. This symbol, reflecting the legal sciences, forensic medical, physical, psychosocial, and nursing sciences, is composed of the scales of justice, the bundle of public service, the caduceus, and the eternal flame of nursing. The flame illustrates enlightenment of humanity and the challenge in nursing to continually evolve and expand into new roles as societal trends demand.

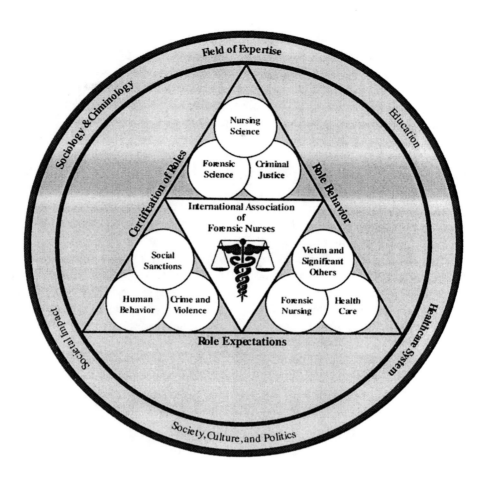

Figure 1-1   Integrated practice model.
Source: Copyright 1990 Virginia Lynch, used with permission.

This enlightenment reflects awareness of the connectedness that the healthcare system has to other social systems. A caduceus represents medical science and, enmeshed in this symbol, the interdisciplinary collaboration that integrates nursing into the multitude of highly specialized scientific psychocultural arenas. The bundle of public service represents the complexity and weight of public service obligations, which all modern systems in our society bear. Finally, the scales of justice emphasize the necessary balance to determine the truth and the notion that patient care must now require the consideration of legal as well as human rights.

The Forensic Nurse

Roles and Relevance

Nurses who apply concepts and strategies of forensic science in their specialty practice include the following:

Clinical Forensic Nurse: Provides care for the survivors of crime-related injury and deaths that occur within the healthcare institution. This specialist has a duty to defend the patient's legal rights through the proper collection and documentation of evidence.

Forensic Nurse Investigators: Employed in a medical examiner's/coroner's jurisdiction and represents the decedent's right to social justice through scientific investigation of the scene and circumstances of death. This role may also include the investigation of criminal behavior in long-term care facilities, institutionalized care, insurance fraud and abuse, or other aspects of investigative exigency.

Forensic Nurse Examiner: Provides an incisive analysis of physical and psychological trauma, questioned deaths, and/or psychopathology evaluations related to forensic cases and interpersonal violence.

Forensic Correctional, Institutional, or Custodial Nurse: Specializes in the care, treatment, and rehabilitation of persons who have been sentenced to prisons or jails for violation of criminal statutes and require medical assessment and intervention.

Legal Nurse Consultant: Provides expert witness testimony and education to judicial, criminal justice, and healthcare professionals in areas such as personal injury, product liability, and malpractice, among other legal issues related to civil and criminal cases.

Nurse Attorney: A registered nurse with a Juris Doctorate degree who practices as an attorney at law, generally specializing in civil or criminal cases involving healthcare-related issues.

Nurse Coroner: A registered nurse serving as an elected officiator of death duly authorized by state and jurisdictional statutes to provide the investigation and certification of questioned deaths; to determine the cause and manner of death, as well as the circumstances pertaining to the decedent's identification and notification of next of kin.

Each of these forensic nursing roles is investigative in nature, requiring specific knowledge of the law and the skill of expert witness testimony. The prevalence of criminal and liability-related trauma indicates a growing need for healthcare providers to intercede on behalf of social justice; to recognize and report crime-related injury and death; to ensure accurate documentation and security of evidence; and to evaluate, assess, and treat offenders.

The Forensic Nurse Examiner

A registered nurse specifically trained to provide comprehensive care in the medicolegal management of forensic patients with demonstrated competency in the performance of the forensic examination and the ability to testify as an expert witness in a court of law can assume the title forensic nurse examiner. Documented nursing and forensic education, certification, clinical performance, and other pertinent credentials determine the nurse's competency.

Forensic nurse examiners will encounter individuals of all ages who present with suspected criminal or liability-related trauma. Physical, psychological, or sexual trauma in both living and deceased patients mandate a forensic evaluation.

Forensic nurse examiners enhance patient care through their expertise, patient education, referrals, and crisis intervention. Forensic nursing services address perceived physical and/or emotional symptoms associated with criminal violence, abuse, and neglect, which are often undiagnosed and may require prompt intervention as well as ongoing investigation of causative factors. The forensic nurse examiner is also responsible for the forensic care of the criminal suspect or offender, providing unbiased, objective assessment and treatment in the clinical or correctional setting.

Forensic nursing care is often episodic, primary, and acute in nature. It is frequently unscheduled, most commonly occurring as the need arises in a specific care setting, such as an emergency department, a mobile unit, a suicide prevention center, the crime scene, the scene of death, or the forensic pathology laboratory. Forensic nurse examiners share a common interest with medicine and law, where scientific knowledge and human caring is applied to the administration of social justice.

Education for the forensic nurse examiner should encompass study of the following:

» Forensic photography
» Nursing and emergency medical technician responsibilities
» Bite mark interpretation and analysis
» Death investigation
» Psychological abuse
» Deviant behavior and psychopathology assessment
» Interpretation of blunt, sharp, or fast (e.g., gunshot) trauma
» Sexual abuse and rape
» Jurisprudence
» Injuries to individuals held in legal custody
» Elder abuse
» Child abuse and neglect
» Substance abuse
» Psychological and physical abuse from occult or religious practices
» Tissue and organ donation

The Forensic Clinical Nurse Specialist

The forensic clinical nurse specialist was the first formal role to incorporate forensic science into nursing practice. The forensic clinical nurse specialist is defined as a nurse educated at the graduate level (master of science in nursing) in a clinical specialist program in forensic nursing at a regionally accredited institution of higher learning. Texas was the first state to address the issue of the forensic clinical nurse specialists as an advanced practice role through the state board of nurse examiners. Advanced practice, credentialed by the state, is still premature without a greater number of practicing forensic nurses with advanced degrees. However, the majority of nurses who first applied forensic science to patient care were registered nurses without advanced education in nursing or forensic science. These nurses were the collective force that established the forensic nursing specialty, showing the commitment and dedication that is the strength of forensic nursing today.

Times change, as science and technology continue to advance and challenge the knowledge and skills of nurses. No physicians, lawyers, scientists, or judges practice their profession without advanced education. Yet these are the colleagues with whom we interface, collaborate, and consult on forensic issues as well as debate within courts of law. Ideally, forensic clinical nurse specialist candidates would hold a bachelor of science in nursing or master of science in nursing degree and have 3–5 years of clinical experience plus a forensic specialization background. As forensic nurses become the standard by which forensic health care is measured, we must step up to the witness stand qualified, certified, and credentialed in our specialty area.

Flexibility is critical in the development of a role that remains in constant evolution based on the needs and demands of society. The role of the forensic nurse will remain flexible and continue to evolve as changing trends in crime and criminality present new challenges.

Forensic Nursing Process

In 1995, the American Nurses Association Congress of Nursing Practice granted specialty status to forensic nursing based on its demonstrated use of the nursing process. The forensic nursing process is client centered and establishes a feedback loop that ensures a dynamic mechanism for the reevaluation and revision of care plans. Collaboration is vital to the forensic nursing process (Lynch, 2006).

The following concepts are among the variables that influence the forensic nursing process:

» Assessment: Identification of forensic situation, potential victims
» Planning: Investigation
» Intervention: Documentation pertaining to the situation, collection of evidence, interviewing, provision of appropriate care, reporting to the appropriate legal agency
» Evaluation: Postintervention review

The forensic nurse also provides traditional nursing interventions such as crisis care for traumatized victims and their families (Lynch, 2006).

Forensic Nursing, Present and Future

International Association of Forensic Nurses

Since its founding in 1992, the **International Association of Forensic Nurses** has promoted the education of forensic nurses and the implementation of forensic nursing roles worldwide. The vision of the founding group was to develop an organization that would encompass a wide and diverse body of those who practice nursing within the arena of the law. Nurses who apply concepts and strategies of forensic science while providing nursing interventions fall within this field of practice. The organization holds the annual Scientific Assembly of Forensic Nurses for the purpose of disseminating knowledge and expertise to members and nonmembers from the United States and abroad.

With the establishment of graduate and undergraduate education programs, role development in forensic nursing in the United States and abroad is recognized as an essential component of antiviolence strategies. The International Association of Forensic Nurses recognizes more than 2000 members in 11 countries and territories. Institutions of higher learning offer formal and informal curricula in Australia, Canada, England, Scotland, Singapore, Brunei, Central America, Italy, South Africa, Sweden, Turkey, Zimbabwe, India, and Japan. South Africa has become the first country to designate forensic nursing as a national priority program. Through the media of the World Wide Web, Internet education and information connects this new frontier in forensic health care with the global community.

Advancing Humanity

One final aspect of forensic nursing science is the issue of human rights. Worldwide, forensic nurses must address the dynamics of archaic cultural traditions and religious practices that continue to pose threats to vulnerable subjects in each society—women, children, the disabled, the elderly, and the poor. An awareness of cultural and traditional practices such as female genital mutilation, honor killings, bride burning, and dowry deaths; criminal issues such as child prostitution and the incarceration of rape victims; and the effects of poverty and lack of education for women must become a part of forensic nursing education.

Within our strategic plan for nursing, we must strive to include issues that the World Health Organization has identified as having the highest priority, not limiting our concerns only to state and national agendas. In addition to basic and advanced forensic studies, a strong emphasis on human rights and international law is an integral part of the educational curricula for forensic nurses. Another critical aspect of their education is a broader focus on transcultural nursing, covering issues unique to immigrants and refugees who are survivors of war or torture, and victims of cultural practices that have maimed and crippled them, physically and emotionally (Lynch, 2006).

Our research, curricula, and practices must address prevention of HIV/AIDS and its direct connection to sexual assault. Forensic nursing must encompass the consequences of disease and death related to the lack of early detection and management of chronic conditions. The need to reduce the abuse of women and children and to curb infant mortality arising from multiple causes must be emphasized. Frank, open, culturally sensitive discussions are imperative for achieving positive responses from victims representing a vast array of social and cultural experiences (Lynch, 2006).

Interpersonal violence and its associated trauma impact all societies. Crimes against women, children, and the elderly are common. In order for forensic nurses to better assist in the management of medicolegal cases, they must be trained in transcultural nursing perspectives, the ethical and moral dimensions of health care, healthcare practices of diverse cultures, and local, national, and international laws as well as the United Nations Declaration of Human Rights.

Challenges and Opportunities

The development of a new field of practice is a challenging experience that brings together diverse professionals who recognize a mutual benefit through collaborative practice, exchange of knowledge, and shared successes in order to reach common goals. We must remain concerned with improving the health care of at-risk populations and advancing the information technologies that are revolutionizing forensic nursing research, clinical care, and education. A partnership must be nurtured between forensic nurses and professionals from all disciplines with similar interests in eliminating threats to health and justice.

Antiquated laws and social policies, restrictive family values, disregard for human equality, and inequalities in healthcare access and delivery must be addressed within the forensic sciences in order to reduce and prevent interpersonal violence. The health and justice challenges that arise from violent crime will not be eradicated for many generations, but it is imperative that the mission is launched within this decade.

Summary

Advances in the forensic and nursing sciences have brought this new discipline to the forefront as one of the four major areas for nursing development in the 21st century. Forensic nursing addresses the manner in which nursing is practiced within various countries, the unique cultures and traditions that influence crimes in each specific locale, the court system and the law, as well as the current and future application of forensic nursing science.

These are extraordinary times for personnel in the health sciences, and both challenges and opportunities abound in every sector of healthcare delivery. The sophisticated capabilities of medical and nursing sciences, rapid transportation, instant communication, and an interdependent world economy have compelled healthcare personnel to reexamine their missions and geographical boundaries of practice. A healthy world cannot be achieved merely within a vacuum of highly industrialized nations. Governments alone cannot meet the immense needs of adults and children who need preventive and restorative health care. Forensic medical and forensic nursing personnel have been among the first to step forward and become involved in the global issues of health care. This involves a broad acumen of knowledge, skills, and attention to justice concerns of the world's peoples (Lynch, 2006).

In achieving an international focus, nurses who have reached out to address human violence and its associated trauma have recognized the similarities of interpersonal crime in all societies. In order for nurses to assist in the forensic assessment and management of medicolegal cases, the incorporation of transcultural nursing perspectives, the ethical and moral dimensions of human care, healthcare practices of diverse cultures, a review of the law—local, national, and international, and an in-depth knowledge of individual human rights are required.

A strong working knowledge of the law promotes interaction with local law enforcement agencies and helps to develop an accurate approach to forensic nursing interventions. Nurses who apply concepts and strategies of forensic nursing science in their specialty practice are becoming recognized as vital resources to the global health and justice system. To meet the healthcare needs of an increasingly diverse population of patients with forensic assessment needs, the establishment of formal and informal education programs, in addition to role development in forensic nursing in the United States and abroad, is recognized as one important component of antiviolence strategies. Individuals who have embraced the challenges of today will provide leadership and solutions for the future.

 QUESTIONS FOR DISCUSSION

1. Describe the historical background of forensic nursing.
2. Why is forensic nursing defined as a specialty within clinical nursing?
3. Describe the various roles inherent within the practice of forensic nursing.
4. Do any new roles suggest themselves in light of the information presented in this chapter?
5. How has the development of the International Association of Forensic Nursing influenced the development of the specialty?
6. How will the implementation of the 2010 Affordable Care Act impact the growth of the forensic nursing specialty?

REFERENCES

American Academy of Forensic Sciences. (2010). Website home page. Retrieved May 5, 2011, from http://www.aafs.org.

American College of Emergency Physicians. (1999). *Management of the patient with the complaint of sexual assault.* [ACEP policy statement No. 400130]. Irving, TX: Author.

American College of Emergency Physicians. (2000). *Child abuse.* [ACEP policy statement No. 400279]. Irving, TX: Author.

American College of Surgeons. (1999). *Resources for optimal care of the injured patient.* Chicago, IL: Author.

American Nurses Association and the International Association of Forensic Nurses. (1998). *Scope and standards of forensic nursing practice.* Washington, DC: Author.

Eisert, P. J., Eldredge, K., Hartlaub, T., Huggins, E., Keirn, G., O'Brien, P., ... March, K. S. (2010). CSI: New York: Development of forensic evidence collection guidelines for the emergency department. *Critical Care Nursing Quarterly, 33*(2), 190–199.

Geberth, V. (1996). *Practical homicide investigation: Checklist and field guide.* Boca Raton, FL: CRC Press.

Joint Commission on Accreditation of Healthcare Organizations. (1995). *Accreditation manual for hospitals.* Oakbrook Terrace, IL: Author.

Koop, C. E. (1988). President and surgeon general condemns violence against women, call for new attitudes, programs. *National Organization Victims Assistance Newsletter,* 13.

Lynch, V. (1990). *Clinical forensic nursing: A descriptive study in role development* (Unpublished master's thesis). Arlington: University of Texas Health Science Center.

Lynch, V. (1991a). Forensic nursing in the emergency department: A new role for the 1990s. *Critical Care Nursing Quarterly, 14*(3), 69–86.

Lynch, V. (1991b). Proposal for a new scientific discipline: Forensic nursing. Presentation to the general section at the annual meeting of the American Academy of Forensic Sciences, Anaheim, CA. Feb 18–23.

Lynch, V. (1993). Forensic aspects of health care: New roles, new responsibilities. *Journal of Psychosocial Nursing, 31*(11), 5–6.

Lynch, V. (1995, September). A new perspective in the management of crime victims from trauma to trial. *Critical Care Nursing Clinics of North America. 7*(3), 489–507.

Lynch, V. (Ed.). (2006). *Forensic nursing.* St. Louis, MO: Elsevier.

Marullo, G. (1995). Keynote address. Annual Scientific Assembly of the International Association of Forensic Nurses, Kansas City, MO. October.

McLay, W. D. S. (1990). *Clinical forensic medicine.* London, England: Pinter.

Mittleman, R., Goldberg, H., & Waksman, D. (1983). Preserving evidence in the emergency department. *American Journal of Nursing, 83*(12), 1652–1656.

National Institute of Health. (1974). Report on National Institute of Child Health and Human Development Research Planning Workshop. *Recognition of infants at risk for sudden infant death: An approach to prevention* (Pub. no. 76-1013). Bethesda, MD: Department of Health, Education and Welfare.

Rooms, R. (2004). *Forensic nursing practice in United States trauma centers* (Unpublished master's thesis). Houston: University of Texas Health Science Center.

Smialek, J. (1983). Forensic medicine in the emergency department. *Emergency Medicine Clinics of North America, 1*(3), 1685.

Smock, W. (1998). Clinical forensic medicine. In P. Rosen (Ed.), *Emergency medicine: Concepts and clinical practice* (pp. 248–262). St. Louis, MO: Mosby.

Smock, W., Nichols, G., & Fuller, P. (1993). Development and implementation of the first clinical forensic medicine training program. *Journal of Forensic Sciences, 38*(4), 835–839.

Taber's cyclopedic medical dictionary (21st ed.). (2010). Philadelphia, PA: FA Davis.

SUGGESTED FURTHER READING

Cashin, A., Newman, C., Eason, M., Thorpe, A., & O'Discoll, C. (2010). An ethnographic study of forensic nursing culture in an Australian prison hospital. *Journal of Psychiatric Mental Health Nursing, 17*(1), 39–45.

Clevinger, R. J. (2010). When your pediatric patient becomes a crime scene. *Emergency Nurse, 36*(1), 53–54.

Gildberg, F. A., Elverdam, B., & Hounsgaard, L. (2010). Forensic psychiatric nursing: A literature review and thematic analysis of staff-patient interaction. *Journal of Psychiatric Mental Health Nursing, 17*(4), 359–368.

Kent-Wilkinson, A. (2009). An exploratory study of forensic nursing education in North America: Constructed definitions of forensic nursing. *Journal of Forensic Nursing, 5*(4), 201–211.

Kent-Wilkinson, A. E. (2010). Forensic psychiatric/mental health nursing: Responsive to social need. *Issues in Mental Health Nursing, 31*(6), 425–431.

Mercer, D. (2009). Research in state institutions: A critical issue for forensic nursing. *Journal of Forensic Nursing, 5*(2), 107–108.

Price, B. (2010). Receiving a forensic medical exam without participating in the criminal justice process: What will it mean? *Journal of Forensic Nursing, 6*(2), 74–87.

Shelton, D. (2009). Forensic nursing in secure environments. *Journal of Forensic Nursing, 5*(3), 131–142.

Sievers, V., & Lechner, M. (2009). Forensic nursing: Evolving practice in response to the epidemic of violence. *Colorado Nurse, 109*(2), 11–12.

Snow, A. F., & Bozeman, J. M. (2010). Role implications for nurses caring for gunshot wound victims. *Critical Care Nursing Quarterly, 33*(3), 259–264.

Williams, T., Richardson, S., O'Donovan, P., & Ardagh, M. (2005). The forensic nurse practitioner role (emergency nursing) — potential response to changing health needs in New Zealand. *Medicine and Law, 24*(1), 111–123.

CHAPTER TWO

Theoretical Foundations for Advanced Practice Forensic Nursing

Anita G. Hufft

This chapter proposes organizing a conceptual framework for forensic nursing to define and establish the relationships among selected concepts identified as relevant to the practice of forensic nursing and to the understanding of the domain concepts of nursing. Such a framework provides opportunities to review relationships between healthcare systems and forensic systems (judicial, correctional, legal) and establish the assumptions upon which these views are based.

CHAPTER FOCUS

» Organizing Forensic Nursing Theory
» Environment/Violence

» Human Beings/Victimization
» Nursing
» Health

KEY TERMS

» assumptions
» caring
» critical thinking
» evidence-based practice
» health

» lived experience
» manipulation
» organizing framework
» revictimization
» violence

Introduction

The nursing profession is based on a specialized body of knowledge that reflects different philosophies and views about those phenomena of interest to nursing. Conceptualized as the science and technology of human **caring**, nursing is concerned with reality-based changing life patterns and experiences of humans (Kenney, 1996; Rodgers & Knafl, 2000). Nursing theory provides a conceptual framework for organizing and relating knowledge for nursing within what are recognized as domain concepts. Health, the environment, human beings, and nursing are the domain concepts of nursing science. When defined and interrelated sufficiently within a specific population or health event, these concepts have the potential to increase our understanding of human experiences within the contexts of their lives (Alligood & Marriner-Tomey, 2006).

A conceptual framework provides a structure by which a discipline can be understood in terms of philosophical **assumptions**, theoretical methods, and developmental influences. Those forces that have shaped the development of forensic nursing occur in the wider context of society and represent the point of contact between healthcare systems and legal systems. Consistent with the framework for nursing, forensic nursing can be described in terms of the domain concepts of nursing as a distinct area of education, practice, and scientific inquiry. A heuristic approach to understanding advanced practice nursing lies in the elaboration of definitions and relationships among the concepts of human beings, environment, health, and nursing.

The forum of medicine and forensic science is an unlikely environment for the development of a nursing specialty if one considers the common conception of nursing as a caring profession that emphasizes holistic understanding of the **lived experience** of persons (Kenney, 2006). Traditional views of nursing place caregivers at the bedside of a sick person, applying the art and science of compassion and healing to the restoration of the human body, mind, and spirit. Contemporary understandings of nursing encompass a wide variety of settings and roles, including the care of society and communities through the identification and prevention of **violence** and traumatic injury (Burgess, Berger, & Boersma, 2004; Sheridan, 2004). A theoretical foundation for forensic nursing establishes linkages between caring constructs and forensic principles.

Current trends in nursing include increased numbers of nurses with graduate preparation and shared experiences with forensic populations. New themes in nursing education stress **critical thinking**, **evidence-based practice**, and theoretical as well as experiential preparation of advanced nurse practitioners (Kenney, 2006; Oberle & Allen, 2001). Observation of phenomena unique and common to forensic experiences, along with emerging prescriptions for nursing interventions specific to forensic populations, signal the need to organize theoretical knowledge applied to forensic nursing.

The general conception of any field of inquiry ultimately determines the kind of knowledge the field develops. The patterns and images that emerge as we observe forensic clients, forensic settings, and the interactions of forensic nurses and colleagues are indicative of the basic understanding we have of our field of work. It is characterized by bias and the influence of other experiences and disciplines, reflecting the nature of existing environments in which forensic nursing takes place (McEwen & Wills, 2002; Meleis, 2006). In addition to empirical knowledge, nursing decisions are based on knowledge derived from our ethics and values, our sense of aesthetics, and our personal experience. The aim of the application of this knowledge is to organize nursing practice by comprehensively assessing clients, recognizing patterns, diagnosing problems, and using selected nursing methods and technology to care for and assist clients and their families, as well as communities, in their responses to those problems. Nurses in forensic practice are obliged to identify an **organizing framework** as the foundation of practice in order to systematically and reliably carry out its aims.

Organizing Forensic Nursing Theory

In order to understand forensic nursing practice as a distinct nursing specialty, a body of knowledge that is unique to this application of nursing must be identified, along with a set of nursing interventions aimed at using this knowledge to *apply the nursing process*.

The value of a conceptual framework for forensic nursing is threefold: (1) It allows for the public debate of philosophical assumptions about the specialty, providing the opportunity for self-evaluation and accountability to the public and to the profession; (2) the development of a conceptual framework provides for the structure of theoretical statements and hypotheses suggesting appropriate and effective nursing interventions; and (3) hypotheses derived from a conceptual framework allow for systematic scrutiny and analysis of emerging care protocols. A conceptual framework also identifies developmental and political influences on the practice of forensic nursing, giving the profession a base from which to determine best practices and best policies for regulation within the field.

Forensic nursing is an evolving entity in search of an identity; it is in competition with and in collaboration with such other disciplines and professionals as forensic psychiatry, forensic psychology, physician assistants, forensic pathologists, emergency room physicians, and medical examiners, to name a few. Major trends in nursing education and nursing practice in the United States include advanced education for nursing practice (nurse practitioners and clinical nurse specialists) and nationally recognized certification in an area of clinical specialization. Other trends include use of specialized bodies of knowledge and skills to deliver research-based or evidence-based practice, use of nontraditional practice sites, and the growth of community-based nursing care. Building on these trends, it is reasonable and prudent for those who identify themselves as forensic nurses to systematically build a body of nursing knowledge by which to differentiate the specialty, providing a framework for basic and advanced nursing education and an agenda for research.

Because this new forensic nursing identity is just emerging, there are very different conceptualizations of it in the United States compared to the United Kingdom and other countries. In Canada and the United Kingdom, the term *forensic nurse* most commonly applies to those nurses working in secure settings with psychiatric patients. In the United States, the term *forensic nurse* is most commonly identified with nurses working in forensic medical settings such as the medical examiner's office and the coroner's office. These nurses, at first appraisal, seem to share nothing but a common term, *forensic,* and the public, along with many in nursing, are confused and at times offended by the association of this name with nursing.

As an applied practice profession, nursing has emerged as a dominant integrator of knowledge applicable to human caring. Nursing borrows from fields of social and biological sciences, as well as the humanities and other applied fields, in order to understand principles explaining health and the nature of human beings. Nursing theory tells us how to apply this knowledge to activities and problems that are distinctly *nursing.*

One can look beyond the stereotype of analyzing the criminal mind or investigating the scene of the crime for a comprehensive role for nursing. The role of a nurse includes the diagnosis and treatment of human responses to actual or potential health problems among clients (individuals, groups, families, or communities) who are victims or perpetrators of crimes, violence, or trauma. Forensic nursing, like so many other nursing specialties, came into being because there was a need that was not being met, in settings where nurses have access, and in which the knowledge and skill set of the nurse could be exploited (Baly, 1995; Oberle & Allen, 2001). Forensic nursing evolved from the caretaking of special populations. Inmates and those accused of crime, along with those victims of crime presenting with mental disorders and other psychological and physical wounds, have long been in the care of nurses. Addressing the needs of these individuals and their families can be developed as an application of general nursing skills and specialized skills from the critical care, emergency room, and women's healthcare settings, along with psychiatric and community health nursing. Over the years, nurses have recognized that the needs of these people required skills and knowledge outside usual nursing preparation. Nurses turned to forensic psychiatry and forensic medicine to acquire information and techniques appropriate to the problems they encountered. Based on disciplines such as these and others, nurses have acquired knowledge to enhance assessment and interventions appropriate to the needs presented in forensic practice (Goll-McGee, 1999; Lynch, 1995).Nurses have always received and cared for victims of crime and trauma. From emergency rooms to schools, nurses have assessed and triaged and planned for and intervened with victims and their families. Law enforcement officers and other representatives of the court intersect with nurses and the healthcare system when evidence collection overlaps with assessment and medical care. Nurses have, out of necessity, looked to forensic science and criminal justice codes as additional sources of knowledge from which to analyze factors affecting client care.

Models of nursing care provided to forensic populations, both perpetrators and victims of crime and their families, have been compared anecdotally and through publications, emphasizing common recurring issues and problems. Observation of phenomena unique and common to forensic experiences, along with emerging prescriptions for nursing interventions specific to forensic populations, signal the need to organize theoretical knowledge applied to forensic nursing.

Environment

Violence is a significant component of understanding environment, particularly in the United States, where violence is more common than in any other industrialized country that is not engaged in a civil war (Gellert, 2002). Consistent with contemporary conceptualizations, violence is viewed as a major public health problem and establishes a context for understanding factors contributing to social resource deficits, political priorities and sensitivities, and acknowledgment or recognition of mental disorders, deviancy, victimization, and trauma (American Association of Colleges of Nursing, 1999; Canadian Public Health Association, 1997). The National Institutes of Health, recognizing the relationship of violence and trauma to mental health, has prioritized research studying acute reactions to trauma and risk for psychopathology, disaster mental health, and mass violence, as well as exposure to domestic and community violence (National Institutes of Health, 2004).

Environments for forensic nursing are viewed as both physical surroundings and social realities that serve as the context for analyzing and understanding the human responses to forensic phenomena of violence and abuse. Crime scenes and settings in which violence has occurred, as well as formal organizational settings such as medical examiner offices and emergency rooms, are environments for forensic nursing. Any event or location where violence or abuse occurs, or where victims or perpetrators of violence or abuse receive care, is potentially an environment for forensic nursing. The unique aspect of environment, as constructed by forensic nursing, is the potential for human suffering or trauma with accompanying interest or involvement of the criminal justice system.

Violence is defined as the intentional use of force to harm a human being; the intended outcome is physical or psychological injury, fatal or nonfatal (Rosenberg, 2002).

Violence takes many forms, from verbal attacks to murder. Both short-term and long-term responses to violence affect individual and group health, including psychological and physical impairment, disintegration of family and community cohesiveness, and destruction of physical and financial bases for social sustainability (American Association of Colleges of Nursing, 1999). Violence is part of the environment, and the experience of individuals and communities in response to violence is a phenomenon of concern to nursing. As society attempts to cope with the growing incidence of violence in individual, group, and societal acts, increased attention is being given to violence as it occurs in everyday life. A growing awareness of limited resources to deal with person-on-person violence has prompted legislators to respond to public demands for action. Violence must be understood in terms of gender, race, culture, and time (Gellert, 2002), and nurses working in forensic settings must be able to construct nursing interventions based on knowledge of violence as a complex environmental concept occurring at every level of social organization, from interpersonal violence among intimate partners to impersonal violence perpetrated as an act of global terrorism.

Growing intolerance for any sort of threat to personal safety and public peace is a stimulus for action and provides a societal need to which nursing has responded by developing forensic nursing roles. Healthcare providers have responded to the issue of violence as a major public health problem, documenting the incidence and impact of violence on the health status of communities through epidemiological research approaches. The conception of violence as a health and medical issue is evidenced by the development of concepts of posttraumatic stress disorder and interventions such as critical incident stress management (Cloitre, Cohen, Edelman, & Han, 2001). Nurses, who use these constructs to develop plans of care for patients, are now being placed in the position of developing effective nursing strategies to respond to the effects of violence and trauma on individuals, groups, and communities (Clements, Vigil, Henry, Kellywood, & Foster, 2003; Glaister & Kesling, 2002). In the absence of a framework for forensic nursing, nurses are challenged to consider diagnoses and interventions related to violence without acknowledgment of the criminal justice system that also intersects with these patients as a result of their involvement in violence related to criminal offense.

Human Beings

A concept related to violence, critical to the understanding of forensic nursing, is victimization. The concept of victim and the field of victimology have traditionally been applied almost exclusively to crime victims who were victimized by individuals. An emerging understanding of victimization includes other forms of harmful behavior that may or may not be criminal and may or may not be perpetrated by one individual upon another. This approach broadens the definition of victimization: A victim is defined as one who is harmed or killed by another; one who is harmed by or made to suffer by an act, circumstance, agency, or condition; a person who suffers injury, loss, or death as a result of an involuntary undertaking; or a person who is tricked, swindled, or taken advantage of. A theoretical exploration of the meaning and impact of victimization relevant to advanced practice forensic nursing is based on defining victim as a recipient of physical and/or psychological trauma. This approach to victimization involves the analysis of the experience of recipients of harm or injury, as well as accompanying issues of guilt, powerlessness, anger, fear, and impaired problem-solving abilities, which so often characterize victims (Campbell & Humphreys, 2003; Elklit, 2002; Fishman, Mesch, & Eisikovits, 2002; Nettlebeck & Wilson, 2002;).

Although considerable data exist reflecting statistics on the incidence and cost of victimization, there is only beginning to be a significant body of literature identifying the process and consequences of victimization. Within a forensic nursing framework, *human beings* are distinguished as either victims or perpetrators of crime or trauma whose care is partially determined by their involvement with and resolution of criminal or justice issues. They are identified as individuals, groups, families, or communities. Relational victimization theory recognizes the commonality of loss experienced by individuals, families, and communities and stratifies victims as primary (actual victims of crime), secondary (families of perpetrators), and tertiary (law enforcement, correctional and criminal justice personnel, and the community at large) (McCarthy & Bruin, 2002). Victims can be survivors or deceased, and perpetrators may also be victims. Nurses working with forensic populations are more likely than not to be caring for a patient who is a victim of crime and abuse. How we evaluate the impact of previous traumatization of an individual or group affects the scope of care we are able to deliver and influences the attitudes we sustain in order to care for these patients. Individuals can assume the role of victim as a learned behavioral response to social and interpersonal cues present in the environment. Many traumatized people expose themselves, seemingly compulsively, to situations reminiscent of the original trauma. These behavioral reenactments are rarely consciously understood to be related to earlier victimization. Behavioral reenactment of a trauma may manifest itself as one or more of three responses, which may involve the individual as victim or victimizer. The responses are:

1. *Harm to others:* Reenactment of victimization is thought to be a major cause of violence. Criminals have often been physically and sexually abused and it is not unusual for inmates to engage in self-mutilating behavior.

2. *Self-destructiveness:* Self-destructiveness is seen frequently in correctional or secure settings. Often a characteristic of borderline personality disorder, self-destructiveness is common in those who have been abused. Self-destructive behaviors, including those acts that deprive an inmate of *privileges or dischar*ge from incarceration, are not primarily related to conflict, guilt, and superego pressure but are related to more primitive behavior patterns originating in painful encounters with hostile caretakers early in life or dependent relationships later in life.

3. *Revictimization:* **Revictimization** is a consistent finding in which rape victims and victims of abuse or violence are more likely to be abused again as adults.

Compliance with an abuser's demands legitimizes those demands, creates an accumulation of repressed anger and frustration in the victim, and creates an environment of violence, threats, degradation, and humiliation. This process deprives the victim of opportunities to build up an effective social support system, and the repressed anger can support continued victimization or lead to acts of aggression or victimization on the part of the original victim.

Information processing of trauma is a theoretical context that identifies victimization behaviors as a neuropsychiatric response (Burgess, Hartman, & Baker, 1995; Walker, Scott, & Koppersmith, 1998). This model assumes the basic constructs of information processing of a living system and that experiences are processed on a sensory, perceptual, cognitive, and interpersonal level. The individual first registers a traumatic experience through the sensory level, after which the perceptual level (within the sensory) begins to classify the event. The cognitive and interpersonal levels further classify the event and give it meaning to the individual.

Posttraumatic Stress Disorder

A general response syndrome to trauma, first described by Horowitz in 1986 occurs in two major stages. First, the disturbing psychological phenomena are presented as a cluster of intrusive and repetitive imagery associated with memory. Second, the victim develops avoidance strategies to keep associations with the trauma out of awareness. Resolution of the event occurs when there is sufficient processing for the information to be stored in distant memory; when the event is remembered, the attendant feelings are neutralized, and the anxiety generated by the event is controlled. When the victim does not resolve the event and it either remains in active memory or becomes defended by a defense mechanism (such as denial, dissociation, or splitting), the diagnosis is generally posttraumatic stress disorder. In this case the individual experiences the trauma both unconsciously and consciously (Burgess, Hartman, & Clements, 1995).

Forensic nursing contains a structure for understanding the tensions and variability among definitions and responses to social deviance and trauma and for caring for those who experience such problems. Using the construct of victimization and the microtheories explaining the process and impact of victimization, forensic nursing applies specific approaches to assessment and planning care specific to the conditions and imperatives determined by the criminal justice system, with whom the patient is also interacting.

Theories of oppression describe the unjust use of authority and provide explanations for deviant human behavior. Oppression is a complex, pervasive social problem emanating from and sustained by oppression of race, class, gender, and even age, as in the application of differential oppression theory to the development of delinquency. In this model, the adult oppression of children is reflected in parents' ability to force children into socially defined and controlled inferior roles. Children's reactions to this oppression are reflected in maladaptive or problem behaviors, one of which is delinquency. In this model, the deviant behavior is actually conceptualized as adaptation through one of four modes: passive acceptance, exercise of illegitimate coercive power, **manipulation** of one's peers, and finally retaliation (Regoli & Hewitt, 2010). Advanced practice forensic nursing applies theoretical knowledge of violence and oppression in relation to social causes of violence. Analyzing health in relation to racism, sexism, classism, and ageism establishes constructs for the prevention of violence and the impetus for social change (Varcoe, 1996).

The experience of *boundary violations* is a theme for understanding victims and perpetrators of crime and abuse. Boundary violations exist when role behaviors of one person are not consistent with the societal norms or personal expectations of another. The degree of boundary violation, and therefore the impact, is determined by the symbolic meaning of the act that is considered deviant, unacceptable, or intrusive. Boundary violation results in emotional or physical discomfort and perceived threat to the person for whom the boundary violation occurs. Boundary violations can occur in terms of space, as when one person touches another or otherwise intrudes upon another's personal space (Cote, 2001; Gutheil & Simon, 2002; Radden, 2001). Boundary violations can also include verbal interruption, speaking for another, or taking away another's opportunity to speak or express ideas. Boundary violations also occur in social terms when one performs an act outside the range of expected or acceptable behaviors, as when a nurse forms a sexual relationship with a patient or when a person deprives another of their personal belongings (theft). When one member of a married couple engages in adultery, he or she invades the roles of his or her spouse, enacting boundary violations on them and their families. Boundary violations also occur when a person unwittingly enters into familiar or inappropriate interaction with another, such as when tourists invade a private social hangout of local inhabitants of a small town and proceed to sit at a regular patron's favorite table, or when a victim of a crime proceeds to find the perpetrator on his own, bypassing the legal system to enact vigilante justice. Any time boundary violations take place, a sense of loss, personal threat, and anxiety occurs. People who are involved with the criminal justice system frequently exert boundary violations, due to either cognitive disorders, social pathology, anxiety, or ignorance.

Every theoretical construct used to define and explain the practice of forensic nursing is dependent upon the understanding of theories of violence and victimization and their application to the nursing process for individuals, groups, and communities, along with social systems and global agencies who are recognized as victims or perpetrators of victimization.

Nursing

Forensic nurses care for those who are victims or perpetrators of crime, violence, or abuse. The nursing process focuses on specific applications of forensic and other sciences and sociocultural sensitivities to the formal assessment, diagnosis, planning, and evaluation of interventions aimed at the resolution of human responses to violence. Forensic nurses must assess boundary violations and intervene to reorient the client to his or her expected role; apply consistent and effective strategies to support the client in recognizing his or her behavior as a boundary violation; recognize where physical, social, and legal boundaries are; and develop a repertoire of skills that enable him or her to maintain appropriate boundaries.

Essential skill sets for forensic nurses include advanced physical and psychological assessment of violence, trauma, and abuse, such as recognition and identification of patterned injury, assessment for risk of violence or self-injurious behavior, differentiation of factitious disorders and manipulation, and delineation of boundaries. Handling, processing, and documenting assessments and interventions as evidence is clearly a distinguishing feature of forensic nursing.

Ethical dilemmas are part of every nurse's role, but the blurred boundaries and conflicting role expectations of nurses working in forensic settings magnify the impact of ethical decision making on forensic nursing outcomes. The intersection of criminal justice with healthcare systems and the balancing of rights between individuals and society are hallmarks of forensic events. The protection of vulnerable individuals' human rights is a common issue addressed in forensic settings, in which nurses are conflicted between the rights of individuals to autonomy and care through a therapeutic and helping relationship and nursing obligations to preserve evidence, security, and control (Grace, Fry, & Schultz, 2003; International Association of Forensic Nursing, 2002; Peter & Morgan, 2001).

The ability to sustain objectivity and a healthy skepticism when assessing individuals and communities in a forensic context often depends on distancing oneself from a relationship with the individual or community. Mastery of the theoretical basis for establishing a trusting professional relationship must incorporate a sound knowledge of legal and ethical principles that serve as boundaries for forensic nursing practice (Austin, 2001; Daly, 2002). Older approaches to nursing ethics—built on contracts, paternalism, and care—are being replaced by a trust approach for nursing ethics (Peter & Morgan, 2001). In this model the ethics of care and justice are integrated, with emphasis on acknowledging vulnerability and the potential for malevolence. The importance of ethical decision-making is clear within the competition for power that exists in events and processes related to the criminal justice system and governments (Austin).

The process and effects of institutionalization and social isolation are factors that determine options in therapeutic interventions for those nurses working with clients in secure settings. Long-term confinements in rigid settings that dictate behaviors narrowly have a profound effect on patients and caregivers alike. Forensic nurses, especially those working in psychiatric settings, need a theoretical base from which to determine the therapeutic value of interventions, particularly when the goal of rehabilitation and wellness held by the nurse may be in conflict with the goal of punishment and retribution held by the institutional staff and the community. The social isolation that often accompanies victims of heinous crimes such as rape or incest can have the same devastating effects as incarceration or confinement in a mental institution. The revictimization that is said to occur often when a victim is processed through the criminal justice system has predictable consequences, which must be taken into account in any understanding of specialized care of these individuals.

Manipulation is a predictable adaptation strategy among clients, and it necessitates prescribed, consistent, and firm responses on the part of the nurse. Dealing with manipulative individuals who may falsify information and fake signs and symptoms or deny them is challenging and exhausting. Recognizing manipulation and dealing with it in a manner that is supportive to the environment in which the client exists is critical to successful forensic nursing.

Health

Defining **health** within a forensic nursing context is a challenging and evolving process, primarily focusing on successful resolution of the effects of traumatization or victimization. Successful applications of different nursing models allow for a pluralistic approach to understanding health, from adaptation to violence to finding meaning in survivorship. A growing body of literature on victimology distinguishes victimization from survivorship, establishing characteristics of successful response to violence, trauma, or abuse (Adkins, 2003; Clements et al., 2003; Cloitre et al., 2001; Gallop, 2002; Gellert, 2002; Lanza, Kazis, & Lee). Assessment of survivor characteristics and implementation of interventions to promote learned behaviors promoting survivorship are essential components of forensic nursing.

Health is constructed in terms of multiple views of human beings and in relation to different contexts or environments in which violence or abuse occurs. Successful resolution of conflicts related to trauma or violence; movement from victim to survivor; and healing of psychological or physical wounds sustained as a result of violence, trauma, or abuse are views of health through a forensic nursing perspective. Promotion of interpersonal or community peace, restoration of family or community integrity, and increasing the resiliency or hardiness of individuals and communities are also indicators of forensic health (Rosenberg, 2002).

An example of the application of forensic health concepts to forensic nursing can be articulated in the nurse death investigator role. The role of death investigator is perhaps the most challenging to relate to traditional definitions of nursing and health. In this situation the patient is the deceased and/or the family or those with whom the deceased had a relationship prior to death. Any unexplained or unexpected death is accompanied by forensic data collection and additional trauma for family and significant others. The forensic nursing model applied to the death investigator role preserves the caring aspect of the nursing relationship with those connected to the deceased and the death event. Rights to nursing care extend beyond death, and this obligation is assumed by the nurse death investigator.

An awareness of the social construction of deviancy provides a foundation for understanding the relative and changing nature of diagnoses and responses to human behaviors associated with crime, trauma, and abuse. The issue of personality disorder as a mental illness is currently being scrutinized. The question of whether someone who has a personality disorder can be treated or whether that person is sick at all or just mean is debated among those who ultimately must either assign care or pay for it (Breeze & Repper, 1998; Gellert, 2002; Mercer, Mason, & Richman, 1999). Nurses must understand that conditions for which we treat individuals can change over time as the nature of public sensibilities in the process of medicalizing human behavior changes. Today, most mental illnesses do not qualify as a defense of innocence for a crime, while being a spouse abuse victim or having premenstrual syndrome may or may not be taken into account as rationale for one's deviant or illegal behavior. A useful nursing framework provides a structure for understanding maladaptive human responses regardless of their standing in the medical/legal system and provides an understanding of appropriate nursing responses. A forensic nursing framework will account for the changing nature of social contexts for care, balancing the need for culturally competent care with universal care needs. Knowledge of the social and criminal justice systems increasingly dictate the conditions under which nurses care for their clients and the resources and priorities assigned to the care of those clients. The conceptual framework for forensic nursing must stand apart from these social systems and propose the range of overlap that best serves the needs of society and the profession.

A conceptual framework for forensic nursing not only must define these considerations, but it also must describe the relationships among the concepts, indicating, among other things, the relationships between the healthcare systems and forensic systems. The social and legal processes by which specific human behaviors and responses are categorized and treated as healthcare problems rather than cruel, evil, or just stupid behavior and the differentiation between victimization and a sense of entitlement must be accounted for as part of the environmental context in which nursing and human health occurs.

Summary

A conceptual framework for forensic nursing is the foundation for education and practice not only for nurses who practice in the specialty, but also for every nurse. A careful examination of the current social and environmental conditions reveals a society that is acutely aware of the relationship between violence and health. Basic education for nursing already includes many areas of content that can be identified as forensic. The value in isolating that content, labeling it as forensic, and incorporating it into the education of the professional nurse is significant. This approach puts a value on forensic knowledge and skills and sets aside specific applications that emphasize the need to raise awareness of the overlap between healthcare systems and criminal justice/forensic systems.

Identifying forensic content in a nursing curriculum lays down the foundation for the recognition of the specialty, encouraging undergraduate experiences in forensic settings. Role socialization for the nurse working in forensic roles begins with a clear conceptualization of the role in basic nursing education. This provides for increased recruitment opportunities of forensic employers, increases the career opportunities for graduates, and supports the nurses working in those settings.

Identification and integration of forensic content into basic nursing education provides a basis for generalist nursing practice inclusive of skills necessary for the care and referral of forensic patients who are cared for in general hospital settings, schools, community settings, and private physician offices. The ability to define concepts central to forensic nursing that differentiate forensic nursing and explain the relationships among those concepts allows nurses to develop a method for organizing our thinking about specialty practice and a guide for evolving as advanced nursing practice. *Forensic nursing* is a term that is emerging in the literature and in practice. Establishing a significant body of theoretical knowledge unique to this specialty will be the challenge of the future.

QUESTIONS FOR DISCUSSION

1. Which nursing interventions impact the health of individuals and communities experiencing violence?
2. What is the process of victimization and how can nursing intervene to prevent, to treat, and to rehabilitate?
   a. What kind of support is necessary for families who participate in the trial, conviction, and execution of the murderer of a family member?
   b. Which clients benefit from reviewing an abusive or victimizing event?
   c. Which nursing interventions can be effective in managing revictimization of patients in incarceration?
3. Which boundary violations characterize perpetrators and victims of crime, trauma, and abuse? How can nurses intervene to promote healthy boundaries among patients?
   a. What is the therapeutic role boundary for a nurse working in a correctional setting?
   b. How does the therapeutic goal for the inmate differ from the patient in a nonsecure setting?
   c. What is the role of the offense in planning and delivering care for persons convicted of crimes?
4. Which processes of institutionalization can be positively impacted by nursing?
5. How does the limitation of citizenship or human rights among offenders affect nursing practice?
6. What is the role of nursing in evidence identification and collection? How does this affect the image of nursing and the public trust?

REFERENCES

Adkins, E. (2003). The first day of the rest of their lives. *Journal of Psychosocial Nursing and Mental Health Services, 41*(7), 29–32.

Alligood, M. R., & Marriner-Tomey, A. (2006). *Nursing theory: Utilization and application.* St. Louis, MO: CV Mosby.

American Association of Colleges of Nursing. (1999). *Violence as a public health problem.* Washington, DC: AACN.

Austin, W. (2001). Relational ethics in forensic psychiatric nursing. *Journal of Psychosocial Nursing and Mental Health Services, 39*(9), 12–17.

Baly, M. (1995). *Nursing and social change* (3rd ed.). London, England: Heinemann Medical.

Breeze, J. A., & Repper, J. (1998). Struggling for control: The care experiences of "difficult" patients in mental health services. *Journal of Advanced Nursing, 28*(6), 1301–1311.

Burgess, A., Hartman, C. R., & Baker, T. (1995). Memory presentations of childhood sexual abuse. *Journal of Psychosocial Nursing & Mental Health Services, 33*(9), 9–16.

Burgess, A., Hartman, C. R., & Clements, P. T., Jr. (1995). Biology of memory and childhood trauma. *Journal of Psychosocial Nursing and Mental Health Services, 33*(3), 16–26; 52–53.

Burgess, A. W., Berger, A. D., & Boersma, R. R. (2004). Forensic nursing: Investigating the career potential in this emerging graduate specialty. *American Journal of Nursing, 104*(3), 58–64.

Campbell, J., & Humphreys, J. (2003). *Family violence and nursing practice.* Philadelphia, PA: Lippincott, Williams and Wilkins.

Canadian Public Health Association. (1997). *Violence in society: A public health perspective.* CPHA Ottawa, Ontario, Canada, issue paper.

Clements, P. T., Vigil, G. J., Henry, G. C., Kellywood, R., & Foster, W. (2003). Cultural perspectives of death, grief, and bereavement. *Journal of Psychosocial Nursing and Mental Health Services, 41*(7), 18–26.

Cloitre, M., Cohen, L. R., Edelman, R. E., & Han, H. (2001). Posttraumatic stress disorder and extent of trauma exposure as correlates of medical problems and perceived health among women with childhood abuse. *Women and Health, 34*(3), 1–17.

Cody, W. K., & Kenney, J. W. (Eds.). (2006). *Philosophical and theoretical perspectives for advanced nursing practice.* Sudbury, MA: Jones and Bartlett.

Cote, I. (2001). A case of pain, factitious disorder, and boundary violations. *Pain Research & Management, 6*(4), 197–200.

Daly, B. (2002). Moving forward: A new code of ethics. *Nursing Outlook, 50*(3), 97–99.

Elklit, A. (2002). Victimization and PTSD in a Danish national youth probability sample. *Child and Adolescent Psychiatry, 41*(2), 174–181.

Fishman, G., Mesch, G. S., & Eisikovits, Z. (2002). Variables affecting adolescent victimization: Findings from a national youth survey. *Western Criminology Review, 3*(2). Retrieved from http://wcr.sonoma.edu/v3n2/fishman.html

Gallop, R. (2002). Failure of the capacity for self-soothing in women who have a history of abuse and self-harm. *Journal of the American Psychiatric Nurses Association, 8*(1), 20–26.

Gellert, G. A. (2002). *Confronting violence: Answers to questions about the epidemic destroying America's homes and communities* (2nd ed.). Washington, DC: American Public Health Association.

Glaister, J. A., & Kesling, G. (2002). A survey of practicing nurses' perspectives on interpersonal violence screening and intervention. *Nursing Outlook, 50*(4), 137–143.

Goll-McGee, B. (1999). The role of the clinical forensic nurse in critical care. *Critical Care Nursing Quarterly, 22*(1), 8–18.

Grace, P. J., Fry, S. T., & Schultz, G. S. (2003). Ethics and human rights issues experienced by psychiatric-mental health and substance abuse registered nurses. *Journal of the American Psychiatric Nurses Association, 9*(2), 17–23.

Gutheil, T. G., & Simon, R. I. (2002). Non-sexual boundary crossings and boundary violations: An ethical dilemma. *Psychiatric Clinics of North America, 25*(3), 585–592.

Kenney, J. W. (Ed.). (2006). *Philosophical and theoretical perspectives for advanced nursing practice.* Sudbury, MA: Jones and Bartlett.

Lanza, M. L., Kazis, L., & Lee, A. (2003). Using the violence prevention community meeting protocol. *Journal of the American Psychiatric Nurses Association, 9*(3), 86–89.

Lynch, V. (1995). Clinical forensic nursing: A new perspective in the management of crime victims from trauma to trial. *Critical Care Nursing Clinics of North America, 7*(3), 489–507.

McEwen, M., & Wills, E. M. (2002). *Theoretical basis for nursing.* Philadelphia, PA: Lippincott, Williams and Wilkins.

Meleis, A. A. (2006). *Theoretical nursing: Development and progress* (4th ed.). Philadelphia, PA: Lippincott.

Mercer, D., Mason, T., & Richman, J. (1999). Good & evil in the crusade of care. Social constructions of mental disorders. *Journal of Psychosocial Nursing and Mental Health Services, 37*(9), 13–17.

National Institutes of Health. (2004). *Health consequences of violence and trauma* (PA-04-075). Department of Health and Human Services. Retrieved from http://grants.nih.gov/grants/guide/pa-files/PA-04-075.html

Nettelbeck, T., & Wilson, C. (2002). Personal vulnerability to victimization of people with mental retardation. *Trauma Violence and Abuse, 3*(4), 289–306.

Oberle, K., & Allen, M. (2001). The nature of advanced practice nursing, *Nursing Outlook, 49*(3), 148–153.

Peter, E., & Morgan, K. P. (2001). Explorations of a trust approach for nursing ethics. *Nursing Inquiry, 8*, 3–10.

Radden, J. (2001). Boundary violation ethics: Some conceptual clarifications. *Journal of the American Academy of Psychiatry and the Law, 29*(3), 319–326.

Regoli, R., & Hewitt, J. D. (2010). *Delinquency in society.* New York, NY: McGraw-Hill.

Rodgers, B. L., & Knafl, K. A. (2000). *Concept development in nursing: Foundations, techniques, and applications.* Philadelphia, PA: WB Saunders.

Sheridan, D. J. (2004). Legal and forensic nursing responses to family violence. In J. Humphreys & J. C. Campbell (Eds.), *Family violence and nursing practice* (pp. 385–406). Philadelphia, PA: Lippincott, Williams & Wilkins.

Varcoe, C. (1996). Theorizing oppression: Implications for nursing research on violence against women. *Canadian Journal of Nursing Research, 28*(1), 61–78.

Walker, G. C., Scott, P. S., & Koppersmith, G. (1998). The impact of child sexual abuse on addiction severity: An analysis of trauma processing. *Journal of Psychosocial Nursing and Mental Health Services, 36*(3), 10–18; 40–41.

SUGGESTED FURTHER READING

Cody, W. K. (2006). *Philosophical and theoretical perspectives for advanced nursing practice.* Sudbury, MA: Jones and Bartlett.

Kim, H. S. (2000). *The nature of theoretical thinking in nursing.* New York, NY: Springer.

Marriner-Tomey, A., & Alligood, M. R. (2005). *Nursing theorists and their work.* Philadelphia, PA: Mosby.

Marriner-Tomey, A., & Alligood, M. R. (2006). *Nursing theory: Utilization & application.* Philadelphia, PA: Mosby.

McCormack, B. (2010). *Person-centered nursing: Theory and practice.* Ames, IA: Wiley-Blackwell.

McEwen, M. (2011). *Theoretical basis for nursing.* Philadelphia, PA: Wolters Kluwer/Lippincott Williams & Wilkins.

Meleis, A. I. (2007). *Theoretical nursing: Development and progress.* Philadelphia, PA: Lippincott Williams & Wilkins.

Pinch, W., & Haddad, A. M. (2008). *Nursing and healthcare ethics: A legacy and a vision.* Silver Spring, MD: American Nurses Association.

Reed, P. G. (2009). *Perspectives on nursing theory.* Philadelphia, PA: Wolters Kluwer Health/Lippincott Williams & Wilkins.

CHAPTER 3

Epidemiology of Violence

Linda C. Degutis

In order to appreciate the range of violent events that may be encountered in the practice of forensic nursing, it is important to understand the various forms of violence that result in injury, as well as the proportions of these events in the population in general, and in specific subgroups of the population. An understanding of the basic principles of epidemiology, with specific reference to injury epidemiology, is also essential.

CHAPTER FOCUS

- » Definition of Violence
- » Description of Types of Interpersonal Violence
- » Sources of Data
- » Epidemiology of Violence
- » Risk Factor for Violence

KEY TERMS

- » assault
- » epidemiology
- » firearms
- » homicide
- » intentional injury
- » intimate partner violence
- » National Violent Death Reporting System
- » suicide
- » terrorism
- » violence
- » war

On any given day, it is possible to read multiple news reports that reinforce the fact that violence is a part of our everyday lives. Dramatic events such as suicide bombings and other acts of terrorism have taken over the front pages of our newspapers, and the common acts of violence such as homicides and assaults that occur around the country are relegated to other parts of the paper. Biases in reporting can lead one to either underestimate or overestimate the number of events that take place in any particular city or state or in any given population subgroup. Putting together the data about all of these events is important in understanding the true nature of violence and its impact on our society.

Violence Defined

Violence has many forms. In this chapter, only physical violence will be discussed in detail. In addition, the standard terms to describe intent with respect to injury will be used. Unintentional injuries are injuries that result from events that have traditionally been thought of as accidents. Some examples of such events are a motor vehicle crash that occurs when a driver fails to stop quickly enough to avoid hitting the car in front of him, an elderly woman tripping and falling over a loose rug in the bathroom, or a toddler who cuts his chin on the sharp edge of an end table. What these events have in common is that they were not intentional—neither the injured person nor another person deliberately caused the event that resulted in an injury.

Intentional injuries or injuries related to violence are the result of a deliberate act that is committed by the person who is injured, or by another person, with intent to cause harm. These events include such things as an overdose of illicit drugs, a fistfight that leads to facial injuries, and a drive-by shooting of two adolescents walking down a street. At times, an intentional act of violence becomes an unintentional act as innocent bystanders, by virtue of being in the wrong place at the wrong time, become the victims.

CASE STUDY 3.1

Innocent Bystanders

In July 2010, a 14-year-old girl was killed by a rain of gunfire as she sat on a safari tourist bus with her relatives in the U.S. Virgin Islands. She was apparently caught in the crossfire between two rival gangs at war. The girl was on an on-shore excursion from a cruise ship that had stopped for the day at Sharma Amalie. Another passenger was injured in the shootout. The girl was found wounded on the bus while the intended victim was found dead in the street near the bus.

Source: CNN. (2010). Teen tourist killed in crossfire in U.S. Virgin Islands. Retrieved from http://news .blogs.cnn.com/2010/07/13/teen-tourist-killed-in-crossfire-in-u-s-virgin-islands

---

The types of violent events that occur and the mechanisms by which they occur can be defined further. **Homicide** is an intentional killing of one person by another. **Suicide** is the deliberate taking of one's own life. **Assault** is the physical attack by one person upon another, which may or may not result in physical injury. **Intimate partner violence** (IPV) is the occurrence of physically violent acts between persons who have an intimate relationship, regardless of their sex. Weapons include any object or body part that is used to inflict physical harm on a person. **Firearms** are handguns, long guns, and any other type of gun that may be used to inflict harm upon oneself or another person. **Terrorism** is the deliberate and planned act of a person or group of people against another person or group of people in order to achieve political or economic gain. **War** is a conflict that results in broad-scale violence against specific groups of people who are sought out because of their religious, political, or social beliefs.

Two particular types of violence that are not discussed in this chapter, as they require more detailed attention, are child abuse and sexual assault. Child abuse includes injuries intentionally inflicted upon a child by a parent, caretaker, or other adult who has responsibility for a child, or who is an intimate partner of the parent or caretaker of a child. Sexual assault is the act of forcing a person, against her or his will, to participate in a sexual act, either actively or passively.

Epidemiology

Epidemiology is the study of the impact of disease and injury on the population. This includes an examination of the distribution of injury and illness, as well as an assessment of the risk factors that contribute to these health problems. The epidemiologic model that takes into account the host, the agent of injury or illness, and the vector by which the injury or illness is transmitted is readily used in the study of injuries and violence. In addition, Haddon (1968) proposed that all injuries, including those resulting from violent acts, could be analyzed using a matrix that includes three phases (preevent, event, and postevent) and three factors (human factors, vehicle/agent factors, and the environment). This matrix can be used to perform an examination of a single event or to evaluate multiple violent events for commonalities and differences. An example of the matrix as applied to a violent event is shown in **Table 3-1**. Applying these types of epidemiologic methods to look at violent events provides information about relationships between various physical and environmental factors and the potential outcomes associated with them.

Sources of Data

Data concerning deaths due to violence as well as nonfatal violence-related injuries may be obtained from a number of sources. However, there is no comprehensive, timely database that provides all of this information in one place. In order to address this problem, at least with respect to violent deaths, the Centers for Disease Control and Prevention has initiated the **National Violent Death Reporting System**. This system is designed to maintain a complete, timely record of violent deaths of residents of 13 states in the United States, as well as any deaths to nonresidents that occur in those states. The cases collected within this system include deaths due to homicide, suicide, undetermined intent, legal intervention, and unintentional firearm injury. Data are obtained from death certificates, medical examiner or coroner records, law enforcement records, and crime laboratories. This system has only recently been initiated, but it shows promise for providing population-based data on deaths due to violence (Paulozzi, Mercy, Frazier, & Annest, 2004). It is expected that all 50 states will be involved in this data collection system in the future.

Various levels of hospital data also are available, but the specific type of data available and degree of complexity vary by state. Hospital discharge data sets are generally based on billing data and can provide information about hospitalizations and sometimes emergency department visits related to violence. National databases that contain information about

TABLE 3-1   Haddon Matrix applied to a violent event

Phases	Factors		
	Human	*Vehicle/Agent*	*Environment*
Pre-event	History of abuse as a child	Firearm stored with bullet in chamber	Violence accepted as a means of settling disagreement
Event	Human body's resistance to energy insults	Hollow-point bullet flattens as it passes through body tissue	Presence of other people during the assault
Post-event	Hemorrhage	Location of bullet fragments	Rapid access to emergency care

treatment for injuries, including those related to violent events, are as follows: the Health-care Cost and Utilization Project data set, which is maintained by the Agency for Health-care Research and Quality and can be queried for specific information (AHRQ 2010); the Emergency Department Internet Query System of the National Hospital Ambulatory Medical Care Survey can be queried by specific International Classification of Diseases -9 code, as well as population subgroup, in order to examine emergency department visits for violence-related injury (McCaig & Burt, 2003).

The Uniform Crime Reports of the Federal Bureau of Investigation provide information about homicide and other crimes, and the National Incident-Based Reporting System provides more in-depth analysis of crime data, which includes homicide and assault information (Uniform Crime Report, 2008). Data about both the perpetrator and victim, which can be useful in investigations and risk assessments, are available.

The Centers for Disease Control and Prevention does provide data on fatal and non-fatal injuries due to various causes in the Web-based injury statistics query and reporting system (CDC, 2010b). This database can be queried in order to identify specific rates of both fatal and nonfatal injury events due to various causes.

Rates

Rates of injuries or deaths due to violence are often reported. In general, the rate is expressed as the rate per hundred thousand of the population of interest. This provides useful information for comparing rates across age groups, sexes, racial/ethnic groups, and other population groups.

The Epidemiology of Violence

Of the approximately 150,000 injury-related deaths in the United States each year, 31% are due to violence. Suicide accounts for 62% of the **intentional injury** deaths, homicide accounts for approximately 37%, and legal interventions account for fewer than 1% (CDC, 2010b). Intentional injuries are one of the leading causes of death for several age groups, as illustrated in **Table 3-2**. Injuries resulting from violence are responsible for approximately 9% of the years of potential life lost prior to age 75. Table 3-2, **Table 3-3**, and **Table 3-4** illustrate the leading causes of death, injury-related death, and violence-related death across the life span for the year 2007.

Suicide

Each year, suicide accounts for approximately 31,000 deaths in the United States. It is important to keep in mind the appropriate terms to use when discussing suicide. A completed suicide occurs when the victim dies. A suicide attempt is an event in which the victim does not die. Suicide disproportionately affects adolescents, young adults, and the elderly. The methods by which these events occur are also important to understand. The instrument most often used in suicide is a firearm. In 2007, 17,352 firearm-related suicides occurred, with the greatest number of these (3,943) in the 65 and over age group (CDC, 2010b). Other means of committing suicide include drug overdose, hanging, suffocation, and carbon monoxide poisoning. **Table 3-5** compares some of the common mechanisms of homicides and suicides.

TABLE 3-2   10 Leading Causes of Death, U.S. 2007, All Races Both Sexes

Age Groups

1–4	5–9	10–14	15–24	25–34	35–44	45–54	55–64
Unintentional Injury 1,588	Unintentional Injury 965	Unintentional Injury 1,229	Unintentional Injury 15,897	Unintentional Injury 14,977	Unintentional Injury 16,931	Malignant Neoplasms 50,167	Malignant Neoplasms 103,171
Congenital Anomalies 546	Malignant Neoplasms 480	Malignant Neoplasms 479	Homicide 5,551	Suicide 5,278	Malignant Neoplasms 13,288	Heart Disease 37,434	Heart Disease 65,527
Homicide 398	Congenital Anomalies 196	Homicide 213	Suicide 4,140	Homicide 4,758	Heart Disease 11,839	Unintentional Injury 20,315	Chronic Low Respiratory Disease 12,777
Malignant Neoplasms 364	Homicide 133	Suicide 180	Malignant Neoplasms 1,653	Malignant Neoplasms 3,463	Suicide 6,722	Liver Disease 8,212	Unintentional Injury 12,193
Heart Disease 173	Heart Disease 110	Congenital Anomalies 178	Heart Disease 1,084	Heart Disease 3,223	HIV 3,572	Suicide 7,778	Diabetes Mellitus 11,304
Influenza & Pneumonia 109	Chronic Low Respiratory Disease 54	Heart Disease 131	Congenital Anomalies 402	HIV 1,091	Homicide 3,052	Cerebrovascular 6,385	Cerebrovascular 10,500
Septicemia 78	Influenza & Pneumonia 48	Chronic Low Respiratory Disease 64	Cerebrovascular 195	Diabetes Mellitus 610	Liver Disease 2,570	Diabetes Mellitus 5,753	Liver Disease 8,004

(continues)

TABLE 3-2 10 Leading Causes of Death, U.S. 2007, All Races Both Sexes (continued)

				Age Groups			
1–4	5–9	10–14	15–24	25–34	35–44	45–54	55–64
Perinatal Period 70	Neoplasms 41	Benign Pneumonia 55	Influenza & Mellitus 168	Diabetes Cerebrovascular 505	Cerebrovascular 2,133	HIV 4,156	Suicide 5,069
Benign Neoplasms 59	Cerebrovascular 38	Cerebrovascular 45	Influenza & Pneumonia 163	Congenital Anomalies 417	Diabetes Mellitus 1,984	Chronic Low Respiratory Disease 4,153	Nephritis 4,440
Chronic Low Respiratory Disease 57	Septicemia 36	Benign Neoplasms 43	Three Tied 160	Liver Disease 384	Septicemia 910	Viral Hepatitis 2,815	Septicemia 4,231

MV = motor vehicle.

Produced by: Office of Statistics and Programming, National Center for Injury Prevention and Control, Centers for Disease Control and Prevention.

Data source: National Center for Health Statistics (NCHS), National Vital Statistics System.

TABLE 3-3 10 Leading Causes of Injury Deaths, United States 2007, All Races, Both Sexes

| | Age Groups | | | | | | | |
	<1	1–4	5–9	10–14	15–24	25–34	35–44	45–54
	Unintentional Suffocation 959	Unintentional Drowning 458	Unintentional MV traffic 456	Unintentional MV traffic 696	Unintentional MV traffic 10,272	Unintentional MV traffic 6,842	Unintentional Poisoning 7,575	Unintentional Poisoning 9,006
	Homicide Unspecified 174	Unintentional MV traffic 428	Unintentional Fire/burn 136	Homicide Firearm 154	Homicide Firearm 4,669	Unintentional Poisoning 5,700	Unintentional MV traffic 6,135	Unintentional MV traffic 6,262

MV = motor vehicle.

Produced by: Office of Statistics and Programming, National Center for Injury Prevention and Control, Centers for Disease Control and Prevention.

Data source: National Center for Health Statistics (NCHS), National Vital Statistics System.

TABLE 3-4 10 Leading Causes of Violence-Related Injury Deaths, United States 2007, All Races, Both Sexes

	Age Groups							
	1-4	5-9	10-14	15-24	25-34	35-44	45-54	55-64
	Homicide Unspecified 174	Homicide Firearm 47	Homicide Firearm 154	Homicide Firearm 4,669	Homicide Firearm 3,751	Suicide Firearm 2,879	Suicide Firearm 3,531	Suicide Firearm 2,786
	Homicide Other Specified, Classifiable 61	Homicide Suffocation 21	Suicide Suffocation 119	Suicide Firearm 1,900	Suicide Firearm 2,306	Homicide Firearm 2,038	Suicide Poisoning 2,015	Suicide Poisoning 1,147
	Homicide Firearm 48	Homicide Cut/pierce 13	Suicide Firearm 53	Suicide Suffocation 1,533	Suicide Suffocation 1,770	Suicide Suffocation 1,839	Suicide Suffocation 1,589	Suicide Suffocation 725

MV = motor vehicle.

Produced by: Office of Statistics and Programming, National Center for Injury Prevention and Control, Centers for Disease Control and Prevention.

Data source: National Center for Health Statistics (NCHS), National Vital Statistics System.

TABLE 3-5   Injury Deaths Classified by Type of Injury

Mechanism	Suicide	Homicide
Firearm	17,352	12,632
Suffocation	8,161	637
Transportation-related	131	30
Poisoning	6,358	85

Source: From WISQARS. WISQARS Leading Causes of Death Reports, 1999– 2007. Retrieved from http://webappa.cdc.gov/sasweb/ncipc/leadcaus10.html

There are multiple risk factors for suicide that may change across the life span. One of the most important risk factors is depression. Other factors that contribute to the risk of suicide include alcohol problems, chronic illness, mental health problems, and impulsive behavior.

Homicide

Homicide accounts for approximately 37% of intentional injury deaths and was responsible for 18,773 deaths in 2007 (CDC, 2010b). The vast majority of homicides in the United States are committed with a firearm; other mechanisms of homicide include knives or sharp objects, assaults with a blunt instrument, fire, or use of a motor vehicle. Although there are fewer homicides than suicides each year, the primary mechanism for each is a firearm, accounting for approximately 55% of these events. Homicide continues to be the leading cause of death for black males between the ages of 15 and 24, as it has been for the past several years. In addition, black females between 10 and 19 experience homicide at a rate that is three times that of white females in the same age group. The homicide rate among black females aged 15 to 45 years has increased over the past several years so that it is now the leading cause of death in this group. Other groups in which homicide is one of the leading causes of death are children between ages 1 and 4, and youth between ages 15 and 19 of all racial groups. Despite this, there has been a steady decrease in the rate of homicide deaths over the past 10 years. This may be attributable to many interventions, and it is difficult to determine exactly what proportion of the decrease is due to these changes.

Intimate Partner Violence

Intimate partner violence (IPV) includes violence between two people of either sex who are currently, or have been, intimate partners. Women who experience IPV are higher utilizers of healthcare services than other women, making more emergency department visits for injuries and medical complaints, as well as more visits to primary care and mental health services (Centers for Disease Control and Prevention, 2010a). Women are victims of IPV far more often than men, and in the United States, women who are homicide victims are most likely to have been killed by a partner. IPV is responsible for approximately 40% of homicides, but only a small percentage of these deaths occur in men.

Generally, homicide in an intimate relationship is not the first act of violence that occurs. Rather, the violence within the relationship escalates over time, with injuries becoming more severe and/or violent episodes becoming more frequent. Estimates are that approximately 1.5 million women are the victims of IPV each year in the United States (Tjaden & Thoennes, 2000). Multiple risk factors contribute to IPV, as well as IPV resulting in homicide. A recent study by Campbell and associates demonstrated that unemployed abusive men were four times more likely to commit femicide than employed men who abused their partners (Campbell et al., 2003). Prior arrest for IPV decreased the risk of femicide, whereas an abuser's access to a firearm increased the risk. Women who left a highly controlling abusive partner were at greater risk of being killed, whereas women who never lived with the abusive partner had a lower risk of femicide.

Dating Violence

Physical violence in a dating relationship has been reported to occur in as many as 32% of relationships in high school and college women (White & Koss, 2003). Sexual assault occurs with some frequency in this age group, as half of sexual assaults against females occur to those ages 12 to 24 (Bachman & Saltzman, 1995). A recent study found a rate of dating violence against young women of 88% (Smith, White, & Holland, 2003). The greatest risk of victimization was in women who had been victimized in childhood and adolescence.

Terrorism

The Code of Federal Regulations defines terrorism as ". . . the unlawful use of force and violence against persons or property to intimidate or coerce a government, the civilian population, or any segment thereof, in furtherance of political or social objectives" (28 C.F.R., 1998, Vol.1, Parts 0-42). Terrorism has been a problem in the United States for many years, with some of the most dramatic examples including not only the events that took place on September 11, 2001, but also events such as the bombing of the Murrah Federal Building in Oklahoma City on April 19, 1995; the intentional poisoning using contaminated food of the citizens of Dalles, Oregon, by a religious cult that sought to take over the town by winning an election; the distribution of weaponized anthrax through the mail and the bombing of the World Trade Center in 1993.

The epidemiology of terrorist events is evolving, as researchers identify methods of collecting data in multiple victim incidents and providing real-time information on the extent of injuries and illness occurring. Some of the particular challenges related to the study of terrorist events include the need to protect sensitive data that may be used in legal actions, and the sheer volume of data that may be necessary in order to include all of the victims of these acts in any analysis. As opposed to the epidemiology of violence-related injury, where there are identifiable specific causes of the incidents, the mechanism of any particular terrorist event may not be predicted, and the temporal nature of these events will be different than that of other types of violence, which focus more on individuals than large groups of people.

War

During a war or conflict, many types of violence may occur, and various population groups may be affected. Military units or civilian groups fighting against one another might be expected to suffer fatal and nonfatal injuries, but civilians who are not part of the conflict may also be injured or killed, either intentionally or unintentionally. In addition, other risks may exist during a conflict or time of little government control, including sexual assaults of women and young girls. Other consequences of war include those related to land mines that are placed during a conflict but left undetonated, which place the population in the area at risk for injury and long-term disability. Forensic nurses are often in a position to care for victims of war and torture, and indeed there are centers in the United States devoted specifically to this purpose. Displaced victims of war and violence frequently find themselves in need of health care in a culture totally foreign to them. The challenge for forensic nursing is to provide care often within the context of memories of horror of the past and extreme anxiety for the future. An understanding of the sufferings and in many cases possible feelings of humiliation, sorrow, and prolonged grieving of this vulnerable population is a unique challenge for forensic nursing.

Workplace Violence

Although workplace violence, an act of physical, verbal or psychological assault by one worker against another, can occur at any place where there is an employer–employee relationship, employee–employee relationship, or, in the case of health care, a client–caregiver relationship, workplace violence within the healthcare setting can be one of the most unpredictable types and therefore the hardest to control. The healthcare sectors lead all occupational settings in terms of the incidence of nonfatal acts of violence (McPhaul & Lipscomb, 2004). Certain risk factors should alert the caregiver staff. These risk factors include a violent episode that precipitated the current hospitalization, substance abuse or mental health instability evident at the time of treatment, a history of violent behavior either by the client or others with him/her, an accident involving children where blame is being argued, and situations involving law enforcement. At other times the simple stress of the situation can cause a seemingly stable individual to act in an erratic and violent manner. Increasingly, healthcare workers—most particularly nurses—are finding themselves the victims of violence that occurs in the workplace. Within healthcare settings, the emergency department of the hospital is one of the most common venues for individuals prone to violent behavior to act out. Other settings such as extended care facilities and critical care units and mental health facilities are also involved. The stressful and sometimes frustrating nature of crises observed in critical settings may trigger aggressive or violent behavior directed at healthcare personnel attempting to provide treatment to friends or relatives of the aggressor. The forensic nurse in these settings may be able to avert disaster by observing each encounter with stressed individuals through a forensic lens and observing simple safety measures such as avoiding arguing with suspected individuals, allowing an escape route from the treatment area, using calming communication skills, allowing limited numbers of individuals in the direct treatment area and soliciting assistance from security personnel before a dangerous situation escalates.

CASE STUDY 3.2

Workplace Violence: Three Examples

An elderly patient verbally abused a nurse and pulled her hair when she prevented him from leaving the hospital to go home in the middle of the night.

An agitated, psychotic patient attacked a nurse, broke her arm, and scratched and bruised her.

A disturbed family member whose father had died in surgery at the community hospital walked into the emergency department and fired a small-caliber handgun, killing a nurse and an emergency medical technician and wounding the emergency physician (NIOSH, 2002, Case reports section).

Source: National Institute for Occupational Safety and Health. (2002). Violence occupational hazards in hospitals. Retrieved from http://www.cdc.gov/niosh/docs/2002-101/#12

Summary

Epidemiology serves as an investigative method that can be used to examine patterns of injury, patterns of circumstances, and patterns of behavior of humans, vehicles, and environments that contribute to violent events. Knowledge of the epidemiology of violence, as well as epidemiologic methods that are used to study injury and violence, can provide a basis for determining the likelihood that specific events are the result of specific causes and circumstances. The consistent use and practice of these methods can enhance the expertise of the forensic investigator and provide excellent tools for practice. Interventions by forensic nurses aimed at changing the behaviors of individuals and families that lead to violence are informed by the nurse's knowledge of where and how violent events are most likely to unfold.

QUESTIONS FOR DISCUSSION

1. How can forensic nursing contribute to the collaborative investigation of violent events?
2. What is the role of forensic nursing in identifying risk factors for violence?
3. What role can forensic nursing play in preventing violence?
4. How can forensic nurses use epidemiology to assist in the investigation of violent events?

REFERENCES

28 C.F.R. (1) § 0–42 (July 1, 1998). From the U.S. Government Printing Office via GPO Access. Retrieved from http://www.gpoaccess.gov/cfr/retrieve.html.

Bachman, R., & Saltzman, L. E. (1995). *Violence against women: Estimates from the redesigned survey* (Bureau of Justice Statistics Special Report NCJ-154348). Washington, DC: U.S. Department of Justice, Office of Justice Programs.

Campbell, J. C., Webster, D., Koziol-McLain, J., Block, C., Campbell, D., Curry, M. A., ... Kathryn Laughon, M. P. H. (2003). Risk factors for femicide in abuse relationships: Results from a multisite case control study. *American Journal of Public Health, 93*(7), 1089–1097.

Centers for Disease Control and Prevention, National Center for Injury Prevention and Control. (2010a). *Costs of intimate partner violence against women in the United States*. Retrieved from http://www.cdc.gov/violenceprevention/pub/IPV_cost.html

Centers for Disease Control and Prevention. (2010b). *Web-based injury statistics query and reporting system (WISQARS)*. Retrieved from http://www.cdc.gov/injury/wisqars/index.html

Haddon, W., Jr. (1968). The changing approach to the epidemiology, prevention and amelioration of trauma: The transition to approaches etiologically rather than descriptively base. *American Journal of Public Health, 58*(8), 1431–1438.

McCaig, L. F., & Burt, C. W. (2003). *National hospital ambulatory medical care survey: 2001 emergency department summary. Advance data from vital and health statistics.* Hyattsville, MD: National Center for Health Statistics.

McPhaul, K., Lipscomb, J. (2004). Workplace violence in healthcare: Recognized but not regulated. *Online Journal of Issues in Nursing, 9*(3). Retrieved from http://www.nursingworld. org/MainMenuCategories/ANAMarketplace/ANAPeriodicals/OJIN/TableofContents/Volume92004/No3Sept04.aspx

National Institute for Occupational Safety and Health. (2002). *Violence occupational hazards in hospitals* (Publication No. 2002-101). Atlanta, GA: Author. Retrieved from http://www.cdc.gov/niosh/docs/2002-101/#12

Paulozzi, L. J., Mercy, J., Frazier, L., & Annest, J. L. (2004). CDC's National Violent Death Reporting System: Background and methodology. *Injury Prevention, 10*(1), 47–52.

Smith, P. H., White, J. W., & Holland, L. J. (2003). A longitudinal perspective on dating violence among adolescent and college-age women. *American Journal of Public Health, 93*(7), 1104–1109.

Tjaden, P., & Thoennes, N. (2000). *Full report of the prevalence, incidence, and consequences of intimate partner violence against women: Findings from the National Violence Against Women Survey* (Report for grant 93-IJ-CX-0012, funded by the National Institute of Justice and the Centers for Disease Control and Prevention). Washington, DC: National Institute of Justice.

United States Federal Bureau of Investigation. Uniform Crime Report. (2008). Retrieved from http://www.fbi.gov/ucr/ucr.htm

White, J. W., & Koss, M. P. (2003). Courtship violence: Incidence and prevalence in a national sample of higher education students. *American Journal of Public Health, 93*(7), 1104–1109.

SUGGESTED FURTHER READING

Carter, A. S., Wagmiller, R. J., Gray, S. A., McCarthy, K. J., Horwitz, S. M., & Briggs-Gowan, M. J. (2010). Prevalence of DSM-IV disorder in a representative, healthy birth cohort at school entry: Sociodemographic risks and social adaptation. *Journal of the American Academy of Child and Adolescent Psychiatry, 49*(7), 686–698.

Cummings, E. M., Schermerhorn, A. C., Merrilees, C. E., Goeke-Morey, M. C., Shirlow, P., & Cairns, E. (2010). Political violence and child adjustment in Northern Ireland: Testing pathways in a social-ecological model including single-and two-parent families. *Developmental Psychology, 46*(4), 827–841.

Cunradi, C. B. (2010). Neighborhoods, alcohol outlets and intimate partner violence: Addressing research gaps in explanatory mechanisms. *International Journal of Environmental Research and Public Health, 7*(3), 799–813.

Curran, V. (2010). Legal. Count the cost of hospital violence. *Health Services Journal, 120*(6207), 24.

Edberg, M., Cleary, S. D., Collins, E., Klevens, J., Leiva, R., Bazurto, M., ... Calderon, M. (2010, July 7). The Safer Latinos Project: Addressing a community ecology underlying Latino youth violence. *Journal of Primary Prevention, 3*(4), 247–257.

Greenfield, E. A., & Marks, N. F. (2010). Sense of community as a protective factor against long-term psychological effects of childhood violence. *The Social Service Review, 84*(1), 129–147.

Harding, D. J. (2009). Violence, older peers, and the socialization of adolescent boys in disadvantaged neighborhoods. *American Sociological Review, 74*(3), 445–464.

Jordans, M. J., Tol, W. A., Komproe, I. H., Susanty, D., Vallipuram, A., Ntamatumba, P., ... de Jong, J. T. (2010). Development of a multi-layered psychosocial care system for children in areas of political violence. *International Journal of Mental Health Systems, 4*(1), 15.

Ludwig, J., & Cook, P. J. (2000). Homicide and suicide rates associated with implementation of the Brady Handgun Violence Prevention Act. *JAMA, 284*, 585–591.

Lueger-Schuster, B. (2010). Supporting interventions after exposure to torture. *Torture, 20*(1), 32–44.

Miles, S. H. (2009). *Oath betrayed: America's torture doctors.* Berkeley: University of California Press.

Murphy, R. A. (2010, June 2). Multi-system responses in the context of child maltreatment and intimate partner violence. *Child Abuse & Neglect, 34*(8), 555–557.

Olofsson, N., Lindqvist, K., Gådin, K. G., Bråbäck, L., & Danielsson, I. (2010, July 9). Physical and psychological symptoms and learning difficulties in children of women exposed and non-exposed to violence: A population-based study. *International Journal of Public Health, 50*(4), 1093–1109.

Schwartz, S., Hoyte, J., James, T., Conoscenti, L., Johnson, R. M., & Liebschutz, J. (2010). Challenges to engaging black male victims of community violence in healthcare research: Lessons learned from two studies. *Psychological Trauma, 2*(1), 54–62.

Wintemute, G. J., Braga, A. A., & Kennedy, D. M. (2010, June 30). Private-party gun sales, regulation, and public safety. *New England Journal of Medicine, 363*(6), 508–511.

Yablonsky, L. (2000). *Juvenile delinquency: Into the 21st century.* Belmont, CA: Wadsworth Thomson Learning.

Yoshii, I., Sayegh, R., Lotfipour, S., & Vaca, F. E. (2010). Need for injury-prevention education in medical school curriculum. *Western Journal of Emergency Medicine, 11*(1), 40–43.

CHAPTER 4

Ethical Considerations in Forensic Nursing

Douglas Olsen

Many definitions and descriptions have been offered for forensic nursing, varying in emphasis on treatment of victims, treatment of offenders, and the nurse's role in developing forensic information (Mason, 2002). This consideration of ethics in forensic nursing will bypass that debate and use Mason's characterization of the discipline, ". . . forensic nursing . . . where crime interfaces with human suffering" (Mason, p. 512). As the field involves crime, which, by definition, involves behavior that society has determined is unacceptable and contrary to the social good, defining ethical comportment in forensic nursing will require careful consideration of the nurse's relationship to both the patient/subject and the community.

 ## CHAPTER FOCUS

» Principles
» Recurring Concepts in Ethical Discourse of Forensic Nursing

» Practice Points of Ethical Tension in Forensic Practice

KEY TERMS

» autonomy
» beneficence
» contextual caring
» distributive justice
» ethical comportment

» ethical tension
» ethics
» fiduciary
» retributive justice
» values-based decisions

Introduction

The study and practice of clinical ethics can be thought of as having two components. First, ethics provides tools for solving dilemmas involving personal or social values, in contrast to clinical decisions based on empirical evidence. For example, whether a nurse should report criminal intent revealed in the context of a clinical relationship is an ethical dilemma because it involves a conflict between the nurse's value of patient confidentiality and his or her value of society's right to safety. In contrast, the decision to withhold or give an antihypertensive medication is made on the basis of clinical data—measurements of the patient's blood pressure, the patient's health history, and knowledge of the efficacy of various interventions. Despite this apparent distinction, the line between **values-based decisions** and clinically based or data-based decisions is anything but clear. Indeed, in a real sense all decisions are values-based, in that clinical nursing practice is based on the value of reducing human suffering; so, in the example of giving or withholding the antihypertensive medication, ultimately the decision is made from the value that a nurse should do good for the patient.

The second aspect of clinical ethics is to guide clinicians in **ethical comportment**. This aspect of ethics is concerned with ongoing moral relationships and behavior. For example, in forensic practice, the development of a therapeutic relationship with a potentially dangerous patient is a question of ethical comportment. Ethical considerations of both types should be used to anticipate problems and to frame problems that do occur in order to design policy.

The discipline of healthcare ethics is related to the law but is not the same as the law. **Ethics** is the study of how one ought to act; it provides rationales as to why one course of action is better than another and finds a basis on which to agree about right and wrong action. Ethics examines values and ways to enact them, as well as ways in which values are not enacted. The language of values includes words that are often avoided in social situations, such as *ought, should, right, wrong,* and *better* (in the sense of more worthy, not more efficacious). The law is presumed to be an attempt to enact the value of fairness and thus often coincides with what we think of as ethical. Further, the law circumscribes what can be done and therefore is vital to ethics as applied to health care. Also, when a recurring situation is identified as unethical, the remedy is often a change in the law. However, the study of how to understand values in health care is different from knowing the law; this chapter will concentrate on ethical and not legal understanding. This distinction needs to be clear in the field of forensic nursing because a detailed understanding of the law is vital to practice; this chapter will help the forensic nurse distinguish how ethics coincides with, differs from, and comments on the law.

An ethical approach to forensic nursing will be proposed by offering five principles (**Table 4-1**) to guide forensic practice; explicating three conceptual areas that occur regularly in ethical discussion of forensic issues; conceiving and labeling pathology and deviance, the nurse–patient relationship, and the assignation of responsibility; and then examining specific points of ethical tension in forensic nursing practice.

TABLE 4-1   Principles Guiding Forensic Nursing Practice

Respect for persons
Beneficence
Distributive justice
Respect for community
Contextual caring

Source: Working Group for the Study of Ethics in International Nursing Research, 2003.

Principles

The principles offered here are intended to assist clinicians both in dilemma situations and in guiding ethical comportment. However, different principles will be more directed toward considering one of the two aspects in particular situations. For example, respect for person is a central consideration in dilemma situations involving the possible need to breach an individual's right of liberty, whereas contextual caring may be more helpful in considering how to respond to a violent patient's depression. However, all five principles have some relevance to all situations.

The articulation of principles has come under criticism in recent years because of fears that certain principles will be applied dogmatically in the manner of rules or laws, without regard to ethically relevant context (Strong, 2000). Many of these problems are avoided by understanding that principles are not prescriptive rules but broad guides in how to consider ethically difficult situations. Such guides can be useful to the nurse attempting to be rigorous in difficult, complex situations, so long as principles are not confused with prescriptions and applied rigidly as rules.

These five principles are adapted from the consideration of ethics in international nursing research because these two situations share several points of similarity, including relationships with legitimate considerations beyond the individual patient/subject, the need for particular attention to the community aside from considerations of resource allocation, and the difficulties of actualizing caring concern in situations of divided obligation.

Respect for Person

The first three principles, respect for persons, beneficence, and distributive justice, are derived from the standard Western canon of ethics as interpreted by Beauchamp and Childress (2001). Respect for person holds that personhood is a privileged category; that is, persons deserve special consideration. The principle of respect for person is based on the irreducible value of personhood, the concept of which reaches an apex of articulation in Kant's second formulation of his categorical imperative, "Act so that you treat humanity, whether in your own person or in that of another, always as an end and never as a means only" (1959, p. 47). Although there is considerable latitude for debate—Is a fetus a person? What is it about being a person that is special? Do any animals have this special quality to some degree?—there is broad social consensus that human life has intrinsic value. Therefore, furthering the respect shown for an individual is a valid ethical justification.

Respect for person incorporates both respect for autonomy and protection of vulnerable persons (National Commission for the Protection of Human Subjects of Biomedical and Behavioral Research, 1979). Granting and respecting personal autonomy is the chief way of expressing respect for person in Western societies. This is because **autonomy**—that is, the ability to rationally self-direct or self-govern—is widely treated as the morally significant and unique feature of being human. If each individual has intrinsic ultimate value and is self-governing, then each person has equal moral worth. It further follows that the right of liberty, as the freedom to pursue those goals without interference, is essential. In everyday social interaction, autonomy is recognized and liberty granted passively by not actively interfering with others. But in health care, clinicians have an ethical obligation to go beyond merely recognizing autonomy and granting liberty to respecting and enhancing the patient's autonomy (Beauchamp & Childress, 2001; Cassel, 1976). *This requires clinicians to take an active role using expert knowledge to make patients more aware of the* possibilities and shortcomings of medical science in defining their goals, and at times, working with patients to define their goals and increase their voice in articulating those goals.

It also follows that if being human has intrinsic value, then those persons who by virtue of some vulnerability, internal (e.g., mental illness) or external (e.g., oppression), cannot govern themselves in their own best interests should be protected. Clinicians need to be highly aware of what conditions—medical, social, and otherwise—interfere with a person's autonomy.

Autonomy and liberty are central concepts in ethical consideration of forensics because limiting liberty is the primary technique for dealing with criminal behavior. Many of the current ethical dilemmas in forensic mental health involve issues of autonomy; for example, implementation of the death penalty with the mentally retarded and children and involuntary restoration of competency. Decisions central to a forensic practice are conceptually based on the work of the Enlightenment-era philosophers (especially Kant and Mill), who held individual autonomy and liberty to be the starting point of ethics. Decisions such as competency, dangerousness, and responsibility are all tied to the belief that autonomous action is central to personhood.

Acts of coercion must be justified as exceptions to the clinician's obligation to respect patient autonomy. The form of currently accepted standards for forcing treatment in psychiatry can be found in John Stuart Mill's *On Liberty*, first published in 1985. The two justifications for denying a patient's choice of treatment are that the patient lacks capacity to make the decision or that the patient's choice could result in harm, either to the patient or others. Mill (1985) gives an example that invokes both criteria. A man is about to walk over a bridge that will collapse under his weight, sending him to his death. A bystander does not have time to warn him and so pushes him out of the way. At first the walker is angry, but when fully informed of the situation, he concurs that pushing him was the proper action.

The legal justification for psychiatric commitment and many other forms of forced treatment in all 50 U.S. states requires the presence of mental illness, which no longer implies legal loss of competence but represents a transformation of Mill's requirement of impaired capacity, coupled with potential danger, either to one's self or others (Tasman, Kay, & Lieberman, 1997). The commitment criterion of gravely disabled is conceptually grounded as an extension of potential danger to self, providing ethical justification of the forced treatment.

In Mill's case, the bystander's assumption that the walker lacked competence is confirmed by the walker's approval of being pushed when he is fully informed of the bridge's condition. This information restores his competence. Thus the walker's liberty was not violated. The analogy in psychiatric treatment is that the noncompetent (i.e., mentally ill) patient who is restrained, committed, or force medicated will concur after a course of treatment has restored the patient to a competent mental state. Allen Stone has labeled this the thank you theory of civil commitment (Alexander et al., 1991).

However, the actual situation of seeking concordance or a thank you regarding both forced treatment and treatment in coercive situations, like prison, presents two problems likely to result in the clinician having an inflated sense of the patient's agreement with the necessity of forcing treatment. First, clinicians believe that they act in a patient's best interest, so they will be biased toward interpreting the patient's discussion of an incident as agreement. The second barrier to assessing the patient's retrospective endorsement of coerced treatment is that asking from the position of the treating clinician, particularly when backed by repressive authority, is inherently coercive. Patients expecting to continue in treatment or gain institutional privileges are likely to feel that their endorsement of the treatment demonstrates cooperativeness and improved health. A study by Soliday (1985) found that patients who endorsed the need for seclusion provoked this response: "Many patients after an episode of solitary confinement will learn that the best way to avoid another is to acknowledge therapeutic benefit, even if this is not how they really feel" (Chamberlain, 1985, p. 290).

The second justification for overruling a patient's stated wishes is to prevent harm. An example is when a homicidal patient refuses inpatient admission and is civilly committed rather than left at liberty in the community.

Autonomy is an essential concept in forensics in a way not found in other areas of health care. The determination of responsibility hinges, in part, on a subject being autonomous, that is, self-directing. People are not considered morally responsible unless they are acting autonomously, and their responsibility may be mitigated if autonomy is felt to be compromised. Forensic nurses may be called upon to assist the court in determining if a person's mental status was compromised to determine the degree of culpability, which may involve appropriate sentencing. In nonforensic practice, nurses are specifically warned that a patient's responsibility for the clinical problem should not influence clinical care. When providing health care, nurses should not determine the degree or type of care a patient deserves based on an assessment of the patient's responsibility (Olsen, 1997a). In some forensic situations, however, the nurse may be assessing a person's mental state in order to help the justice system determine what conditions and handling are just and deserved by the person. Nurses need to be clear with patients/prisoners when they are in a situation where the nurse's assessments may be used to determine responsibility—such as an evaluation prior to sentencing—and when those assessments are for clinical purposes. For example, in prison nursing, as in nonforensic health care, the patient's responsibility for either the crime or the clinical problem should not influence a patient's/prisoner's nursing care. Because relationships are part of good nursing care, these also should not be negatively affected by responsibility. For example, smokers with emphysema should not receive inferior care, either in terms of physical care or in terms of the quality of the nurse–patient relationship. Although this is relatively clear and easy for most clinicians to implement in the case of smokers, forensics can present special difficulties, such as a child molester with depression or a surly gang member with a knife wound. In summary, patient responsibility for problems should never be a consideration in giving health care, except as an adjunct for self-healing. However, assessments regarding responsibility may be a consideration in certain forensic situations to help the justice system determine appropriate responses to criminal behavior.

Beneficence

Beneficence is the principle that one should act for the benefit of others, maximizing positive good and minimizing or preventing harm (Beauchamp & Childress, 2001). In nonforensic health care, many ethicists posit a fiduciary relationship with patients. A **fiduciary** is one in whom a person has placed special trust and confidence and who is required to watch out for the person's best interests. Such a relationship acknowledges a differential in power and knowledge requiring special loyalty on the part of the clinician. Many of the ethical dilemmas in health care are framed as a conflict between respect for a patient's autonomy and the duty to act beneficently toward the patient, that is, in the patient's best interests. This conflict is particularly pertinent to mental health as a specialty because many of the disorders encountered include denial of disorder or dysfunction as an integral aspect of the disorder. Much of the mental health clinician's effort is often directed toward having the patient acknowledge the problem and commit to working toward change. This takes on an added dimension in forensic practice where people are often forced into treatment situations.

Justice

Distributive justice is the principle dealing with the fair distribution of goods and resources. The goal of this principle is to determine just ways to distribute goods and resources and to develop polices for determining distribution. Frankena says, "The paradigm case of injustice is that in which there are two similar individuals in similar circumstances and one of them is treated better or worse than the other" (1973, p. 49). As with other ethical principles, the difficulty is often in how key terms are interpreted. In Frankena's definition, many decisions hinge on what are considered the ethically relevant features of treatment and circumstances to determine similarity. For example, gender is no longer considered ethically relevant in determining the appropriate level of education a child should receive, but historically gender was considered a relevant circumstance in determining education.

Another form of justice is **retributive justice**—the ethics of determining just punishment. Punishment is not a part of healthcare ethics, but is an integral concept of the criminal justice system. The use of certain healthcare techniques, such as administering a lethal injection to carry out the death penalty, and the denial of health care are not appropriate forms of punishment, and corrections nurses should never be involved in these actions (American Nurses Association, 1995).

Respect for Community

The fourth ethical principle suggested for forensic nursing practice, respect for community, departs somewhat from standard Western canon. This principle suggests that a wider context of concern than the individual should come under consideration.

Although ethics in nursing always requires attention to the clinical relationship, the consideration of the community as a context in the forensic situation has unique features, including: (1) Persons who have committed crimes are not always easy people with whom to form relationships that nurses consider ethically ideal or therapeutic (Peternelj-Taylor & Johnson, 1995); (2) the community has substantial legitimate interests that may conflict with the patient's wishes and perceived interests; (3) the nurse may have substantial personal safety concerns; (4) therapeutic interaction or community interests may require nurses to go beyond simple advocacy in working with victims; (5) diagnostic entities common in the forensic situation are often blurred by social conceptions of the meanings and implications of deviance and volition; (6) forensic nurses often work with society's outcasts in marginalized institutions; and (7) some roles confer legitimate obligations to the community that conflict with an offender's perceived best interests.

Ethical actions in forensic practice should consider a community's self-conception, how perceptions outside the community might be altered, and policy questions arising from particularly difficult situations. These considerations go beyond justice because they are not simply questions of the distribution of goods and services. The consideration of any effect on the community has become increasingly important in today's climate of media coverage where particular crimes capture the imagination of the entire nation. These situations often go beyond news coverage and influence policy, as in the case of such named laws as Megan's law or the Amber alert legislation. The interactions and interdependency of forensic nursing, the media and public policy are discussed in a subsequent chapter.

Contextual Caring

The final guiding principle, **contextual caring**, entreats the forensic nurse to interact with each patient, whether criminal or victim, as a person within an ethical relationship of caring concern grounded in the nurse's personal values. This differs from beneficence, where the actions are abstractly guided by the principle of acting in the patient's best interest. In contextual caring, the nurse acts in accord with personal caring concern for the concrete specific other within the context of a particular relationship. Caring is more difficult to prescribe than beneficence because it is more closely bound to the nurse's emotional reactions; however, there is increasing recognition that emotion is inextricably bound to moral good (Nortvedt, 1996; Vetlesen, 1994). The principle of caring concern encourages the consideration of what good can and may be done for the patient to whom one is responsible beyond the obligatory dictates of patients' rights (Benner & Wrubel, 1989; Gastmans, 1999; Gastmans, Dierckx de Casterlé, & Schotsmans, 1998). Although all health care should be guided by a caring concern for the specific patient, care as a guide to practice has special import in forensic practice because of the patient and the type of problems encountered. First, there is the difficult question of how one cares for a patient who either denies the problem, seems to takes a volitional role in the problem, or is threatening or belligerent. Second is the other side of this issue: Should victims receive special caring and concern in their health care? (For a comparison between clinical and forensic application of these principles, see **Table 4-2**.)

Recurring Concepts in Ethical Discourse of Forensic Nursing Practice

In examining ethical practice and dilemmas in forensic practice or in creating policy to anticipate dilemmas and foster ethical practice, three conceptually dense quandaries repeatedly recur. First is the problem of diagnostic labels and their meanings, which define what is considered pathology, what is deviance, and what these distinctions should mean in terms of responsibility, culpability, clinical treatment, and treatment by the justice system. The second issue is that of relationship. This is an especially complex issue in forensics because of the difficult population served and because some forensic roles have legitimate concerns other than the patient's welfare. The last is the issue of responsibility, which has two aspects, the determining of individual responsibility for acts and the effect on the nurse of the offender's responsibility. These issues are too large and complex to be completely separate; discussion of each includes aspects of the other two.

Labeling Issues

Labeling issues are of particular concern to forensics because many legal decisions, particularly those relating to culpability and punishment, are influenced by social assumptions regarding the nature of disease. Mental health experts may be called upon to report

TABLE 4-2   Comparison of Ethical Principles in Clinical Relationships and in Relationships in Forensic Evaluation

Principle	Clinical Relationship	Forensic Evaluation
Respect for autonomy	Patient sets treatment goal.	Person is made aware of the purpose of the evaluation.
Justification for overriding autonomy; beneficence	Patient's best interests when competence is impaired. Do the best thing for the patient.	Compelling offenders to undergo evaluation is justified by their potential for harm to society. Person should not be deliberately harmed nor any potential for benefit from the evaluation minimized.
Justice	1. Fair access to health care.	1. Due process in ordering the evaluation and the use of the information.
	2. Fair distribution of healthcare resources.	2. Qualified evaluators.
Goal	Best treatment for individual patient.	Benefit society by: 1. Minimizing harm that person might cause. 2. Helping to determine justly deserved treatment.
Nature of relationship; offender's motivation	Assistive. Meet healthcare goals.	Coercive. 1. Evaluation may help person. 2. Person may be actively opposed to evaluation.
Nurse's motivation	Help individual patients.	Benefit society through the court.

the existence of various disorders and their relationship to a person's mental status in determining an individual's culpability. **Figure 4-1** diagrams in simplified form the implications of distinctions between problem behavior arising from illness and that arising from badness.

Society is increasingly alert to the relationship between psychiatric issues and the work of the justice system, both sides showing concern about inappropriate use of mental disorder to avoid responsibility and the alarming rate at which the mentally ill are being incarcerated for minor crimes (though the latter gets bigger headlines).

Despite advances in understanding the biology of the brain, diagnosis in psychiatry remains phenomenological. Patients are given diagnostic labels based on what the clinician sees, what the patient reports, and what is reported about the patient. As of yet there are no objective (observable physical criteria that are relatively uninfluenced by the desires and volition of the patient) or laboratory tests for mental disorders, although there are known statistical differences between normal people and those with certain disorders. For

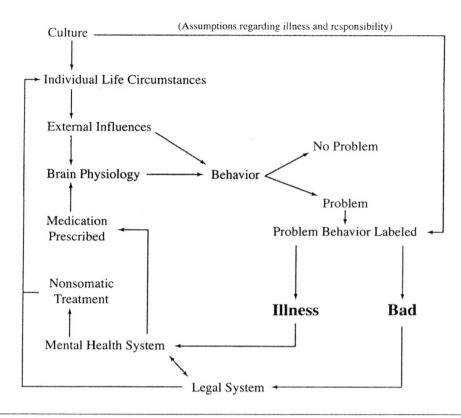

Figure 4-1   Schematic of behavior, culture, and treatment.

example, it is well known that, on average, people with schizophrenia exhibit ventricular volume abnormalities (Andreasen et al., 1990).

Mental health care provides three rationales for labeling a person as having psychopathology — distress, dysfunction, and deviance. None of these alone serves as a complete guide to identifying psychopathology in an individual. Distress can be thought of as personal discomfort or pain. The patient complains and wants the condition changed. However, all forms of mental distress are not mental disorders: grief, for example, is not a disorder and should not be treated as such. The example of prisoners reporting feelings of depression highlights the difficulty of diagnostic issues in forensics, because one expects prisoners to experience distress, indeed for many in our society this is the purpose of incarceration. Thus, more than distress must go into the determination of pathology in a context where distress is anticipated as normal.

Dysfunction can be thought of as an impaired ability to perform one's social or family role. The person may complain of the condition causing dysfunction, as with distress, or the person may deny the condition but others who interact with the person, like an employer or family member, may report dysfunction related to the condition. Many mental disorders are characterized by the person's denial of the disorder or any associated dysfunction, for example, alcohol dependence and mania. In some cases the person denies both the disorder and the dysfunction, whereas in other cases the person attributes the dysfunction to other causes. Although denial is inherent to the nature of some disorders, the tendency to deny and minimize is severely exacerbated by the stigma society puts on mental illness, causing many people with more distress-based disorders, like depression, to deny and actively resist the possibility that their problems are a mental disorder.

Deviance can be thought of as behavior outside accepted social norms. The family, employer, police, or members of the general public may complain about the deviant person's behavior. In those cases where the deviant behavior causes distress, the person may complain. However, in many cases, the deviant behavior is pleasurable or is perceived by the person as creating an advantage. Deviance as a determinant of psychopathology brings the field of mental health close to forensics because criminal behavior is deviant behavior. Some psychiatric diagnoses, including antisocial personality disorder, substance abuse disorders, and conduct disorder, are closely related to criminal behavior. Although deviance is an essential aspect of identifying psychopathology, it must be viewed cautiously because not all deviant behavior is criminal or pathologic. Simple deviation from accepted norms is not sufficient to define criminality or mental disorder. As Altman (1982) points out, "There is no such thing as a value-free concept of deviance; to say homosexuals are deviant because they are a statistical minority is, in practice, to stigmatize them. Nuns are rarely classed as deviants for the same reason, although if they obey their vows they clearly differ very significantly from the great majority of people" (p. 5). A society that values personal freedom and harbors a strong concept of individual rights could never equate deviance with mental illness and conformity with mental health. Deviance as a determinant of pathology underscores the inevitable element of social construction in defining pathology. Society cannot give up its function in defining acceptable and unacceptable behavior, because this is one function of the community. Therefore there is a social responsibility to make moral decisions regarding what are acceptable and unacceptable variations in behavior, and whether the unacceptable behavior is an illness or criminal. Current Western society is based on the concept that free and open discussion of the issues combined with power sharing throughout the population will result in fair and reasonable norms and humane categorization of deviance.

Relationship

There are two different reasons for focusing on nurse–client relationships in forensic practice—the often difficult nature of the population and the fact that clinicians have legitimate goals other than the welfare of the person under consideration. The patient population in forensic practice has, by definition, some involvement with crime either as perpetrators or victims, and each group presents relationship problems.

Working with Offenders

For many nurses, a forensic practice means working directly with convicted criminals, persons accused of a crime, persons who committed crimes but are found not guilty by reason of insanity, or persons who are believed to have committed crimes but are incompetent to bring to trial. The criteria for some DSM-IV (Diagnostic and Statistical Manual of Mental Disorders, 4th edition) diagnoses specify criminal or violent behavior, whereas in others it is easily inferred. Antisocial personality disorder is the most well-known diagnosis, but the implication of criminal or violent behavior is also found in the criteria for conduct disorder, some impulse control disorders, intermittent explosive disorder, and some paraphilias. In addition to antisocial personality disorder, other Cluster B personality disorders (narcissistic, borderline, and histrionic) can be expected among people who exhibit violent or criminal behavior, because these disorders consist mainly of difficulties with interpersonal relations. Further, many individuals without clear personality disorders rely on some immature and dysfunctional personality traits like intimidation and spitting. Peternelj-Taylor and Johnson (1995) are quite discouraging regarding the possibility of the usual nurse–patient relationship in an institutional setting, stating, "the relationships that are formed are dubious at best; offenders regard the professional as a friend or confidant when requests are approved, and as a member of the establishment or the system when requests are denied" (p. 16).

One could even argue that the nature of forensic settings like prisons encourage anti-social traits as a survival mechanism. In addition, the connection between the lifestyle involved in substance abuse and criminal activity is well established, although criminal behavior is not inherent in the DSM diagnostic of substance abuse disorder. The U.S. Department of Justice reports that 19–37% of violent crimes between 2002 and 2008 were committed by someone under the influence of alcohol (Rand, Sabol, Sinclair, & Snyder, 2010), and one study showed that 64% of adult males arrested had one of five drugs in his blood: cocaine, marijuana, opiates, methamphetamine, or phencyclidine (Arrestee Drug Abuse Monitoring Program, 2000).

One concern when working with a criminal population is the potential for violence. Nurses certainly have the right to safety in their working environment. At the same time, even potentially violent individuals have a right to health care.

Many measures intended to ensure the safety of the community and healthcare staff in an institution are repressive to the inmates. As with other forms of security, such measures will be unnecessary much of the time for most individuals. In many cases, when security serves a preventive function, one cannot know of specific incidences of violence that were averted. Retrospective analysis showing an overall reduction of incidents is the only way to evaluate specific techniques for reducing violent incidents and other breaches of security. Airport security provides a good illustration of this problem. Very few of the people searched will be terrorists, and no one knows how many prospective terrorists are deterred by airport searches, but most agree that searches are needed. (The analogy is not perfect because incidents of violence in a prison can be expected to be far more frequent than incidents of terrorism on airplanes.) This essential overdone quality of security makes it feel repressive to the recipient, conveying a lack of trust and certainly reinforcing the power differential between staff and inmate. Again, it is similar to the case when typical business travelers are pulled out of line while boarding a plane for a more extensive search. Such travelers know that they are not terrorists and that the search is a waste of time, at least as far as the threat from them. It requires some degree of maturity on the part of such travelers to acknowledge that although they are not threats, tight security benefits everyone through prevention, including them. This maturity is much more difficult for an inmate inside a prison, where the message of distrust and lack of power is not a one-time event but a continuous feature in all aspects of life. Also, inmates with personality disorders and other forms of mental disorder may lack the maturity and foresight to see repressive security as a benefit to them by deterring others. Beyond the effect of any diagnoses on particular prisoners, many inmates come from oppressed segments of society where messages of power and distrust, such as racial profiling by police and the extreme security in many inner-city stores, are rampant. Indeed, the issue of diagnosis and effect of social repression are not separate and additive but interactive. People raised in oppressive or traumatic circumstances will develop ways of surviving that may be labeled as pathological or deviant by the dominant society; further, such individuals may interact with the larger society in ways that become labeled symptomatic. People who perceive themselves as outsiders to a dominant, more powerful group will often act in ways that are labeled paranoid.

The need to ensure safety must be balanced with the inmate's right to health care and a desire to show respect to the individual. Stringent security measures during the provision of health care should be driven only by the degree of actual threat and not by an impulse to punish the offender. The appropriateness of punishment as a motivation for harsh measures elsewhere in prison life is a separate and controversial issue.

Another difficult ethical question occurs at the level of the individual. Clinicians and authorities must decide the proper response to the individual who has used violence or intimidation in dealing with clinicians. The consideration of an ethical response to violence by the patient will vary depending on how certain controversial ethical issues are viewed. For example, consider the question of whether health care for inmates is considered a privilege or a basic right. Some aspects of health care, such as prevention, may be seen more as privilege, whereas other aspects, such as wound care, are more concerned with basic rights. In some cases intimidation may be an issue of respect for autonomy. If intimidation is used to refuse a treatment, then clearly the treatment is unwanted and perhaps autonomy should be respected by allowing the person to refuse. This is more complex in cases where the person's competence and understanding of the treatment is questionable or where the treatment is psychiatric medications that help maintain the competency needed for an autonomous refusal. Clearly, respect for autonomy is not an issue where intimidation is being used to obtain medications that the clinician has determined are not needed.

Security and care need to be balanced in terms of the environment, but a nurse providing health care in that environment is left with an even more difficult balance to resolve. Nurses working with intimidating and potentially violent persons still need to develop a clinical relationship in as ethical and therapeutic a manner as possible despite the considerable constraints to good relations. Constraints can be external, like a security environment conducive to distrust; internal, such as patients with personality structures/disorders that make connection difficult; and social, as in the culture of oppression and bias from which many inmates originate.

In nursing, therapeutic and ethical relationships are generally held to involve an empathetic regard for the patient. In seeking to form such relationships with perpetrators, nurses in forensic practice face the obstacle of an intrinsic social bias against feeling sympathetic toward persons believed to have caused the problem. One need only reflect on certain everyday formulations of expression to see how deeply embedded is the assumption that it is correct to feel less sympathy when a person is responsible for their troubles. Consider, for example, the mother who scolds a child running at poolside, "Don't come crying to me when you fall; I told you not to run," or when a person asked his or her feelings regarding the plight of another responds by saying, "She brought this on herself." This formulation of responsibility is so commonly understood to convey a negative feeling that reflection is required to realize that it is not an expression of feeling at all.

Nurses are not immune to this way of thinking. In one study, 50% of nurses specifically stated that their empathetic regard for patients was tied to their sense of the patient's responsibility for the clinical problem (Olsen, 1997b). In nonforensic practice it is clear that the clinician's role never involves deciding whether and how much care a patient deserves based on the patient's responsibility. Nurses are quite clear that smokers with lung cancer don't deserve any less care, including empathetic regard, than nonsmokers with lung cancer. However, a forensic practice with offenders can push this boundary because of the extremity of the acts committed. Some mental disorders found in criminal offenders actually involve harm to others; for example, pedophilia, by definition, involves either having harmed children or wanting to harm children, and other disorders like anti-social personality imply the possibility of harm to others as part of the disorder. Personal feelings about acts like murder, rape, and child molesting are much harder for the nurse to put aside in the name of an abstract duty to care for all, regardless of how they came to need care, than feelings about smokers and those with a poor diet.

Nurses working with offenders have an ethical duty to reflect honestly on their feelings and strive for personal growth in their regard for others. Nurses working in this environ-ment are cautioned against a facile use of the concept of the nonjudgmental attitude. The first problem is that the formulation, nonjudgmental attitude, can easily become a ratio-nalization for perfunctory physical care given to personally distasteful patients without reflection on the patient's suffering and ways to help. The second problem with a non-judgmental attitude is that when behavior related to a mental disorder is morally wrong, healing for the patient means facing and accepting responsibility for the behavior and for changing it. The Alcoholics Anonymous philosophy provides an excellent example of how personal responsibility can be construed in the context of a disease model. Nurses should not be judgmental or condemn patients, but they should be able to tolerate the moral eval-uation of behavior by the patient. It may seem odd to suggest simultaneously that nurses should not be judgmental and that nurses should not rely on the concept of the nonjudg-mental attitude, but as these terms are commonly used, they are not diametric. Judgmental implies a critical and dismissing attitude that is certainly not a good attitude for clinicians, whereas nonjudgmental implies the acceptance of all patient behaviors as morally equal. That the latter is not humanly possible provides another argument against the overreliance on the concept.

An overinterpretation of the nonjudgmental attitude can be problematic when com-bined with the social bias of connecting sympathetic regard to responsibility. The nurse may mitigate a patient's responsibility in an attempt to develop a more positive connec-tion with the patient than is possible if the patient is seen as responsible. The result is an inability to hear and accept the patient's own moral assessment of the behavior, which, if accurate, is a needed step to change. The attitude recommended here is to break through social bias and separate a moral assessment of the patient's behavior from concern for the person's suffering. One must try to simultaneously understand the moral weight of the offender's behavior, which is clinically essential, and empathize with the person's real suf-fering, which is essential for therapeutic and ethical relations.

Working With Victims

A patient's status as victim presents related problems in developing helpful relationships. One's natural sympathy for people harmed through no fault of their own or even actively wronged by another should not be allowed to interfere with what is best for the person. One must tread a fine line and not blame the victim while simultaneously not being blind to any role the victim's behavior may have played. Further, the nurse must understand the particular role he or she plays in the victim's treatment. Even when a victim's behavior has played a significant role in current troubles, that aspect is generally not the initial focus with a victimized individual, and harm can be done if this concept is introduced clumsily or at the wrong time.

In working with victims, social advocacy can be seen as the enactment of one's respect for the community. When working with a victim population, the nurse will gain inside knowledge of the social condition of victims and of problems leading to certain types of crimes. This knowledge leads to a responsibility to act on one's knowledge and expertise in advocating changes for the community's benefit. For example, nurses counseling rape victims may be thought of as having an obligation to use their expertise for the benefit of the larger community.

Community advocacy may be needed when working with either victims or perpetrators. Social conditions such as poverty, inequitable treatment, and oppression create an environment that enhances the possibility of specific types of individuals becoming perpetrators. When this happens, it is often members of that same community who are victimized. This is amply demonstrated by the overrepresentation of African Americans in both the prison population and the victim population (U.S. Department of Justice, 2000, 2009). Many forms of social advocacy don't require a distinction between victim and perpetrator to argue for community change that will help decrease the incidence of both. Understanding that social conditions are linked to the incidence of crime does not necessarily mitigate any specific individual's responsibility; this is a controversial argument that has well-meaning adherents on both sides. However, nurses can advocate for social change without the implication that individual responsibility is lessened.

Special Forensic Relationships

In some roles, nurses working in a forensic practice will bring clinical techniques, particularly assessment skills, to bear on individuals where the goal of the encounter or intervention is not the person's welfare. This is drastically different from normal clinical nursing practice where there is broad consensus that ethical conduct demands that the patient's welfare be the nurse's primary and overriding goal. Even in those cases where patient autonomy is denied, the justification rests on the patient's being unable to choose in his or her best interest.

There are at least two specific instances where forensic practice has legitimate goals that are not necessarily the same as the patient's and may actually work to harm the patient, at least from that person's perspective: court-ordered evaluation and restoration to competency.

There are many reasons why a court may order an evaluation of a person's mental status, including to determine the person's competence to stand trial, to help evaluate not guilty by reason of insanity claims, and to help determine appropriate sentencing and disposition. The nurse's primary obligation in performing an evaluation for the court is to serve the needs of society as determined by the court. The nurse is not performing the evaluation for the person's benefit, and may make assessments that the person and the person's legal counsel feel are against the person's interests.

The nurse makes an assessment of such a person based strictly on observations and reports it to the court. These assessments may favor the person's position or not. However, in these situations, nurses are specifically charged to use their clinical skills to benefit society and not to be acting solely in the person's interests. Therefore, the usual strictures of privacy are not in effect with regard to the court. The nurse is acting as an extension of the legal system, which is balancing society's safety, society's interest in just treatment of the offender, and the person's rights and interests. Although the goal of the evaluation is not the person's benefit, people under evaluation must still be shown respect as people and so should be aware of the circumstances and purpose of the evaluation (American Academy of Psychiatry and the Law, 1995).

Another situation requiring coercive treatment that is done at the behest of the legal system is competency restoration, particularly in cases where the person is refusing the treatment. In these cases, people may not wish to be declared competent because that will allow them to stand trial, or they may not want treatment because they lack the insight needed to see that treatment is required or that they are acting on delusional beliefs. (See Table 4-2 for a comparison of the application of ethical principles between clinical and forensic care.)

The nurse in forensic practice needs a grasp of the conceptual basis of responsibility for three reasons. The first reason is because court evaluations and expert testimony are often part of the court's attempt to determine responsibility or assign the appropriate degree of responsibility for an offender's action. Although the nurse may not be asked directly to assign the degree of responsibility, the court's determination will likely be influenced by the evaluation. Many aspects of mental status sought by courts bear directly on the formulation of the offender's responsibility, for example, irresistible impulse and reduced mental capacity. The formulation not guilty by reason of insanity directly connects mental state and moral responsibility for a criminal act. Beecher-Monas and Garcia-Rill stress the connection between psychiatry and responsibility determinations, saying, "Mental state is such an important facet of our understanding of criminal responsibility that judges need to be open to the new ideas emerging in the field of brain science" (1999, p. 260).

The second reason is the effect the patient's responsibility can have on the clinical relationship. Although nurses should work to keep notions of responsibility separate from caring concern in the clinical relationship, this will best be accomplished if the nurse understands the nature of responsibility. Further, only through understanding can the forensic nurse take the lead with other clinicians to examine the effect of the patient's responsibility and formulate an ethical approach.

The third reason is clinical: Patients who are offenders will need to examine and accept responsibility for their actions as part of healing. Forensic nurses can only act as a guide and help in this process through understanding the nature of responsibility.

The concept of personal responsibility forms a fundamental background assumption to personal relations in the same way gravity is a background concept in our understanding of how to handle physical objects. However, a slight scratch of the surface shows responsibility to be a difficult, controversial topic—the nature of which has been debated throughout history. Plato felt bad action resulted from ignorance, stating, "But if justice be power as well as knowledge—then will not the soul which has both knowledge and power be the more just, and that which is the more ignorant be the more unjust" (1926, p. 425)? Aristotle, however, felt that bad actions could be willful: ". . . the virtues are voluntary (for we are ourselves somehow partly responsible for our states of character . . .), the vices also will be voluntary; for the same is true of them" (1935, p. 215).

The first distinction to address in understanding responsibility is that between being responsible *for* (that is, liable or culpable) and responsible *to* (that is, owing an obligation). Although there is a distinction, the two in a sense are related in that when one is responsible for a negative or harmful act, one is often thought of as also being responsible to the person harmed and sometimes to society at large. In the case of a crime, an offender is held to be responsible *for* committing the act that is the offense, and in committing the act the offender has breached a responsibility *to* society and the victim—that is, the responsibility to honor the rights of others. In some cases, victims will even stake a legal claim on the offender's social obligation through civil action. We intuitively sense responsibility as occurring on a continuum, with the severity of our moral condemnation corresponding to the assessment of degree. Responsibility can be seen to be shared with another person or persons, acts of nature, or society and culture. Indeed, most sophisticated assessments of responsibility are multifactorial. However, in Morse's estimation, the law has difficulty accounting for partial responsibility, saying, "Although insanity defense rules do draw such an (admittedly blurry) 'bright' line, in principle and in fact rationality is distributed along a continuum in the population at large" (1999, p. 160).

Another inherent aspect of the concept of responsibility is the connection to consequences. One test of responsibility is to see what and where consequences actually lie and where one feels they should lie. Our intuitive sense of responsibility is tied to the sense that responsible parties ought to bear the consequences. Our sense that consequences are closely tied to responsibility is so strong that people often must be reminded that you cannot work backward from all consequences to reveal responsibility. People must be reminded that bad things happen to good people without apparent reason (Kushner, 1997). Much early religion is based on the notion that one's fortune in life, including health, is tied to the morality of one's character.

Consequences have two sources, natural and imposed. Emphysema is a natural consequence of smoking; time in prison is an imposed consequence for burglary. When consequences are imposed, the legitimacy of the imposing agency is vital. In the legal system, the imposition of consequences is an issue of retributive justice or deservedness, but there are other forms of consequence imposition. For example, "sin taxes" are a consequence imposed on smokers and drinkers, and other financial incentives are manipulated by the government to alter behavior.

This shows one aspect of the ethical reasoning behind not penalizing smokers in their health care. Smokers bear the burden of the consequences of their actions by getting ill; to impose consequences beyond those that occur naturally would require greater justification in the realm of retributive justice, showing that smokers deserved more consequences than those inherent in the act.

Hans Jonas (1984) provides a straightforward set of criteria for determining the responsibility for particular actions:

1. *Causality:* The act must cause the consequence.
2. *Control:* The agent must control the act.
3. *Foresight:* The agent must foresee the consequence.

All three conditions must be met to consider a person responsible for a specific act. Many legal tests of criminal responsibility can be related to these criteria. For example, the irresistible impulse standard used in about five states (Levine, 1998) for determining insanity clearly echoes Jonas's control criteria. Also, the M'Naghten test for insanity, which requires that the defendant lack the capacity to appreciate the difference between right and wrong, coincides with the Jonas requirement of foresight for responsibility (Slovenko, 1998). In this case, foresight is understood as the ability to see a moral wrong occurring as a consequence of the act. The model penal code for determining insanity in the United States combines both these criteria (Slovenko). An interesting additional test of insanity used only in New Hampshire, called the Durham test (Levine), finds that "a person is relieved of liability if his unlawful act is the product of a mental disease or defect" (Bienstock, 2003, p. 482), which essentially repeats Jonas's causality criteria by separating the

TABLE 4-3   Autonomy and Responsibility

Criteria for: Autonomy	Informed Consent	Responsibility	Criminal Responsibility	Comments
		Causality	Did the person perform the act? *Actus Reus* (bad action)	Criteria of autonomy and criminal responsiblity bear on teleologic cause (i.e., intention)—why an act was done.
Intentional (competence)	Competent and gives authorization	Foresight	*Mens rea* (bad intent)	More knowledge confers greater responsibility. However, as the severity of consequences increases we tend to imbue more responsibility at lower levels of understanding.
With understanding	Clinician gives proper disclosure		Appreciation of wrongfulness	
Without coercion	Without coercion	Control	Irresistible impulse Act a product of mental disorder Under duress?	The less influence, the more autonomous the decision. (That one's decisions cannot be entirely without influence is a critique autonomy; to decide is to sort among influences.)

person from his or her disorder. Using this standard, the mental disease is responsible, not the person.

The concepts of autonomy and responsibility are closely related. Beauchamp and Childress (2001) state that for a decision to be considered autonomous, it must be intentional, occur with understanding, and be made without controlling influences. In these criteria, intention, which requires rationality and thus competence, is internal to the person, whereas understanding and lack of influence are essential in the decision environment. Understanding is internal, but the information must be provided from the outside; the ability to understand and form intentions (that is to be competent) is internal. Responsibility requires competence to achieve foresight and lack of coercion to achieve control. Essentially, one must be acting autonomously to be responsible for an act. (See **Table 4-3** for a comparison of the Jonas criteria with the criteria for autonomy and various criteria used to determine criminal responsibility. The elements of informed consent are also included in Table 4-3 because informed consent is the principle means for respecting autonomy.)

Points of Ethical Tension in Forensic Practice

The principles and concepts presented in this chapter can be used to identify and categorize points needing discussion and clarification when facing specific situations or dilemmas or when formulating policy. In the scope of forensic practice there sometimes exists an **ethical tension**; The forensic nurse must sometimes choose between alternative courses of action that each have ethical implications and impacts, such as treatment v. containment, privacy v. safety, and treating v. placating. In ethics, one proceeds by clarifying who the interested parties are; their interests, which can be based in the five principles; and precedent practice, and then discerning distinctions that need to be made using the key concepts. For example, for ethical justification of decisions regarding how much and what types of control are needed to maintain safety in specific situations with prisoners, a nurse may need to be able to distinguish between those who are dangerous and nondangerous, responsible and nonresponsible, and competent and noncompetent, as well as behavior indicating disorder from other kinds of bad behavior. This section will review some situations where an ethical tension impacts forensic practice.

Treatment vs. Containment

Power is not equally distributed in the clinical relationship; the nurse has the power of greater knowledge and experience, whereas patients control specific knowledge of their condition and the emotional character of encounters. In addition to the usual power held by clinicians, mental health and forensic nurses can also bring socially sanctioned forms of physical force to bear. Although the nurse has most of what is considered the traditional power in the clinical relationship, the patient retains certain types of power that are always available to oppressed people. The patient can cooperate and create a situation where the encounter runs smoothly or the patient can be difficult and passive aggressive, making the encounter difficult from the nurse's perspective. Although it seems counterproductive for patients to make life difficult for the clinician helping them, patients are often not willing participants, especially in mental health and forensic situations. Further, mere recognition of being in the lower position of an encounter is often enough to evoke an exertion of whatever power one does have available. Compliance issues can be viewed in this way.

In all clinical situations, nurses are continuously making assessments regarding how much and what types of influence are appropriate to exert. Titrating the proper amount of influence is a central concern in mental health practice, where patients are habitually considered to have an impaired ability to make rational decisions in their own best interests, and so coercive treatment is routine. The concern over coercion is compounded in forensic practice with criminals because the severe coercion of incarceration is considered essential to community safety. Forensic nurses in prisons and similar settings must not only balance respecting patients'/inmates' autonomy with a duty to act in their best interests and with a sense of caring concern, but also consider the safety interests of the community, including the prison community, which may be most at risk from an inmate's poorly controlled behavior. A further complication is that patients/inmates are in an exceptionally oppressive environment prior to and surrounding the clinical encounter. This environment colors and pervades all encounters in the prisoner's life, health related and otherwise. So although the nurses have some control over the amount of influence that can be brought to bear depending on their clinical assessment and judgment, the patient/inmate remains in a highly coercive environment.

A relational approach can help the nurse examine a wide variety of factors that bear on the decision of how much influence is appropriate in specific situations. Briefly, the relational approach is a shift in emphasis onto the maintenance of an ethical relationship entailing positive obligation to the patient extending beyond simple honoring of patient rights. The relational approach makes these assumptions:

» *Influence is inherent in the clinical relationship:* The patient cannot be without influence from the clinician. If the focus is set too narrowly on respect for autonomy and liberty rights, then all forms of influence seem negative. However, *a wider focus on clinical relations recognizes that patients want the nurse to use influence for their* benefit. Influence is inherent in the concept of treatment. This confers a responsibility on the nurse to wield such influence ethically.

» *The factors relevant to treatment decisions and the use of influence are continuous, not dichotomous:* A too-narrow focus on preserving patient rights forces clinicians to consider relevant factors dichotomously. For example, competent patients have a right to refuse treatment, so to honor this right one must know whether the patient is competent or incompetent; no answer in between will do. Of course, this is not the way mental status and competence occur. To maintain an ethical relationship, the nurse must recognize and balance competence and all other ethical factors as they occur on a continuum without imposing false dichotomy.

» *All decisions are subjective, and so the clinician, as a person, is a fundamental component of the situation:* Decisions made with a narrow focus on rights have the character of objectivity. In the relational approach, the application of influence in clinical relations arises from a particular relationship between that provider and that patient. Thus, determining ethical action is connected to the personhood of the clinician in the context of each unique relationship, highlighting the need to include the principle of caring concern (Olsen, 2003).

In many situations, a nurse must consider increasing or decreasing the degree of influence exerted; in the prison setting, influence may be contemplated for clinical care or for security. For example, finding that a patient/inmate who was previously undiagnosed with a mental disorder is now psychotic but declining treatment would prompt the nurse to bring increased influence to bear with the goal of better clinical treatment. In contrast, assessing that a patient/inmate with antisocial personality felt violent toward another inmate would prompt increased influence for security purposes. Assessing that a patient/inmate with schizophrenia had decompensated, possibly to a point where fellow inmates were at risk from delusional violence, would require the nurse to bring some influence to bear for both clinical and security reasons. A list of factors that can be brought to bear in considering the ethical justification of clinical decisions is found in **Table 4-4** and discussed next.

» *Strength and nature of clinical relationship:* This provides the context within which all other factors are evaluated. Decisions made by a clinician who has just met a patient and spent an hour assessing him or her are different contextually from those made by a primary care provider who knows the patient well. In the relational approach, all considerations are embedded in the actual relationship. Too strong a focus on

TABLE 4-4   Ethical Justification of Clinical Decisions

Strength and nature of clinical relationship

The patient's mental state

The patient's willingness to participate

Potential for harm if treatment is not instituted

Degree of benefit from an intervention

Intensity of restriction or intrusion from the intervention

Intensity of the method used to exert influence

Degree of confidence in the intervention's efficacy

patient rights deemphasizes differences in relationships, seeking a right answer that would apply regardless of the specific relationship.

» *The patient's mental state:* Greater impairment in a patient's mental status provides more justification for overriding a patient's decision. This is an area where the quality of the clinical relationship makes a critical difference. The nurse must take care to distinguish poor judgment due to impaired mental function from decisions with which the nurse disagrees. The greatest ethical error regarding this factor is to equate sound judgment with the agreement with the treatment plan.

» *The patient's willingness to participate:* More intensive interventions are justified when patients are willing recipients. Even restraint, the most restrictive intervention, can be applied without ethical conflict if the patient desires the intervention. This excludes cases where the intervention is clinically inappropriate or the patient's motives are not congruent with the therapeutic use of the intervention. However, assessing willingness must be an ongoing, open process because of the coercion inherent in clinical relationships and clinicians' bias to perceive patients as willing.

» *Potential for harm if a treatment is not instituted:* The greater the potential for harm, the more intensive the influence that is justified. This includes harm to the patient, others, and the community.

» *Degree of benefit from an intervention:* The greater the benefit, the more intense the influence that is justified.

» *Intensity of restriction or intrusion from the intervention:* More intrusive treatment requires stronger justification. A rough hierarchy of intensity of influence follows:
  ■ Body movement (e.g., four-point restraint)
  ■ Movement in space (e.g., seclusion rooms)
  ■ Decisions of daily life (e.g., food, television, when to smoke, with whom to socialize, what to keep private)
  ■ Meaningful activities (e.g., housing, work)
  ■ Treatment choice (e.g., court-mandated treatment)
  ■ Control of resources (e.g., use of money)
  ■ Emotional or verbal expression (e.g., censorship, social expectation) (Olsen, 1998)

Restraint is the most intensely restrictive and intrusive intervention available to the clinician, so it requires the highest level of justification.

» *Intensity of the method used to exert influence:* More intensive forms of exerting influence require a higher level justification. A rough hierarchy of intensity in methods used to influence a patient might be:
  ■ Physical force.
  ■ Manipulation of resources (e.g., access to privileges).
  ■ Manipulation of social forces (e.g., access to other inmates, telling inmates that compliance with treatment reflects well on them).
  ■ Social pressure (e.g., arranging peer pressure, men wear neckties and not skirts); some mental disorders might be seen as an insensitivity to this influence.
  ■ Advice (e.g., psychotherapy) (Olsen, 1998).

Again, as the most restrictive measure, physical force requires the strongest justification, usually imminent substantial harm to specific persons.

» *Degree of confidence in the intervention's efficacy:* The lower the probability of an intervention's beneficial effect, the less justification for coercion.

In making a decision regarding the increase or decrease in the use of influence, including extreme forms of coercion, seclusion from others, restraint, or forced medication, all relevant factors should be considered. In this list of relevant factors, the patient's position on the continuum represented by each factor bears on the justification of an intervention exerting influence, but no single factor is definitive. Nor is a simple formula sufficient when factors are seen as continuous rather than dichotomous. The balance of all relevant factors should be weighed. The list presented here is not necessarily exhaustive. Each use of influence changes the moral tone of the relationship. So although putting a patient/inmate in restraints may be justified, the nurse must maintain an ethical relationship with that person. The nurse bears the moral weight of the responsibility inherent in holding great power over others and the charge to use that power for their good.

Privacy vs. Safety

The two broad areas where privacy is considered are privacy of information and privacy of person. Privacy of information, also referred to as confidentiality, is most closely tied to respect for autonomy because it is maintained by giving patients control over the flow of information about them. Privacy of person is closely tied to contextual caring in that the bodily exposure and exposure of the most intimate and personal aspects of daily life, such as excretion and bathing, that occur in nursing care require the nurse to extend deep personal trust, at times compelling a type of closeness the patient will have with few others.

Control over personal presentation is a central mechanism of identity, serving as a basis for social relations (Bok, 1983; Goffman, 1973). Thus some privacy of person is needed to develop and maintain a sense of personhood (Reiman, 1984). Privacy provides a boundary between self and others and allows limitations and controls to be placed on what is presented publicly and what is shown to intimates. Private time and space allows expression of characteristics and desires that one does not wish to reveal publicly. When others view what the society considers private, embarrassment and shame are experienced (Levy, 1983; Lynd, 1958). An inability to maintain some secrecy about aspects of the self can result in a profound loss of identity (Bok). The experience of shame and embarrassment from public exposure of the private is a cross-cultural phenomenon (Levy), and virtually all cultures have some accommodation for individual privacy (Moore, 1984).

Although prisoners may have issues with privacy of information, it is privacy of person that is especially compelling during incarceration. Prison is extraordinary in the degree to which privacy of person is denied. Indeed, extreme denials of privacy have been used as a method of breaking down political prisoners (Caplan, 1982).

As with other constraints on forensic practice, nurses working in prisons will make ethical decisions regarding patient privacy embedded within a context of unusually little privacy of both information and person. This will influence not only the nurse's decisions, but also the way the nurse's behavior is viewed by the patients/inmates. The forensic nurse will want to maintain privacy of person to the greatest degree feasible as a sign of respect for the patient. However, this will be significantly curtailed from what is expected in nonforensic clinical encounters. Patients/inmates may be required to undergo searches or observation by nonclinicians that would be unthinkable in nonforensic practice.

Incursions on privacy can be considered a form of influence because the exposure of person or revelation of information that a patient/inmate prefers to keep private denies autonomy and restricts choices. This means the guide to considering other forms of influence can be used. Anticipation is the best way to keep losses of privacy respectful and for the loss of privacy to be distributed fairly among the entire prison population. All parties should be aware in advance what information and in what situations the patient/ inmate can expect privacy to be maintained, the extent and types of exposure that will occur during clinical encounters, and what information the nurse will feel compelled to report.

Treating vs. Placating

Incarcerated people have higher rates of diagnosable mental illnesses, including depression and anxiety disorders, than the general population (Baillargeon, Black, Pulvino, & Dunn, 2000; Teplin, 1990). In the United Kingdom, 16% of inmates were found to suffer from depression (Mitchison, Rix, Renvoize & Schwiger, 1994). Further, the rate of treatment for those with depressive disorders in prison was found to be higher than the treatment rate in the general population (Baillargeon, Black, Contreras, Grady, & Pulvino, 2001).

However, the circumstances resulting in incarceration and the situation of the imprisonment itself can be expected to produce reactions much like many of those described in DSM-IV for the identification of a depressed patient—difficulty sleeping, irritability, depressed mood, alterations in weight, feelings of worthlessness, and difficulty concentrating (American Psychiatric Association, 2000). The current recommendation regarding the diagnosing of depression is to treat the disorder where the symptoms exist, even in the context of extreme life circumstances such as terminal illness (Massie, Gagnon, & Holland, 1994).

Patients/inmates may want to take medications for a variety of reasons—to cure or ameliorate symptoms, which is the usual socially accepted motivation; to relieve boredom; or to continue a pattern of using substances as a panacea begun and reinforced by participation in a drug-abusing subculture. Simply raising the issue creates awareness that there is no firm line between symptoms and reactions to life circumstances. Further, particularly in regard to mental disorders, reactions to life circumstances may be the disorder. Indeed, this is the definition of posttraumatic stress disorder (APA, 2000).

The epistemological position that real illnesses are biological is unsatisfactory because all behaviors, even malingering, reflect biologically distinct brain states (Olsen, 2000). This controversy has been avoided by some managed care companies in reference to decisions about what treatment for aberrant behaviors should be reimbursed as mental disorders by saying that real disorders are those found in the DSM (Sabin & Daniels, 1994).

The forensic nurse confronted with a request for psychotropic medications may sense that the patient desires the drugs for inappropriate reasons, particularly when certain categories of medications, such as benzodiazepines, are requested. The nurse faces several difficult issues in distinguishing appropriate from inappropriate motivations— respecting the patient's autonomy; demonstrating care for the patient despite denying a request; beneficence, in the sense that the nurse wants to address any underlying problem; and care of the community, because overly easy or restrictive access to medications will adversely affect the entire inmate population.

As discussed earlier, the nurse should be willing to examine his or her own feelings about whether perception of patient volition in creating or bringing about the clinical circumstances affects judgments regarding the reality of the condition. Fabrication of symptoms should not result in medicating the fabricated symptoms, but the nurse should remain aware that the motivation to fabricate symptoms is itself a cause for concern and possibly a legitimate disorder—just not the one the patient is reporting. Unfortunately, many cases will be clouded—not complete fabrication, but not fully forthright disclosure. Further, the nurse should be aware that some reports may result from differing assumptions between the nurse and the patient/inmate regarding the level and type of distress for which medication is appropriate, particularly symptoms like anxiety or insomnia that are ubiquitous problems and are often identified as disorders by degree of severity.

The Unhappy Prisoner

The following case brings together many of the issues discussed in this chapter: the balance of respect for autonomy and beneficence, deciding the correct degree of coercion in treatment, contextual caring in the face of difficult or even repulsive behavior, the effect on the clinician of feeling the patient/inmate is deliberately causing a problem, what is illness and what is bad behavior, and honoring or denying a patient's/inmate's request for medications. This case is not far-fetched, unusual, or exotic, and it is drawn from actual practice. There are no easy answers, but reflection on the events in light of the issues raised in this chapter will help the reader to clarify his or her feelings about the issues.

CASE 4.1

The Unhappy Prisoner

Johnny was a 25-year-old black Haitian man who was in the custody of a State Department of Corrections for 3 years following a conviction on a robbery charge. His incarceration ended with suicide 2 months after being transferred to the state's oldest and most secure facility. Prior to transfer he was prescribed psychotropic medication; following transfer medication was discontinued.

Johnny had two prior arrests on unknown charges. He was also in and out of treatment at his local community mental health center and had three documented inpatient psychiatric admissions for unknown diagnoses. Shortly after his arrest he was sent to the State Hospital for the Criminally Insane. He spent 2 months at this facility. His discharge diagnoses were depression, alcohol abuse, cocaine abuse, opioid abuse, malingering, and borderline personality with histrionic and narcissistic traits.

Johnny's time in prison was marked by severe behavioral and social problems. He frequently demonstrated intimidation, violence, self-mutilation, threats of self-mutilation, and feigned symptoms. His prison record reveals numerous offenses for which he was disciplined. Over a period of 2.5 years there were 35 infractions, including:

Five assaults
Seven fighting
Six destruction of property
Six self-mutilation
Two arson
Disobedience
Malingering
Theft
Contraband

The 6 months prior to his death were a particularly difficult period. He spent most of this time in isolation. His record while in isolation reflects numerous requests for medication and behavioral acting out. He was frequently noted in the medical record to be feigning symptoms, including extrapyramidal symptoms and psychosis. He often refused medications in whole or in part.

When his wishes were not gratified he would lash out at staff with spiteful anger, for example, ripping up his isolation mattress or defecating on the floor. Staff's attitude is illustrated in the following nurse's note, "He likes to whine a lot and tries to get other people to feel sorry for him."

During the period prior to his transfer to maximum security, an effort was made to keep him compliant by tying medications to privileges. Despite this, his compliance was sporadic and the medications became the focus of intense struggle. Johnny sometimes reported that the medications helped him calm down.

During this period the nurse practitioner supervising his care, Ms. Green, repeatedly documented that the vigor of his acting out was significantly less when on medication. In the medical record, she stated:

- *"Pt. has been compliant to meds for at least 48 hours. He now reports being aware of his aggression and impulsivity and articulates that his meds help this."*
- *"He becomes more impulsive and more assaultive the longer he is non-compliant to prescribed medication regimen including Klonopin [clonazepam], Tegretol [carbamazepine] or a neuroleptic. . . ."*

  After transfer to the maximum-security facility his new clinician, Ms. Blue, PNP, made the following notations in the medical record:
- *At transfer: "I think that routine, somewhat impersonal, handling might help this individual grow up."*
- *A month later and a week prior to his suicide on a form titled, "Prisoner Request for Mental Health Services": "Meds discontinued due to noncompliance. Will monitor off meds and make appropriate diagnosis."*

Summary

Forensic practice is by necessity very close to legal matters, but the forensic nurse should remain mindful that ethics and law, although closely related, are different. Lawful practice requires knowing the laws and following them. Ethical practice is a process best conducted by knowing and using the available tools, principles, and concepts to guide daily behavior and clinical relationships, and to reason through and justify actions and solutions. Memorizing what is right and what is wrong and then acting in accordance will not do; one must engage in the process. The best approach to creating an ethical practice environment is to anticipate problems and react to the inevitable occurrence of problems. This can be done by widely discussing the social and personal values and ethical issues either in advance or as they arise within an agreed-on, fair procedure for achieving consensus regarding how specific situations will be approached within that practice environment, creating policies where needed.

QUESTIONS FOR DISCUSSION

1. If caring concern for patients is one of the benefits of good nursing care, are there potential barriers to achieving this when caring for forensic patients? And how might a nurse overcome the barriers?
2. What are some problems that might occur when applying Western bioethical principles to persons from non-Western cultures?
3. How does recognition that psychiatric diagnosis is, at least in part, socially constructed inform the practice of forensic nursing?
4. How would you balance the community's need for security and the individual's right to treatment in the case of the unhappy prisoner found at the end of this chapter?
5. Use the factors for considering the ethical justification of clinical decisions to discuss the decisions made about the unhappy prisoner.
6. How would you use ethical principles and justifications in deciding on a course of action in the case of a patient making a questionable request for medication?

REFERENCES

Alexander, V., Bursztajn, H., Brodsky, A., Hamm, R., Gutheil, T., & Levi, L. (1991). Involuntary commitment. In T. Gutheil, H. Bursztajn, A. Brodsky, & V. Alexander (Eds.), *Decision making in psychiatry and the law* (pp. 89–107). Baltimore, MD: Williams & Wilkins.

Altman, D. (1982). *The homosexualization of America.* New York, NY: St. Martin's Press.

American Academy of Psychiatry and the Law. (1995). *Ethical guidelines for the practice of forensic psychiatry.* Bloomfield, CT: AAPL.

American Nurses Association. (1995). *Position statement: Nurses' participation in capital punishment.* Washington, DC: American Nurses Publishing.

American Psychiatric Association. (2000). *Diagnostic and statistical manual of mental disorders* (4th ed., text rev). Washington, DC: American Psychiatric Association.

Andreasen, N., Swayze, V., Flaum, M., Yates, W., Arndt, S., & McChesney, C. (1990). Ventricular enlargement in schizophrenia evaluated with computed tomographic scanning. Effects of gender, age, and stage of illness. *Archives of General Psychiatry, 47,* 1008–1015.

Aristotle. (1935). *Aristotle.* (P. Wheelwright, Trans.). New York, NY: Odyssey Press.

Arrestee Drug Abuse Monitoring Program. (2000). *Annual report 2000.* Washington, DC: U.S. Justice Department. Retrieved from http://www.ncjrs.org/pdffiles1/nij/193013.pdf

Baillargeon, J., Black, S., Contreras, S., Grady, J., & Pulvino, J. (2001). Antidepressant prescribing patterns for prison inmates with depressive disorders. *Journal of Affective Disorders, 63*(1–3), 225–231.

Baillargeon, J., Black, S., Pulvino, J., & Dunn, K. (2000). The disease profile of Texas prison inmates. *Annals of Epidemiology, 10,* 74–80.

Beauchamp, T., & Childress, J. (2001). *Principles of biomedical ethics* (5th ed.). New York, NY: Oxford University Press.

Beecher-Monas, E., & Garcia-Rill, E. (1999). The law and the brain: Judging scientific evidence of intent. *The Journal of Appellate Practice and Process, 1,* 243–277.

Benner, P., & Wrubel, J. (1989). *The primacy of caring.* Menlo Park, CA: Addison-Wesley.

Bienstock, S. (2003). Mothers who kill their children and postpartum psychosis. *Southwestern University Law Review, 32,* 451–499.

Bok, S. (1983). *Secrets: On the ethics of concealment and revelation.* New York, NY: Vintage.

Caplan, A. (1982). On privacy and confidentiality in social science research. In T. Beauchamp, R. Faden, R. Wallace, & L. Walters (Eds.), *Ethical issues in social science research* (pp. 315–325). Baltimore, MD: Johns Hopkins Press.

Cassel, E. (1976). What is the function of medicine? In S. Gorovitz, R. Macklin, A. Jameton, J. Oconnor, & S. Sherwin (Eds.), *Moral problems in medicine* (2nd ed., pp. 73–78). Englewood Cliffs, NJ: Prentice-Hall.

Chamberlain, J. (1985). An ex-patient's response to Soliday. *The Journal of Nervous and Mental Disease, 173,* 289–290.

Frankena, W. (1973). *Ethics* (2nd ed.). Englewood Cliffs, NJ: Prentice-Hall.

Gastmans, C. (1999). Care as a moral attitude in nursing. *Nursing Ethics, 6,* 214–223.

Gastmans, C., Dierckx de Casterlé, B., & Schotsmans, P. (1998). Nursing considered as moral practice: A philosophical-ethical interpretation of nursing. *Kennedy Institute Ethics Journal, 8,* 43–69.

Goffman, E. (1973). *The presentation of self in everyday life.* Woodstock, NY: Overlook Press.

Jonas, H. (1984). *The imperative of responsibility: In search of an ethics for a technological age.* Chicago, IL: University of Chicago Press.

Kant, I. (1959). *Foundations of the metaphysics of morals.* (L. Beck, Trans.). New York, NY: Macmillan. (Original work published 1785.)

Kushner, H. (1997). *When bad things happen to good people.* New York, NY: Schocken Books.

Levine, A. (1998). Denying the settled insanity defense: Another necessary step in dealing with drug and alcohol abuse. *Boston University Law Review, 75,* 78–103.

Levy, R. (1983). Self and emotion. *Ethos—Journal of the Society for Psychological Anthropology, 11*(3), 128–134.

Lynd, H. (1958). *On shame and the search for identity.* New York, NY: Harcourt Brace.

Mason, T. (2002). Forensic psychiatric nursing: A literature review and thematic analysis of role tensions. *Journal of Psychiatric and Mental Health Nursing, 9,* 511–520.

Massie, M., Gagnon, P., & Holland, J. (1994). Depression and suicide in patients with cancer. *Journal of Pain & Symptom Management, 9*(5), 325–340.

Mill, J. (1985). *On liberty.* New York, NY: Penguin.

Mitchison, S., Rix, K., Renvoize, E. & Schweiger, M. Recorded psychiatric morbidity in a large prison for male remanded and sentenced prisoners. *Medicine, Science and the Law, 34*(4), 324–330.

Moore, B. (1984). *Privacy: Studies in social and cultural history.* Armonk, NY: M. E. Sharpe.

National Commission for the Protection of Human Subjects of Biomedical and Behavioral Research. (1979). *The Belmont report: Ethical principles and guidelines for the protection of human participants of research.* Washington, DC: OPPR Reports. A6-14. Retrieved from http://videocast.nih.gov/pdf/ohrp_belmont_report.pdf

Nortvedt, P. (1996). *Sensitive judgment: Nursing moral philosophy and the ethics of care.* Oslo, Norway: Tano Aschehoug.

Olsen, D. (1997a). The development of an instrument measuring the cognitive structure used to understand personhood in patients. *Nursing Research, 46,* 78–83.

Olsen, D. (1997b). When the patient causes the problem: The effect of patient responsibility on the nurse–patient relationship. *Journal of Advanced Nursing, 26,* 515–522.

Olsen, D. (1998). Toward an ethical standard for coerced mental health treatment: Least restrictive or most therapeutic? *Journal of Clinical Ethics, 9,* 235–246.

Olsen, D. (2000). Policy implications of the biological model of mental disorder. *Nursing Ethics, 7,* 412–424.

Olsen, D. (2003). Influence and coercion: Relational and rights based ethical approaches to forced psychiatric treatment. *Journal of Psychiatric and Mental Health Nursing, 10,* 705–711.

Peternelj-Taylor, C., & Johnson, R. (1995). Serving time: Psychiatric mental health nursing in corrections. *Journal of Psychosocial Nursing, 33*(3), 12–19.

Plato. (1926). *Plato: Cratylus, Parmenides, Greater Hippias, Lesser Hippias* (H. Fowler, Trans.). (Loeb Classical Library, No 167). St. Edmundsbury, Suffolk, UK: St. Edmundsbury Press.

Rand, M., Sabol, W, Sinclair, M., & Snyder, H. (2010). Alcohol & crime: Data from 2002 to 2008. U.S. Department of Justice. Retrieved from http://www.ojp.usdoj.gov/bjs/content/acf/ac_conclusion.cfm

Reiman, J. (1984). Privacy, intimacy, and personhood. In F. Schoeman (Ed.), *Philosophical dimensions of privacy* (pp. 330–316). London, England: Cambridge University Press.

Sabin, J., & Daniels, N. (1994). Determining "medical necessity" in mental health practice. *Hastings Center Report, 24*(6), 5–13.

Sharpe, M. E., & Morse, S. (1999). Craziness and criminal responsibility. *Behavioral Sciences & the Law, 17*(2), 147–164.

Slovenko, R. (1998). The mental disability requirement in the insanity defense. *Behavioral Sciences & the Law, 17,* 165–180.

Soliday, S. (1985). A comparison of patient and staff attitudes toward seclusion. *The Journal of Nervous and Mental Disease 173,* 282–286.

Strong, C. (2000). Specified principlism: What is it, and does it really resolve cases better than casuistry? *The Journal of Medicine and Philosophy 25*(3), 323–341.

Tasman, A., Kay, J., & Lieberman, J. (1997). *Psychiatry.* Philadelphia, PA: Harcourt Brace.

Teplin, L. (1990). The prevalence of severe mental disorder among male urban jail detainees: Comparison with the epidemiologic catchment area program. *American Journal of Public Health, 80,* 663–669.

U.S. Department of Justice. (n.d.). Retrieved from http://www.ojp.usdoj.gov/bjs/pub/pdf/ac.pdf

U.S. Department of Justice. (2000). *Jail populations by race and ethnicity, 1990–2000.* Retrieved from http://www.ojp.usdoj.gov/bjs/glance/tables/jailracetab.htm

U.S. Department of Justice. (2009). *Violent crime rates by race of victim.* Retrieved from http://bjs.ojp.usdoj.gov/content/glance/race.cfm

Vetlesen, A. (1994). *Perception, empathy, and judgment: An inquiry into the preconditions of moral performance.* University Park: Pennsylvania State University Press.

Working Group for the Study of Ethics in International Nursing Research. (2003). Ethical considerations in international nursing research: A report from the International Centre for Nursing Ethics. *Nursing Ethics, 10,* 122–137.

SUGGESTED FURTHER READING

Alyegbusi, A., & Clarke-Moore, J. (2009). *Therapeutic relationships with offenders.* Philadelphia, PA: Jessica Kingsley.

Corley, M. C., Minick, P., Elswick, R. K., & Jacobs, M. (2005). Nurse moral distress and ethical work environment. *Nursing Ethics, 12*(4), 381–390.

Maeve, M. K. (2001). Nursing with prisoners: The practice of caring, forensic nursing or penal harm nursing? *Advances in Nursing Science, 24*(2), 47–64.

Rowan, R. (2008). A global basis for nursing ethics in a culturally complex world. In V. Tschudin & A. Davis (Eds.), *The globalization of nursing* (pp. 41–50). Milton Keynes, United Kingdom: Radcliffe Publishing.

Williams, D. (2009). Distributive justice in a bad economy: Some thoughts on ethics of care. *Journal of Forensic Nursing, 5*(3), 183–184.

CHAPTER 5

Sociocultural Diversity

Nathan Light

Forensic nurses practice in cultural contexts that are far more complex, diverse, and challenging than those that most other nurses will encounter in their work. Forensic nursing clients bring widely varied backgrounds and expectations; victims, offenders, and psychiatric patients have radically different needs and ways of engaging in the nurse–client relationship. Even if clients come from similar cultural and social backgrounds, those who suffer from crimes, those who may have committed them, and those with psychologic difficulties will be involved in very different institutional processes, and their concerns and responses to treatment will vary widely. To properly treat people with such complex and varied backgrounds and issues, nurses must develop a sensitivity to the cultural and social factors that shape each nurse–client interaction.

Forensic nurses will rarely be able to carry out all their work solely within a single institution, such as a hospital, without some understanding and engagement with the cultures and institutional practices of other concerned organizations and their differing goals. Law enforcement, parole boards, correctional institutions, courts, and victim or substance abuser support groups are a few of the organizations that may become involved in a forensic nurse's work, in addition to the more familiar medical, family, and community contexts. Each context has its own cultural particularities, and offenders and victims will experience institutional interactions differently. They may deal with the same police, prosecutors, and medical personnel along the way, but their social roles and the significance of these contacts will differ greatly. Each client will move from crisis and separation from ordinary life through redress and reintegration into social life, but the actual processes will vary widely.

This chapter will introduce concepts needed to understand and deal effectively with culturally and socially diverse people and institutional contexts and will offer models for understanding the particular cultural contexts in which forensic nurses will find themselves. This chapter will also describe the ways that cultural processes shape socialization so students will understand how childhood establishes the vital permanent connections between culture and the person who make transcultural nursing skills so important. To understand how and why client socialization affects behavior and thinking, this chapter provides a detailed discussion of the processes and effects of learning culture.

This chapter will also familiarize students with the ethical principles that guide transcultural nursing in order to better serve clients through communication and consideration of cultural preferences and concepts. The institutional contexts of nursing will be expanded to show how all clinical situations include transcultural elements, and how understanding this contributes to nursing practice.

CHAPTER FOCUS

- » Culture and Health
- » Cultural and Social Diversity
- » Transcultural Communication
- » Transcultural Nursing
- » Dominant and Minority Cultures
- » Prejudice and Discrimination
- » The Institutional Cultures of Forensic Nursing

- » Ritual Process (Separation, Liminality, Reintegration)
- » Cultural Issues in Forensic Nursing
- » Ideas and Practices Related to Institutions
- » Ideas and Practices Related to Illness
- » Ideas and Practices Related to Trauma
- » Ideas and Practices Related to Mental Illness

KEY TERMS

- » cultural pain
- » culture-bound conditions
- » ethnicity
- » gender
- » institutional culture
- » institutional discrimination
- » interpretation
- » macroculture
- » microculture
- » minority

- » organizational subcultures
- » personal prejudice
- » race
- » situational identity
- » stereotypes
- » tolerance
- » transcultural communication
- » transcultural nursing
- » Vega model

The Experience of Culture

For practitioners of forensic nursing to work effectively in a multicultural society such as the United States, they must understand sociocultural diversity from a scientific perspective. Without an objective understanding of culture and social organization, professionals in positions of power tend to accept dominant European American middle-class values and norms and expect clients and colleagues to conform with them. Medical personnel may judge deviation from dominant culture expectations and values as social, emotional, intellectual, or medical failings.

In the medical and legal contexts within which forensic nurses work, many institutional values and practices are based on dominant culture expectations. If forensic nurses do not objectively understand the sociocultural processes in these institutions, they may provide inadequate service to clients because dominant culture assumptions about thinking, emotion, and behavior lead nurses to ignore, misunderstand, or reject a client's concerns.

This section will explain what culture is, how people experience it, and how these concepts can be applied to understanding the issues of sociocultural diversity in the context of forensic nursing.

Tradition and Innovation in Culture Support Transcultural Communication

Culture is acquired through learning meaningful patterns among associated experiences and behaviors. Because each person creates his or her own associations and understandings, culture does not exist separately from the work of individuals to learn it. Culture is not a fixed set of unchanging practices or beliefs passed as a whole from parent to child, but part of the ongoing process of making sense of the world. Cultural innovation makes **transcultural communication** possible.

In culture contact situations, new cultural forms that help people deal with cultural difference emerge. Understanding cultural differences depends on cultural values and cultural practices that facilitate such understanding. Transcultural understanding, like all interpersonal understanding, requires creative work and has to be nurtured. In most of the world, cultural values that stress hospitality, aid, and respect for others provide the foundation for creating **tolerance** and mutual understanding. When people do not show respect and hospitality towards others, they communicate less and create fewer of the shared understandings that facilitate tolerance.

Despite the widely varying lifeways and worldviews learned in sociocultural groups, because humans are creative, they can invent new ideas and ways of communicating. People can creatively accomplish understanding, but only if they create the conditions for such understanding. The essential element is the will to understand, because when someone wants to understand and tries to understand, she calls upon her ability to creatively respond to others, and creative response creates meaningful associations. Each person can learn how others experience the world. Cultural creativity is regulated by cultural concepts and practices, just as values about respect and hospitality regulate contact.

Applying Transcultural Understanding in Forensic Nursing

Although nursing science has developed a fairly comprehensive understanding of how to deliver nursing care when working with socioculturally diverse populations (Leininger & McFarland, 2002), the special concerns of forensic nurses have been far less carefully researched with respect to sociocultural diversity. We need a much more detailed understanding of cultural ideas about violence and culturally shaped responses to physically and mentally traumatic experience. This section will develop a discussion of the major issues within forensic nursing, as they relate to health practices, cultural care and dealing with trauma and violence.

Health Practices Within Cultural Life

Cultural health practices are complex and ubiquitous, and because they are only partially explained discursively, they are subconscious to a significant degree. Most discussions of health practices in a particular culture focus on those that are consciously recognized by participants in that culture, while the importance of other practices remains unrecognized until **cultural pain** and careful exploration of the issue bring out the underlying expectations that lead to the discomfort (Leininger, 1997).

From conception and pregnancy through birth, postnatal care, and throughout life, human existence in all cultures is guided by health concepts and practices. These include techniques for maintaining physical and mental health, preventing injury and disease, and restoring bodily and mental functioning when they are disrupted. Diet, movement, rest, body manipulation, cleanliness, security, warmth, and contamination avoidance are all part of daily health practices that are learned during childhood. Around the world people have widely varying beliefs about even simple substances such as air and water. Some people see night air as dangerous, others make sure they have adequate ventilation when they sleep; some people believe in daily washing, whereas others, such as Tibetan nomads, associate water washing with potential illness. Most Han Chinese avoid cold water and other cold drinks as potential sources of illness. Some Muslims in Central Asia believe that running water is pure and will not drink from bodies of standing water. Historically, people in Europe believed moonlight could cause mental illness, while in China the moon was valued as a reminder of distant loved ones, and in Persia it became a metaphor for great beauty.

Some of these beliefs have a certain validity—boiled water will not transmit intestinal illnesses and washing in cold water at the high altitudes where Tibetans live can be a threat to health—but the strongest motivation for these and many other beliefs is that maintaining consistent cultural practices helps maintain a sense of control and familiarity within life, and when such practices are changed, uneasiness and cultural discomfort often result.

Since these practices start at the beginning of life, they are deeply embedded within understandings of a proper and balanced life, and it is difficult to separate health maintenance from food ways, bodily practices, and ideas about purity and contamination, which often include supernatural components. Most culturally shaped activities involve elements that are believed to injure health if not conducted properly. Sociocultural health practices also include the processes of learning and maturation that are believed to create the properly adjusted and developed adult.

Health Practices and Nursing Communication

As mentioned earlier, the most important way to explore differing health practices and their effects on personal comfort and needs for care is through communication. The first goal of a nurse should be to facilitate communication concerning the client's emotional state and concerns, because this will usually reveal the earliest evidence of discomfort. Communication is very important in nursing, and every effort should be made to determine how to improve it. This includes assessing linguistic skills in English and in other languages, finding family or friends who can help a client communicate and help support the client in raising issues that he or she is reluctant or embarrassed to discuss, and finally, exploring what aspects of the clinical setting, activities, and personnel cause concern to the client.

Once effective means of communication have been established, the nurse should explore with the client any cultural discomforts he or she is experiencing and attempt to identify the sources of those discomforts. As mentioned earlier, many aspects of cultural care are not consciously recognized but will affect how someone feels about the care he is receiving in the clinical context. In order to adequately support the client's needs, open-ended exploration of sources of vague discomfort or unease will help him to describe and understand how his cultural expectations are being thwarted (American Medical Association, 1999; Galanti, 1997; Luckmann, 1999).

A number of issues should be kept in mind in transcultural communication. First, recognize that ways of speaking to clients readily convey attitudes and prejudices. Because health-care workers have the authority of institutionalized medical practices, they often establish power relationships through hierarchical modes of communication. Styles of speech that condescend to a client, especially minorities, women, and children, can effectively close off communication (Waitzkin, Cabrera, deCabrera, Radlow, & Rodriguez, 1996).

Just as derogatory **stereotypes** and condescending attitudes have to be avoided to promote open communication, so too do ethnocentric and nationalist assumptions about history and tradition. The common identification of Mexicans as immigrants to the United

States reveals a gap in many Americans' historical understanding. At the end of the U.S. Mexican War in 1848, Mexico ceded California, Arizona, New Mexico, Texas, and parts of Colorado, Nevada, and Utah, to the United States. Mexicans living in these areas became American citizens but were then confronted with violence, discriminatory voting laws, and fraudulent treatment that pushed them off their land. In the Southwest, the border moved, not the Mexicans. Obviously, assuming that a Mexican has immigrated might only serve to remind one of the discrimination and ignorance perpetuated by some non-Mexicans in the United States.

Transcultural Nursing

The concepts and practices of **transcultural nursing** are widely used, but often in ways that imply that some nursing is not transcultural. In fact, all nursing should be seen as transcultural to the extent that the client is not a part of the healthcare community, and thus only partially shares the knowledge, expectations, and ways of thinking that are shared among medical personnel. When a patient from the dominant culture receives health care, the transcultural dimension remains largely unnoticed because healthcare workers accommodate dominant cultural expectations.

For instance, although nurses and doctors understand the biological differences between viral, bacterial, fungal, and parasitic infections, they do not expect the general public to make such clear distinctions, and they make allowances for this lack of understanding when they explain why an antibacterial drug is useless or even harmful in treating a viral or fungal infection. Likewise, although personal sanitation in the dominant culture of the United States involves certain shared concepts and practices—such as the germ theory of disease and the use of soap and disinfectants to control germs—the inpatient sanitation procedures in a hospital require additional explanation. These procedures are not part of the dominant culture's understanding, so they must be learned in order to participate properly as a patient in the hospital community. But the same courtesy is not automatically extended to people who do not bring dominant culture expectations with them when they arrive for health care. In such cases, nurses have to make sure that dominant culture assumptions about care are not getting in the way of proper treatment or causing cultural discomfort.

To perform the social role expected of a patient in a hospital, he or she acquires specialized knowledge from nurses and doctors, just as nurses and doctors acquire specialized knowledge to fulfill their roles. The patient goes through a necessarily transcultural socialization process when entering a hospital, although if caregivers assume that a patient shares their dominant cultural background, they will only explain how the hospital context differs from other dominant culture contexts and resist seeing that this is a transcultural interaction. Because all patients are potentially new to the culture of the clinical context they have just entered, transcultural nursing is an integral part of explaining and carrying out healthcare procedures in cooperation with the patient. Communicating and explaining carefully are very important, and the patient's level of understanding must be closely monitored. Assumptions should always be made overt and tested so they do not cause misunderstandings.

Cultural Pain Interferes With Communication

Culture helps people maintain meaningful and orderly social relations through shared understandings and expectations. When one person's social expectations and communicative practices do not conform to those of another, mutual avoidance may result because each feels that the other is a source of disorder. The only way to overcome the sense of alienation or unease someone feels when confronting the unexpected is to become aware of cultural sources of discomfort and to communicate about them. Nurses have to help people recognize when they are experiencing cultural discomfort, or what Madeleine Leininger calls cultural pain (1997; Leininger & McFarland, 2002, p. 52), and understand ways to both cope with and reduce it. Coping with the unease resulting from differing cultural expectations can be particularly difficult in institutional contexts where one person has a lower status and is less respected, and thus has difficulty being heard when attempting to communicate about cultural discomfort. When an authority figure such as a nurse, doctor, or police officer assumes that their practices are not merely culturally distinct, but somehow more rational or moral, coping with cultural miscommunication becomes even more difficult.

Reducing Cultural Pain and Communication Barriers by Understanding Diversity

Properly understanding what sociocultural diversity means for healthcare practitioners is complex and cannot be reduced to contrasts between the dominant culture and **minority** cultures. In fact, every person is a member of multiple cultures because ethnic and racial groups do not define the totality of cultural and social experiences. All people participate in a number of groups, from family and friends to local communities, to schools and places of work. Those people develop shared identities based on work, play, skill, age, handicap, sexual preference, participation in social organizations, and so forth.

A useful way to understand sociocultural diversity is to think of each individual as a member of multiple partially overlapping groups, as in **Figure 5-1.** Because most social groups that shape someone's identity consist of people who spend time together and have experiences in common, they develop shared cultural understandings and expectations. Communicative interaction and shared experience are the basis for any cultural sharing. Different sociocultural contexts have different emotional values for participants, and people usually become more attached to and deeply rooted and comfortable in culture learned within their family and community and often less attached to the culture of their schools or workplaces, which are less encompassing experiences.

Although a person's identity is often reduced to social categories known to sociologists as master statuses, such as **ethnicity**, **race**, age, or **gender**, human identities are complex products of experience in and affiliation with multiple communities and social contexts. Social scientists now recognize that identities are situational and strategic, and people can define themselves differently in different contexts by using relevant aspects of their background. In one situation, someone may identify himself as African American, while in another he may say he is a New Yorker, and in yet another he may identify himself as a Red Sox fan. The **situational identity** someone chooses as salient in a social context depends on how he wants to be perceived, what he is there for, and what he wants to accomplish at any given moment. Very few people live within a single ethnic, class, or occupational identity without creating more differentiated and individualized identities within their families and among groups of friends or coworkers.

Nonetheless, most of us know that people assign us to groups by behavior, clothes, skin color, or language before they even know us, and they make guesses about our background, lifestyle, economic status, and so on from this flimsy evidence. Such labels become

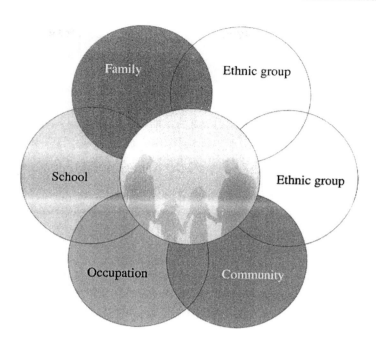

Figure 5-1 Some social contexts of socialization; through interactive participation the individual develops personal identity and culture.

part of our experience and we come to share more with people in the same ascriptive category, regardless of what we share in terms of other experience, simply because we are treated similarly in society. Obviously, such treatment can be negative and discriminatory, such as that often experienced by racial, ethnic, or sexual minorities or low-status workers. The underlying motivation is understandable; it is difficult to recognize and get to know every person as a distinct individual. It is much simpler to reduce the many dimensions of experience, personality, and identity to obvious and socially salient categories. This is particularly the case when the relationship one has with other people is the result of occupational duties. People try to limit and simplify job responsibilities by creating routines and categories.

When nurses or other healthcare workers feel they can assign people to particular categories, they may feel this increases their control and efficiency in clinical relationships. The risk is that such categories become self-fulfilling prophecies, as stereotypes fill in for real knowledge about a client gained through communicative interaction. Understanding people requires that they be seen as complexly connected to multiple groups and multiple intersecting sets of cultural experiences and beliefs. External markers should not be allowed to serve as indicators of identity or cultural patterns. Each patient has to be approached as an individual whose social and physical reality can be explored only through open communication.

Racial Categories Are Socially Constructed

As most students should already recognize, race is not a valid category within biological science, because it has no consistent genetic meaning. Race imagined as a biological category has no place in medical physiology and epidemiology (Cooper & David, 1986). The much-vaunted associations between race and conditions such as sickle-cell anemia only work when race is used as shorthand for assessing population genetics. Statistically in the United States, many African Americans have West African ancestors and are thus somewhat more likely to have the sickle-cell trait. But West African ancestry is the genetic reason and has no consistent expression in body type or skin color. Many people with West African ancestry are identified socially in the United States as white, and many people without West African ancestry are identified as black (including East Africans, South Africans, South Asians, and Pacific Islanders). In addition, the sickle cell trait is found in other population groups from other parts of the world without recent genetic connections to West Africa (Cavalli-Sforza, Menozzi, & Piazza, 1994).

All human groups have widely ranging traits and have to be diagnosed according to standard procedures, not guesses about genetic background. Race is a social category defined according to cultural principles. Often in the United States, the principle of hypo-descent—a social rule, whereby children of a union between members of different socio-economic groups are automatically placed into a less privileged category—causes people to be identified as members of a nonwhite race when they are known to have any ancestor from that group (Harris, 1974). This illustrates that the genetic significance of socially defined race is very limited.

Even the argument that race can be used as a proxy measure that stands in for cultural and social factors that affect health leads to careless assumptions because of the enormous range of cultural and social experience; Asian American, African American, or Native American experiences and lifestyles vary widely from place to place and depend upon income, urban or rural living, and geographic origins. Except for the very broadest statistical generalizations, racial categories are not useful in medicine. Instead, more precise characterizations of sociocultural and genetic groups should be used when attempting to construct groups for statistical study (Ikemoto, 1997; Krieger & Fee, 1994). When this is done, it is possible to make useful correlations among sociocultural background, culturally shaped health practices and ideas, and environmentally influenced health patterns. Otherwise, the genetic, environmental, cultural, and individual patterns cannot be usefully disentangled, and attempted generalizations based on race or sociocultural experience risk leading to prejudice and discrimination.

Prejudice and Discrimination

Racial attributions and ideas do affect treatment of people within hospital, court, school, and other public contexts. Although biological functioning and cultural behavior have no firm correlation with socially defined categories such as race, racism and discrimination do influence health. When someone's perceived racial identity affects how others treat her in social life or in clinical contexts, this may affect her health and the outcomes of medical care (Barbee, 1993). Similar effects result from the differing treatment people encounter because of their ethnicity, gender, sexual identity, age, or handicaps.

The **Vega model** offers great insight into the workings of racism and discrimination in American society (Martin, 1992; Vega, 1978). The Vega model describes the intersection of three dimensions of social relations: (1) cultural bias, (2) **personal prejudice**, and (3) **institutional discrimination**. In order to accurately understand how institutions discriminate, one must understand how cultural biases shape images of people who belong to recognized social groups. Cultural bias can arise from any representations or ascriptions of particular behaviors and abilities to people because of their social identity. When such images become widespread, a cultural bias that leads to personal prejudice emerges.

For instance, if I hear from people I know or from media reports that Gypsies are involved in various petty crimes and I never know any Gypsies (properly known as Rom) from personal social experience—outside of institutional contexts that perpetuate biased interactions—I may form broad prejudices linking them to criminal activities. Rather than recognizing that rumor, media stereotypes, and outsider perspectives have biased my ideas about Gypsies, such ideas will replace the ignorance that I would otherwise have to acknowledge. Most people do not question their received cultural biases and hearsay knowledge, but often rely upon it and end up discriminating against people about whom they know nothing.

To avoid contributing to institutional discrimination, each individual must vigorously question the cultural biases to which they are exposed. Cultural biases are widespread, and individuals cannot avoid being exposed to them, but people can prevent themselves from acting upon them or perpetuating their circulation. Individuals within an institution who carry out its policies and procedures should recognize that institutional discrimination remains potent in many contexts because people have failed to take responsibility for changing the ways that cultural bias, prejudice, and discrimination reinforce each other.

Examples of cultural biases that lead to prejudice and institutional discrimination are easily found. The witch trials in colonial New England and the Inquisition in Europe both resulted from Christian cultural biases about non-Christian religious practices that were interpreted as being evidence for dealings with Satan. The dominant cultural model provided biased **interpretations** of all non-Christian and heterodox religious activities as satanic practices, and the practitioners were punished and even executed, although they explained that their beliefs and practices had nothing to do with Satan and were for the good of their community. Because of cultural bias, only the dominant official culture model of caring for a community's spiritual health was accepted, and practitioners of minority beliefs were harshly discriminated against and suppressed (Ginzburg, 1983).

Such witchcraft trials are not as far off as one might imagine; in the 1980s and early 1990s in the United States, Britain, and Australia, a panic about satanic ritual abuse led to widespread mobilization of legal and psychologic professionals against the perceived threat of a worldwide network of satanic cult members systematically attacking children. Despite the fact that there was never evidence for such a network, and many of the events were testified about by witnesses who had been coached by so-called experts or were the work of teenagers using imagery borrowed from rock lyrics, hundreds of people were accused and many brought to trial. The mobilization against this supposed plague included many counselors, consultants, and police advisors who created a systematic cultural model of satanic rituals. Because they persuaded people these practices were ubiquitous, evidence was easy to bring together into the narrative they created—rock lyrics, kids' pranks on Halloween, communal lifestyles, and the practices of followers of beliefs such as Wicca and Santería were no longer seen as separate events, but as integral parts of a systematic satanic religion. The following quotes from two news stories show how easily law enforcement jumped from identifying a minority group to accusing them of satanic ritual abuse of children:

> Six unidentified children taken from two men believed to be members of a satanic cult were moved from a shelter when officials there received threatening phone calls, police said Saturday. The cult, known as the Finders, was suspected of engaging in human trafficking of the members' children. (Birk, 1987a)

Six days later, the police retreated from their accusations based in the cultural model of satanic ritual abuse determining that situation was nothing out of the ordinary for this rural area of the country (Birk 1987b).

Working from a biased cultural model, hypothetical narratives, and a few shreds of evidence, people can readily put things together into a believable explanation. The human mind strives to make narrative sense of the world, and people are often not willing to stop and question received models because the comprehensive explanation seems more reliable and enables decisive action. For this reason justice and science have to rely heavily on skepticism and the benefit of the doubt. Culturally biased models and stereotypes become traps, especially if based on hearsay and stories, because people frequently pass on stories without believing them simply for their entertainment value, and often encourage others to give them credence (Dégh, 2001). One person's funny story becomes another's truth. An excellent example of this is the wide credence people give to the obviously culturally biased stories about pets disappearing into the kitchens of Chinese restaurants.

The crack baby panic of the 1980s was similarly framed as a problem of poor minorities. Cultural biases against minorities led to discrimination that resulted in jail penalties for crack cocaine use that were more than 10 times as long as for noncrack cocaine, despite the lack of scientific evidence that crack was more destructive than other forms of cocaine (Hartman & Golub, 1999; Litt & McNeil, 1997). One has to assume that such moral panics will happen again and thus use critical thinking to resist urban legends and supposed news stories that promote cultural bias, because these will lead to personal prejudice and to participation in institutional discrimination (Goode & Ben-Yahuda, 1994).

In addition to cultural biases against people who are not members of the dominant culture, cultural biases can also provide images of positive behavior by members of the dominant culture. Pediatric doctors are more likely to assess nonwhite children for abuse injuries (Lane, Rubin, Monteith, & Christian, 2002), although white offenders are more likely than nonwhite offenders to commit violence against children (Finkelhor & Ormrod, 2001, p. 4). The positive dominant culture image of middle-class, Anglo-American families reduces education and healthcare professionals' willingness to recognize abuse when it occurs within such families. Child sexual abuse is common in all ethnic groups and social classes (Finkelhor, 1993), but biased intervention and prosecution tend to facilitate denial or concealment of abuse and the protection of dominant culture offenders, which in turn perpetuates the belief that such cases are less common. Assumptions about the infrequent occurrence of and the milder consequences for child sexual abuse by female perpetrators likewise motivates social workers and the police to provide less protection to victims of such cases (Hetherton & Beardsall, 1998).

Clearly institutional cultures are important places to prevent discrimination through systematic questioning of the biases and stereotypes that shape personal prejudice. The following section will consider some of the ways that **institutional cultures** form, and how these affect client experiences.

Institutions Create Their Own Cultures

Much of what people feel to be the shared and unspoken cultural understandings of a group are often quite weakly shared. People usually assume they can make themselves understood to people who share their language, but within organizations interaction can be complex for outsiders who do not understand the organizational culture very well. Any complex institution, such as a university, bank, or hospital, develops complex systems and specialized language, whether about research procedures, insurance, mortgages, or medical procedures. Even straightforward procedures are highly technical in unsuspected ways. When someone wants to know why the bank has not processed a check yet, she discovers the complexities of financial processes. Every institution has complex procedures that are obscure to outsiders pursuing their particular goals, and insiders may take the procedures so completely for granted that they cannot explain them to outsiders.

Expert knowledge consists of both the formal and explicit systematic knowledge of how to practice a particular skill, such as nursing, as well as extensive informal knowledge acquired piecemeal through experiences that would be difficult to systematize and explain. This kind of sociocultural knowledge develops through long participation in a work context.

Upon arriving for the first day of a new job in a healthcare institution, such as a hospital, one begins a very steep learning curve of discovering its formal and informal culture. Over the course of weeks and months one builds a fairly accurate knowledge of job responsibilities and social expectations in most circumstances. But only over the course of years does one become aware of the political, historical, and institutional forces shaping the policies, attitudes, and practices of the hospital. Like any large institution, hospitals are complex social systems with diverse cultures that outsiders know little about. Wards, departments, and offices within a hospital develop idiosyncratic patterns. The people within the hospital bring characteristic modes of behavior from their prior experiences into their present interactions with others, creating patterns sometimes described as **organizational subcultures** (Brooks & MacDonald, 2000; Costello, 2001; Jermier, Slocum, Fry, & Gaines, 1991; Louis, 1980; Mason, 2002; Secker et al., 2004; Walker, 1967).

A client's arrival in a new medical context is likewise a complex learning experience. New clients do not know what to do, what to expect, who to ask for information, or how they will be treated. They will likely expect some highly structured bureaucratic and medical procedures that bestow patient status on outsiders, and they will understand that attaining this new status is a prerequisite for getting the diagnosis and treatment that they came for, but the power and knowledge differential makes a productive clinical experience problematic. The rituals of entering a new organization and negotiating to resolve concerns are important components of care-seeking processes (Lock & Scheper-Hughes, 1996; Rimal, 2001).

Madeleine Leininger points to many ways that different cultures arise in clinical and hospital contexts, and that differences between the cultures of nursing and medicine can lead to conflicts within nurse–physician interactions and hierarchies. The recognized authority and expertise of physicians facilitates their professional autonomy and exercise of decision-making power. "Physicians tend to communicate that they 'always know what is best' for the client" (Leininger, 1997, p. 33) despite seeing the client only briefly in care settings and hospitals. Leininger argues that most hospitals and physicians rely on a technoscientific model of disease treatment and symptom management and finds that problems arise when the nurses do not retain their own autonomy in care and instead allow the physicians' model to be imposed on them. Further, public media support the dominance of the physicians' model, so "nursing's unique and valuable discoveries" (Leininger & McFarland, 2002, p. 202.) to healing and well-being remain little noted, and the hegemonic practices of medicine perpetuate clients' "cultural pain and distrust" (Leininger & McFarland, 2002, p. 202). The physician model of technoscientific medicine significantly impedes client treatment when it overwhelms or leads to rejection of client concerns. The symbolic rituals of technoscience tend to subordinate client needs to those of the institution and its procedures. Studying these rituals has become an important part of overcoming obstacles that prevent culturally sensitive client care.

The Ritual Process of Medicine

The conflicts between technoscience and care models may be largely invisible to clients, who tend to perceive the institution's staff and their policies and activities as integrated parts of a homogeneous and impenetrable system. In fact, the client experience of medical institutions usually revolves around the ritualized aspects of admission, treatment, and discharge, which have been interpreted from the perspective of Arnold van Gennep's theory of rites of passage (Davis-Floyd, 1992). Using this approach, filling out forms, changing into a hospital gown, transportation by wheelchair, submission to an admission physical, and being assigned to a room and a bed serve as the ritual stage of separation during which the client leaves the everyday world of individuated identities to become one of many patients under the care of authoritative ritual experts whose tutelage they must follow for successful treatment and transition back to the everyday world.

Many aspects of hospital treatment have more to do with controlling patient individuality, freedom, and options, and enforcing their obedience to ritual specialists than with medically necessary activities. Sitting in a wheelchair for transport, bodily exposure and accessibility enforced by the hospital gown, and catheterization with a saline drip just in case intravenous access is needed are all examples of rendering the body the object of technoscientific ritual and taking away comfort and freedom. Such practices remind the patient that she is there to wait, to suffer, and to be passive (all root meanings of the word *patient*).

The ritual and symbolic aspects of hospital technoscience have been extensively documented by Robbie Davis-Floyd in her study of the technocratic model of birth; she finds that the hospital birth ritual treats the mother as if she is suffering from a dangerous condition and is dependent on medical technology to avoid the impending disaster threatened by a natural body. The patient is expected to subordinate her needs to those of the hospital staff, who often seem to want childbirth to be a calm and well-managed affair, like other institutional procedures. The mother's body is subjected to an unnatural birth position for the convenience of the doctor and for many years the mother was expected to undergo anesthesia in order that her experience of pain would not disturb the doctor's concentration (Davis-Floyd, 1992, p. 52).

Davis-Floyd's description can be expanded to include other interventionist medical procedures; hazardous screening tools such as X-rays, computed tomography scans, and procedures requiring anesthesia are routinely ordered merely to eliminate unlikely conditions. Inadequate risk-reward analysis plagues medical diagnostic procedures. The dominant interpretation of technology as solving problems overwhelms the recognition of the risks and possibility of medical error that come with its use. Risk assessment is rarely carried out despite the incidence of complications with even the most routine medical procedures and prescriptions. When a patient rejects a treatment as too invasive or dangerous, strong pressure is often applied to encourage compliance.

The patient experiences treatment rituals imposed from outside with few choices about the process. It is taken for granted that the doctor's expertise outweighs patient concerns or preferences, so the patient's role is often reduced to consenting to the treatment plan presented. After the *liminal* period in which the treatment and its outcome, and hence the patient's health status itself, remain indefinite and monitored, the healing process begins, and the patient gradually transitions back to normal social roles through rituals of *reintegration*, such as removal from intravenous or breathing support, or starting physical therapy. The passage through ritual separation, liminal uncertainty in which the patient's body is subjected to symbolic domination by technologic and bureaucratic means, and finally the declaration that one is healing and can be reintegrated back into ordinary life, are all part of the technoscientific control of medical crisis, and as Davis-Floyd (1992) points out, such rituals function to reinforce social values.

It is important to understand how client experience involves ritual processes because technoscientific medical training and clinical practices often deny the sociocultural effects of medical ritual and rely primarily on medical and institutional necessities to legitimize procedures. But ritual techniques are used in all cultures for giving a sense of control over uncertain or dangerous processes (Glicksman, 2003; Gmelch, 2003; Malinowski, 1948). Although the uncertainties of medical diagnosis and treatment involve many complex and demanding ritual practices, the psychosocial effects are subordinated to more objective demands such as sterility, standardization, rational procedures, and the catch-all placebo effect. The concept of the placebo effect has the added benefit of implying that only patients may be influenced by rituals while practitioners preserve their scientific rationality. Even the broadest studies of so-called context effects in healing situations avoid examining how treatment rituals may influence the caregivers themselves to reduce anxiety and improve outcomes (e.g., Christakis, 2003; Di Blasi, Harkness, Ernst, Georgiou, & Kleijnen, 2001; Kaptchuk, 2002).

It seems obvious that medical rituals reassure both patients and practitioners that the best possible treatments are being identified and carried out in the best possible way. Rituals create a sense of control that alleviates anxieties about injury, trauma, pain, illness, and outcomes that can promote recovery in patients and preserve a sense of effectiveness in practitioners. Research on pain shows that pain is subjectively experienced as much worse when the patient does not know how long and how painful a condition will become. If a patient has some certainty about the duration and severity of the pain that he or she will feel, he or she actually feels less pain (Goldberg & Remy-St. Louis, 1998). Similarly, physicians who focus their attention and work in controlled and ritualized contexts "with well-defined sequences of actions," "precise expectations," and limits on sources of variation are able to feel confident and effective (Delle Fave & Massimini, 2003; p. 335; see also Csikszentmihalyi, 2000).

Forensic nursing clients experience multiple crises and encounter numerous institutional procedures that are meant to help them regain control. Understanding how these processes involve elements of ritual (especially separation, liminality, and reintegration) will aid communication with and treatment of clients. Medical procedures not only serve to restore physical and mental health, but also can support or impede the psychosocial recovery process by helping clients make sense out of traumatic and disabling events and regain control over their lives.

Client Experiences in the Institutional Contexts of Forensic Nursing

The forensic nursing client faces complex institutional involvements that are not limited to nursing and medicine, but can include police, courts, and therapists, among others. This added complexity is less common in other fields of nursing; the different organizational cultures of these institutions place demands on both the client and the nurse. The nurse will often have to mediate and explain these demands for clients, because the client will not understand the various institutional expectations.

In order to understand client experiences of the overlapping cultural processes pertaining to a victim of domestic violence or sexual assault, one needs to think of the ways that each social context has its own culture. The shared dominant culture within which these groups exist can be described as a **macroculture**, with each professional group having its own **microculture** within that macroculture. The client will have to interact with and learn the concerns, rules, and expectations of the unfamiliar cultures of police, doctors, courts, and nurses, among others. In addition, they have to maintain relations with their family and community while in a period of crisis that will profoundly affect expectations and interactions. The assault itself and any court proceedings will bring victims into contact with the offender, and the healing process will potentially bring the victims into contact with other victims. One way of understanding how these intersecting microcultures are experienced is represented graphically in **Figure 5-2.**

To understand the relationship of macroculture and these microcultures, it is best to see the macroculture as the shared national culture, including all the general expectations and understandings of the roles of the police, doctors, nurses, and courts; the sense of a shared project of maintaining social order; and even the exploitative ideologies that contribute to violence or sexual assault as antisocial attempts to attain culturally idealized power. The macroculture cannot be said to be as deeply learned or completely shared by its members, but brings general understandings and language, while each microculture develops more specific cultural expectations as well as ways of using language.

Similar diagrams for understanding the interacting sociocultural contexts for incarcerated or psychiatric clients can be seen in **Figures 5-3** and **5-4**. These diagrams only suggest the complexity of intersections among these contexts because in many there will be more than the three subcultures or identities overlapping.

A Cultural Process Model of Recovery

Understanding the client experience in terms of overlapping institutional contexts, each with their own cultural models of events, methods, and goals, can guide practitioners who wish to promote integration and communication among these processes. Despite the great differences among these institutions and their goals, the overall processes are comparable. Understanding these processes will help the forensic nurse understand the situation of the clients he or she works with and will facilitate supporting clients in dealing with these overlapping institutional cultures.

The Model

In forensic nursing, the client is generally in a crisis or has undergone traumatic experiences that make trust and communication difficult. In any sociocultural context, crisis creates an unexpected and dangerous situation that cannot be dealt with by ordinary means—by its very nature there are few cultural responses and expectations to draw upon because culture consists of familiar and usual social activities. To gain sociocultural control over unusual natural or social crises or disasters depends upon specialists. In U.S. society, these specialists can include police, firefighters, emergency medical technicians, Red Cross personnel,

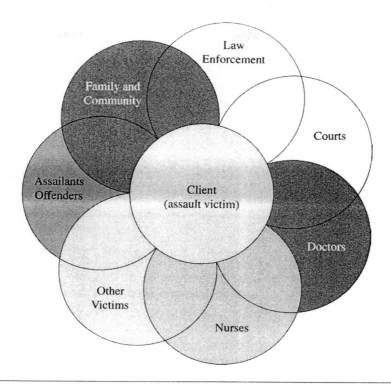

Figure 5-2   The interacting sociocultural contexts for a victim client with the larger macroculture in the background.

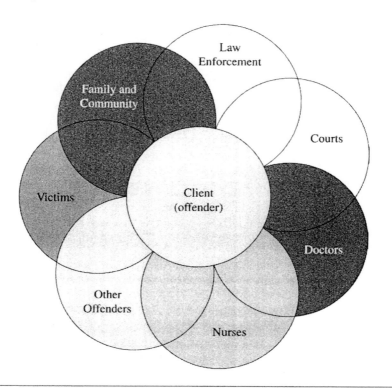

Figure 5-3   The interacting sociocultural contexts for an incarcerated client.

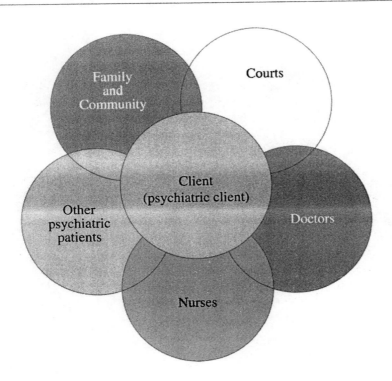

Figure 5-4 The interacting sociocultural contexts for the psychiatric client.

the National Guard, news reporters, politicians, and nurses and doctors (Vaughan, 1999; in press).

These specialists are responsible for identifying the components of the crisis, seeking out its causes, healing its symptoms, and resolving long-term consequences. As can be seen from **Table 5-1**, in a medical emergency involving a crime victim, each specialist not only focuses on particular aspects of crises, but also provides certain kinds of remedies and redress. Although the client is the central subject of the remedies and redress of a crisis, he or she generally knows little about the roles and work of these specialists and must discover the procedures and expectations as the specialists do their work. Although overlapping in many ways, the client's concerns can be quite different from those of the specialists.

The sociocultural process that a client undergoes as part of a traumatic experience can be narrated as a sequence consisting of a prehistory of relative normalcy and meaningful participation in a familiar social order, followed by a personally disruptive event or events that occur with little or no warning and disconnect the client from meaningful and orderly existence. The client is thrown into a liminal or crisis period in which expectations about social relations and physical experience break down. The changed behavior or concerns of significant others and the unfamiliar language of crisis specialists can add to the sense of separation and result in loss of stability, safety, and trust.

Coping with a crisis has to include institutional processes of redress, psychosocial processes of reestablishing familiarity and trust, and sociocultural processes of reclaiming one's former roles, relationships, and identity. The social complexity of these overlapping processes indicates the degree of importance society places on controlling such events and

TABLE 5-1   The Culturally Shaped Concerns of Client and Specialists Through the Course of the Trauma and Recovery Process; the Client Is a Sexual Assault Victim in This Example (see also Helman, 2000)

Identity and Institutions	Pre-event Social Life	Trauma or Crisis Event	Identify Events, Causes, Agents, Models	Apply Models in Planning Redress	Perform Redress	Resolve Remaining Issues	Reintegrate into Social Life
Client (victim of assault)	Meaningful multidimensional participation in a variety of social groups and contexts	Injury and confusion about what, how, and why Seek safety Emotions: fear, stress, anxiety, frustration, feel trapped by event and aftermath of violated privacy Potential culturally-shaped feelings: guilt, shame, anger, hatred, or distrust of others	Seek reasons, causes, responsibility, models, and understanding Flashbacks to events Identify sources of social and emotional support; seek narrative knowledge from others with similar experiences Begin to identify as "victim of this event"	Engage with significant others; explore physical, emotional, and legal solutions; use others' narrative knowledge to develop a probable course to recovery; develop a narrative of this new identity; develop symbolic representations of this "trial," this "burden," this "chaos"	Find support; rebuild trust in others Pursue medical, emotional, legal redress Attempt to follow models of recovery Find more positive, active symbolic identity to separate from event	Separate more fully from the event Return to other identities and roles Rebuild integrity and stability of social relations Return to social participation and to self-concept from before the event	Come to see self as once again having multidimensional social identity within one's community
Police (from client perspective)	Facilitate and organize daily community life; enforce laws and court orders	Emergency response	Identify and investigate crime; identify suspects	Build case against suspects; attempt to arrest suspect	Incarcerate offender; monitor offenders in the community	Inform and educate community to help avoid similar events; provide continuing protection	Promote safety and order; facilitate community activities

(continues)

TABLE 5-1 The Culturally Shaped Concerns of Client and Specialists Through the Course of the Trauma and Recovery Process; the Client Is a Sexual Assault Victim in This Example (see also Helman, 2000) (continued)

Identity and Institutions	Pre-event Social Life	Trauma or Crisis Event	Identify Events, Causes, Agents, Models	Apply Models in Planning Redress	Perform Redress	Resolve Remaining Issues	Reintegrate into Social Life
Courts and prosecutors (from client perspective)	Carry out justice procedures	Limited role	Determine legal issues; identify suspects	Develop case; prosecute suspect; hold trial	Reach judgment; sentence and punish culprit	Restrict offender's recidivism potential; consider victim's concerns	Carry out justice procedures
Medical personnel (from client perspective)	Promote health; identify and resolve medical issues	EMTs; emergency room treatment: return client to physical and mental integrity	Diagnose medical condition; identify concerns	Determine treatments; alleviate symptoms	Apply medical remedies; support bodily healing; evaluate prognosis; plan management	Psychological support and counseling for emotional recovery and reintegration; aid in restoring social integrity	Promote health; identify and resolve medical issues
Nurses (from client perspective)	Promote health; facilitate prevention; mediate contact with physicians	Relieve trauma; carry out SANE protocol; convey and gather vital information; understand client needs	Determine client care needs; Identify cultural, social, personal issues; Begin to provide culturally congruent care	Expand communication with client and explain procedures and resources; help find narrative understanding; Monitor and help resolve patient concerns about physical, mental, and social situation	Perform procedures; support bodily, social, and emotional healing; facilitate interaction with physicians and with significant others	Monitor client's healing; educate about issues and options; facilitate contact with psychological support staff	Promote health; facilitate prevention; mediate contact with physicians

finding multiple kinds of redress for these disruptions. Social order and cultural consistency are highly valued by most members of society. Violence, trauma, crisis, and disaster that threaten sociocultural order must be dealt with as effectively as possible. The work of specialists involves discovering the causes and resulting symptoms of the crisis to remedy them and applying specialist cultural models to restore order and stability. Victims generally have fewer models and must rely on others to provide explanatory narratives that help make sense of the crisis. **Figure 5-5** offers one way to understand this process in overview for victims of violent trauma, and Table 5-1 shows the many different specialist roles and activities that can be identified within each stage of the process.

Table 5-1 helps us to understand that the complexity of experiencing violent trauma is only one generalized model of the experience, but it suggests the value of seeing it as a multilayered process. Its complexity is even more pronounced when the client is not a member of the dominant culture or is unfamiliar with the cultural patterns of personnel in these institutions. If the client has to have everything translated into his or her native language and learn unfamiliar interaction patterns and expectations, cultural pain can be added to already existing trauma.

When we add these stages to the earlier discussion of the ways in which the ritual process is experienced in the hospital as a loss of control to technoscientific procedures, we can begin to understand why the cultural and symbolic meanings of the experience can be as important as the physical reality of the trauma itself. The ritual helps bring a sense of control over a crisis, but at the cost of relinquishing personal control to ritual specialists to whom we turn when we cannot deal with a crisis as individuals. One result of Table 5-1 is that we see that the opportunity to take time planning redress is more pertinent to the doctor, therapist, and prosecutor roles, while the police, emergency medical technician, emergency room doctor, and nurse roles require that more immediate care be given to a client. Despite these differing orientations, a planned, integrated, and systematic organization of treatment within an environment of open communication with the client will be extremely helpful in healing and regaining a sense of control over her life.

This model is not comprehensive because every situation is different, but the processes of healing body, mind, and social relations are central to recovery. In fact, these are overlapping phases rather than the tidy stages represented in the table. But healing requires not simply a return to prior bodily, mental, and social wholeness; it also requires finding

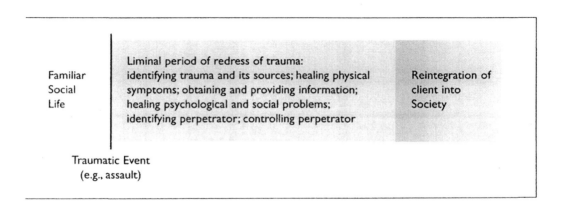

Figure 5-1   The overall sociocultural model of the trauma process.

labels, explanations, and resolutions to use to give meaning to traumatic experience. The resolution of disorder involves identifying and naming the pieces of that disorder, explaining the causes and effects, and beginning to resolve ongoing problems with normal social functioning.

Trauma Process and Ethnomedical Techniques in Folk Healing

The trauma process model can help understanding of healing rituals in other cultures. One of the most important steps in healing is the diagnosis. In technoscientific medicine, this is presented as a way to systematically classify and describe the etiology and symptoms of a condition, but more generally this serves to label and explain the problem. The ritual process moves beyond disorder and ambiguity by labeling and explaining the condition and then seeking remedies. In the case of many healing traditions, diagnosis includes identifying supernatural explanations for a condition. However, the diagnosis of the cause is usually less important than characterizing the severity of the injuries and the probable prognosis for treatment and healing. Such diagnosis moves patient and medical staff from a condition of lacking information to one of having a somewhat elaborate description of the condition that helps return the patient to the meaningful world of cultural understandings.

The feeling that a bodily or mental crisis has brought loss of control can begin to be overcome as soon as the mysterious is put into familiar and *culturally congruent* terms. When Madeleine Leininger advocates culturally congruent care, she means not only care that fits within patient expectations and experiences, but also care that begins by making culturally reasonable sense of the condition from which the patient suffers (Leininger & McFarland, 2002). Within forensic nursing, the conditions of uncertainty and crisis that a nurse will likely provide care for clearly extend beyond medical or psychologic to the social liminality that crime victims, offenders, and psychiatric patients all experience in one way or another. An important aspect of care is labeling and explaining the condition in order to promote healing. This involves finding answers to the following questions: What happened? Why has the event disconnected the client from society? What processes of recovery and reintegration will be most effective? These questions arise in all medical treatment because all clients need to be reassured about when they will get out of the hospital, but the multi-institutional nature of victim and offender experiences makes the uncertainties greater in their cases, as they deal with intersecting processes.

Cultural care techniques from many different societies have been described for illnesses and psychiatric conditions, but there are far fewer studies of traditional healing methods used for injuries. Thus it is rather difficult to describe in much detail examples of techniques with which clients may be familiar. Beyond ethnomedical rituals that assist in injury diagnosis, treatments for injuries can include plant or other substances, ritual recitations, offerings, and so on. The trauma itself will be less important than engaging and appeasing the supernatural forces that allowed it to happen so that they do not allow further injury, as well as seeking supernatural aid to promote healing. Ideas about dealing with the evil eye, making offerings to helpful spirits, or warding off witchcraft are often part of traditional medical practices and should not be interfered with because they often provide clients with a sense of added security in the face of uncertainty.

Although folk healing techniques for dealing with injuries are not very highly elaborated and have not been studied adequately in most cases, the techniques for dealing with psychologic conditions are often quite complex and may well be encountered by forensic nurses. Beliefs about supernatural influences or strong emotions leading to **culture-bound**

conditions such as *locura* (psychosis), *susto* (fright illness), and *nervios* among Hispanics; *ceeb* (fright illness) and soul wandering among the Hmong; *shenkui* (panic with somatic conditions) among Chinese; and *zar* (spirit possession) among people from North Africa and the Middle East (Simons & Hughes, 1985). It has been pointed out that hypoglycemia has similarly entered popular thinking as an ambiguous and flexible illness construct because those who claim to suffer from it far outnumber those who have been clinically diagnosed with it (Hunt, Browner, & Jordan, 1990).

All of these conditions can be diagnosed and treated by folk healers using a variety of ways to gain information about supernatural and emotional events that influence a person. Extensive studies have explored how shamans in Native American, Siberian, Hmong, Korean, and Balinese societies, among many others, provide important diagnostic and healing practices to help cure a wide range of mental and physical conditions, ranging from infertility to epilepsy (Connor, Asch, & Asch, 1986; Grim, 1983; Thao, 1989). Most shamans rely on knowledge gained through interaction with spirits, who diagnose the problem in terms of bodily, supernatural, or social causes, and then prescribe treatment. Such consultation of the spirits often involves the shaman going into a trance and inviting spirits to speak through him or her as a medium or channel. When the shaman comes out of the trance, he or she often has to ask those present what the spirit has said. Thus the shaman does not claim medical expertise, but has authority that comes from intimate connections with spirits who can explain unseen causes and effects (Kendall, 1985).

It is very important to recognize that although shamans and other healers are generally expert in interaction with the supernatural, they do not necessarily have a narrow medical specialization or a consistent style of performing their rituals. Each shaman and supernatural healer develops his or her own relationship with particular spirits, and they tend to expand their repertoire of supernatural services to deal with almost all problems or concerns clients might bring, from explaining the causes of bad luck and preventing further bad luck to predicting the future to providing healing services. Although any given culture will have certain patterns of interaction and typical kinds of conditions that healers can treat, there is extensive personal variety, especially in larger societies and more urban settings where many different traditions come together and healers tend to pick and choose among practices that they feel work best. For instance, the Balinese medium and healer Jero Tapakan both goes into trances, so that clients can ask for speech from the spirits to determine the source of medical problems and misfortunes, and provides therapeutic massage and medicines to heal people after they have been diagnosed by the spirits. In contrast to the traditions of *curanderismo* in Latin America, where the *curandero* usually does diagnose and prescribe based on personal expertise (Press, 1971), Tapakan could not herself diagnose a problem or prescribe medicine. When asked the diagnosis for one patient she says, "In my opinion—well, I don't know anything, but according to my guardian deity, the Balinese diagnosis is called *babai*. But I don't know, it's not visible." On the other hand, Tapakan does display extensive traditional knowledge about bodily forces and channels when she discusses her clients' conditions and treats them by massage (Connor, Asch, & Asch, 1986, p. 202).

These are only a few examples of the endless array of healing alternatives available in any urban setting around the world. As Irwin Press describes for residents of Bogota, there are healers who diagnose through bodily examination, divination, pseudoscientific instruments, and religious practices. Treatments can include homeopathy, patent medicines, charms, amulets, prayer and saints' images, holy water, injections, and prescriptions to restore humoral imbalance (Press, 1971). One mile from the university where I am writing this in the yurvedic United States, I can walk into a health food store and ask one of the several prescribing salespeople about any condition I might believe I have, and they will offer me a vitamin, mineral, herb, or extract that they believe will cure or alleviate it. I could just as easily consult with nearby chiropractors, and would not have to go much further to find fortune-tellers or faith healers who would suggest other treatments. Many people in North America rely on practitioners of Wicca and religious healing systems derived from West African traditions, including Santería, Vodun, and Candomblé. Or I could go to one of the two local hospitals, both less than two miles from here, that rely on biomedical principles. The human capacity to feel ill or otherwise out of balance far exceeds the ability of medical science to manage, and people rely on many treatments that seem to offer control over the complex uncertainties of bodily and mental life, as long as the practices are culturally congruent with their understanding of the connections among themselves, their society, and the world around them.

In addition to many curing processes that include supernatural components or placebo effects, research has revealed that many folk remedies prove to be effective therapies in double-blind studies and thus offer alternatives to more expensive patented medicines. Such substances rarely find a place in technoscientific medicine because the drug approval process is very costly and hence only worthwhile for companies when they know they can make a profit from patent-protected drug innovations. Since it is not possible to patent natural products, these are rarely shepherded through the FDA approval process, and thus remain folk or herbal remedies that people rely on as alternatives to high-priced drugs.

Sociocultural Concerns in Treating Injuries

Perhaps because they have less mysterious origins and heal with somewhat less mystery than bodily and mental illness, injuries are more often the subject of self-care, which is not as well studied as the practices of professional healers. There are few descriptions in the literature of techniques used to diagnose injuries, trauma, blood loss, and the like, but many medical techniques used to treat them.

Traditional treatments for injury and trauma include applying mineral, plant, and animal products; rituals and incantations; mechanical treatments; and bodily manipulation. A comprehensive review of the literature on the botanical pharmacopeia used in yurvedic medicine (from India) showed that only 8% of the 166 plants described had uses for controlling pain and inflammation, and none were described as being used to aid treating other trauma (Khan & Balick, 2001). In eastern Indonesia, palm oil, betel nut, turmeric, and papaya are all used to treat wounds. Papaya is similarly used by Native Americans (Dweck, 1997). Aloe vera has also been used to treat wounds in some areas, but research shows it has little effectiveness. Acupuncture is an alternative therapy with considerable effectiveness for treating pain.

Although many injury treatments that will be part of the cultural repertoire of many patients are little known, there has been considerable study of how people from different cultural backgrounds respond to and express pain (Edwards, Fillingim, & Keefe, 2001). This is an important dimension of nursing because pain sensations have important effects on well-being and healing and serve to alert caregivers to problems that may need further assessment. The clinical assessment of pain and its cultural variability have been extensively studied. Many examples of how people in different societies cope with pain have been combined into a model that attempts to predict the experience and expression of pain in terms of cultural values and social conditioning that influence choices among the options of stoicism versus expression, extroversion versus introversion, anticipatory anxiety about pain, emotional state, accurate understanding of the probable degree of pain, and narrative understanding and explanation of pain (Goldberg & Remy-St. Louis, 1998).

There is also complex literature on the many biologic pathways that generate pain. It shows that although there are no fundamental biologic differences in pain experience around the world, culture does profoundly shape pain sensations. It has also been found that in many treatment contexts in the United States, minorities are not given adequate pain management, especially if they receive care from people who do not share their native language (Lasch, 2002). Pain assessment clearly depends heavily upon culturally sensitive communication and empathy, including the willingness to find the means to communicate in the client's native language so that full and open assessment of pain can be attained (Davidhizar & Giger, 2004).. In addition, nurses should be sensitive to client behaviors and expressions such as limping or grimaces that indicate pain.

Cultural Practices and Forensic Nursing

A few issues remain about the connections between forensic nursing and cultural practices. Although there has been very little systematic study of the legal and medical dimensions of the wide variety of religious, educational, ritual, and folk healing practices, a number of relevant examples have been studied by anthropologists and medical researchers.

Folk medical practices can be fairly invasive and often result in injuries or leave lasting marks on the body. Since medical practices are often done to children by adults, some instances result in injury that may lead to questions about child abuse. In one case, an infant who died of unknown causes later ascribed to SIDS was examined and found to have healing clavicular fractures. The parents were initially suspected of child abuse, but further investigation revealed that the child had been treated by an unlicensed chiropractor 3 or 4 weeks before the death (Sperry & Pfalzgraf, 1990). In rare cases, injuries have resulted from acupuncture techniques, and these might be more likely in small children because the needle depth would have to be adjusted to account for smaller body size. Another Asian medical tradition, moxibustion, has also been misinterpreted as child abuse because it can leave burn marks (Feldman, 1984).

Faith healing and Christian Science practices raise deep questions about parental rights to refuse medical treatment to a child and generate numerous legal cases each year, when states try to impose treatment by having a parent declared negligent and then taking custody of the child, or when a state presses criminal charges against a parent for not seeking medical treatment for a child who suffers permanent harm or death.

Although there were legal statutes that protected the rights of Christian Scientists to provide alternative medical care without being considered negligent, most have been eliminated in the past few decades, so it is now easier for states to prosecute parents for neglect when they do not seek medical care for children (Merrick, 1994, 2003; Swan, 1983).

Another dimension of religious healing involves practices that are designed to eliminate supernatural causes of possession. This can take many forms, including the shamanism described earlier. In the case of certain forms of faith healing based on the Christian Bible, people can be subjected to physical practices that can cause harm and even death. A recent example from Milwaukee concerns a faith-healing service to rid an autistic boy of spirits. The healing practices allegedly involved physical restraint that resulted in the boy's death (McCord, 2003). Religious worship can also involve other hazardous practices such as snake handling, fire walking, or piercing the body to show imperviousness to pain due to supernatural protective powers. In general, such practices are not protected religious expression if they result in harm to a child, so investigation and prosecution are standard responses in the United States. Another example of practices that can result in injury include some of those that are used to rid a child of the influences of the evil eye (Bottoms, Shaver, Goodman, & Qin, 1995).

In general, however, religious and faith-healing practices involve little threat to the body or mind and do not result in injury. There are a number of initiation rituals that can easily involve injury to a child, especially those that involve physical modification of the body such as circumcision. Already widely recognized are the dangers of female genital cutting in many parts of the world. Less well publicized are the dangers of male circumcision and subincision. Other ritual practices involve body modification, scarification, and tattoo. As with religious healing practices, there are cultural and religious motivations for these practices that make it difficult to interfere without being accused of discriminatory treatment. In general, there has to be a risk of serious harm before legal sanctions can be used to challenge a traditional custom. Worldwide, the campaign against more extreme forms of female genital mutilation has only been successful when people from the local culture are enlisted to support changes to the practice. One positive aspect of changing such rituals is that often the initiation aspect of the rite of passage can be accomplished symbolically without significant body modification. Few people consider the standard circumcision of male babies after birth in the United States to be a major body modification—although it is not medically necessary—so there is little effort to change it. Female genital cutting rituals are being replaced in Africa and elsewhere by less extreme symbolic acts, with role models provided by activists who publicly reject the practices and promote the alternatives.

Summary

Dealing with client experiences and ideas about cultural and social dimensions of life are complex responsibilities that depend upon caregivers' sensitivity, skillful and attentive communication, and open-minded willingness to understand clients' concerns. Healthcare practitioners have to be careful to avoid bringing their own cultural biases or personal prejudices into their institutional practices.

Physical and mental experience do not exist outside of the cultural interpretations, concepts, and needs that people begin learning in early childhood, and continue to develop throughout their lives. Effective, nondiscriminatory communication about emotional, physical, or cognitive experience, and cultural meanings requires creative work to bridge the gap between those different experiences. This is particularly true with transitions into new organizational subcultures, such as those found in hospitals.

In addition to trauma experienced before arriving at an institution, the clinical experience itself, along with encounters with law enforcement and the courts, can contribute to separation of the patient from ordinary social functioning. Treatment has to take into account psychosocial needs in order for the patient to deal with this new state of liminality. Through complex ritual processes, many specialists will participate in aiding a patient in accomplishing redress and reintegration with society at large.

Biomedical procedures—like those of most healing traditions—depend upon ritual practices to help control anxiety and uncertainty. Although there has been extensive work on how healthcare provider rituals can influence patient experiences and outcomes, there remains a reluctance to consider the ways rituals in the healing situation also significantly affect practitioners. Acknowledging the significant contribution that ritual processes make to controlling uncertainty and restoring social order in the face of crisis would go a long way towards linking patient experiences more closely to physician and nurse experiences and in adding to our understanding of the complexity of these social processes.

Perhaps the most important influences on caregiving interactions are the aspects of technocratic and bureaucratic ritual and symbolism that prevent effective therapeutic communication. The hierarchical effects of depending on medical technology and procedures to control uncertainty in the clinical context can suppress the mutual respect that will help a client regain control over his or her situation.

In addition, patients' own care traditions should be understood and respected as techniques that help them introduce familiar cultural order in unfamiliar situations. Practitioners should work to be aware of the variety of different cultural practices and communicate openly with patients about the effects and concerns of alternative treatments.

Cultural concepts and expectations about communication, health, food, and bodily comfort are diverse and have a deep impact on the feelings of people made vulnerable by the conditions or experiences that bring them into forensic healthcare settings. Forensic healthcare patients should be understood as individual members of a number of different subcultures that shape complex sociocultural concerns in ways that must be explored through attentive interaction and caregiving.

QUESTIONS FOR DISCUSSION

1. What are class, race, and ethnicity, and what role do they play in social life?
2. How and when do people use culture in daily life to communicate, judge, make choices, and act?
3. How do people respond to violations of cultural norms and values?
4. How do institutions create, propagate, and use culture?
5. What cultural patterns and practices will be encountered in forensic nursing?
6. When, why, and how will cultural assumptions have to be made overt in forensic nursing?
7. What tools can you use to visualize cultural and social domains?
8. How can one evaluate cultural knowledge, expectations, and communication strategies?
9. How can one recognize when cultural differences are distorting communication?
10. How do rituals and cultural models shape the practice of medicine?

ACKNOWLEDGMENTS

I wish to thank Barbara Chesney, Lynne Hamer, and Seamus Metress for discussing this chapter with me and suggesting issues and resources I should include.

REFERENCES

American Medical Association. (1999). *Cultural competence compendium*. Chicago, IL: American Medical Association.

Associated Press. (1988, April 1). *Devil getting unwarranted publicity in McComb*. Associated Press wire story. Retrieved from Lexis/Nexis database.

Barbee, E. L. (1993). Racism in U.S. nursing. *Medical Anthropology Quarterly, New Series, 7*(4), 346–362.

Birk, E. (1987a, February 14). Authorities tone down description of Finders. Associated Press wire story. Retrieved from Lexis/Nexis database.

Birk, E. (1987b, February 8). *Threats phoned to tattered kids; Police on alert*. Associated Press wire story. Retrieved from Lexis/Nexis database.

Bottoms, B. L., Shaver, P. R., Goodman, G. S., & Qin, J. J. (1995). In the name of God: A profile of religion-related child abuse. *Journal of Social Issues, 51*, 85–111.

Brooks, I., & MacDonald, S. (2000). "Doing life": Gender relations in a night nursing sub-culture. *Gender, Work and Organization, 7*(4), 221–229.

Cavalli-Sforza, L. L., Menozzi, P., & Piazza, A. (1994). *The history and geography of human genes*. Princeton, NJ: Princeton University Press.

Christakis, N. A. (2003). On the sociological anxiety of physicians. In C. Messikomer, J. Swazey, & A. Glicksman (Eds.), *Society and medicine: Essays in honor of Renée C. Fox* (pp. 135–144). New Brunswick, NJ: Transaction.

Connor, L. H., Asch, P., & Asch, T. (1986). *Jero Tapakan: Balinese healer, an ethnographic monograph*. Cambridge, UK: Cambridge University Press.

Cooper, R., & David, R. (1986). The biological concept of race and its application to public health and epidemiology. *Journal of Health Politics, Policy and Law, 11*(1), 97–116.

Costello, J. (2001). Nursing older dying patients: Findings from an ethnographic study of death and dying in elderly care wards. *Journal of Advanced Nursing, 35*(1), 59–68.

Csikszentmihalyi, M. (2000). *Beyond boredom and anxiety: Experiencing flow in work and play*. San Francisco, CA: Jossey-Bass.

Davidhizar, R., & Giger, J. N. (2004). A review of the literature on care of clients in pain who are culturally diverse. *International Nursing Review, 51*(1), 47–55.

Davis-Floyd, R. (1992). *Birth as an American rite of passage*. Berkeley: University of California Press.

Dégh, L. (2001). *Legend and belief: Dialectics of a folklore genre*. Bloomington: Indiana University Press.

Delle Fave, A., & Massimini, F. (2003). Optimal experience in work and leisure among teachers and physicians: Individual and bio-cultural implications. *Leisure Studies 22*, 323–342.

Di Blasi, Z., Harkness, E., Ernst, E., Georgiou, A., & Kleijnen, J. (2001). Influence of context effects on health outcomes: A systematic review. *Lancet, 357*(9258), 757–762.

Dweck, A. C. (1997). Ethnobotanical use of plants. Part 4. The American continent. *Cosmetics and Toiletries, 112*(11), 1–12. Retrieved from http://www.dweckdata.com/Published_papers/American_Indians.pdf

Edwards, C. L., Fillingim, R. B., & Keefe, F. (2001). Race, ethnicity and pain. *Pain, 94*(2), 133–137.

Feldman, K. W. (1984). Pseudoabusive burns in Asian refugees. *American Journal of the Diseases of Children, 138*, 768–769.

Finkelhor, D. (1993). Epidemiological factors in the clinical identification of child sexual abuse. *Child Abuse and Neglect, 17*(1), 67–70.

Finkelhor, D., & Ormrod, R. (2001). *Offenders incarcerated for crimes against juveniles*. Washington, DC: U.S. Department of Justice, Office of Juvenile Justice and Delinquency Prevention. Retrieved from http://www.unh.edu/ccrc/pdf/offendersincarcerated.pdf

Galanti, G. (1997). *Caring for patients from different cultures: Case studies from American hospitals*. Philadelphia: University of Pennsylvania Press.

Ginzburg, C. (1983). *Night battles: Witchcraft and agrarian cults in the sixteenth and seventeenth centuries*. Baltimore, MD: Johns Hopkins University Press.

Glicksman, G. G. (2003). It couldn't hurt: An ethnographic study of a ritual for healing. In C. M. Messikomer, J. Swazey, & G. Glicksman (Eds.), *Society and medicine: Essays in honor of Renée C. Fox* (pp. 59–68). New Brunswick, NJ: Transaction.

Gmelch, G. (2003). Baseball magic. In J. Spradley, & D. M. McCurdy (Eds.), *Conformity and conflict: Readings in cultural anthropology* (pp. 348–357). Boston, MA: Allyn and Bacon.

Goldberg, M. A., & Remy-St. Louis, G. (1998). Understanding and treating pain in ethnically diverse patients. *Journal of Clinical Psychology in Medical Settings, 5*(3), 343–356.

Goode, E., & Ben-Yahuda, N. (1994). *Moral panics: The social construction of deviance.* Cambridge, UK: Blackwell.

Grim, J. (1983). *The shaman: Patterns of Siberian and Ojibway healing.* Civilization of the American Indian Series (Vol. 165). Norman: University of Oklahoma Press.

Harris, M. (1974). *Patterns of race in the Americas.* New York, NY: Norton.

Hartman D. M., & Golub, A. (1999). The social construction of the crack epidemic in the print media. *Journal of Psychoactive Drugs, 31*(4), 423–433.

Helman, C. G. (2000). Ritual and the management of misfortune. *Culture, Health and Illness* (4th ed., pp. 156–169). Boston, MA: Butterworth-Heinemann.

Hetherton, J., & Beardsall, L. (1998). Decisions and attitudes concerning child sexual abuse: Does the gender of the perpetrator make a difference to child protection professionals? *Child Abuse & Neglect, 22*(12), 1265–1283.

Hunt, L. M., Browner, C. H., & Jordan, B. (1990). Hypoglycemia: Portrait of an illness construct in everyday use. *Medical Anthropology Quarterly, 4*(2) 191–210.

Ikemoto, L. C. (1997). The fuzzy logic of race and gender in the mismeasure of Asian American women's health needs. *University of Cincinnati Law Review 65*(Spring), 799–824.

Jermier, J. M., Slocum, J. W., Fry, L. W., & Gaines, J. (1991). Organizational subcultures in a soft bureaucracy: Resistance behind the myth and facade of an official culture. *Organization Science, 2*(2), 170–194.

Kaptchuk, T. J. (2002). The placebo effect in alternative medicine: Can the performance of a healing ritual have clinical significance? *Annals of Internal Medicine, 136*(11), 817–825.

Kendall, L. (1985). *Shamans, housewives, and other restless spirits: Women in Korean ritual life.* Honolulu: University of Hawaii Press.

Khan, S., & Balick, M. J. (2001). Therapeutic plants of Ayurveda: A review of selected clinical and other studies for 166 species. *The Journal of Alternative and Complementary Medicine, 7*(5), 405–515.

Krieger, N., & Fee, E. (1994). Man-made medicine and women's health: The biopolitics of sex/gender and race/ethnicity. *International Journal of Health Services, 24*(2), 265–283.

Lane, W. G., Rubin, D. M., Monteith, R., & Christian, C. W. (2002). Racial differences in the evaluation of pediatric fractures for physical abuse. *Journal of the American Medical Association, 288*(13), 1603–1609.

Lasch, K. (2002). Culture and pain. *Pain: Clinical Updates, 10*(5). Retrieved from http://www.iasp-pain.org/PCU02-5.html

Leininger M. (1997). Understanding cultural pain for improved health care. *Journal of Transcultural Nursing, 9*(1), 32–35.

Leininger, M., & McFarland, M. R. (2002). *Transcultural nursing: Concepts, theories, research and practice.* New York, NY: McGraw-Hill.

Litt, J., & McNeil, M. (1997). Biological markers and social differentiation: Crack babies and the construction of the dangerous mother. *Health Care for Women International 18*(1), 31–41.

Lock, M., & Scheper-Hughes, N. (1996). Critical-interpretive approach in medical anthropology: Rituals and routines of discipline and dissent. In C. F. Sargent, & T. M. Johnson (Eds.), *Medical anthropology: Contemporary theory and method* (pp. 41–70). Westport, CT: Praeger.

Louis, M. (1980). Surprise and sense making: What newcomers experience in entering unfamiliar organizational settings. *Administrative Science Quarterly, 25,* 226–251.

Luckmann, J. (1999). *Transcultural communication in nursing.* Albany, NY: Delmar.

Malinowski, B. (1948). *Magic, science, and religion.* Garden City, NY: Doubleday.

Martin, R. J. (1992). A model for studying the effects of social policy on education: Gauging the impact of race, sex, and class diversity. *Equity & Excellence, 25,* 53–56.

Mason, T. (2002). Forensic psychiatric nursing: A literature review and thematic analysis of role tensions. *Journal of Psychiatric and Mental Health Nursing, 9,* 511–520.

McCord, M. (August 25, 2003). *Autistic boy dies during prayer service; man arrested in connection with death.* Associated Press wire report.

Merrick, J. C. (1994). Christian-Science healing of minor children–spiritual exemption statutes, first-amendment rights, and fair notice. *Issues in Law & Medicine, 10*(3), 321–342.

Merrick, J. C. (2003). Spiritual healing, sick kids and the law: Inequities in the American healthcare system. *American Journal of Law & Medicine, 29*(2–3), 269–299.

Press, I. (1971). The urban curandero. *American Anthropologist, New Series, 73*(3), 741–756.

Rimal, R. (2001). Analyzing the physician–patient interaction: An overview of six methods and future research directions. *Health Communication, 13*(1), 89–99.

Secker, J., Benson, A., Balfe, E., Lipsedge, M., Robinson, S., & Walker, J. (2004). Understanding the social context of violent and aggressive incidents on an inpatient unit. *Journal of Psychiatric & Mental Health Nursing, 11*(2), 172–178.

Simons, R. C., & Hughes, C. C. (1985). *The culture-bound syndromes: Folk illnesses of psychiatric and anthropological interest.* Dordrecht, the Netherlands: D. Reidel.

Sperry K., & Pfalzgraf, R. (1990). Inadvertent clavicular fractures caused by "chiropractic" manipulations in an infant: An unusual form of pseudoabuse. *Journal of Forensic Science, 35*(5), 1211–1216.

Swan, N. R. (1983). Faith healing, Christian Science, and the medical-care of children. *New England Journal of Medicine, 309*(26), 1639–1641.

Thao, P. (1989). *I am a shaman: A Hmong life story with ethnographic commentary.* (D. Conquergood & X. Thao, Trans.) Minneapolis: Southeast Asian Refugee Studies Project, Center for Urban and Regional Affairs, University of Minnesota.

Vaughan, D. (1999). The dark side of organizations: Mistake, misconduct, and disaster. *Annual Review of Sociology, 25,* 271–305.

Vaughan, D. (in press). Organizational rituals of risk and error. In B. Hutter, & M. Power (Eds.), *Organizational encounters with risk.* Cambridge, UK: Cambridge University Press.

Vega, F. (1978). *The effect of human and intergroup relations education on the race/sex attitudes of education majors.* (Unpublished doctoral dissertation). University of Minnesota, Minneapolis.

Waitzkin, H., Cabrera, A., deCabrera, E. A., Radlow, M., & Rodriguez, F. (1996). Patient–doctor communication in cross-national perspective—A study in Mexico. *Medical Care, 34*(7), 641–671.

Walker, V. H. (1967). *Nursing and ritualistic practices.* New York, NY: Macmillan.

SUGGESTED FURTHER READING

Aboul-Enein, B. H., Aboul-Enein, F. H. (2010, spring). The cultural gap delivering health care services to Arab American populations in the United States. *Journal of Cultural Diversity, 17*(1), 20–23.

Chege, N., & Garon, M. (2010). Adaptation challenges facing internationally educated nurses. *Dimensions of Critical Care Nursing, 29*(3), 131–135.

Gertner, E. J., Sabino, J. N., Mahady, E., Deitrich, L. M., Patton, J. R., Grim, M. K., ... Salas-Lopez, D. (2010). Developing a culturally competent health network: A planning framework and guide. *Journal of Healthcare Management, 55*(3), 190–204.

Hunter, J. L., & Krantz, S. (2010). Constructivism in cultural competence education. *Journal of Nursing Education, 49*(4), 207–214.

Im, E. O. (2010). Current trends in feminist nursing research. *Nursing Outlook, 58*(2), 87–96.

Kramer, L. W. (2010). Generational diversity. *Dimensions of Critical Care Nursing, 29*(3), 125–128.

Mendonca, L., Minchella, L., Selser, K., Soria, S., Teskey, C., Wattigny, C., & Butler, S. (2010). Immigrant and refugee youth. Challenges and opportunities for the school nurse. *NASN School Nurse, 24*(6), 250–252.

Piki, E. S. (2010). Cultural diversity. *Nursing Standard, 24*(29), 59–60.

Sharpnack, P. A., Griffin, M. T., Benders, A. M., & Fitzpatrick, J. J. (2010). Spiritual and alternative healthcare practices of the Amish. *Holistic Nursing Practice, 24*(2), 64–72.

CHAPTER 6

Vulnerable Populations

Barbara Moynihan

This chapter will identify and focus on the special needs of those who comprise the population of at-risk or vulnerable groups. The charge to the forensic nurse is to identify and address the unmet and ever-changing complexities inherent in providing services to this population.

 ## CHAPTER FOCUS

» Vulnerable Populations
» Characteristics of Vulnerable Populations
» Forensic Nursing Practice Interventions
» Evolving Deficits in the Healthcare Response to Vulnerable Populations
» Development of Appropriate Interventions Specific to This Population

» Theoretical Foundations Specific to the Unique Needs of At-risk Vulnerable Populations
» Predisposing Factors to Vulnerability

KEY TERMS

» assessment
» cultural sensitivity
» disenfranchised population

» marginalized
» vulnerability

The quality of mercy is not strain'd,
It droppeth as the gentle rain from heaven
Upon the place beneath: it is twice blest;
It blesseth him that gives and him that takes.

—William Shakespeare, *The Merchant of Venice,*
Act IV, Scene I: Portia's Speech (pg. 242)

Introduction

There are many facets to forensic nursing practice that are consistent with nursing practice in general but are specific to the specialized expertise of the forensic nurse. The neediest, the disenfranchised, and the least powerful comprise a population that may become invisible within the healthcare system. **Table 6-1** lists some of the vulnerable population groups of special concern to the forensic nurse. These groups do not represent all vulnerable groups, however. "Vulnerable populations are defined as social groups who have an increased relative risk or susceptibility to adverse health outcomes"

TABLE 6-1   Vulnerable Population Groups

- Poor/disadvantaged people
- Homeless people
- Pregnant adolescents
- Undocumented workers
- Mentally ill individuals
- Substance abusers
- Abused people
- People with communicable disease(s)
- People who have the hepatitis B virus or sexually transmitted diseases or who are HIV positive

Source: Stanhope, M. & Lancaster, S. (2000). *Community & public health nursing* (p. 639). St. Louis, MO: Mosby.

Risk Factors	Client	Support systems
Age	(individual/family/	formal/informal
Gender	community)	external/internal
Environment	Resource Factors	Sociocultural
Occupation		Environment
Race/ethnicity		Occupation
Sociocultural		Economic/financial
Economic/financial		Education
Genetic		Resiliency/hardness
Other		(challenge/commitment/
		control)
		Other
		Buffering Activities
		(counterbalancing)

Figure 6-1   The web of causation model.

Source: Lundy, K., & Janes, S. (2001). *Community health nursing* (5th ed.) (p. 579). Sudbury, MA: Jones & Bartlett.

(Flaskerud & Winslow, 1998, p. 69). According to the web of causation model of health and illness shown in **Figure 6-1** (Lundy & Janes, 2001), the interaction among numerous causal variables creates a potent combination of factors that predisposes an individual to risk. This model can be used by nurses to understand the relationships among various factors that contribute to health status and vulnerability. Based on their skills as nurses and as forensic experts, forensic nurses have the potential to identify vulnerable populations and to assist with the development of services for the most disadvantaged. The scope and standards of forensic nursing practice are both broad and comprehensive, and they provide an extensive frame of reference within which the forensic nurse can flourish. Due to ever-increasing concerns regarding national and international vulnerability and risk, assessment and interventions related to local as well as global populations are essential. Violence is rooted in the social, cultural, and economic fabric of human life. These factors interact with family, community, and other external factors to create a feeling of vulnerability among certain populations. These vulnerable, invisible populations suffer not only from a climate of oppression, which is compounded by a lack of resources, but also from feelings of helplessness and hopelessness. Consider the factors that contribute to an individual seeing himself or herself as invisible, as being isolated, or as excluded from or denied services and resources for a variety of reasons. The reasons for this sense of invisibility have many causes; included among those reasons is not even being recognized as needy.

Predisposing Factors to Vulnerability

The vulnerable represent all segments of society and are not a homogeneous group. Vulnerable populations are a subgroup that shares common risks or combinations of risk factors; one that is pervasive is poverty or low socioeconomic status (U.S. Department of Health and Human Services, 1998, 2000). Poverty, which is a growing problem in the United States, has been noted by some as a primary cause of vulnerability (Northam, 1996; Pesznecker, 1984). According to the landmark study by the World Health Organization (2002), poverty is a major factor internationally as well. This study also shows that poverty is linked to all types of violence. Although the topic of violence is discussed in another chapter, it should be noted that the linkages between vulnerability and violence are clear and compelling. Other factors that contribute to risk and vulnerability noted among all countries studied include family dynamics, substance abuse, and a lack of resources. Of the U.S. population, 37 million or 12.6% live below the official poverty line (Center for American Progress, 2007). In addition, approximately 24.5% of America's children live in poverty (National Coalition, 2007). Within this context, a lack of understanding on the part of the nurse or other healthcare providers can add to the formidable barriers that already exist and prevent those in need of services from receiving them. The fears, misconceptions, and biases that are communicated by caregivers due to perceived conflicts in values, lifestyles, and so on result in even deeper feelings of oppression and powerlessness already possessed by the client. Vulnerable populations among the poor include people with special needs, the unemployed, the homeless, and the disenfranchised.

There are many factors related to vulnerability and many consequences associated with this status. Health-related issues include limited access to care, higher infant mortality rates, trauma-related injuries and death, substance abuse, and chronic illness. The physically, emotionally, or mentally challenged are at significant risk for being underserved. Not only does vulnerability result in poor health care and access to services, but the risk factors associated with vulnerability often lead to violence. That violence may involve the vulnerable person as either a victim or a perpetrator. Family, school, community, sociocultural, and cultural factors all influence coping skills of young people and their ability to deal with their community. This is another arena in which the forensic nurse, who is able to understand the relationships among social factors as they contribute to vulnerability and violence, may be able to reduce or interrupt the downward cycle that poverty, family stress, and lack of supports create within the vulnerable population.

Populations currently experiencing poor health status are increasing, while those experiencing good health status are decreasing. According to some experts, this disparity in health status created by socioeconomic, racial, and ethnic differences is great and is on the rise in the United States. When elements of racism, poverty, and community converge, greater overall threats to health develop. The health risks within these vulnerable populations were recognized in the objectives identified by the U.S. Department of Health and Human Services document, *Healthy People 2020* (2009). The objectives included increasing the composition of racially and culturally appropriate programs that address substance abuse, mental health services, violence, and unintentional injuries, as well as nutrition, exercise, and stress management. By utilizing a theoretical framework of holism and caring, the forensic nurse is well positioned to intervene in addressing the inequities in both health care and social services among vulnerable populations. Identifying the underserved, developing **cultural sensitivity**, and creating a climate of acceptance and safety contribute to reversing the cycle of vulnerability and risk. Primary prevention, however, may not always be possible; when primary prevention is not feasible, secondary or tertiary prevention may be significant in breaking the cycle.

It is beyond the scope of this chapter to review all populations who are vulnerable or at risk; however, a brief overview of selected populations has been included. Chapters in this text regarding policy, nursing leadership, and other topics are the threads that address the comprehensive network of forensic nursing practice as it applies to vulnerable populations.

Vulnerable Populations

Vulnerability implies that, when compared with the general population, some people are more sensitive to certain risk factors that can negatively impact their health. Those who are vulnerable are particularly sensitive to risks that originate from economic, physical, social, biologic, and genetic factors along with their lifestyle behaviors. Rarely does one factor act in isolation, as illustrated by the web of causation shown earlier. The interaction of multiple risks results in increasing vulnerability to other factors, which also can negatively impact an individual's health (Sebastian & Bushy, 2000). Trauma, violence, chronic illness, natural disasters, and the possibility of terrorism can all result in increasing vulnerability.

The Homeless

Who are the homeless? There are many definitions used for various reasons. In general, a person is considered to be homeless if he or she lacks a fixed regular address and adequate sleeping arrangements. Homeless people include those whose primary nighttime residence is a supervised publicly or privately operated shelter, an institution that provides a temporary residence (a halfway house), or a public or private place not designated for sleeping (a park bench). This definition addresses those people who are literally homeless (e.g., living under bridges or in shelters), but does not include those who are living with relatives or in substandard housing (Scholler-Jaquish, 2000). Since the 1980s the number of homeless people has surpassed that of the Great Depression (Sebastian and Bushy, 2000). The face of this new homeless population is more varied than the unemployed male who dominated the Great Depression homeless. This new era of homelessness includes women, children, adolescents, whole families, immigrants, substance abusers, the elderly, the chronically and mentally ill, and war veterans. The causes of homelessness are many. Homelessness in the United States leads to major health problems that fall into three basic categories: health problems that contribute to homelessness, health problems that are a consequence of homelessness, and treatment of health problems that are complicated by homelessness (Institute of Medicine, 1988). The vicious cycle of poverty, isolation, and limited access to resources, including health care, contributes to overwhelming stressors for many homeless people. Chronic stressors, physical and sexual abuse, lack of family supports, poverty, domestic violence, street violence, overcrowding, poor hygiene, and poor nutrition often lead to substance abuse, the development of depression, infant mortality, child abuse, poor parenting, and a myriad of other predictable outcomes of poverty, unemployment, poor education, and homelessness.

Undocumented Residents

Many undocumented residents enter the United States through the nation's southern border with Mexico. The majority of these who are workers are men who rarely return to their native country. Because of tougher immigration laws after the September 11, 2001 terrorist attacks, higher travel expenses, and tighter restrictions at border crossings, moving between the United States and Mexico is difficult for migrant workers. This is especially true if they are undocumented. If the workers do leave the United States, they may not be able to return. Undocumented residents rarely present for health care; when they do, depression and substance abuse are common. Medical problems often are untreated until they become acute and complex (National Advisory Council on Migrant Health, 1998). A number of factors, including language barriers, work demands, work environment, and fear related to being undocumented, interfere with timely access to medical care for this population. The difficulties of daily life, with implications for resulting healthcare issues, are illustrated in a variety of opinions expressed by migrant workers presented in **Figure 6-2**.

Health and Health Care
"What we have to do is reeducate our people and let them know that we have many rights to live and work and to educate and to have health care. And without health care, we cannot have the other three."
Unidentified male farm worker, California

Work Conditions
"We're used to working. We don't want to be given things; we just want to be respected and to be paid the salaries."
Teresa, California
"Right now, because I'm here today (testifying at a hearing on work conditions), I may not have my job. Possibly I may not have my job tomorrow."
Jose, California

Housing
"My slogan is, there must be a way to build houses. I believe we have the right to live in a decent way. We are the labor force. It's like we are foreigners—I am a U.S. citizen.
Margarita, California
"The foremen even charged [the farmworkers] for sleeping under the trees."
Teresa, California

Women
". . . Another thing I would like to mention is the way we are treated as women. As women we are discriminated with our coworkers because they see us as insignificant beings. The men think that they are superior."
Maria, California

Children and Youth
". . . [the children] go out to the fields. They lay under the trees and there is a residue falling on the children. They are picking grapes, what happens? The sprayers are there with the residue falling on the children."
Irma, Oregon

Figure 6-2 Workers' comments on migrant life.
Source: Stanhope, M., & Lancaster, S. (2000). *Community & public health nursing* (p. 703). St. Louis: Mosby. Citing Galarneau C. (Ed.). (1993). *Under the weather: Farm worker health.* Austin, TX: National Advisory Council on Migrant Health, Bureau of Primary Health Care, USDHHS.

Undocumented residents are at high risk for suicide, as well. The suicide rate for men is four times that of women (Archives of Internal Medicine, 2000). Other health risks include tuberculosis and other infections due to poor living conditions, diabetes, depression, pesticide exposure, and occupational injuries (National Center for Farmworker Health, 2010).

The undocumented resident may also be among the hidden homeless because once employment ends, housing may become a serious issue. There are a myriad of complex issues to consider when addressing the needs of the illegal resident. These include the needs of families who often accompany the worker to the new location, including housing; sanitation; health care for women, infants, and children; education for children; and work-related injuries or diseases. The infant mortality rate among migrant workers' children is 25 times that of the national average. Deaths from tuberculosis, influenza, and pneumonia are 25% higher than the general population, and the life expectancy for migrant workers is 49 years compared with a national average of 75 years (Sandhaus, 1998). Successful programs have included mobile clinics, convenient time schedules, cultural sensitivity, and bilingual workers (Lundy & Janes, 2001).

Disenfranchised Populations

Disenfranchisement refers to feelings of separation from the mainstream of society (O'Connor, 1994; Sebastian & Bushy, 2000; U.S. DHHS, 1998, 2000). When these feelings occur, the individual or group does not experience an emotional connection with the rest of society. The **disenfranchised population** includes the chronically mentally ill, the homeless, immigrants, refugees, and people with HIV/AIDS. Those who are disenfranchised or **marginalized** may be treated as though they are insignificant; thus, these people begin to believe that this is their status—insignificant. Once they acquire such a belief, the disenfranchised may develop behaviors that further contribute to isolation, a sense of being invisible, and serious healthcare issues.

The Severely Mentally Ill

The severely mentally ill individual is at high risk to join the ranks of the powerless, marginalized, and disenfranchised population. The numbers of homeless individuals residing in public shelters has increased, in part, because some of these individuals do not have the capacity to perform the activities that support independent living. The deinstitutionalization of the mentally ill did not result in the simultaneous development of comprehensive community services in every community; thus, the severely mentally ill person was on his/her own when seeking health care or other related services. Many of these individuals lived in institutions for years and had no idea how to live independently. Deinstitutionalization led to unforeseen increases in homelessness and incarceration. Ineffective means to monitor the mentally ill have led to lack of proper medication, monitoring, and increases in substance abuse (Bachrach, Leona, Lamb, & Richard, 2001).

Women

Millions of people, particularly women, do not have access to the basic resources necessary to achieve a state of health. Although women live longer than men, they are often less healthy. This difference is often related to poverty. Women *represent 70% of the people in the world who live in poverty* (Craft, 1997). In spite of this fact, the issue of gender is often overlooked in the prevention of health problems. The magnitude of intimate partner violence, sexual assault, and sexual harassment contributes to the development of both physical and emotional health problems for women who are victims of these offenses. Unwanted pregnancies as well as limited access to health care result in women being at high risk for developing stress-related conditions and even HIV/AIDS. About 26% of women in the United States are members of racial and ethnic minority groups. The life expectancy for minority women is 76.6 years, whereas the life expectancy for white women is 80.6 years (NCHS, 2006). The problem of women's health was noted in *Healthy People 2010* (DHHS, 2000), which called for a reduction in health disparities between the majority population and special populations in the United States, particularly for people of color (Hamburg, 1998).

Children and Adolescents

Although the number of adults and the elderly living in poverty has decreased in recent times, the number of children living in poverty has significantly increased. Nearly 40% of those living in poverty are younger than 18 years of age, whereas 11% of those living in poverty are older than 65 (DHHS, 1998, 2000). Those living in single-parent families are twice as likely to fall into this group, while African American children represent one third of poor children. Native American children are among the poorest and most likely to live in substandard housing and on reservations (National Center for Health Statistics, 1999; U.S. Bureau of the Census, 1997). Dr. Jocelyn Elders, a former U.S. surgeon general, stated that many of these children were members of the 5-H Club; they are "hungry, homeless, hugless, hopeless and without health care" (Elders, 1997, p. 583). Disadvantaged adolescents are also at significant risk for developing criminal behaviors, dropping out of school, developing substance abuse behaviors, and becoming parents at an early age (National Center for Health Statistics, 1998; National Rural Health Association, 1994, 1998, 1999).

American Indian and Alaska Native Populations

American Indians and Alaska Natives are people having origins in any of the original peoples of North and South America, including Central America, and who maintain tribal affiliation or community attachment. According to the 2000 U.S. Census, those who identify themselves as only American Indians/Alaska Natives constitute 0.9% of the U.S. population, or approximately 2.5 million individuals According to the 2010 U.S. Census, those who identify themselves as only American Indians/Alaska Natives constitutes .9% of the U.S. population or approximately2.7 million individuals. The Census Bureau projects modest growth within the next few decades, exceeding 5 million individuals by the year 2065. The greatest concentrations of these native populations are in the West, Southwest, and Midwest, especially in Alaska, Arizona, Montana, New Mexico, Oklahoma, and South Dakota (U.S. Bureau of the Census, 2010). There are 569 federally recognized tribes and an unknown number of tribes that are not federally recognized. Each tribe has its own culture, beliefs, and practices. American Indians/Alaska Native populations have a unique relationship with the federal government because of historic conflict and subsequent treaties. Federally recognized tribes are entitled to health and educational services provided by the federal government. However, because U.S. Census (U.S. Bureau of the Census, 2000) statistics show that more than half of these people do not reside on a reservation, native populations have limited or no access to Indian Health Services, an organization charged with serving the health needs of these populations. Geographic isolation, economic factors, and suspicion toward traditional spiritual beliefs are some of the reasons why health among native groups is poorer than other groups. Other factors include cultural barriers, poor housing, and poor sewage disposal.

The relationship between **vulnerability** and at-risk behaviors is apparent in reviewing some of the information relating to the 10 leading causes of death of youth among the Native American and Alaska Native populations. According to the Indian Health Services, part of Health and Human Services (2002-2003) suicide rates are 2.5 times higher than the national average and is the second leading cause of death among Native Americans and Alaska Natives ages 15–24. Automobile accidents are the leading cause of death for Native American children. HIV/AIDS was 1.6 times higher in the Native American/ Alaska Native adolescents than for non-Hispanic whites; the death rate from AIDS was 4.9 per 100,000 Native Americans compared to 3.32 for whites. Barriers to care include fewer emergency services, ambulances, and life support services; long distances to hospitals; and inadequate and inconsistent health care through Indian Health Services. Another contributing factor is that health care through Indian Health Services is nontransferable. Additional barriers to care for native populations include lack of prevention education and few disease prevention programs, as well as a lack of understanding and respect for Native American culture. Few, if any, health education programs exist for youth.

This population represents a different type of challenge to the culturally naive forensic practitioner. Values clarification, cultural sensitivity, and an understanding of the history of oppression, discrimination, and exploitation specific to this population are critical if intervention is to be both allowed and effective.

Assessment of vulnerable populations must also include the assessment of grief and loss. The Native American population in particular has lost a great deal, not only in terms of material goods, but also in terms of identity. This may be a prevailing theme among those who are suffering from a variety of losses and for whom identity has been shattered. The forensic nurse can no longer assume that he or she will not be asked to interact with this underserved population It is incumbent on those who are providers of care for Native Americans to develop the knowledge and skills necessary to effectively provide care to those who may present at your facility. The following case study reflects some of the difficulties that may be encountered when providing comprehensive treatment to a Native American teenager.

CASE STUDY 6.1

Eric

Eric, a 16-year-old Native American, comes to the walk-in clinic that you staff. Your clinic is managed by Indian Health Services; however, Eric does not live in an authorized and recognized reservation. He was involved in an altercation the previous evening and presents with bruises and a cut on his arm that would have required sutures if he presented earlier. Steri strips were applied and tetanus toxoid was administered. A 10-day supply of antibiotics was given to the patient, due to concerns that he might not have funds to pay for a prescription. Your assessment includes a psychosocial component and you discover that Eric is very depressed, has been abusing alcohol, and his 15-year-old girlfriend is pregnant.

There are many challenges inherent in this situation that require extensive explora-
tion and collaboration in order to meet this young man's needs. Assessment is one of
the most critical skills that nurses possess. For forensic nurses, the ability to see through
a "forensic lens" enhances completeness and comprehensiveness in order to develop
more accurately a realistic treatment plan. Healthcare providers working within sys-
tems may encounter limited resources and formidable barriers to comprehensive care.

Summary

It is essential that the forensic nurse listen and try to understand the relationships between lifestyle and vulnerability and the resulting, often predictable, health consequences. Understanding requires knowledge of the client's culture, beliefs, and lifestyle without further alienating an already compromised population (Kudzma, 1999; Leninger, 1997). Nurses, particularly forensic nurses, can play an important role as agents of change, both nationally and globally. Effective delivery of care requires culturally appropriate, knowledge-driven, holistic, and humane practices. Influencing the delivery of care to the most needy populations (the vulnerable) can begin to break or interrupt the cycle that imprisons the neediest in the United States and in the rest of the world as well. In addition, the power of legislation to address inequities and gaps in services to the most vulnerable cannot be overlooked. The forensic nurse, with his/her knowledge of statutes and the legal process, could not be in a better position to assist with or develop legislation to meet these needs. He or she can take the lead in breaking the barriers that continue to exist, whether within the system or due to a lack of effective legislation that addresses the issues important to the disenfranchised.

This chapter has focused on identifying and addressing vulnerable and at-risk populations. We have defined vulnerability and discussed the relationship between these terms. If issues contributing to vulnerability are not addressed, inevitably at-risk behaviors will develop in direct relationship to the causes of vulnerability, such as poverty, violence, crime, unemployment, and the lack of education, among other factors. Essential considerations for the forensic nurse include rigorous inquiry regarding personal biases and beliefs. If the nurse believes that people in need exploit the system or take advantage of resources, or if he or she utilizes a "we and them" attitude, the cycle of hopelessness will continue. We must adhere to the forensic nursing standards of practice (American Nurses Association [ANA], 2001), which include assessment, diagnosis, outcome identification, planning, implementation, and evaluation. Professional performance that includes quality of care, performance appraisal, education, collegiality, collaboration, research, and resource utilization is essential. In addition, consistent with collaborative practice are mutual trust and mutual respect for cultural diversity, shared planning, and so forth (ANA).

Florence Nightingale described nursing as an "art that requires as exclusive a devotion and as hard a preparation as any painter's or sculpture's work" (1969/1859, p. 52). This could not be truer than in the practice of forensic nursing in general, and with vulnerable populations in particular. In forensic nursing we have the privilege of utilizing one or more theoretical frameworks that have been developed by nursing professionals. For example, Barbara Dossey's theory of holism (Dossey, Keegan, & Guzzetta, 2000), Betty Neuman's systems model (Neuman & Young, 1972), and Jean Watson's theory of caring (1995) are available as tools and references to guide forensic nursing practice. Promoting a healing and caring environment is essential in all areas of nursing practice, regardless of the behavior that precedes entry into the forensic nursing practice arena; this is especially true with the vulnerable.

During the 21st century, the forensic nurse should be the standard bearer for excellence in nursing practice, as well as an agent for change in the treatment of those who comprise the neediest of populations who present for care.

QUESTIONS FOR DISCUSSION

1. Who are vulnerable populations?
2. What are the health risks specific to selected at-risk groups?
3. What is the role of poverty in increasing the risk of vulnerability?
4. What are the links between various types of vulnerability?
5. What groups are the most vulnerable?
6. How can the forensic nurse influence the resources and treatment of vulnerable populations?

REFERENCES

American Nurses Association. (2001). *Scope and standards of forensic nursing practice.* Washington, DC: American Nurses Publishing.

Archives of Internal Medicine. (2000). *Depression, coronary heart disease and death in males.*

Center for American Progress. (2007). *The poverty epidemic in America by the numbers.* Washington D.C. Author.

Clark, G., & Wright, W. A. (1931). *The Complete Works of William Shakespeare.* New York, NY: Grosset & Dunlap.

Craft, N. (1997). Women's health: A global issue. *British Medical Journal, 315*(7116), 1154.

Dossey, B., Keegan, L., & Guzzetta, C. (2000). *Holistic nursing: A handbook for practice* (3rd ed.). Gaithersburg, MD: Aspen.

Elders, J. (1997). *Health United States.* Washington, DC: U.S. Government Printing Office. As cited in K. Lundy & S. Janes. (2001). *Community health nursing.* Sudbury, MA: Jones and Bartlett.

Flaskerud, J. H., & Winslow, B. J. (1998). Conceptualizing vulnerable populations health related research. *Nursing Research, 47*(2), 69.

Hamburg, M. (1998, July/August). Eliminating racial and ethnic disparities in health: A response to the presidential initiative on race. *Public Health Report, 113,* 372.

Indian Health Service. (2002–2003). Regional differences in Indian health. Washington, D.C.: U.S. Government Printing Office.

Institute of Medicine. (1988). *Homelessness, health and human needs.* Washington, DC: National Academy Press.

Kudzma, E. (1999). Culturally competent drug administration. *American Journal of Nursing, 8,* 46–52.

Leninger, M. (1997). Transcultural nursing research to transform nursing education and practice: 40 years. *Nursing Research, 29*(4), 341–347.

Lundy, K., & Janes, S. (2001). *Community health nursing* (5th ed.). Sudbury, MA: Jones & Bartlett.

National Advisory Council on Migrant Health. (1998, May 13–17). National Farm Workers Health Conference, Houston, TX.

National Center for Farmworker Health, Inc. (2010). *Farmworker health.* Retrieved from http://www.ncfh.org/?pid=4&page=7

National Center for Health Statistics. (1998). *Health United States.* Hyattsville, MD: U.S. Public Health Service.

National Center for Health Statistics. (1999). *Health United States.* Hyattsville, MD: U.S. Public Health Service.

National Coalition for the Homeless. (2007). *Why are people homeless?* Fact sheet No. 1. Washington, DC: Author.

National Rural Health Association. (1994). *A shared vision: Building bridges for rural health access; Conference proceedings.* Kansas City, MO: Author.

National Rural Health Association. (1998). *Bringing resources to bear on the changing care system: Conference proceedings for 2nd annual rural minority health conference.* Kansas City, MO: Author.

National Rural Health Association (1999). *A national guide for rural minority health.* Kansas City, MO: Author.

Neuman, B., & Young, R. S. (1972). A model for teaching total person approach to patient problems. *Nursing Research, 21,* 264–269.

Nightingale, F. (1969/1859). *Notes on nursing: What it is and what it is not.* New York, NY: Dover.

Northham, S. (1996). Access to health promotion, protection and disease prevention among impoverished individuals. *Public Health Nursing, 12*(5), 353.

O'Connor, F. (1994). A vulnerability stress framework for evaluation interventions in schizophrenia. *The Journal of Nursing Scholarship, 26,* 231–237.

Pesznecker, B. (1984). The poor population at risk. *Public Nursing, 4*(1), 237.

Sandhaus, S. (1998). Migrant health: A harvest of poverty. *American Journal of Nursing, 98*(9), 52–54.

Sebastian, J. G., & Bushy, A. (2000). *Special populations in the community.* Gaithersburg, MD: Aspen.

Stanhope, M., & Lancaster, S. (2000). *Community & public health nursing.* St. Louis, MO: Mosby.

U.S. Bureau of the Census. (1997). *Population profile of the United States.* Washington, DC: U.S. Government Printing Office.

U.S. Bureau of the Census. (2000). *Population profile of the United States.* Washington, DC: U.S. Government Printing Office.

U.S. Bureau of the Census. (2010). *Population profile of the United States.* Wasington, DC: U.S. Government Printing Office.

U.S. Department of Health and Human Services. (1998). *Update to the recommendation of the National Advisory Council on Migrant Health.* Austin, TX: National Migrant Resource Program.

U.S. Department of Health and Human Services. (2000). *Healthy people 2010* (Conference ed.). Washington, DC: U.S. Government Printing Office.

U.S. Department of Health and Human Services. (2009). *Healthy people 2020* (Conference ed.). Washington, DC: U.S. Government Printing Office.

Watson, J. (1995). *The philosophy and science of caring* (pp. 9–10). Boulder: Colorado Associated University Press.

World Health Organization. (2002). *World report on violence and health.*

SUGGESTED FURTHER READING

Aday, L. A. (2010). At risk in America: The health and health care needs of vulnerable populations in the United States. New York, NY: John Wiley.

Andrews, M., & Boyle, J. (2008). *Transcultural concepts in nursing care.* Philadelphia, PA: Lippincott Williams & Wilkins.

Burbank, P. M. (2006). *Vulnerable older adults: Health care needs and interventions.* New York, NY: Springer.

De Chesnay, M. (2005). *Caring for the vulnerable: Perspectives in nursing theory, practice, and research.* Sudbury, MA: Jones and Bartlett.

Katz, P. R. (2004). *Vulnerable populations in the long term care continuum.* New York, NY: Springer.

McFarland, M., & Leininger, M. (2006). *Culture care diversity and universality: A worldwide nursing theory.* Sudbury, MA: Jones and Bartlett.

Pender, N. J. (2011). *Health promotion in nursing practice.* Upper Saddle River, NJ: Pearson.

Shi, L., & Stevens, G. D. (2005). *Vulnerable populations in the United States.* Newark, NJ: John Wiley.

Stanhope, M. (2008). *Vulnerable populations.* Philadelphia, PA: Saunders.

CHAPTER 7

Sexual Offenders: Who Are They and Why Do They Commit Sexual Abuse?

David A. D'Amora, Ted Brandhurst, and Randall Wallace

Forensic nurses are critical collaborators in the management of situations involving sexual deviancy. A clear understanding of the dynamics underlying the thinking and behavior of sexual offenders is critical to providing holistic, caring interventions to both current and potential victims and offenders. Without such understanding, preventive measures designed to protect vulnerable populations from becoming victims or offenders cannot be realized. Forensic nurses, armed with an informed basis for understanding the genetic and environmental complexities that come together to result in an act of sexual deviancy, are key players in proposing effective intervention strategies.

CHAPTER FOCUS

» What is Sexual Abuse?
» Informed Consent
» Theories of Sexual Offender Behaviors
» Psychodynamic Model
» Psychosocial Model
» Addiction Theory
» Family Systems Model
» Sociopolitical (feminist) Theory
» Biologic Theory

» Social Learning Theory
» Behavioral Theories
» Cognitive Behavioral Model
» Theory Integration
» Sexual Offense Typologies
» Typology of Rapists
» Crossover
» Etiological Considerations for Adult Sex Offenders

KEY TERMS

» age of consent
» attachment theory
» coercion
» crossover
» differential association
» Electra complex
» informed decision

» modeling
» Oedipal complex
» pedophilia
» role reversal
» sexual abuse
» typology
» volition

What Is Sexual Abuse?

Although the fine points of what constitutes sexually abusive behavior may vary from state to state, country to country, and culture to culture, sexually abusive behavior can be defined as any sexual interaction between person(s) of any age that is perpetrated: (1) against the victim's will; (2) without consent; or (3) in an aggressive, exploitative, manipulative, or threatening manner (Ryan, 1997). Another definition of sexually abusive behavior posited by the National Task Force on Juvenile Sexual Offending (1993) states that such behavior occurs without consent, without equality, or as a result of **coercion**.

Central to any definition of sexually abusive behavior is the concept of consent. Just as the constituents of sexually abusive behavior may be defined differently in various milieus, consent usually is composed of several key elements (see **Table 7-1**).

There must be an understanding of the nature of the sexual act that is proposed (e.g., vaginal, oral, or anal sex, or even sadomasochistic acts). There must also be a knowledge of societal standards for what is proposed (e.g., incest, cultural expectations, and taboos). An awareness of potential consequences and alternatives (e.g., health concerns, pregnancy) must be present. There is an assumption that agreement or disagreement will be respected equally (e.g., one party's right to say, "no" to the sex act at any point). It is a voluntary decision to engage in a particular sex act; there is an assumption that all parties in a consensual sex act are not having sex against their will. The act of **volition** assumes that there is no coercion by alcohol, drugs, intimidation, or force. Mental competence assumes that the individual is capable of making an **informed decision** about engaging in a sexual act. People with severe mental illness or developmental disabilities who may not emotionally or intellectually be able to make informed consent fall into this category.

Finally, age and sexual maturity must be appropriate. The **age of consent** to engage in sexual acts varies widely. In the United States, the age for all consensual sexual acts can range from 16 in Connecticut to 18 in California. There is a further age delineation in a number of states for sexual acts depending on whether they are heterosexual or homosexual. For instance, in the state of New Hampshire the age of consent for heterosexual acts is 16, whereas the age for homosexual consent is 18. In countries such as Mexico, the legal age of consent for heterosexual acts is 12, but for homosexual acts the age is 18. In Saudi Arabia all sexual acts outside of marriage are considered illegal regardless of the age or sex of the persons engaging in them. In countries such as Armenia, the age of consent for heterosexual sex is 16 whereas homosexual acts at any age are illegal.

TABLE 7-1   Elements of Consent

Understanding the nature of the act

Knowledge of societal standards

Awareness of potential consequences

Assumption of respected agreement/disagreement

Mental competence

Age and sexual maturity appropriateness

Theories of Sexual Offending Behaviors

Psychodynamic Theories

Psychodynamic theories describe sexually abusive behavior as a direct reflection of a form of character disorder. Sigmund Freud's psychodynamic theory of the human psyche is divided into three categories (id, ego, and superego) that he believed are in a constant battle in the mind for domination. The ego is the sense of consciousness created by the interaction between the id and the superego; the superego serves as the conscience and modulator of the id; and the id is buried deep in the unconscious mind, with its primitive sexual and atavistic urges operative in each human. According to this theory, a person's mental health is determined by how well he or she reconciles these opposing forces.

Using Freud's model, psychodynamic clinicians suggest that sexual offenders may have very weak consciences (superegos) that allow the overpowering sexual drives (ids) to drive their actions. Initially Freud (1923) discussed reported cases of childhood **sexual abuse** in a lecture to the Society for Psychiatry and Neurology of Vienna in April 1896. His lecture was entitled, *The Seduction Theory.* He abandoned this position the next year after strong resistance from his peers and his personal belief that the many instances of childhood sexual abuse he encountered were more likely to be fabrications of his patients. From this revised stance, Freud initiated his theories of the **Oedipal complex** and **Electra complex** to try to reconcile himself to the times and cultural expectations of Victorian Austria. His development of an elaborate schema of defense mechanisms and complexes looked at sexual abuse of children in a context of intra psyche as opposed to extra psyche modes. Freud also expanded the idea of the unconscious (those mental processes that are buried deep within the mind and accessible only through psychoanalysis) and described numerous defense mechanisms to protect the ego.

The defense mechanisms delineated by Freud are still used to explain behavior in clinical circles. These are mechanisms of denial (this is not really happening, it doesn't really exist), displacement (this is happening outside of me, someone else is responsible), and projection (uncomfortable feelings are placed upon someone else).

The psychodynamic model places great emphasis on the mother–son relationship, suggesting that the mother–son relationship is qualitatively different in sexual offenders than in nonoffenders. The seductive mother is one who, though she does not have a sexual relationship with her son, treats him as her spouse or lover. The conflict that arises in the son from this type of mothering can lead him into sexual deviancy later in life due to a variety of feelings of anxiety and inadequacy, both sexual and interpersonal, that interact with aggression directed at the victim as a substitute object for the mother, thus producing a sexual assault.

Psychodynamic theories have been influential with respect to discourse on sexual offending, but not with respect to treatment or prevention due to a lack of empirical support.

Psychosocial Model

Finkelhor (1984) proposes a psychosocial model of child sexual abuse. This model proposes primary factors occurring as *preconditions* (see **Table 7-2**). Finkelhor maintains that four conditions must be present before child sexual abuse can occur:

TABLE 7-2 Finkelhor's Preconditions for Sexual Abuse

Motivation

Overcoming internal inhibition

Overcoming external impediments

Undermining or overcoming a child's resistance

1. There must be *motivation* for the offender to abuse from some internal reason, such as projecting emotional needs onto the child victim or the perpetrator's deprivation of sexual gratification.
2. *Internal inhibitions* are not present or are diminished through the use of alcohol or drugs, by stress, by rationalizations, through the lowering of societal sexual taboos, through subculture norms, or by mental disorders.
3. *External inhibitions* must be lacking or weakened. Examples can involve poor parental/caretaker supervision, isolation, or overcrowding.
4. The *child's resistance* must be overcome. The offender may accomplish this by trickery or manipulation, by using a child's emotional instability, or by garnering the trust of the child. Threats, physical power, and authority roles also can be part of the process to undermine a victim's resistance to sexual abuse (Jackson, Karlson, & Tzeng, 1991).

Addictions Theory

In addictions theory, the origins of sexual deviancy are found in dysfunctional family patterns and have many similarities with chemical dependency and gambling behaviors. Patrick Carnes, PhD, defines sexual addiction as a process where "the addict substitutes a sick relationship to an event or process for a healthy relationship" (2001, p. 4). He goes on to state,

> Sexual addiction can be understood by comparing it to other types of addictions. Individuals addicted to alcohol or other drugs, for example, develop a relationship with their "chemical(s) of choice"—a relationship that takes precedence over any and all other aspects of their lives. Chemically addicted individuals find that they need drugs merely to feel normal. (Carnes,, p. 14)

In sexual addiction, a parallel situation exists. Sex—like food or drugs in other addictions—provides the high, and addicts become dependent on this sexual high to feel normal. They substitute unhealthy relationships for healthy ones. They choose temporary pleasure rather than the deeper qualities of normal intimate relationships. Sexual addiction follows the same progressive nature of other addictions. Sexual addicts struggle to control their behaviors, and experience despair over their constant failure to do so. Their loss of self-esteem grows, fueling the need to escape even further into their addictive behaviors. A sense of powerlessness pervades the lives of addicts (Carnes, 2001).

Carnes (2001) has developed an addictive systems model of sexual deviancy that defines sexual deviancy as the result of messages that the individuals tell themselves and how these are acted upon. This model posits the idea of *core beliefs, which are derived* from the person's experiences in life. According to Carnes (pp. 112–115), the common core beliefs of the sexual addict are:

» I am basically a bad, unworthy person.
» No one would love me as I am.
» My needs aren't going to be met if I have to depend on others.
» Sex is my most important need.

The sexual addict takes these core beliefs and reshapes them into distorted thinking patterns. Some of the distorted thoughts often seen in sex offenders may be:

» Since I can't get sex through regular means, I'll make people have sex with me.
» She really wanted me and really didn't mean it when she said, "no."
» She got me to have sex with her because she needed a man.
» She's just too uptight about sex and has sexual hang-ups.

Distortions such as those listed can provide justification for an offender's deviant sexual behavior (Carnes, 2001, p. 17).

Carnes's addiction cycle has four components:

1. *Preoccupation:* This is characterized by obsessive/compulsive sexual thoughts and fantasies.
2. *Ritualization:* To further sexual stimulation, the sexual addict will often engage in rituals that lead up to sexually acting out, such as cruising, using sexual toys, or wearing women's undergarments to heighten the sexual experience.
3. *Compulsivity:* This is the level at which preoccupation and ritualization become unmanageable and the sexual addict commits a deviant sexual act.
4. *Despair:* At this stage guilt, regret, or hopelessness sets in (Carnes, 2001, pp. 19–20).

As the addictive cycle continues, the sexual addict becomes more and more out of control. His or her obsession with deviant sex may take a toll on his or her family as more and more of his or her time is devoted to deviant addiction. He or she may lose his or her job because of time spent cruising for sex partners or an ever-deepening interest in pornography and strip clubs. The addictive cycle feeds on itself and the sex addict continues a downward spiral. Carnes (2001) states that the sexual addict will go through three stages of this downward spiral if not treated. The first stage is marked by compulsive masturbation, promiscuity, pornography, and use of prostitutes. The second stage is punctuated by exhibitionism, voyeurism, and indecent phone calls. The third and most problematic stage may include child molestation, incest, or rape. Although there is a strong element of compulsivity in many sex offenders' behaviors, most researchers and clinicians in the field of sex abuse treatment and research do not find the global explanations of addictions theory applicable to the adjudicated sex offender.

Family Systems Model

In addition to the sexual addiction system, Carnes (2001) has adapted the circumplex marital and family systems model (Olson, 1989) to describe the effects of family on sexually abusive persons. Olson and Craddock (1980) contend that 16 types of families can be described by their relative positions on two intersecting continua. The first continuum concerns dependency issues and has the extremes of chaotic *family structure* and *rigid family* structure. The second continuum deals with intimacy issues, with the extremes being a disengaged family structure and an enmeshed family structure.

The chaotic family system can be described as having no accountability for sexual behavior, discrepancies between values and behavior, parental sexual unmanageability and inconsistencies, and consequences. Frequently, **role reversals** around sexual behavior are apparent. The chaotic family system does not have any clearly defined rules or expectations and the children often are dealt with as though they are authoritatively equal with the parents. Moralistic black and white standards, extreme efforts to control child sexual behavior, punishment for sexual behavior, and unreachable expectations about sexuality are common elements in the rigid family system. As a result of the extreme structure and high expectations, the child is unable to develop his or her own system of self-regulation. The child may respond to the authoritarian parent through rebellious direct acting out behavior.

On the other continuum, the disengaged family structure can be described as having elements of abandonment, having tension and distance around sexual matters, lacking in physical or sexual closeness, and evading sexual issues. The disengaged system views sex as something to be discovered by the individual and not to be discussed. The child in the disengaged family is likely to feel alone and without support.

The opposite of the disengaged family system is the enmeshed family structure. In this family system, a lack of boundaries is evident. The enmeshed family can also be described as having anxiety about a family member's sexual behavior reflecting on the family, secrecy preserved at all costs from outsiders, covert and overt sexual abuse, and limited sexual privacy. Children in the enmeshed system do not develop a self-identity. They tend to develop a communal identity with few boundaries drawn clearly. According to Carnes (2001), most sexual addicts come from chaotically enmeshed families.

Sociopolitical (or Feminist) Theories

Sociopolitical theorists view rape as a pseudosexual act that is predominantly motivated by male sociopolitical dominance. Sex role stereotypical beliefs, adversarial sexual beliefs, and acceptance of interpersonal violence are critical factors. Women and children in such environments are seen as property or as an extension of the male to do with as he chooses. There is a growing body of research that indicates acceptance of rape myths and the mythology of machismo contribute greatly to rape behavior. Interpersonal violence is a critical factor.

Biologic Theories

Biologic theories posit that genetic, hormonal, chromosomal, or neurologic causes create sexual violence. Sociobiologic theory in particular suggests that males in general have learned throughout time to become more aggressive and dominant toward women in particular. This would be due to successful reproduction and passing on the male's genetic material. The more aggressive males continued to pass on those genes while at the same time learning from prior generations. Prehistoric women were monogamous by nature—they needed men to assist them during and after childbirth. Without the assistance of men, the mortality rate for women and children would be substantially higher. The more sexually aggressive males mated much more frequently than passive males, and therefore those genes kept evolving. In many respects the human sexual drive and behavior is very similar to that of other mammals. Though our brains have advanced throughout time, our inherent drive to reproduce has not. This theory is put forward as a way to partially account for rape, but fails to address child molestation. Supporters of this theory point to the fact that males commit most sexual crimes. However, there is little research to support these premises, and such a theory does not account for an individual's control over cognitive processes.

The biomedical model suggests that sexual offenders produce more testosterone than nonoffenders and is similar to the sociobiologic theory. Sexual deviancy is viewed as a response to overproduction of testosterone in the testes. The removal of the testes either surgically or chemically reduces or eliminates testosterone. Numerous studies suggest significant reductions in recidivism rates in those who have been castrated. There is a possibility that some type of genetic, hormonal, chromosomal, or neurologic process is responsible for sexually aberrant behavior.

Social Learning Theory

Social learning theory looks at the concepts of **differential association**, reinforcement, and modeling. It suggests that an offender has somehow learned the sexual deviancy from his or her environment. This theory also incorporates **modeling**, the idea that the offender learned the behavior from watching someone else behave in a similar fashion, or even by his or her own sexual abuse. Studies have suggested that a number of offenders have been sexually abused themselves in the past, and proponents of this theory view that fact as credible evidence to support this theory. However, there are many sexual offenders who report they have never been sexually abused and never witnessed sexual abuse in the past. Many offenders do appear to be continually learning and advancing in their sexual deviancy. They learn how to obtain victims more effectively, learn how far they can go, learn what deviant sexual behaviors arouse them, and learn how to avoid or escape detection.

There are a number of subtheories, including the dynamics of posttraumatic stress disorder, **attachment theory**, and so forth. Many sex offenders, both adult and juvenile, appear to share the same symptomology, including low self-esteem, poor self-perception, depression, isolation from their peers, and difficulty achieving and maintaining intimate relationships. Social cognitive research results suggest that rapists misinterpret the interpersonal cues from women (e.g., negative mood) and overperceive hostility and seductiveness (e.g., friendliness versus seductiveness). Rapists may hold greater adversarial beliefs leading to the belief that women accept and even enjoy male domination.

Behavioral Theories

Behavioral theories suggest that sexual deviance results from classical conditioning, possibly from either sexual assault or covert seduction during childhood, or negative modeling. An example of classical behavioral theory would be the experiment of Pavlov and his dog. Pavlov paired the introduction of meat powder with the ringing of a bell. Soon, just the ringing of the bell was enough to get the animal to salivate. However, these theories do not explain the cognitive progression necessary to behave inappropriately, and human beings have a significantly more complex thinking process than animals.

Cognitive-Behavioral Theories

The proponents of the cognitive-behavioral model state that for a sexual assault to occur, the offender must go through a progression of cognitive distortions and behavioral

TABLE 7-3 Cognitive Progression of Criminal Thinking

The idea to commit the sexual assault.

The distorted view that most of society is unjust and uncaring and that he or she is a victim and this is an unjust system.

Justifications, excuses, rationalizations, and distortions give the permission to commit the offense.

Fantasies about irresponsible use of power over weaker persons for pleasure.

The plan to successfully commit the offense.

The belief that the sexual offense can be accomplished without repercussions and the consequences resulting from this belief.

The immediate decision to commit the offense when the first six steps have been accomplished.

---

stages that involve the accumulation of unique behaviors and characteristics and must be defended internally or externally by the offender. According to Nichols and Molinder (1984), a cognitive progression of criminal thinking occurs even before the sexual offense is committed (see **Table 7-3**).

This cognitive progression may take a matter of a few days or several years to develop. Closely related to the cognitive progression is a behavioral progression (Nichols & Molinder, 1984), during which the offender hunts for his or her victim(s). This hunt may include cruising, stalking, or manipulating a situation. The second stage of the behavioral progression is the offender's playing with the victim. This playing may include any behavior that intensifies the sexual experience for the offender such as verbal abuse, winning a child over with gifts, or playing out a role with the potential victim. The last stage of the behavioral progression is the actual sexual assault, which may also expose the victim to direct physical assault.

Sexually deviant individuals must defend their deviancies in order for the deviancies to be maintained (Nichols & Molinder, 1984). This defending usually takes some combination of forms: (1) deception through dishonesty, (2) deception through distortion, and (3) deception through denial. In deception through dishonesty, the offender attempts to manipulate the truth through a system of omissions of details and additions to the truth. Deception through distortion occurs when the perpetrator attempts to defend his or her behavior by utilizing cognitive distortions and justifications such as "He/she came onto me for sex," "We had a true romance that no one understands," "I was just taking his temperature with an anal thermometer because I thought he had a fever," "She/he had sex before me." Deception through denial occurs when the offender admits to others his or her guilt but attempts to deceive him- or herself about being aroused by sexually deviant desires.

Cognitive-behavior theories explore how thoughts create or mitigate actions. Offenders set up negative emotional states through negative thinking; to relieve the negative mood states, they preoccupy themselves with deviant sexual fantasies. The deviant behaviors are then justified, rationalized, or explained away.

The cognitive-behavior theories suggest that irrational beliefs and cognitive distortions help to initiate sexual deviancy. Soon after this initial step, the offender becomes conditioned to negative sexual stimuli, with orgasm being the reinforcement. These constructs combined (cognitive/behavioral) create persistent patterns on how the offender behaves as well as views the world. The secrecy, among other constructs, soon becomes part of the conditioned response and perpetuates the deviancy. Learning theory is also a significant component of this approach. Children who are sexually abused learn sex through inappropriate means, and if exposed enough, children may internalize this learned behavior. Male sex offenders do appear to view the world differently than normal men—they perceive women, children, sex, and arousal qualitatively differently. When this occurs after a long period of time, the offender begins to behave accordingly. Many times the male or female sexual offender suffers from chronic low-grade depression, has very low self-esteem, has been ridiculed his or her entire life, and so forth. These traits tend to distort the offender's view of the world, and the molester may find comfort and acceptance in the children he or she so desires. Immaturity is a trademark of the child molester. This appears to occur due to the fact that he or she has not advanced emotionally since adolescence.

Toward Theory Integration

A significant number of commonalities are shared by many adult sex offenders, including early life damage to the ability to develop affectional and/or attachment bonds, negative models of behavior, and/or actual abuse. Further, data suggest that supports for sexually abusive behavior through sex role stereotyping and cultural supports for violence play a role in the creation of sexually abusing behavior. Add to this inappropriate and/or deviant coping mechanisms that develop with accompanying cognitive distortions to normalize the behavior in sex offenders' minds, and you have a recipe for sexually abusive behavior. One of the most current integrated or multifactorial theories was developed by Ward and Hudson (1998). They state that every sexual offense has both distal, or historical, factors and proximal, or recent, factors. Additionally, they state that every sexual offense involves the following five factors:

1. Intimacy deficits
2. Deviant sexual scripts
3. Emotional dysregulation
4. Antisocial cognitions
5. Multiple dysfunctional pathways to the offense

Sexual Offense Typologies

Typologies categorize offenders into distinct and understandable groups or subtypes. Ideally they provide guidance regarding distinct and specific treatment needs and interventions; however, they can limit our thinking, lead to pigeonholing, and inadvertently lead to overlooking individual needs. Some examples of noteworthy typologies include those in the following sections.

Child Molester and Rapist Typology

The first typology for adult male sex offenders was developed by Dr. Nicholas Groth in 1979; the second, known as the FBI typology (developed by Kenneth Lanning), is based upon Dr. Groth's work; and the third (the Knight-Prentky typology) takes Dr. Groth's work and validates the different types statistically. The Groth typology breaks down adult male sex offenders into two categories—the child molester and the rape offender.

Child Molester

Child molesters often utilize persuasion and/or manipulation to perpetrate the sexual abuse. They typically begin their involvement with children by using grooming behavior. Grooming behavior is intended to make the victim or potential victim or victim's guardians feel comfortable with the molester and even interested in interacting with him. In addition, the molester often convinces himself that the child wants to be involved in a sexual relationship with him and that his involvement with the child will meet his adult emotional needs. The molester is usually not interested in hurting the child and wants the child to enjoy the experience. The molester often projects thoughts and feelings he wants the child to have about him onto the child. He interprets the child's positive responses to the grooming and manipulation as acceptance of his behavior and convinces himself that the abusive behavior is not hurtful or damaging.

According to the Groth typology, there are two different types of child molesters, fixated/pedophile and regressed/situational. **Pedophilia** is a clinical diagnosis that appears in the *Diagnostic and Statistical Manual of Mental Disorders*, 4th edition (DSM-IV). A diagnosis of pedophilia is made when an individual who is over the age of 16 has a primary or overarching sexual attraction to prepubescent children. An individual does not have to act on his primary or overarching sexual attraction to prepubescent children in order to be diagnosed as a pedophile. It may be helpful to think of this type of child molester as a fixated child molester. In fact, there may be times when someone is considered to be a fixated molester even though he may not fully meet the complex DSM-IV criteria.

When we describe people as fixated child molesters, we are describing men who have a primary or overarching sexual attraction to children. These offenders often see their attractions as permanent and report that they have had them for as long as they can remember. Often the interests began when the offenders reached puberty. More often than not, the victims of fixated molesters are young males (however, there are fixated molesters who abuse both males and females, and those who abuse only females). A fixated child molester's offenses tend to be planned and carefully carried out over a period of time. In other words, these offenders do not act impulsively or without forethought. Fixated child molesters engage in a variety of sexually abusive activities with children. Typically, however, the activities do not include intercourse or penetration. Fondling, masturbation, and other kinds of sexual stimulation are the most typical behaviors exhibited by fixated molesters. They focus on sexually stimulating both their victims and themselves; they view their behavior as a way to meet their own emotional and social needs. Fixated child molesters usually perpetrate their abuse without using alcohol or other mood-altering substances.

According to the Groth typology, the second type of child molester is known as a regressed (or situational) child molester. His primary sexual attraction is to adult females. That is, if you asked him the question about the ideal sexual partner, he would more than likely describe an age-appropriate female. The regressed or situational offender's sexual involvement with children often develops as a result of responses to external stress and situational difficulties that they experience. In other words, these molesters usually turn to children as a way to cope with the stress they are dealing with in their lives—as a way to feel better about their situations and themselves. Unlike fixated child molesters, regressed molesters may go for months or even years without molesting, depending on their ability to deal with stressors in their lives. In many instances, these individuals replace the conflicted and problematic relationships they are having with adult women by becoming sexually involved with children. They place pseudoadult status on their victims and then view them as they would their peers.

Unlike the victims of fixated molesters, the victims of regressed/situational molesters are usually female. Most, though not all, incest offenders fit the description of regressed/ situational molesters. In general, regressed/situational molesters' victims may be a little older than those of the fixated molester. In addition, although the sexually abusive behavior may begin prior to the time when the victim enters puberty, it may continue after the victim enters puberty. Also, and unlike the fixated molester, the regressed molester typically is involved in consensual, age-appropriate sexual behavior, or has been at some point in his life. A fixated molester's attention is overwhelmingly focused upon the arousal of the child. A regressed/situational molester's focus is primarily upon his own arousal and release. Regressed/situational molesters are also more likely to use alcohol or other illicit drugs as a part of their offense pattern.

Rapist

Rape is a violent act, but also a sexual act, and it is this fact that differentiates it from other crimes. Further, it is illogical to argue, on the one hand, that rape is an extension of normative male sexual behavior and, on the other hand, that rape is not sexual.

> . . . [R]ape is not less sexual for being violent, nor is it necessarily true that the violent aspect of rape distinguishes it from legally "acceptable" intercourse. . . . It is unfortunate that the rather swift public acceptance of the "rape as violence" model, even among groups who otherwise discount feminist arguments, has unintended implications. . . . [E]mphasizing violence—the victim's experience—is . . . strategic to the continued avoidance of an association between "normal" men and sexual violence. Make no mistake, for some men, rape is sex—in fact, for them, sex is rape. The continued rejection of this possibility, threatening though it may be, is counterproductive to understanding the social causes of sexual violence (Scully, 1990).

The other major form of sexual assault behavior is rape, in which the victims are usually, *though not exclusively*, postpubescent. Rape is associated with very aggressive, though not necessarily physically violent, behavior on the part of the perpetrator. He attacks, threatens, and uses hostility and/or physical force to intimidate and overpower his victim. Although this type of offender may use physical force, he may also use threats and intimidation as a method of forcing his victim into sexual activity. It is important to understand this because, as we discussed earlier in our discussion of victims, rape behavior often does not result in physical injury. When an individual commits rape, he is interested in overpowering and possessing complete control and dominance over his victim. Victims are often viewed by the rapists as weak and easily dominated. Rapists do not care about the emotions of their victims (as some child molesters do), and their primary interests are self-gratification, dominance, and control. Another difference between child molesters and rapists is that some rapists will victimize an individual once, then move on to others, which is much less likely with child molesters. Finally, rapists engage in penetration or specific sexual acts with their victims, as opposed to the high incidence of fondling that is commonly associated with child molestation.

Groth (1979) identified the following three different kinds of rapists in his typology:

1. Anger rapists
2. Power rapists
3. Sadistic rapists

Anger rapists, as one would assume, are very angry men. Although they may be angry at women in general, or may react angrily to specific behavior of their victim, they are more often angry about a variety of issues in their lives. They cannot and will not face the difficult issues in their lives directly and in a prosocial manner. Anger rapists tend to use a significant amount of physical force when they subdue their victims—in most cases, far more force than is necessary to perpetrate the abuse. This often leaves victims severely battered and bruised on various areas of their bodies. Anger rapists also tend to be verbally abusive during their assaults, which are short in duration and very explosive in nature.

Anger rapists tend not to plan their specific offenses. Rather, they act impulsively to take advantage of situations that have presented themselves. Victim choice depends solely upon whom anger rapists see as vulnerable and available at the moment they decide they want to offend. Between 25% and 40% of known rapes are committed by men who are considered anger rapists.

The second type of rapist in the Groth typology is the power rapist. Power rapists—like anger rapists—use sexual assault as a way to feel powerful and in control. They do not, however, discharge anger during their offenses and they only use the physical force necessary to perpetrate the offense. If power rapists can gain control through threat and psychological coercion (rather than physical intimidation) they will do so. As a result, the physical injuries usually associated with anger rapists are less common with power rapists. Power rapists tend to make demands and give orders to their victims. They are not, however, as verbally hostile as anger rapists. The offenses themselves may last over a longer period of time than those committed by anger rapists, and they may be repetitive in nature. Domestic violence offenders who commit sexual assaults against their partners are often power rapists.

Like anger rapists, power rapists often look for potential victims who seem vulnerable. Unlike anger rapists, however, they consider how much intimidation and force are necessary to gain control. Their preference is to attack potential victims who are both physically vulnerable and relatively easy to intimidate. Power rapists usually plan their offenses and may fantasize about how they are going to look and feel.

Both anger and power rapists may have weapons available when they commit their offenses. Anger rapists are more likely to use them to hurt their victims, while power rapists are more likely to use weapons to threaten their victims and thereby decrease the need to physically overpower them. Between 60% and 70% of known rape offenders fit into the power rapist category.

Sadistic rapists are individuals who eroticize power, anger, or violence. Sadistic rapists engage in very compulsive, sometimes very ritualized sexual assault behavior. Because they have an erotic response to power and control, extreme violence and torture often characterize their assaults. In many cases, victims of sadistic rapists are murdered during the assaults. Unlike all of the other types of sex offenders in Dr. Groth's typology, sadistic rapists often have very significant psychiatric difficulties that may have a direct relationship to the offense behavior. It is fortunate, given the high degree of violence and significant likelihood of victim death, that there are relatively few known sadistic rapists. Estimates are that approximately 2–5% of all rapists are sadistic in nature. It is also fortunate that once apprehended, sadistic rapists are usually removed from the community for many, many years, or life.

Clinicians do not know how to treat sadistic rapists. Nothing that the treatment community has tried with this population has reduced the likelihood that they will offend again.

In addition, if they are not apprehended, they are more likely than child molesters or other types of rapists to continue their brutal assaults.

Noncontact Offenders

The Groth typology does not include perpetrators of noncontact forms of sexual abuse, such as voyeurs and exhibitionists. These types of offenders are important to keep in mind, as their recidivism rates are very high, and many noncontact offenders have perpetrated, or go on to perpetrate, more serious contact types of offenses. This information reminds us that there is no one-size-fits-all response to sex offenders, and it gives us insight into how to use the information we get from and about individual offenders, in determining the best way to supervise them.

Knight and Prentky Typology

Knight (1988) and Prentky, Knight, Rosenberg, and Lee (1989) have proposed one of the most comprehensive and most validated taxonomic systems to date. This model proposes six types of molesters (interpersonal, narcissistic, exploitative, muted, sadistic, and nonsadistic aggressive) and four types of rapists (compensatory, exploitative, displaced anger, and sadistic) based upon the degree of physical injury incurred by the victim and the meaning of the motivation of the offender. This rape typology further defines nine types that come from four basic categories (opportunistic, pervasively angry, sexual, and vindictive).

Types include the overtly sexual, sadistic, antisocial person who plans the offense; the covert sadist with little antisocial history who plans the offense; the individual who rapes for sexual gratification, has little sadism and high social competence, and engages in offense planning; the individual who rapes for sexual gratification, has little sadism and low social competence, and engages in planning; the vindictive type who focuses anger on women and has low social competence; and another vindictive type, as the previous type, but with high social competence. In categorizing child molesters, Knight (1988) determined the following dimensions to be significant: the amount of contact with children, the meaning of contact, and the amount of physical damage of aggression. Both interpersonal molesters and narcissistic molesters desire high levels of contact with children. Interpersonal molesters are described as wanting interpersonal contact with others' children for a caring relationship that becomes sexual. Narcissistic molesters appear to be primarily concerned with personal sexual gratification and seek out children for this purpose. For the remaining four types of molesters, the primary distinction is in the amount of permanent damage done and the motivation for the aggression (Knight). Exploitative and muted sadistic molesters usually do not do much physical damage to victims. Nonsadistic aggressive and sadistic molesters usually do significant damage to their victims.

Prentky and colleagues (1989) have placed rapists into four categories based on two dimensions. The first dimension is the degree of physical injury incurred by the victim. The second dimension is the meaning of the aggressive motivation intended by the offender at the time of the victimizing event. In category one, the compensatory offender is attempting to make up for his or her inadequacies and typically uses a minimal amount of violence. The exploitative offender also uses a minimal amount of violence and is seeking sexual gratification; he or she is using the victim as a sexual object. With the displaced anger offender, the motivation is to release pent-up anger. The displaced anger offender may use a range of violence from almost no violence to a violent outburst to release this anger. The sadistic offender is seeking to hurt for the sake of hurting the victim. The sadistic molester causes extreme physical or psychological harm to the victim.

The muted sadistic offender has more control than the sadistic offender and usually uses humiliation and degradation rather than physical damage to the victim.

Crossover

Most offenders have some preference for a particular victim or type of behavior. This might lead one to believe that an offender would be less of a danger to those potential victims who do not match his or her preference. Research has demonstrated, however, that although **crossover** rates vary among different populations of sex offenders, a significant percentage of offenders engage in more than one type of abuse. In 1987, Abel and colleagues examined crossover behavior in sex offenders and found that nearly 50% of the subjects in the study had engaged in multiple sex-offending behaviors. Another study conducted in 1998 (Ahlmeyer, English, & Simmons, 1999) reports significant crossover with respect to the gender and age of victims. This research has significant implications regarding the need to restrict access to a very wide range of potential victims (all ages, both genders, etc.) when a sex offender is placed under community supervision.

Etiological Considerations for Adult Sexual Offenders

Table 7-4 identifies factors that are considered to play an etiological role in the development of sexual offenders. However, none of these factors is correlated strongly enough such that the existence of that factor would indicate increased risk.

Summary

Sexual offenders hurt others through their behavior, have ongoing empathy deficits, have deficits in emotional expression, have cognitive distortions/thinking errors that make it easier to behave in an abusive fashion, commit more offenses than those for which they are apprehended, and are a heterogeneous group with a need for a variety of interventions. They do not all commit their offense for the same reasons or to try to meet the same

TABLE 7-4   Etiological Factors Contributing to the Evolution of the Sexual Offender

Exposure to violence, aggressive role models	Social competency deficits
Cultural/societal influences	Empathy deficits
Substance abuse	Emotional regulation difficulties
Esteem deficits	Coping skills deficits
Psychopathy	Sexual victimization
Abuse-supportive attitudes	Etiological considerations for juvenile sexual abusers
Attachment difficulties	
Intimacy deficits	Child maltreatment
Physiological/hormonal factors	Exposure to pornography
Deviant sexual arousal	Poor impulse control

types of needs. They pose varying degrees of risk and dangerousness and have widely varied rates of recidivism, although the overall average recidivism rate tends to remain below 20%.

QUESTIONS FOR DISCUSSION

1. What criteria determine an instance of sexual abuse?
2. Discuss the most significant elements of the concept of informed consent.
3. How can knowledge of the dynamics of sexual abuse be used to propose strategies aimed at prevention?
4. Who are the most vulnerable potential victims/offenders in the case of sexual abuse?
5. Propose some measures that might be useful in the prevention of sexual abuse.
6. Describe the role of the forensic nurse in relation to the current management of sexual abuse.
7. Discuss the potential for collaboration between forensic nurses, other healthcare professionals, and the criminal justice system in the management of sexual abuse.

REFERENCES

Abel, G. G., Becker, J. V., Cunningham-Rathner, J., Mittlemann, M., Murphy, W. D., & Rouleau, J. L. (1987). Multiple paraphilic diagnoses among sex offenders. *Bulletin of the American Academy of Psychiatry and the Law, 16,* 153–168.

Ahlmeyer, S., English, K., & Simmons, D. (1999). *The impact of polygraphy on admissions of crossover offending behavior in adult sexual offenders.* Presentation at the Association for the Treatment of Sexual Abusers 18th Annual Research and Treatment Conference, Lake Buena Vista, FL.

Carnes, P. (2001). *Out of the shadows: Understanding sexual addiction.* Center City, MN: Hazelden.

Finkelhor, D. (1984). *Child sexual abuse.* New York, NY: The Free Press.

Freud, S. (1923). *The ego and the id.* London, England: Hogarth Press.

Groth, A. N. (1979). *Men who rape: The psychology of the offender.* New York, NY: Plenum Press.

Jackson, J. W., Karlson, H. C., & Tzeng, O. C. S. (1991). *Theories of child abuse and neglect: Differential perspectives, summaries, and evaluations.* New York, NY: Praeger Publishers and U.S. Department of Health.

Knight, R. A. (1988). A taxonomic analysis of child molesters. In R. A. Prentky & V. L. Quinsey (Eds.), *Human sexual aggression: Current perspectives* (pp. 2–20). New York, NY: New York Academy of Sciences.

National Task Force on Juvenile Sexual Offending. (1993). *Final report.* Denver: University of Colorado Health Sciences Center.

Nichols, H. R., & Molinder, L. (1984). *Multiphasic sex inventory.* Tacoma, WA: Author.

Olson, D. H. (1989). *Circumplex model of family systems VIII: Family assessment and intervention.* In D. H. Olson, C. S. Russell, & D. H. Sprenkle (Eds.), *Circumplex model: Systemic assessment and treatment of families* (pp. 7–26). New York, NY: Haworth Press.

Olson, D. H., & Craddock, A. E. (1980). Circumplex model of marital and family systems: Application to Australian families. *Australian Journal of Sex, Marriage and Family 1,* 53–69.

Prentky, R. A., Knight, R. A., Rosenberg, R., & Lee, A. (1989). A path analytic approach to the validation of a taxonomic system for classifying child molesters. *Journal of Quantitative Criminology, 6,* 231–257.

Ryan, G. (1997). *Juvenile sexual offending: Causes, consequences and correction.* New York, NY: John Wiley and Sons.

Scully, D. (1990). *Understanding sexual violence* (pp. 142–143). New York, NY: Routledge.

Ward, T., & Hudson, S. M. (1998). The construction and development of theory in the sexual offending area: A metatheoretical framework. *Sexual Abuse: Journal of Research and Treatment, 10,* 47–63.

SUGGESTED FURTHER READING

Levenson, J. S., Becker, J., & Morin, J. W. (2008). The relationship between victim age and gender crossover among sex offenders. *Sex Abuse, 1,* 43–60.

Levenson, J. S., D'Amora, D. A., & Hern, A. L. (2007). Megan's law and its impact on community re-entry for sex offenders. *Behavioral Science Law, 25*(4), 587–602.

Palermo, G. B. (2007). The mind of the sexual predator. *Current Opinions in Psychiatry, 5,* 497–500.

Patrick, C. (2007). *Handbook of psychopathy.* New York, NY: Guilford.

Ramsey-Klawsnik, H., Teaster, P. B., Mendiondo, M. S., Marcum, J. L., & Abner, E. L. (2008). Sexual predators who target elders: Findings from the first national study of sexual abuse in care facilities. *Journal of Elder Abuse and Neglect, 20*(4), 353–376.

Rogers, R., & Jackson, R. L. (2005). Sexually violent predators: The risky enterprise of risk assessment. *Journal of the American Academy of Psychiatry Law, 33*(4), 523–527.

Wolak, J., Finkelhor, D., Mitchell, K. J., & Ybarra, M. L. (2008). Online "predators" and their victims: Myths, realities, and implications for prevention and treatment. *American Psychologist, 63*(2), 111–128.

CHAPTER 8

Forensic Implications of Intimate Partner Violence

Daniel J. Sheridan, Catherine R. Nash, Shadonna L. Hawkins, Jennifer L. Makely, and Jacquelyn C. Campbell

Intimate partner violence has become one of the primary areas of interest for forensic nursing. Early screening, identification, and treatment of intimate partner violence patients can help break often serious and deadly cycles of violence. The scope of practice in the area of intimate partner violence has also grown with awareness of the many aspects of this problem. The forensic nurse who works with victims of domestic violence must be well equipped to recognize and document any injuries. In addition, the forensic nurse must maintain appropriate relationships with representatives of various community services to best serve the needs of this population.

CHAPTER FOCUS

» Development of Hospital-based Domestic Violence Programs
» Screening Tools for Domestic Violence

» Identifying Injuries and Wounds
» Written Documentation
» Photographic Documentation

KEY TERMS

» abrasions
» abuse
» avulsions
» contusions
» cuts/incisions
» domestic violence
» ecchymosis

» laceration
» partner violence screen
» pattern of injury
» patterned injuries
» petechiae
» strangulation

Development of Hospital-Based Domestic Violence Programs

In the late 1970s and early 1980s, nurses conducted some of the earliest and now classic research that identified battering against women by intimate partners as a major health problem and a public health problem (Drake, 1982; Parker & Schumacher, 1977). As early as 1975, during the foundational years of the battered women's advocacy movement, Betty Cavanaugh, an emergency department nurse at the Hennepin County Medical Center (located in Minneapolis, Minnesota), created the Women's Advocacy

Program (Jackson, 1992; Sheridan, 1998). Approximately 30 years later, the program still exists as the Battered Women and Men's Advocacy Services.

Susan Hadley, a community-based women's advocate, is credited with developing the first comprehensive, nationally recognized, hospital-based **domestic violence** service program (Hadley, 1992; Hadley, Short, Lesin, & Zook, 1995). In early 1986, Hadley (1992) registered WomanKind, Inc., Support Services for Battered Women as a tax-exempt non-profit corporation in Minnesota. She then convinced administrators at Fairview Southdale Hospital (located in the greater Minneapolis area) to allow WomanKind staff and volunteers to provide victim advocacy to abused patients and domestic violence education to the healthcare staff. WomanKind, Inc. eventually merged into the Fairview Health System as a separate department, and its staff continues to provide a variety of advocacy and educational services at numerous Fairview Health System hospitals (Hadley et al.).

On July 1, 1986, the primary author of this chapter created the Family Violence Program at Chicago's Rush-Presbyterian St. Luke's Medical Center (Sheridan & Taylor, 1993). The Family Violence Program, as its name implies, was designed to provide specialized advanced practice nursing services to survivors of all forms of family violence. Within a few weeks of its inception, the Family Violence Program inherited the training, administrative, and fiscal responsibility for the medical center's fledgling volunteer-based Rape Victim Advocacy Program. In addition to victim advocacy and domestic violence training of health professionals, the nurses and social workers employed in the Family Violence Program (primarily from grant funding) provided direct patient care assessments, nursing, and/or social work care, including thorough written and photographic documentation. It did not take long before hundreds of patients had been served. Within a few months of providing services, the Family Violence Program staff began to be subpoenaed to testify in a variety of criminal and civil cases that resulted from the reported **abuse**.

In 1991, the primary author created a similar nurse-coordinated domestic violence intervention team at Oregon Health Sciences University Hospital in Portland, which focused primarily on assessment, interventions, and documentation of intimate partner and elder abuse patients who presented anywhere within the medical center's inpatient system. Again, it did not take long before hundreds of patients had been served and the program staff was being called into a variety of courts.

Nationally, hospital-based family violence programs were providing forensic nursing services to survivors of child abuse/neglect, intimate partner violence, and elder abuse years before such services were identified as forensic nursing. The International Association of Forensic Nurses was not created until 1992. Its creation gave a name to the type of nursing being practiced by innovative nurses all over the country who provided increasingly specialized care to a wide variety of patients who had been victimized in criminal acts.

During the early 1990s the number of hospital-based domestic violence programs slowly increased. In 1994, Susan Dersch, a nurse-advocate, created the Assisting Women with Advocacy, Resources, and Education (AWARE) program at Barnes and Jewish Hospital in St. Louis (Sheridan, 1998). The Assisting Women with Advocacy, Resources, and Education program is unique compared to most hospital-based family violence programs in that it is *not* focused on *nor* housed in an emergency department. Rather, the program recognizes domestic violence as an issue that primarily affects the health of all women who present throughout the healthcare system. Although the Assisting Women with Advocacy Resources, and Education program collaborates closely with the emergency department, the majority of its referrals are from routine screening for abuse that is conducted by staff throughout the Barnes and Jewish Hospital system.

In recent years, the number of hospital-based domestic and family violence programs has grown exponentially. Many of the programs are advocacy based, staff education focused, and managed via a wide variety of partnerships with community-based domestic violence service providers. Other domestic violence healthcare-based programs are being developed as natural extensions of the rapidly growing number of sexual assault nurse examiner programs. The Family Violence Prevention Fund is collecting data on existing hospital-based family violence programs and offers a treasure of health system–related materials (many free and some for nominal cost) on its website (www.endabuse.com).

Screening Tools for Domestic Violence

There are several published, reliable, and valid intimate partner violence screening tools used in clinical healthcare settings. Among the best known are varying-length versions of the Abuse Assessment Screen (AAS) and the three-question Partner Violence Screen (PVS).

Helton (1986) developed the first version of the Abuse Assessment Screen as a nine-question screen that was published by the March of Dimes (see **Figure 8-1**). In 1988, the Nursing Research Consortium on Violence and Abuse modified the original AAS to a six-question screen (see **Figure 8-2**) for use in clinical and clinical research settings. This version of the AAS asks about three nonphysical forms of domestic abuse: (1) experiencing fear during arguments with a partner; (2) feeling like the partner is trying to emotionally hurt the woman; and (3) feeling like the partner is trying to control the woman. The six-question AAS version has been used very effectively in numerous clinical settings by the primary author. However, using a six-question screen raised concerns about staff time. Therefore, the Nursing Research Consortium on Violence and Abuse developed a three-question version of the AAS that was used in a large prospective study that screened for battering during pregnancy in a population of about 700 women (McFarlane, Parker, Soeken, & Bullock, 1992; Parker & McFarlane, 1991) that established baseline reliability and validity. The three questions focused on if and when the partner was physically abused and the form that abuse took. The three-question AAS received further reliability and validity when used in a larger study (N = 1,203) (Parker, McFarlane, Soeker, Torres, & Campbell, 1993). A two-question version of the AAS also has been developed, tested, and shown to have reliability and validity (McFarlane, Greenberg, Weltge, & Watson, 1995).

The Partner Violence Screen (Feldhaus et al., 1997) uses one item from the AAS (being hit, kicked, punched, or otherwise hurt by someone) and also asks if a former partner is making the woman feel unsafe. Those with clinical experience know that many women are being abused (or at risk of being abused) by current and former intimate partners.

McFarlane et al. (2001) added two questions about withholding services or care to people with physical disabilities to the two-question AAS to create the Abuse Assessment Screen—Disability (AAS-D), which was tested on over 500 women at public and private specialty clinics. The AAS-D detected a 9.8% prevalence rate of abuse, with the perpetrator of physical or sexual abuse being most often an intimate partner.

Many emergency departments have tried to reduce their screening process to one question on their intake forms. No published studies have found a one-question screen to be a reliable and valid intimate partner violence screening tool. A one-item screening question for intimate partner violence that has *not* been particularly clinically useful is, "Do you feel safe in your home?" Patients may not feel safe in their homes for any number of reasons, including living in a high-crime neighborhood.

1. Do you know where you would go or who could help you if you were abused or worried about abuse? Yes ❑ No ❑

   If yes, where _____

2. Are you in a relationship with a man who physically hurts you?
   Yes ❑ No ❑ Sometimes ❑

3. Does he threaten you with abuse? Yes ❑ No ❑ Sometimes ❑

4. Has the man you are with hit, slapped, kicked, or otherwise physically hurt you?
   Yes ❑ No ❑ Sometimes ❑

5. If yes, has he hit you since you've been pregnant?
   Yes ❑ No ❑ Not applicable ❑

6. If yes, did the abuse increase since you've been pregnant?
   Yes ❑ No ❑ Not applicable ❑

7. Have you ever received medical treatment for any abuse injuries?
   Yes ❑ No ❑ Not applicable ❑

8. If you have been abused, remembering the last time he hurt you, mark the places on the body map where he hit you.

9. Were you pregnant at the time? Yes ❑ No ❑ Not applicable ❑

Figure 8-1 Abuse assessment screen—original version.

Source: Helton, A. (1986). *Protocol of Care for the Battered Woman*. Houston, TX: Houston chapter of the March of Dimes.

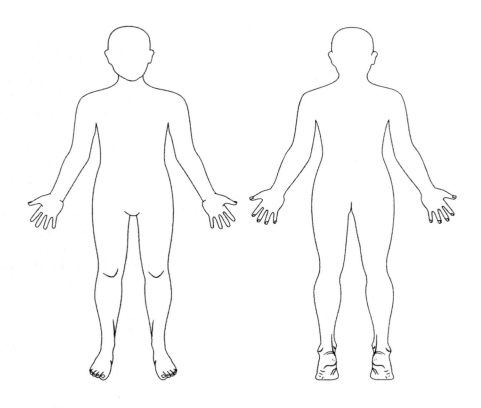

Figure 8-2 Abuse Assessment Screen—NRCVA Version (1988)

Intimate Partner Violence–Related Homicide

Early screening, identification, and treatment of intimate partner violence patients can help break often serious and deadly cycles of violence. Intimate partner violence–related homicide is identified as the leading cause of death in the United States among African American females between the ages of 15 and 45 and as the seventh leading cause overall in premature deaths of young women (Campbell et al., 2003b).

Campbell states:

> In 70 to 80 percent of intimate partner homicides, despite which partner was killed, the man physically abused the woman before the murder. Thus, one of the primary ways to decrease intimate partner homicide is to identify and intervene promptly with abused women at risk (2003a, p. 18).

In response, a recent study spanning 11 cities was completed to identify risk factors pertaining to intimate partner homicide, specifically femicide, the homicide of women (Campbell et al., 2003b). The study was completed using control design methodology. Data was collected from two main sources: femicide cases (dead women) and abuse victims who had similar profiles to the deceased. The data were analyzed from various disciplinary vantage points including domestic violence advocates, police enforcement, and medical examiners. Common themes throughout data analysis were identified as risk factors.

Risk factors that were categorized as putting a female at high risk for domestic violence homicide include:

1. A perpetrator's access to a gun with previous threats of weapon use
2. A stepchild of the perpetrator living in the home
3. Estrangement of the victim from the perpetrator (Campbell et al., 2003b)

In addition, the researchers found that a past history of stalking, forced sex, and abuse during pregnancy increased risk for femicide. The leading socioeconomic factor linked to increased risk of domestic homicide was the abuser's lack of employment (Campbell et al., 2003a, 2003b).

Various intimate partner violence, dangerousness, and harassment tools were used in Campbell's study, including the Danger Assessment (DA) and select items from the HARASS (Harassment in Abusive Relationships: A Self-Report Scale) tool. All of the items on the DA (see **Figure 8-3**) and the HARASS (see **Figure 8-4**) are positively correlated with increased risk of homicide. Therefore, whenever one has a positive screen for intimate partner abuse, the patient should be asked to complete the DA and the HARASS. Both tools are self-report scales and can be completed by the patient while the forensic nurse is completing other tasks in or outside the patient's room. The DA will produce better results if completed in conjunction with a calendar where the woman can mark the dates or approximate dates of abusive episodes. The calendar serves as a memory trigger. The data from the DA and the HARASS can guide the forensic nurse in discharge and/or admission to the hospital for safety planning. In addition, when abused women answer the questions on the DA and the HARASS, it lowers their ability to minimize the seriousness of the abuse in the relationship.

Several risk factors have been associated with increased risk of homicides (murders) of women and men in violent relationships. We cannot predict what will happen in your case, but we would like you to be aware of the danger of homicide in situations of abuse and for you to see how many of the risk factors apply to your situation.

Using the calendar, please mark the approximate dates during the past year when you were abused by your partner or ex-partner. Write on that date how bad the incident was according to the following scale:

1. Slapping, pushing; no injuries and/or lasting pain
2. Punching, kicking; bruises, cuts, and/or continuing pain
3. "Beating up"; severe contusions, burns, broken bones
4. Threat to use weapon; head injury, internal injury, permanent injury
5. Use of weapon; wounds from weapon

(If **any** of the descriptions for the higher number apply, use the higher number.)

Mark **Yes** or **No** for each of the following. ("He" refers to your husband, partner, ex-husband, ex-partner, or whoever is currently physically hurting you.)

_____ 1. Has the physical violence increased in severity or frequency over the past year?

_____ 2. Does he own a gun?

_____ 3. Have you left him after living together during the past year?

   3a. (If you have *never* lived with him, check here____)

_____ 4. Is he unemployed?

_____ 5. Has he ever used a weapon against you or threatened you with a lethal weapon? (If yes, was the weapon a gun?____)

_____ 6. Does he threaten to kill you?

_____ 7. Has he avoided being arrested for domestic violence?

_____ 8. Do you have a child who is not his?

_____ 9. Has he ever forced you to have sex when you did not wish to do so?

_____ 10. Does he ever try to choke you?

_____ 11. Does he use illegal drugs? By drugs, I mean "uppers" or amphetamines, speed, angel dust, cocaine, "crack," street drugs, or mixtures.

_____ 12. Is he an alcoholic or problem drinker?

_____ 13. Does he control most or all of your daily activities? For instance: does he tell you who you can be friends with, when you can see your family, how much money you can use, or when you can take the car? (If he tries, but you do not let him, check here: ____)

_____ 14. Is he violently and constantly jealous of you? (For instance, does he say "If I can't have you, no one can.")

_____ 15. Have you ever been beaten by him while you were pregnant? (If you have never been pregnant by him, check here: ____)

_____ 16. Have you ever threatened or tried to commit suicide?

_____ 17. Has he ever threatened or tried to commit suicide?

_____ 18. Does he threaten to harm your children?

_____ 19. Do you believe he is capable of killing you?

_____ 20. Does he follow or spy on you, leave threatening notes or messages on your answering machine, destroy your property, or call you when you don't want him to?

_____ Total "Yes" Answers

Thank you. Please talk to your nurse, advocate, or counselor about what the Danger Assessment means in terms of your situation.

Figure 8-3   Danger assessment.

Source: Jacquelyn C. Campbell, PhD, RN, Copyright 2003, www.dangerassessment.com.

Identifying Injuries and Wounds

Great importance is placed on accurately identifying and documenting injuries. Many healthcare providers consistently misuse medical forensic terms, and this can have a profound effect on the legal outcome of an assault. The following sections present important terms and their appropriate use as determined by several authors and leaders in the field of forensic medical science and authors of medical dictionaries (Brockmeyer & Sheridan, 1998; DiMaio & DiMaio, 2001; Miller & Keane, 1978; Sheridan, 2001; Venes & Thomas, 2001).

Injury Patterns

Patterned injuries present identifiable markings that allow a provider to discern (with reasonable certainty) that they were caused by a specific or unknown object, and/or by a specific mechanism of injury. Examples of such include fingertip-*like* contusions from being grabbed, cord-*like* contusions and abrasions from being whipped with a corded object, and fingernail scratch-*like* abrasions around the neck from being strangled. Note the appropriate use of the word *like* to describe what the provider identifies as the most likely cause of these patterned injuries.

Injuries in various stages of healing are referred to as a **pattern of injury**. The term can be used in describing both cutaneous and orthopedic injuries. It should be noted that in other forensic science circles this term may be used to mean patterned injuries.

Abrasions

Often called scrapes by the lay public, **abrasions** to the skin are superficial injuries that are caused by the friction or rubbing of the skin against a rough surface or object. The rougher the surface, the more severe the abrasion will be. An important point to remember is that abrasions, especially abrasions that have not been thoroughly cleaned, can be an excellent source of trace physical evidence. Care should be taken to collect any material found in or around the wound and surrounding clothing that may have come from the surface or object that was scraped, prior to cleaning and dressing the wound. The clothing should also be secured and labeled as evidence.

Avulsions

Avulsions refer to skin or other tissue that has been completely torn away by blunt and/or shearing force energies. Frequently occurring over bony prominences, forearms, and hands, blunt and/or shearing force energies can result in partial avulsions (often called skin tears).

Bruises/Contusions

Created by either a blunt or compression force trauma, bruises/**contusions** are wounds resulting in discoloration in the skin or other organs caused by the breaking of blood vessels. The terms bruise and contusion can be used synonymously. Both contusions and cuts (defined in a later section) are frequently seen along the upper and outer aspects of the upper extremities in defensive posturing when attempting to protect oneself during an assault.

There have been several research studies to assess the accuracy of dating bruises. The findings have been consistent — there is *no* scientific basis to accurately date bruises either by looking at photographs of injuries or by viewing the injuries directly (Bariciak, Plint,

Gaboury, & Bennett, 2003; Langlois & Gresham, 1991; Wilson, 1977). Forensic health professionals caution all health professionals to not date injuries by their general appearance (DiMaio & DiMaio, 2001; Sheridan, 2001, 2003). However, in general, bruises go through a relatively predictable color changing process (from red to black and blue, to bluish-green, to greenish-brown, to brownish-yellow, to yellow, to light yellow, and then to fade), but the time between each stage varies from person to person (Sheridan, 2003). The pigmentation of the victim's skin can also make it difficult to document, either through photographs or visually. The forensic nurse may be able to determine if the bruise is from relatively recent trauma or from older trauma. In addition, the forensic nurse may be able to testify if the age of the bruise is consistent or not consistent with the history provided.

Ecchymosis

Ecchymosis is a frequently misused term often incorrectly used as a synonym for a bruise/contusion that is caused by trauma. **Ecchymosis** refers to subcutaneous, hemorrhagic blotching under the skin often caused by a medical/hematological condition or indirectly caused by trauma. Ecchymotic lesions are usually nonpainful and nonindurated (not hard or firm) in nature. However, it would be forensically accurate to describe a spread of discoloration from a directly traumatized area as ecchymosis. For example, a person who is punched to the mid-forehead right above the nose will almost certainly develop bilateral, periorbital ecchymoses (swelling and discoloration to both eyes). The trauma was to the forehead and the blood seeped or leaked downward into the orbital area. In contrast, if a person was punched directly to one eye with resulting swelling, pain, and discoloration to the point of impact, that injury would be most accurately called a bruise/contusion. The color changes related to the resolution of ecchymotic lesions will parallel the color changes of bruising, but the etiology of the bleeding under the skin or other body organs are different.

Lacerations

The word **laceration** is probably the most mistakenly used term when providers are describing wounds. Laceration refers to the tearing or splitting of tissue from blunt and/or shearing injuries. Lacerations are often to the skin; however, it is not uncommon to receive a laceration to the liver from a blunt or squeezing force trauma. Unlike cuts to the skin from sharp injuries, lacerated wounds typically have a jagged edge or edges and occur most often over bony prominences. A bruise or contusion is also often present embedded around the torn or ruptured tissue.

Cuts/Incisions

Unlike lacerations, cuts or incisions typically have a smooth edge to them and are caused by a sharp instrument or object. The depth of **cuts/incisions** is also consistent, whereas for lacerations they may be varying. It should be noted that when a provider is in doubt as to whether an injury is a laceration or cut, the term *wound* should be used with an accompanying description.

Petechiae

Petechiae, tiny, nonelevated, purplish hemorrhagic spots, are frequently seen in the face and eyes of victims of **strangulation** (either manual, ligature, or mechanical). Other medical conditions, such as severe vomiting, severe coughing, severe sneezing, strenuous bowel movements, and platelet deficiency can also cause them. Women giving vaginal birth may develop facial petechiae from pushing, and children have developed impressive facial petechiae from severe screaming.

Traumatic Alopecia

Often overlooked, traumatic hair loss (alopecia) can occur when the victim is pulled or dragged by his or her hair. This alopecia is painful and can be difficult to photograph. If hair pulling has been reported, the forensic nurse may be able to run a comb through the patient's hair to secure large numbers of pulled hairs as evidence to support traumatic alopecia.

Slap Injuries

Slap injuries usually initially present as raised, reddened, painful welts to the skin. As the swelling subsides there are often patterned linear parallel bruises outlining the edges of the perpetrator's fingers. If hit hard enough to the head, a punch or slap can rupture a victim's eardrums. This can sometimes be the only presenting sign of injury from a slap.

Strangulation

Manual and ligature strangulation is a frequent injury inflicted by perpetrators of intimate partner violence onto their partners. Physical findings range from ligature-induced patterned bruising and/or abrasion, to fingernail scratch-like abrasions to the neck, to petechiae of the face or eyes. However, most victims of strangulation present with no physical signs (Strack, McClane, & Hawley, 2001). The danger lies in healthcare providers under-appreciating the health risks associated with strangulation and its delayed effect on one's breathing. Even without signs of dyspnea, a victim of strangulation should at a minimum be hospitalized and frequently assessed for 24 hours with continuous pulse oximetry (Kuriloff & Pincus, 1989). A study found that strangulation is an assault that occurs late in an abusive relationship, thereby placing the victim at increased risk of significant injury or death (Wilbur et al., 2001). Long-term symptoms from repeated strangulations include neck and throat injury, neurological disorders, and psychological disorders (Smith, Mills, & Taliaferro, 2001).

Firearm Injuries

Victims of firearm injuries are frequently seen by healthcare providers in an acute emergency setting. In addition to lifesaving measures, efforts should be made to secure and save clothing and to carefully document the location and size of the wounds. Protocols for the collection of evidence should be present in every healthcare facility that may come into contact with victims of violence. Individual pieces of clothing should be placed in labeled paper bags to dry. Bullet fragments should each be placed in separate containers. No attempt should be made with multiple openings to ascertain whether a bullet wound is an entrance or an exit. Studies have shown that physicians are rarely correct (Randall, 1993).

Bite Marks

Bite marks can occur almost anywhere among victims of domestic violence, but are often seen in sexual areas, especially the breast (Vale & Noguchi, 1983). The unique characteristics of these patterned injuries provide opportune evidence and may be able to be matched to the perpetrator by forensic odontologists if documented appropriately. Again, protocols should be in place at the facility to help make the process easier. Close-up photographs should be taken using a right-angle ruler developed by the American Board of Forensic Odontology (Sheridan, 2001).

Sexual Assault

Typically overlooked in intimate partner abuse, nearly half of all cases of domestic violence involve forced sexual assault (Campbell, 1989, 1998). Forensic nurses should follow protocols for the collection of sexual assault evidence that are in place within their jurisdictions, keeping in mind that valuable biologic information has been obtained after the traditional 72-hour time frame.

Written Documentation

When documenting histories of intimate partner violence, the forensic nurse should try to be as verbatim as possible with the stated details of the actual reported assault. The nurse should not sanitize statements made by the patient even if the statements include curse words or write a progress note that reads as if the patient were using accurate medical terms when, in fact, the patient was using slang to describe body parts. The patient's demeanor should also be documented. As with sexual assault patients, patients experiencing intimate partner violence will present for care with a wide variance of emotions. It is critical that the forensic nurse encourage the provider (nurse practitioner, physician, or physician's assistant) to list as one of the discharge or admission diagnoses something like, "reported domestic violence" or "reported adult maltreatment syndrome." If the provider only lists S/P assault, medical records coders would not know to use the appropriate International Classification of Diseases, 9th Revision, Clinical Modification code for adult maltreatment syndrome (995.80). Failing to use an appropriate code for intimate partner violence could present problems during site visits by the Joint Commission. As part of chart audits for compliance with documentation of abuse, if a site surveyor asks the hospital to produce records on 15 intimate partner violence patients, it will be difficult to tease out domestic violence assaults from the scores of nonintimate violence assaults seen by the emergency department and/or clinics.

Photographic Documentation

Forensic photographs are critical pieces of medical documentation of all forms of family and interpersonal violence and can be used as evidence in a criminal or civil case. Forensic photography implies that the photograph may be used in a legal proceeding (Besant-Matthews & Smock, 2001). A photograph gives visual evidence of an observed or treated wound that the healthcare provider assessed on the day of the exam. In addition, a photograph documents injuries or conditions before and after medical treatment and shows detail of a wound or injury that may have been overlooked by a visual inspection. In conjunction with the written medical documentation, the forensic photograph may be able to substantiate a victim's story or, in some cases, exonerate a suspect. When on the witness stand, the forensic nurse needs to become comfortable saying the injuries depicted in the photographs are true and accurate likenesses of the wounds seen and treated on the day of care. The following discussion reviews some of the important aspects of photography to consider when documenting the effects of partner violence. In some jurisdictions, the police department may be called in to document the injuries for evidentiary purposes. A detailed overview of forensic photography can be found in Appendix 2.

Before forensic photographs can be taken, a signed consent for forensic photography must be obtained in most medical settings. The healthcare provider should explain to the patient the reasons why the photographs are being taken, as well as the risks and benefits, and also ask if the photographs can be used for educational purposes. If the patient is unconscious and the injuries are secondary to a potentially litigious situation, take the picture and get consent later (Pasqualone, 1996).

In the past, the gold standard for forensic photography was the 35-mm camera. Digital cameras have essentially replaced the standard SLR 35-mm camera. Issues related to the use of digital images are also discussed in Appendix 2. The long-term storage of digital images should be considered and hospital policies should be formulated to address this issue. It is important to know your hospital's and legal jurisdiction's policies regarding photographic and digital evidence.

The following is a summary of the various factors that must be taken into account when taking a forensic photograph. See Appendix 2 for a more detailed discussion of these principles.

1. *Lighting.* According to Besant-Matthews and Smock (2001), a general principle is to mimic or add to existing light or create your own lighting according to your preference and the nature of the subject. For example, fluorescent lighting, which gives off green light not visible to the eye, can produce an artificial greening effect to bruises, which may suggest the bruise being photographed is older than it actually is. Another important factor is background. The lens is also an important factor. Some lenses have a focal length that allows you to clearly see detail as close as 2 feet, whereas with a higher powered lens may photograph objects as close as 1.5–2 inches away with great detail. In cases where trace evidence may be in a dirty wound, it becomes important to show this detail in the photograph.

2. *Scales.* A scale should be used in at least one of the photographs of every individual injury. If the scale covers a part of the body, another photograph of the injured area should be taken without using the scale. The scale gives an exact measurement or size to the wound. The preferred scale is the ABFO scale, which will indicate any distortion, angle or curvature in the photograph.

3. *Sequence of photographs.* According to Pasqualone (1996), the first photo should be a full body photo of the patient in order to establish the documented injuries were found on this patient. The second photograph should be mid-distance, and the third should be a close-up shot. A minimum of two close-up photographs should be taken of each injury, one with a scale to show injury size and another without to show that the scale did not obscure information (Pasqualone). This photographic principle is a common practice by scene investigators and is often referred to as the rule of threes (Sheridan, 2001).

    A series of photographs should be taken over time to demonstrate progression of injury. This is often referred to as serial photography.

4. *Labels on photographs.* Once your photographs are completed, it is important to place identifying information such as patient name, patient hospital number, patient date of birth, name of photographer, case number (*if indicated*), *and most importantly, the date and time the photo was taken and your initials/name. Photographs

H arassment in
A busive
R elationships:
A
S elf-report
S cale

Many women are harassed in relationships with their abusive partners, especially if the women are trying to end the relationship. You may be experiencing harassment. This instrument is designed to measure harassment of women who are in abusive relationships or who are in the process of leaving abusive relationships. By completing this questionnaire, you may better understand harassment in your life. If you have any questions, please talk with the service provider who gave you this tool.

Harassment is defined as: *a persistent pattern of behavior by an intimate partner that is intended to bother, annoy, trap, emotionally wear down, threaten, frighten, terrify, and/or coerce a woman with the overall intent to control her choices and behavior about leaving an abusive relationship.*

There are no right or wrong answers. Do not put your name on the form. The instrument takes about 10 minutes to complete.

For each item, circle the number that best describes how often the behavior occurred. Next, rate how distressing the behavior is to you. If the behavior has never occurred, circle 0 (NEVER) and go to the next questions. If the question does not apply to you, circle NA (NOT APPLICABLE). If you are still in the relationship please circle MY PARTNER. If you have left the relationship, please circle MY FORMER PARTNER.

	0 = Never 1 = Rarely 2 = Occasionally 3 = Frequently 4 = Very Frequently NA = Not applicable	0 = Not at all distressing 1 = Slightly distressing 2 = Moderately distressing 3 = Very distressing 4 = Extremely distressing NA = Not applicable
THE BEHAVIOR **MY PARTNER MY FORMER PARTNER** (circle one)	**How often does it occur?**	**How distressing is this behavior to you?**
1. Frightens people close to me	0 1 2 3 4 NA	0 1 2 3 4 NA
2. Pretends to be someone else in order to get to me	0 1 2 3 4 NA	0 1 2 3 4 NA
3. Comes to my home when I don't want him there	0 1 2 3 4 NA	0 1 2 3 4 NA
4. Threatens to kill me if I leave or stay away from him	0 1 2 3 4 NA	0 1 2 3 4 NA
5. Threatens to harm the kids if I leave or stay away from him	0 1 2 3 4 NA	0 1 2 3 4 NA
6. Takes things that belong to me so I have to see him to get them back	0 1 2 3 4 NA	0 1 2 3 4 NA
7. Tries getting me fired from my job	0 1 2 3 4 NA	0 1 2 3 4 NA
8. Ignores court orders to stay away from me	0 1 2 3 4 NA	0 1 2 3 4 NA
9. Keeps showing up wherever I am	0 1 2 3 4 NA	0 1 2 3 4 NA
10. Bothers me at work when I don't want to talk to him	0 1 2 3 4 NA	0 1 2 3 4 NA
11. Uses the kids as pawns to get me physically close to him	0 1 2 3 4 NA	0 1 2 3 4 NA
12. Shows up without warning	0 1 2 3 4 NA	0 1 2 3 4 NA
13. Messes with my property (For example: sells my stuff, breaks my furniture, damages my car, steals my things)	0 1 2 3 4 NA	0 1 2 3 4 NA
14. Scares me with a weapon	0 1 2 3 4 NA	0 1 2 3 4 NA
15. Breaks into my home	0 1 2 3 4 NA	0 1 2 3 4 NA
16. Threatens to kill me if I leave or stay away from him	0 1 2 3 4 NA	0 1 2 3 4 NA
17. Threatens to harm our pet	0 1 2 3 4 NA	0 1 2 3 4 NA
18. Calls me on the telephone and hangs up	0 1 2 3 4 NA	0 1 2 3 4 NA
19. Reports me to the authorities for taking drugs when I don't	0 1 2 3 4 NA	0 1 2 3 4 NA
Additional harassing behaviors not listed above:		
20. _____	0 1 2 3 4 NA	0 1 2 3 4 NA
21. _____	0 1 2 3 4 NA	0 1 2 3 4 NA

Please answer a few additional questions:

_____ Your age in years

Check the statement that best describes you:

u Married, living with an abusive partner
u Single, living with an abusive partner
u Married, living apart from an abusive partner
u Single, living apart from an abusive partner.

How long were you in the above relationship? _____
Are you still in the relationship? u Yes u No
If you have left the relationship, how long have you been out? _____
What is your approximate annual income? _____
How many years of school have you completed? _____

Check the statement that best describes you:

u Asian/Pacific Islander
u Black/African American
u Caucasian/White
u Hispanic
u Native American/American Indian
u Other _____

Figure 8-4   HARASS Scale.

of injuries taken at differing points in time on the same day may look markedly different.

Once the photographs have been properly labeled and documented, it is important to follow your agency's chain of confidentiality and/or chain of custody policy to make sure the photographs are secured properly.

Summary

Assessing for domestic violence with a reliable and valid intimate **partner violence screen** is now considered a nursing standard of care. With any positive finding of abuse, the forensic nurse should have immediate access to the Danger Assessment and HARASS tools to further explore for risk of domestic homicide. Written and photographic documentation must be accurate, thorough, and unbiased. The forensic nurse needs to have excellent command of all basic forensic terms and knowledge. This includes being able to discriminate between a cut and a laceration, a bruise and ecchymosis, etc. Intimate partner violence is a major public health problem. Forensic nurses can and should be key members of multidisciplinary coordinated community responses whose focus is to break the cycle of domestic violence through the development and utilization of specific and comprehensive assessment tools as described herein, as well as to focus on prevention and early identification of risk.

 QUESTIONS FOR DISCUSSION

1. What are the factors that place women at high risk for domestic violence? In what ways might this categorization assist the forensic nurse in assessment of a client's risk? In what ways might this hinder the identification of those at risk?
2. Which assessment tools are useful in identifying the risk of partner violence?
3. What roadblocks may be encountered when working with a client who does not fit the common conception of the victim of domestic violence? What strategies may be useful to overcome some of these problems?

REFERENCES

Bariciak, E. D., Plint, A. C., Gaboury, I., & Bennett, S. B. (2003). Dating of bruises in children: An assessment of physician accuracy. *Pediatrics, 112*(4), 804–807.

Besant-Matthews, P. E., & Smock, W. S. (2001). Forensic photography in the emergency department. In J. S. Olshaker, M. C. Jackson, & W. S. Smock (Eds.), *Forensic emergency medicine* (pp. 257–282). Philadelphia, PA: Lippincott Williams & Wilkins.

Brockmeyer, D. M., & Sheridan, D. J. (1998). Domestic violence: A practical guide to the use of forensic evaluation in clinical examination and documentation of injuries. In J. C. Campbell (Ed.), *Empowering survivors of abuse* (pp. 214–226). Thousand Oaks, CA: Sage Publications.

Campbell, J. C. (1989). Women's response to sexual abuse in intimate relationships. *Women's Health Care International, 8*, 335–347.

Campbell, J. C. (1998). Making the health care system an empowerment zone for battered women: Health consequences, policy recommendations, introductions, and overview. In J. C. Campbell (Ed.), *Empowering survivors of abuse: Health care for battered women and their children* (pp. 3–22). Thousand Oaks, CA: Sage.

Campbell, J. C., Webster, D., Koziol-McLain, J., Block, C. R., Campbell, D., Curry, M. A., ... Wilt, S. (2003a). Assessing risk factors for intimate partner homicide. *NIJ Journal, 250,* 14–19.

Campbell, J. C., Webster, D., Koziol-McLain, J., Block, C., Campbell, D., Curry, M.A., ... Laughon, K. (2003b). Risk factors for femicide in abusive relationships: Results from a multi-site case control study. *American Journal of Public Health, 93*(7), 1089–1097.

DiMaio, V. J., & DiMaio, D. (2001). *Forensic Pathology* (2nd ed.). Boca Raton, FL: CRC Press.

Drake, V. K. (1982). Battered women: A health care problem in disguise. *Image, 14*(2), 40–47.

Feldhaus, K. M., Koziol-McLain, J., Amsbury, H. L., Norton, I. M., Lowenstein, S. R., & Abbott, J. T. (1997). Accuracy of 3 brief screening questions for detecting partner violence in the emergency department. *Journal of the American Medical Association, 277*(17), 1357–1361.

Hadley, S., Short, L., Lesin, N., & Zook, E. (1995). WomanKind: An innovative model of health care response to domestic abuse. *Women's Health Issues, 5*(4), 189–198.

Hadley, S. M. (1992). Working with battered women in the emergency department: A model program. *Journal of Emergency Nursing, 18*(1), 18–23.

Helton, A. (1986). *Protocol of Care for the Battered Woman.* Houston, TX: Houston chapter of the March of Dimes.

Jackson, H. C. (1992). The Hennepin County Medical Center's Women's Advocacy Program: Sixteen years of service. *Journal of Emergency Nursing, 18*(1), 27A–30A.

Kuriloff, D. B., & Pincus, R. L. (1989). Delayed airway obstruction and neck abscess following manual strangulation injury. *Annals of Otology, Rhinology, and Laryngology, 98,* 824–827.

Langlois, N. E. I., & Gresham, G. A. (1991). The ageing of bruises: A review and study of the colour. *Forensic Science International, 50,* 227–238.

McFarlane, J., Greenberg, L., Weltge, A., & Watson, M. (1995). Identification of abuse in emergency departments: Effectiveness of a two-question screening tool. *Journal of Emergency Nursing, 21*(5), 391–394.

McFarlane, J., Hughes, R. B., Nosek, M. A., Groff, J. Y., Swedland, N., & Mullen, P. D. (2001). Abuse Assessment Screen-Disability (AAS-D): Measuring frequency, type, and perpetrator of abuse toward women with physical difficulties. *Journal of Women's Health and Gender-Based Medicine, 10*(9), 861–866.

McFarlane, J., Parker, B., Soeken, K., & Bullock, L. (1992). Assessing for abuse during pregnancy. *Journal of the American Medical Association, 267*(3), 3176–3178.

Miller, B. F., & Keane, C. B. (1978). *Encyclopedia and dictionary of medicine, nursing, and allied health* (2nd ed.). Philadelphia, PA: WB Saunders.

Parker, B., & McFarlane, J. (1991). Identifying and helping battered pregnant women. *Public Health Nursing, 17*(6), 443–451.

Parker, B., McFarlane, J., Soeker, K., Torres, S., & Campbell, D. (1993, May/June). Physical and emotional abuse in pregnancy: A comparison of adult and teenage women. *Nursing Research, 42*(3), 172–178.

Parker, B., & Schumacher, D. N. (1977). The battered wife syndrome and violence in the nuclear family of origin: A controlled pilot study. *American Journal of Public Health, 67*(8), 760–761.

Pasqualone, G. (1996). Forensic RNs as photographers: Documentation in the ED. *Journal of Psychosocial Nursing, 34*(10), 47–51.

Randall, T. (1993). Clinician's forensic interpretations of fatal gunshot wounds often miss the mark. *Journal of the American Medical Association, 269*(16), 2058–2061.

Sheridan, D. J. (1998). Heath care-based programs for domestic violence survivors. In J. C. Campbell (Ed.), *Empowering survivors of abuse: Health care for battered women and their children* (pp. 23–31). Thousand Oaks, CA: Sage.

Sheridan, D. J. (2001). Treating survivors of intimate partner abuse. In J. S. Olshaker, M. C. Jackson, & W. S. Smock (Eds.), *Forensic emergency medicine* (pp. 203–228). Philadelphia, PA: Lippincott Williams & Wilkins.

Sheridan, D. J. (2003). Forensic identification and documentation of patients experiencing intimate partner violence. *Clinics in Family Practice, 5*(1), 113–143.

Sheridan, D. J., & Taylor, W. K. (1993). Developing hospital-based domestic violence programs, protocols, policies, and procedures. *AWHONN's Clinical Issues in Perinatal and Women's Health Nursing, 4*(3), 471–482.

Smith, D. J., Mills, T., & Taliaferro, E. H. (2001). Frequency and relationship of reported symptomology in victims of intimate partner violence: The effect of multiple strangulation attacks. *Journal of Emergency Medicine, 21*(3), 323–329.

Strack, G. B., McClane, G. E., & Hawley, D. (2001). A review of 300 attempted strangulation cases. Part I: Criminal legal issues. *Journal of Emergency Medicine, 21*(3), 303–309.

Vale, G. L., & Noguchi, T. T. (1983). Anatomical distribution of human bite marks in a series of 67 cases. *Journal of Forensic Science, 28*(1), 61–69.

Venes, D., & Thomas, C. L. (Eds.). (2001). *Taber's cyclopedic medical dictionary* (19th ed.). Philadelphia, PA: Lippincott-Raven.

Wilbur, L., Higley, M., Hatfield, J., Surprenant, Z., Taliaferro, E., Smith, D. J., & Paolo, A. (2001). Survey results of women who have been strangled while in an abusive relationship. *Journal of Emergency Medicine, 21*(3), 297–302.

Wilson, E. F. (1977). Estimation of the age of cutaneous contusions in child abuse. *Pediatrics, 60*, 750–752.

SUGGESTED FURTHER READING

Arosarena, O., Fritsch, T., Hsueh, Y., Aynehchi, B. & Haug, R. (2010). Maxiollofacial injuries and violence against women. *Archive of Facial Plastic Surgery, 12*(5), 284–365.

Duma, S., & Ogunbanjo, G. (2004). Forensic documentation of intimate partner violence in primary health care. *Clinics in Family Practice, 46*(4), 37–40.

Johnston, B. (2006). Intimate partner violence screening & treatment: The importance of nursing caring behavior. *Journal of Forensic Nursing, 2*(4), 184–188.

Moracco, C., Runyan, J., Bowling, M., & Earp, J. (2007). Women's experience with violence: A national study. *Women's Health Issues, 17*(1), 3–12.

Walthan, C. N. (2008). Who is identified by screening for intimate partner violence? *Women's Health Issues, 18*(6), 423–432.

CHAPTER 9

Child and Adolescent Sexual Abuse

Frederick Berrien

The sexual abuse of a child or adolescent is a complex experience that is very different from the sexual assault of an adult. The way children and adolescents experience the abuse depends upon their age and development, the circumstances of the abuse, their relationship to the offender, and the response of their environment to the abuse. This chapter will explain the clinical and forensic approach to children and adolescents who have been sexually abused. The evaluation described in this chapter applies to all prepubescent children who have had sexual contact and to those adolescents who have been involved in abusive sexual relationships. A caring and competent forensic clinical examiner is critical to the appropriate assessment and management of these evaluations.

CHAPTER FOCUS

- » Epidemiology Manifestations of Sexual Abuse
- » Psychodynamics of Sexual Abuse
- » Multidisciplinary Issues
- » Physical Evaluation of the Child
- » Medical Evaluation of the Child
- » Testing for Sexually Transmitted Diseases
- » Forensic Evidence Collection
- » Treatment Considerations
- » Medical Treatment
- » Mental Health
- » Family Support
- » Judicial Proceedings

KEY TERMS

- » Children's Advocacy Center
- » colposcope
- » consensual sexual activity
- » *guardian ad litem*
- » nonpredatory
- » sexual abuse
- » sexual assault
- » statutory rape

From a medical perspective, **sexual abuse** is any contact involving the breast, genitalia, anus, and inner thighs that is nonconsensual, usually perpetrated by an individual in a position of power or influence over the child. These forms of sexual abuse usually involve a perpetrator who is significantly older than the victim; however, such sexual contact can involve children of similar age. These contacts among children of similar age require an extensive psychological evaluation to determine if such activity is abusive or is generated by other emotional needs.

Participation in pornography or forced exposure to sexually explicit materials is another form of sexual abuse that can cause psychological harm. These forms of sexual abuse require a full investigation and possibly judicial procedures, but rarely require a medical evaluation.

In contrast to **sexual assault**, sexual abuse is often regarded by the child as a part of a continuum of affectionate interactions with the perpetrator. The perpetrator has usually established emotional ties with the child and, therefore, the child is not necessarily inclined to resist the physical contact. The child is emotionally very vulnerable, often experiencing a complicit role in the sexual abuse and feeling ambivalent about his or her relationship with the perpetrator.

It is important in working with adolescents to distinguish sexual abuse from other types of sexual contact that may be inappropriate and potentially harmful, but not necessarily abusive. **Consensual sexual activity** among adolescents as young as 13 is not uncommon (Connecticut Department of Public Health, 2010); however, the age difference between the partners should be assessed in the context of their power differential. Consensual sexual relationships among youth with significant age differences are defined by most states as **statutory rape**. These cases may require investigation; however, a clinical approach should be used by the healthcare clinician. The appropriate approach to these cases is to provide reproductive health and psychological care according to the adolescent's health and developmental status and circumstances of the sexual contact. It is also important to distinguish cases of rape from sexual abuse or consensual sexual relationships. Occasionally, adolescents who are discovered by an adult to be engaged in sexual relationships will initially disguise it as a sexual assault. It is important that the clinician give the adolescent the latitude to provide an accurate account of the sexual activity. Evaluation of a rape in an adolescent requires procedures that address forensic and emotional issues that, although similar, are different than those of an abuse victim. See Chapter 18 for details of the rape evaluation.

Children can also offend sexually, usually with younger children. However, it can be difficult to distinguish normal, healthy sexual behaviors that are exploratory and **nonpredatory** from problematic behavior that requires a clinical evaluation to determine their significance. Friedrich, Fisher, Broughton, Houston, & Shafran (1998) developed an inventory of childhood sexual behaviors to assist in making this distinction. This inventory has been standardized with several preadolescent populations. In general, sexual acts among children that appear premeditated, involve force or coercion, or involve penetrating or insertive acts should be considered potentially abusive and should be evaluated from the perspective of abuse. Mutual fondling, excessive masturbation, and looking at genitals or breasts are possible indications of stress or other psychological problems that should be evaluated by a child psychologist or pediatric behavioral specialist familiar with sexual development.

Epidemiology

An estimated 772,000 children were the victims of maltreatment in the United States in 2008, and of those, 9.1 % were the victims of sexual abuse according to U.S. Department of Health and Human Services Administration for Children and Families (2010). These data are based upon confirmed cases of sexual abuse. Many cases of sexual abuse are never reported, and many cases are not confirmed by investigation, so these incidence data are regarded as very conservative. Based upon many surveys of adults who have experienced sexual abuse during their childhood, the prevalence of this problem is estimated to be at least 20% for females and conservatively estimated to be 5–10% for males (Finkelhor,

1994). Although sexual abuse rates have declined in the past few years, the decline appears to be leveling off and possibly rising again. The reasons for the changes in case rates are unknown.

Sexual abuse is found in all socioeconomic groups and in all cultures. There appears to be higher incidence among low-income populations, which may be a result of limited options for ensuring safe care arrangements for children. Clearly children brought up in households with substance abuse are at greater risk of sexual abuse due to the loss of inhibition and respect for boundaries. Children who are disabled also are found to have a higher incidence of sexual abuse due to vulnerabilities based on mobility and communication limitations. For reasons that remain obscure, it is common to find that children who have been sexually abused have been raised by nonoffending parents who were also sexually abused (Wurtele & Miller-Perrin, 1992).

Manifestations of Sexual Abuse

Sexual abuse is most commonly detected when a child makes a disclosure to a family member, a friend, or a trusted adult. Young children may make a disclosure that is vague, such as statements that express dislike for a person or being in a particular situation. Sensitive follow-up questions then raise the possibility of abuse. With adolescents, the initial disclosure is often to a peer who encourages a report to an adult.

If a child presents with medical symptoms such as genital pain, bleeding, or discharge, questions to parents and children regarding possible genital or anal contact are indicated to determine if abuse may be an underlying cause. Enuresis and encopresis are sometimes associated with sexual abuse and therefore should prompt questions to explore the possibility of sexual abuse.

Changes in behavior and mood are associated with sexual abuse; however, there are many potential causes of these changes. Sexualized behaviors always raise concern about sexual abuse. These behaviors need to be assessed in the context of normal sexual development behavior (Friedrich et al., 1998) and exposures that children have to sexual materials. Children who have been sexually abused may become aggressive, appear depressed, experience eating disorders, have sleep disturbances, or perform poorly in school, so it is important to consider abuse as one of the possible reasons for these problems.

Psychodynamics of Sexual Abuse

Sexual abuse is the result of the interaction among the child, the perpetrator, and the environment. Finkelhor (1984) described four preconditions for sexual abuse to occur. The two preconditions that apply to the perpetrator are motivation and ability to overcome internal inhibitions toward sexual abuse. The third applies to the environment in which external barriers to sexual abuse must be overcome. The last precondition is a child who is unable to resist abuse.

The primary factor in sexual abuse is the perpetrator. The motivations of the perpetrator may emanate from a variety of conditions. The true pedophile is a person whose lifelong sexual orientation has involved children; however, the true pedophile accounts for a relatively small number of sexual abuse cases. The more common type of perpetrator is a person who uses children for sexual satisfaction while also having adult sexual relationships. The reasons for a perpetrator's need to have sexual contact with children vary but usually relate to disordered relationships resulting in deficits in coping abilities, which are compensated with child sexual contact. In some cases these disordered relationships may be a response to the perpetrator's sexual or physical abuse victimization during childhood. For some perpetrators, a lowering of internal inhibitions with alcohol or drugs may permit them to engage with children when they otherwise would not. In essence, the perpetrator's motivation for sexual satisfaction with children comes from a distorted relationship with a child and/or use of psychoactive substances to overcome internal inhibitions.

The environment must permit the contact between child and perpetrator to occur, allowing the perpetrator to carry out the acts without others being aware. This requires that the perpetrator plan the sexual activities in locations or at times when others are not present. In some situations, the perpetrator may distort the perceptions of others present such that the acts are not interpreted as abuse. In some situations, the perpetrator will create an environment in which the child perceives the acts as acceptable; for example, the perpetrator may tell the child, "This is what people do when they love each other." As children become aware of the taboos against sexual contact, the perpetrator will resort to coercion or threats. These environmental conditions contribute strongly to the secretive nature of sexual abuse. For example, leaving a preschool child in the care of a sexual offender for regular periods of time each day creates an environment that excludes witnesses and permits the offender to distort the sexual contact as special attention; this will be reinforced by rewards such as presents or privileges as long as it remains a secret. For the older child, the abuse may initially appear innocent, but evolves for the child into sexual acts associated with shame or fear that the child will conceal to avoid exposure. In these situations, the environment not only permits the abuse to occur but also inhibits the child from disclosing the abuse.

The child is generally regarded as a passive participant in the sexual abuse. However, if we look more carefully at the position of children in this dynamic with the perpetrator and the environment, we recognize that the child has some characteristics that may be protective and others that make the child more susceptible. For example, depending on age, knowledge, and cognitive ability, children are aware that sexual contacts are socially prohibited for children. This is a protective resource for the child. On the other hand, a child's smaller size and strength is usually regarded as characteristics that make them more susceptible. Similarly, the notion that children don't always tell the truth or cannot be believed again leaves children more vulnerable to sexual abuse. In viewing a child's protective and susceptible characteristics, it is recognized that children's participation in sexual abuse is in part determined by these characteristics.

Sexual abuse usually is progressive, with the perpetrator first simply engaging the child during innocent circumstances. The experienced perpetrator will identify the vulnerable child and the proper environment where the circumstances permit a trusting relationship to develop with the child. The child will accept the initial contacts as signs of caring and affection, often not understanding the progression of contact as unusual. For younger children the sexual activities involve fondling, exposure, and masturbation. These sexual acts are usually not painful and may not be regarded by the child as particularly harmful.

Digital penetration of the anus and genital to genital contact are not unusual; however, actual vaginal penetration is not common with prepubescent girls. Nevertheless, children frequently experience these activities as genital penetration, although physical evidence of vaginal penetration is not often found. Frequently the children do not experience pain or discomfort, and in some cases may find the sexual contact to be pleasurable. To maintain the secrecy of the abuse, children are often given rewards to reinforce the secrecy or the perpetrator may threaten the child with abandonment or physical harm.

Children will decide to disclose sexual abuse for a variety of reasons. The child may be questioned by a trusted adult who has concerns. A young child may innocently disclose in reference to a discussion about touching. Sometimes the disclosure statements of young children are indirect, such as a general expression of dislike for a specific person or place; follow-up questions may lead to abuse concerns. Older children and adolescents often will want to protect nonoffending parents from knowing about the abuse and choose to disclose to a trusted person outside the immediate family.

Statements of children who suggest sexual abuse must be acknowledged and appropriately explored. In most cases, parents and other inexperienced adults should not ask children detailed questions. Rather, it is the role of adults to support the disclosure, clarify the spontaneous statements of children, and seek out experienced professionals to explore the meaning of children's statements.

Most children do not anticipate the magnitude of distress that such a disclosure will create. The disruption created in a family may lead to a recantation of allegations by children. This is more common with older children who believe that once the abuse has been exposed that it will stop without legal intervention. Unfortunately, families unfamiliar with the magnitude of problems associated with sexual abuse may suppress the allegations with the expectation that the problem can be managed within the family. These approaches to child sexual abuse usually perpetuate the problem, leading to chronic stress, unresolved trust issues, and revictimization.

Multidisciplinary Issues

Successful investigation and management of sexual abuse cases involves a full understanding of the child, the perpetrator, and the environment. Multiple disciplines are required to assess and understand each of these components to achieve successful outcomes. Successful outcomes include the diagnosis and treatment of the child's medical problems, restoration of the child's mental health, development of appropriate family relationships, protection of the child from further abuse, and prosecution of the perpetrator. To optimize the possibility of successful outcomes, a collaborative relationship among the disciplines is a necessity.

The disciplines required for this work to proceed successfully include health care, child protection services, victim advocacy, law enforcement, and mental health. In addition, the attorneys who are actively involved in the management of these cases, such as the prosecutor and attorney representing the child, are often an essential component of this collaboration. In each community, specific services contribute to the management of child abuse cases; in particular, service providers who specialize in mental health or family relations issues should be a part of this collaboration.

Each discipline has a specific role in the management of sexual abuse; however, the procedures necessary to accomplish their specific roles are often similar and can overlap. This may lead to interference or unnecessary duplication unless care is taken to maximize collaboration. Effective collaboration among the disciplines, including a clear understanding of roles, expectations, and limitations, will avoid conflict and promote efficiency.

Child protection services (CPS) focuses its investigation on what happened to a child and how to prevent it from happening again to that child and others in the family. To accomplish this, the CPS investigation must include an understanding of the family and the circumstances of the sexual abuse. This includes assessing for high-risk situations such as substance abuse, domestic violence, and history of prior sexual abuse in the family. Interviews of everyone in the family, particularly other children in the family, are an important part of the CPS investigation. CPS often must present this information to the family and juvenile court system to allow appropriate protection.

Law enforcement's role is to undertake a criminal investigation leading to prosecution. Although the criminal investigation focuses on the alleged perpetrator of the abuse, the evidence available from the child victim is critical to a successful prosecution. Law enforcement usually requires a high standard or quality of evidence to effect a successful prosecution. This requires all interviews of children to be forensically appropriate and properly documented.

At the same time, the medical and mental health status of the child must be assessed, not only for clinical purposes, but also for evidentiary purposes. The details of the medical evaluation are explained in the next section. A specific mental health assessment is necessary to determine the degree to which the child's behavior and cognitive abilities have been affected by the abuse. To fully assess the child's mental status, the child must be viewed within the context of the family and the abuse conditions. CPS usually provides much of this information and uses the mental health assessment in determining the requirements for restoration of healthy relationships within the family.

A major challenge for the investigation is obtaining a credible history from a child whose perception of events and ability to describe them are often different than those of an adult. In addition, children are often under pressure to recant their disclosure of abuse. Because there are rarely witnesses to these events and physical evidence is not frequently found, the statements of the child and an effective investigation of the suspected perpetrator become the paramount components of a forensic investigation.

In the midst of a major family disruption there is a vulnerable child from whom specific and accurate information must be elicited. To obtain this essential information effectively, all of the aforementioned disciplines must collaborate. The **Children's Advocacy Center** (CAC) model has been successfully established in many communities in the United States for the multidisciplinary evaluation of child sexual abuse victims. The core service of the CAC model is the collaborative interview; in this interview, a single trained and experienced member of the team interviews the child in an age-appropriate manner using forensically appropriate techniques to elicit essential details of the abuse. With this approach, the child only gives the story once, the interview is appropriately documented by recording or transcript, and all the appropriate disciplines have an opportunity to obtain necessary information. This approach minimizes the emotional trauma to the child and avoids the chance of conflicting information arising from multiple interviews involving different interviewing techniques.

The CAC model also includes medical and mental health components as well as services for the nonoffending members of the family. Ideally, these services are all located at a single site, providing for the child and family a facility that is secure, child friendly, and familiar. However, if all services are not available at a single site, the cornerstone of the CAC model is collaboration among all of these disciplines.

Communities that do not have a CAC model may have a multidisciplinary team that provides a structure for collaborative investigation and management similar to the CAC model, but without the single-site facility and formalized interviewing process. Generally these community-based teams have a lead agency, which may be the mandated child protection agency, a mental health agency, or another agency involved with family issues.

Another model of multidisciplinary teams is the child protection team, which may be based within an institution such as a school or hospital. These teams are composed of the disciplines involved with child abuse within the institution and may include outside agencies. Generally their purposes are to ensure that cases of abuse are appropriately handled within the institution and to advocate for children and families under their care.

Physical Evaluation

The purposes of the medical evaluation are to: (1) identify medical problems that may affect the health of the child or adolescent; (2) identify evidence associated with the sexual abuse; and (3) provide reassurance to the child or adolescent and his or her family regarding his or her medical integrity.

The type and extent of the examination depends upon the nature of the sexual abuse and the circumstances of the examination. If the complete history of the sexual abuse is known, the determination of the proper examination is clear. For older children and adolescents, the history is clearer and therefore the extent of the sexual abuse better understood. In general, the examination is determined by the interval between the last sexual contact and the proposed examination (see **Table 9-1**).

The purpose of the immediate forensic examination is to document evidence of trauma and recover semen for identification of the perpetrator. Therefore, if time has elapsed since the sexual contact such that there is little likelihood of recovery of semen, generally after 72 hours, it is possible to defer the examination to a time and place that best meets the needs of the child.

Whenever possible, a child should be examined by a clinician who is familiar with pediatric and adolescent genital development. This examination should be conducted in a setting that is supportive of the child and nonoffending parents. Staff providing this evaluation should have time and experience that they use to help the child through this new and stressful procedure. In many emergency departments where these children first present,

TABLE 9-1   Medical Evaluations

Time Interval Since Last Sexual Contact	Type of Sexual Contact	Type of Evaluation	Timing of Examination
(up to) 72 hours	Contact with male genitalia or semen	Complete medical evaluation with evidence collection	Immediate
(up to) 72 hours	No contact with male genitalia or semen	Complete medical evaluation	As soon as possible with an experienced examiner
(up to) 72 hours	Any sexual contact involving victim's genitalia, mouth, or anus	Comprehensive medical evaluation	As soon as possible with an experienced examiner

these conditions do not exist; therefore, if the immediate examination is not necessary, the exam can be deferred to a facility where the needs of the child can be better addressed.

The medical evaluation of a child who has been sexually abused starts with a history. The history includes details of the sexual abuse including when it occurred, who was involved, and what parts of the perpetrator's and victim's anatomy were involved. This information may be available through a forensic interview or from adults who accompany the child or adolescent. If this information is not available from either of these sources, focused, nonleading questions should be asked by the examiner with recording of both questions asked and responses of the child or adolescent. Additional details of the abuse involving the context of the abuse should be obtained by trained interviewers (see "Multidisciplinary Issues" earlier in the chapter for a discussion of forensic interviews).

Additional necessary medical history includes symptoms frequently associated with the abuse including anal and vaginal discharge, anal and vaginal bleeding, dysuria, urinary frequency, urinary tract infections, and sore throat. If these symptoms are current and significant, a focused examination should be performed regardless of the other determinates of the examination type. It is also useful to have a history of other injuries involving the genital or anal region because such injuries may result in scars or other findings that could be misinterpreted.

Behavioral symptoms may include phobias, fears, sleep disturbances, changes in eating habits, emotional outbursts, and mood changes. If any of these behavioral symptoms are severe, they should be evaluated as soon as possible by a mental health professional; a mental health evaluation may provide additional forensic information as well as assist the child and family in dealing with the sexual abuse and the secondary symptoms.

A medical history is important to identify specific genital or anal problems including injuries, constipation, or other causes of bleeding or trauma (see **Table 9-2**). In addition, major medical problems that may affect the outcome of the examination should be identified.

Proper preparation of the child and adolescent for the examination is essential for a successful assessment. The preparatory phase of the evaluation is time-consuming but necessary to accomplish a complete examination with a minimum of fear for the child. The parent or other adult who is present to support the child or adolescent during the examination should be fully informed of the procedures in advance. Older children and

TABLE 9-2   Components of the Medical History

Focused details of the abuse	Behavioral changes
Who was involved?	Specific fears
What parts of the body were involved?	Emotional outbursts
When was last sexual contact?	Mood changes
Genital and anal symptoms	Eating habits
Bleeding	Aggressiveness
Discharge	Sleep patterns
Pain	School performance
Dysuria	Past medical history
Constipation	Injuries
Prior injuries	Chronic or recurrent illnesses
	Surgery
	Allergies

adolescents should be given the option of having the procedure without such a support person. The child should be informed in advance regarding the details of the procedure according to their age and ability to understand the information provided. In all cases, the child or adolescent should be told in age-appropriate language that the examination will involve their genitalia and anus, but be reassured that the examination is not expected to cause any pain.

The examination of a child or adolescent includes a general medical examination. This examination will identify conditions such as trauma, which may relate to the sexual abuse. In addition, this part of the examination provides the examiner an opportunity to establish rapport with an anxious child and observe the reaction of the child to a standard examination prior to the more sensitive genital and anal examination. For very young children, particularly those under 3 years of age who may be uncomfortable with any form of examination, the general physical exam may be minimized.

The genital and anal examination on a child or adolescent may include the use of a **colposcope** or other device that permits the magnification and photo documentation of the findings. These devices are an adjunct to the exam but are not necessary if the examiner is familiar with the appearance of the genitalia of children and adolescents at various stages of development and the signs of abuse.

Proper positioning and use of exposure techniques are very important to obtain good visualization of a girl's genitalia. An assistant who is familiar with the examination procedure is usually essential for positioning of the child and handling specimens. Young children who are anxious may be examined on their mother's lap, as illustrated in **Figure 9-1**. Girls whose legs are too short for use of stirrups can assume a frog leg position for good exposure. Older girls and adolescents are usually examined in stirrups. In addition, both males and females may be examined in the knee-chest position (see **Figure 9-2**) to obtain better exposure of the anus as well as an alternative view of the female genitalia. This position is usually necessary to confirm abnormalities of the hymen.

The technique of exposing girls' genitalia involves labia separation and labial traction. Labial separation is simple separation of the labia majora laterally, usually with the thumb or forefinger of the examiner or assistant (see **Figure 9-3**). This permits observation of the labia majora, labia minora, clitoral hood, and possibly the hymen. Initially care should be taken to observe for posterior labial agglutination, which is often friable and easily lysed, causing pain. To get better exposure of the inner aspect of the labia majora, vaginal vestibule, and hymen, labial traction is used. This is accomplished by grasping the labia majora with the thumb and forefinger and gently pulling the labia toward the examiner.

The examiner should first identify the major landmarks on the genitalia of girls. These include the clitoral hood and adjacent labia minora. These structures define the anterior and lateral boundaries of the vaginal vestibule. The posterior border of the vaginal vestibule is the posterior commissure (fourchette). Penetrating trauma usually involves the vaginal vestibule and in particular the navicular fossa, which is the posterior portion of the vaginal vestibule. Using the techniques noted, the examiner can usually easily identify the hymen at the proximal end of the vaginal vestibule.

The hymen changes over time (Berenson, 2002; Berenson, Heger, & Andrews, 1991) and its appearance varies with position and technique (McCann, Wells, Simon, & Voris, 1990). The hymen may be annular, surrounding the hymeneal opening, or there may be no anterior portion of the hymen, which is described as crescent shaped. The hymen may be redundant and evert into the vestibule, making definition difficult in the lithotomy

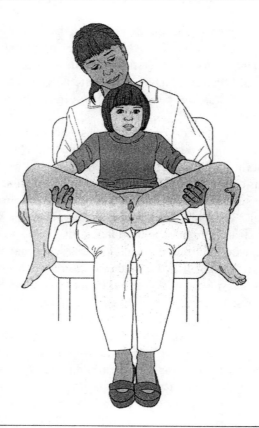

Figure 9-1 Prepubertal child positioned in the lap of accompanying adult for genital and anal examination.

Source: Reece, R. M., & Ludwig, S. (2001). *Child abuse: Medical diagnosis and management.* Philadelphia, PA: Lippincott, Williams & Wilkins.

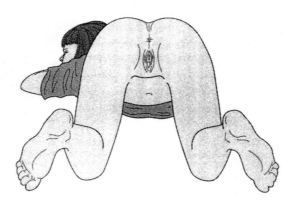

Figure 9-2 Knee-chest position for genital examination of the prepubertal child.

Source: Reece, R. M., & Ludwig, S. (2001). *Child abuse: Medical diagnosis and management.* Philadelphia, PA: Lippincott, Williams & Wilkins.

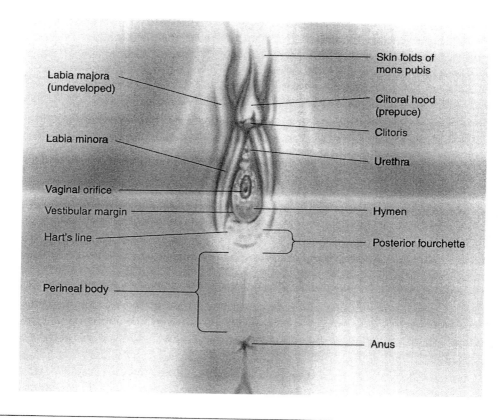

Figure 9-3 The prepubertal vulva.

Source: Heger, A., & Emans, S. J. (1992). *Evaluation of the sexually abused child: Medical textbook and photographic atlas.* New York, NY: Oxford University Press.

position. A young girl's redundant hymen may fold and overlie, resulting in unusual appearances. In young girls, the hymen may appear to cover the entire hymeneal opening, making observation of the hymeneal border difficult. It is essential that the examiner be familiar with the variety of hymeneal appearances through supervised examinations and access to published atlases that provide examples of normal anatomy.

Speculum examination should not be performed in prepubescent girls and usually is not necessary in young adolescents who have not experienced vaginal penetration. If there appears to be intravaginal injury in a prepubescent child or early adolescent, an examination under anesthesia may be indicated with preparation for surgical repair.

An older adolescent or younger adolescent who has experienced vaginal penetration should have a speculum exam if possible to observe for injuries to the vagina and for obtaining appropriate specimens.

Genital findings in girls that are consistent with acute sexual contact include abrasions, ecchymoses, and lacerations (see **Table 9-3**). Abrasions may be small and might be appreciated only with magnification. Lacerations are usually noted in the posterior aspects of the vestibule (navicular fossa) and hymen; using the face of the clock, they are usually found between 3 and 9 o'clock.

Indications of nonacute trauma are less definitive. It is known that acute injuries heal relatively rapidly, and traumatic defects to the hymen can heal with almost complete

TABLE 9-3 Significant Physical Findings

Acute sexual contact
Nonacute contact
*Ecchymoses
Absent hymen
*Presence of semen
Deep hymeneal notches
*Lacerations
Pregnancy
*Abrasions
Minimal hymen
Anal scars
Absence of rugal folds

restitution of normal appearance in some cases. In general it is accepted that a healed defect, referred to as a notch or cleft, that extends through at least 50% of the hymen is an indicator of prior hymeneal injury (Berenson, Chacko, Wiemann, Mishaw, Friedrich, & Grady, 2000). Minimal hymeneal rim is considered significant by some examiners. A minimal hymeneal rim is defined as less than 1 mm of hymen when compared to a previous exam in which the width of the hymen was greater (APSAC, 1995). It is not common to have successive examinations that permit this comparison. The hymen often has irregularities to its margin or edge resulting in bumps or mounds; these are usually variants of normal and are considered abnormal only if they are associated with a deep cleft or notch (> 50% of the hymeneal width).

The examination of the genitalia on the male victim of sexual abuse consists of inspection of the penis, scrotum, and adjacent areas. Significant findings include abrasions, contusions, lacerations, bite marks, and other signs of trauma. In the uncircumcised male it is important to examine under the foreskin.

The anal examination consists of an inspection of the anus to observe for signs of trauma or laxity of the anal sphincter. This examination is ideally accomplished in the knee-chest position, holding the position for up to 2 minutes for complete relaxation; however, many children and adolescents become anxious in that position and alternative positions such as lateral decubitus or prone may be used.

Acute signs of anal trauma include lacerations, ecchymoses, and abrasions. Signs of healed anal trauma may include deep fissures or loss of normal rugal folds. It is important to be aware of smooth, pale areas midline at the 12 and 6 o'clock positions, which may be slightly depressed; this is considered a normal finding in most cases. Anal dilation up to 2 cm has been found in nonabused children (McCann, Voris, Simon, & Wells, 1989); therefore, anal dilation must be greater than 2 cm to be considered significant.

Testing for Sexually Transmitted Diseases

Testing for sexually transmitted diseases (STDs) in prepubescent children depends upon a number of risk factors associated with the abuse. When a child has a discharge, bleeding, or other signs of inflammation associated with the abuse, testing is indicated. Testing would also be indicated if the abuse was perpetrated by a person known to have an STD. Because there is increasing likelihood of an STD in postpubescent victims, it is generally agreed that testing for postpubescent girls is appropriate in most cases with or without symptoms (Hammerschlag & Guillén, 2010; Whaitiri & Kelly, 2010). Many tests are available for chlamydia and gonorrhea. There is concern that nonculture methods such as enzyme-linked immunosorbent assays and nucleic acid amplification tests are not sufficiently specific for forensic purposes in children, resulting in a significant rate of false positive results, thereby invalidating the results. However, for clinical purposes these results may be valid; if nonculture techniques are used, all positive results should be repeated with a culture prior to treatment.

Obtaining vaginal specimens in girls requires good technique to avoid contact with the prepubescent hymen, which is very sensitive to pain. The hymeneal opening is usually only a few millimeters wide, so the use of a small calcium alginate applicator rather than the larger cotton applicator can often permit specimen collection from the vagina with minimal trauma. When the child has a crescent-shaped hymen, inserting the applicator against the anterior surface of the vagina, avoiding the urethra, will usually not induce pain. If it is not possible to obtain a vaginal specimen, collection from the vaginal vestibule may be adequate. Care should be taken in obtaining these specimens because the vestibule is a sensitive area as well. Cervical specimens are not necessary in prepubescent girls. In pubescent and adolescent girls, cervical specimens are desired, but a speculum examination may be difficult, in which case a vaginal specimen may be adequate. A wet mount examination of vaginal secretions will identify bacterial vaginosis and *Trichomonas.*

An examiner might need urethral specimens from a male victim if symptoms or exposure suggest that he could have acquired an STD. Because obtaining these specimens is painful, collection of these specimens should be determined according to clinical indicators and the child's ability to understand and tolerate the procedure.

Serologic testing for HIV, syphilis, and hepatitis C are recommended if the sexual abuse includes potential exposure to those infections. For many families and children, such testing may be reassuring even when the risk of exposure is negligible. These serologic tests should be appropriately timed to ensure that the negative test will not convert at a later point in time. In general, testing for HIV 3 months postexposure should be adequate. However, it is advisable to have baseline testing shortly after the exposure to demonstrate that the child did not acquire the infection prior to the alleged sexual exposure in question.

The most commonly observed STD in young children is genital or venereal warts *(condylomata acuminata)* caused by human papillomavirus (HPV). However, HPV can be transmitted to a child congenitally, by cutaneous contact, or by sexual contact. When this virus is congenitally acquired, it can remain latent for months or years. Mothers carrying HPV in their genital tract may be asymptomatic. Other mothers may have evidence of HPV with an abnormal Pap smear or symptomatic genital warts. Most congenital genital warts will appear within the first 2 years; however, it is believed that it is possible for the virus to remain latent for many years. HPV can also be transmitted from cutaneous warts to the genitalia, particularly prior to a child being toilet trained. These multiple modes of transmission in addition to sexual transmission create a dilemma for forensic evaluations of HPV infections. For children less than 2 years of age, if investigation does not identify other indicators of sexual abuse, it is acceptable to attribute the infection to congenital acquisition. For children over 2 years of age it is more likely that the infection is caused by sexual contact. In children over 5 years of age, it is virtually certain that sexual contact is the mode of transmission.

Many STDs require a clinical assessment to determine their significance to sexual abuse. These include chlamydia, herpes, HIV, and hepatitis B and C. Chlamydia is known to be acquired at the time of birth and has the ability to persist without signs of illness for weeks or months. Therefore, the significance of genital chlamydia infections in the first year of life must be evaluated within the context of possible congenital acquisition. Herpes simplex types 1 and 2 can be found on the genitalia as a result of sexual contact or contamination from other sites, such as the mouth. In cases of contamination, the virus may be autoinoculated from a lesion on the victim or from a lesion on a person providing care for an infant or toddler. Distinguishing between herpes simplex types is not clinically or forensically significant unless you are comparing viruses between the victim and an alleged perpetrator. Because HIV and hepatitis B and C are transmitted in body fluids, as well as congenitally, it is important to understand all of the possible exposures if testing indicates infection possibly related to sexual contact. Congenital infections of herpes simplex, syphilis, and gonorrhea are usually diagnosed in the neonatal period or early infancy with very characteristic manifestations. See **Table 9-4** for the clinical significance of bacterial vaginosis and *Trichomonas*.

Forensic Evidence Collection

Forensic evidence collection should be considered in all cases seen within 72 hours of the last sexual contact. Because the primary focus of this collection is the recovery of semen, this collection is only necessary to pursue if there has been contact with male genitalia. However, in many cases, children are not aware of the extent of genital contact or are unable to initially disclose complete details. Therefore, when the circumstances indicate the possibility of contact with male genitalia, the collection should be undertaken. The collection procedure for a child and adolescent is a modification of the procedures used with adults (see Chapter 18). The modifications are dictated by the circumstances of the abuse and the need to minimize physical and emotional trauma to children. In most cases, sexual abuse of children and adolescents, in contrast to adults, is not a violent physical assault; sexual abuse involves emotional manipulation combined with dominating power and authority. Therefore, findings associated with resistance or injuries to other areas are not usually found.

TABLE 9-4   Significant Sexually Transmitted Infections

Infection	Methods of Infection	Specificity for Sexual Abuse
Gonorrhea	Congenital, sexual	High
Syphilis	Congenital, sexual	High
HIV	Congenital, blood, sexual	Needs clinical assessment
Chlamydia	Congenital, sexual	Needs clinical assessment in first year of life
HPV	Congenital, cutaneous, sexual	Needs clinical assessment
Herpes simplex	Congenital, casual contact, sexual	Needs clinical assessment
Hepatitis B and C	Congenital, blood, sexual	Needs clinical assessment
Trichomonas	Sexual, fomites	Moderate
Bacterial vaginosis	Sexual and other	Low

It is essential to obtain specimens from the appropriate orifice whenever there is reason to think that the sexual contact involved the mouth, anus, or vagina. The technique for obtaining female genital specimens is similar to that used for STD specimens described in the previous section. Specimens from the labia of girls and intergluteal areas may provide additional evidence. Although fluorescence with the Wood's lamp examination is not very specific for semen, such an examination indicates areas of possible semen contamination. In young children who are anxious about the examination, hair plucking and blood sampling can be deferred until such time as it becomes essential for distinguishing the source of positive evidence. With adolescent victims, the full evidence collection procedure may be indicated depending on the circumstances of the abuse and the physical and emotional maturation of the victim.

A study conducted by Christian, Lavelle, DeLong, Loiselle, Brenner, & Joffe (2000) showed that bed linens and clothing are the most likely sources of positive evidence. Because most sexual abuse of children does not involve penetration, it is less likely that semen will be detected from the orifices. In this study of 273 completed examinations, positive evidence from the child's body was found only when the exam was completed within 24 hours of the sexual contact.

Treatment Considerations

Medical Treatment

If a child has experienced serious trauma to the genitalia or anus, surgical repair may be necessary. Proper attention to pain control and risks of infection are a component of management of this type of trauma. Fortunately, superficial trauma will heal without medical or surgical intervention.

Unless exposure to an STD is evident from history or a physical, STD treatment is usually not provided to prepubescent children due to the relatively low risk of infection. In adolescents, treatment for syphilis, gonorrhea, and chlamydia is often given depending upon the extent and likelihood of significant exposure to STDs and the ability to follow up with the adolescent. This treatment would consist of a cephalosporin such as ceftriaxone and a macrolide such as azithromycin, which have the advantage of requiring only a single dose administered at the time of evaluation. In addition, consideration should be given to administering hepatitis B immunization if the child or adolescent has not completed the series. If *Trichomonas* or bacterial vaginosis is of concern, metronidazole may be prescribed. Routine postexposure prophylaxis for HIV infection is generally not recommended due to the potential side effects of the medications. However, if there is good reason to expect exposure to the virus, immediate consultation with an appropriate infectious disease specialist is indicated to determine the best regimen.

Adolescent girls should be evaluated for pregnancy if there is the possibility of contact with semen. This should include an acute evaluation and follow-up in approximately 2 weeks. If an adolescent is not pregnant and is seen within 72 hours of exposure to semen, emergency contraception is an option.

Mental Health Treatment

At the time of disclosure, children must feel supported through a process that they often perceive to be frightening and confusing. Initially, the child needs to understand that disclosure was the correct thing to do. In addition, the investigation needs to be explained in terms and details that prepare, but not overwhelm, the child. Family distress and unfamiliarity with the investigation process may limit family members' ability to provide this support to their child, so the professionals need to ensure that this support is provided. In many communities, sexual assault crisis services are available to support children at this phase of their disclosure and investigation.

The emotional trauma experienced by child and adolescent victims of sexual abuse can have long-lasting effects extending into adulthood. Sexual abuse has been associated with smoking, alcohol and drug abuse, chronic pain, suicide attempts (Felitti et al., 1998), personality disturbance (Wonderlich et al., 2001), depression, and sexual dysfunction (O'Leary, Coohey, & Easton, 2010). In general, the more violent, threatening, and intrusive the abuse, the greater the emotional trauma; however, at initial evaluation, the full extent of the abuse is often not disclosed. It is essential to have a mental health evaluation that addresses the types of trauma the child has experienced, the behaviors of the child, and the current environment of the child. This evaluation will then determine the type and extent of the treatment required.

Family Support

The nonoffending members of the child's family are usually the greatest source of support for child and adolescent victims. However, the family members are also traumatized by these events and need assistance to deal with their concerns as well as those of the child or adolescent.

Because most abuse involves trusted individuals known to the child and family, everyone involved struggles with the issues of deceit and must reexamine the formation of trusting relationships. One approach is to provide nonoffending parents with an understanding of how sexual abuse evolves and progresses. With this information, families are better prepared to move ahead, develop healthy relationships, and protect their children from additional abuse.

In a situation in which the nonoffending parent had an intimate relationship with the offender, it will be important for the nonoffending parent to address his or her anger and ambivalence related to the abuse and disclosure. If the victim is an adolescent, the nonoffending parent may question the complicity of the adolescent in the sexual activity. In these situations, immediate work with nonoffending parents and the adolescent separately is particularly important in order to understand the concerns of all involved.

If the sexual abuse is within the family, there will be changes in the life of the family. This may mean that some members of the family may need to leave the household. This could mean interruption in the financial support for the family or added financial burden. If one child has sexually offended against another child within a family, parents will need to cope with their ambivalence toward the child who committed the offense; this may require placing one child out of the home or providing 24-hour surveillance of the children's activities.

For most families, this is the first time they must deal with law enforcement, child protection, and other aspects of the legal system. Families need to know the roles of each of the agencies and become familiar with the individuals involved with the investigation. The apparent redundancy of investigations, slowness of resolution, and failure to achieve expected outcomes are major frustrations for many families.

Sexual abuse appears to be a multigenerational problem in many families. Often the nonoffending mothers and/or fathers of the child victims were victims themselves. Many of these parents have never adequately dealt with their own victimization. This compromises their ability to help their children. These parents should be seeking treatment for themselves.

Judicial Proceedings

The judicial proceedings for child abuse involve two separate systems, one for the protection of the child and one for the criminal justice system. Both systems are dependent upon the information and evidence collected during the assessment of a child. The two systems may use the information and evidence somewhat differently and impose different standards on the verifiability of this information and evidence.

The judicial system for child protection proceeds in either a family or juvenile court. Compelling, complete, accurate, and verifiable information is necessary to arrive at decisions that reflect the best interests of the child. This information is presented by an attorney who represents the investigating agency (CPS), as well as an attorney who represents the child. The latter may represent the child as a *guardian ad litem*. A judge is usually the individual who makes decisions based on material presented in hearings. In most states these decisions are made on the basis of the preponderance of the evidence. These decisions affect the immediate life of the child, so they must be accomplished over a short period of time, usually involving weeks and months. Once a child is under the custody of the state for a child abuse problem, there will be periodic hearings until a permanency plan is activated. This plan may include reunification with the child's family of birth or adoption. Although all child protection systems are determined by individual state statutes, the federal government imposes expectations of such systems through regulations accompanying federal funding sources.

The criminal court system depends upon the same information and evidence as applies to the child protection courts, but in this case the information is used to prevent the offender from committing additional abusive acts. The evidence is presented by a prosecuting attorney who must convince a jury or judge beyond a reasonable doubt that the offender committed the crime. In general, conviction in the criminal court system requires a higher standard of verifiable evidence than applies in the child protection court. Usually the criminal court proceedings occur months or years after the allegations of abuse are made. In many cases when the evidence is strong, the defendant will agree to a plea arrangement, which eliminates the need for a court trial. The defendant does not contest the evidence and receives a sentence that is less harsh than if convicted in a trial. Because a child's testimony in these trials is often very traumatic, it may be in the best interests of the child not to testify when a plea arrangement can be made.

In either court system it is essential for witnesses to be adequately prepared by the attorney who subpoenas them. This preparation should include a clear understanding of the questions to be asked and the anticipated answers. The attorney should also anticipate the questions that will come from the other parties at the hearing or trial. These questions are often the ones that make the witness most vulnerable to presenting evidence and information in a confusing and contradictory manner. However, a well-prepared witness will understand the basic aspects of his or her testimony and will be able to present the basic testimony concisely and cogently to all parties.

Summary

Sexual abuse is a potentially devastating experience for children, adolescents, and their families. The forensic clinician is an important part of the team of professionals investigating the abuse and assisting the children and families to recover and prevent reoccurrence of abuse. This will be accomplished when the clinician works collaboratively with the team and is sensitive to the needs of the child.

The role of the forensic clinician is to obtain history, make physical observations, document findings, obtain forensic specimens, address medical concerns, assess the significance of evidence, and ensure that the child and family have access to other members of the team. The forensic clinician who is evaluating children must be familiar with child and adolescent physical and emotional development. Each child and adolescent presents with unique circumstances that must be evaluated in the context of his or her baseline development. Correct interpretation of observations and findings depends upon an understanding of the dynamics of physical and emotional development.

The goal of a forensic evaluation is to provide convincing information that will contribute to the safety of an individual child and decrease the risks that the perpetrator of abuse can harm other children. This must be performed in a manner that will minimize trauma to the child or adolescent and provide maximum support for nonoffending family members. This can be accomplished by a well-informed clinician who is comfortable with child and adolescent concerns and has knowledge and experience with the components of the evaluation.

The role of the forensic nurse in the evaluation of child sexual abuse is evolving. With sufficient training and experience, the forensic nurse may be the primary examiner and evaluator of the child. In other situations, the nurse may serve as a consultant to a primary pediatric healthcare provider; in this role the forensic nurse will help to guide the inexperienced examiner through an unfamiliar, complex, and detailed examination. The forensic nurse may also be a resource for nonhealthcare investigators who need the forensic medical expertise to understand and interpret the results of a sexual abuse evaluation.

 QUESTIONS FOR DISCUSSION

1. How does sexual abuse of a child or adolescent differ from the sexual assault of an adult?
2. What is the difference between statutory rape, sexual abuse, and sexual assault?
3. What are the special considerations in evaluating an adolescent victim of sexual abuse or rape?
4. How do children and adolescents who are victims of sexual abuse usually present in the healthcare setting?
5. What is the most effective method of obtaining a full disclosure of sexual abuse from a child?
6. Which disciplines are involved with the management of sexual abuse?
7. What determines the extent of a physical examination in a sexually abused child?
8. What are the components of the sexual abuse examination?
9. What techniques assist visualization of girls' genitalia?

10. What are some actions that can be taken during the examination of a child or adolescent victim of sexual abuse or sexual assault to avoid retraumatization?
11. What are the usual findings in acute and nonacute sexual contact?
12. What determines the need for STD testing?
13. When should forensic evidence collection be performed?
14. What are the judicial proceedings that may follow a physical examination?
15. What factors do you think might account for the recent rise in the reported rates of sexual assault?
16. What conditions in an environment pose a risk for the sexual abuse of a child or adolescent?

REFERENCES

American Professional Society on the Abuse of Children. (1995). *APSAC practice guidelines: Descriptive terminology in child sexual abuse medical evaluations.* Charleston, SC: Author.

Berenson, A. B., Chacko, M., Wiemann, C., Mishaw, C. O., Friedrich, W. N., & Grady, J. J. (2000). A case-control study of anatomic changes resulting from sexual abuse. *American Journal of Obstetrics and Gynecology, 182*(4), 820–834.

Berenson, A. B., Heger, A., & Andrews, S. (1991). Appearance of the hymen in newborns. *Pediatrics, 87*(4), 458–465.

Christian, C. W., Lavelle, J. D., DeLong, A. R., Loiselle, J., Brenner, L., & Joffe, M. (2000). Forensic evidence findings in prepubertal victims of sexual abuse. *Pediatrics, 106*(1), 100–104.

Connecticut Department of Public Health. (2010). *Voices of Connecticut youth 2003.* Hartford, CT: Author.

Felitti, V. J., Anda, R. F., Nordenberg, D., Williamson, D. F., Spitz, A. M., Edwards, … Marks, J. S. (1998). Relationship of childhood abuse and household dysfunction to many of the leading causes of death in adults. *American Journal of Preventive Medicine, 14*(4), 245–258.

Finkelhor, D. (1984). *Child sexual abuse: New theory and research.* New York, NY: Free Press.

Finkelhor, D. (1994). Current information on the scope and nature of child sexual abuse. In R. Behaman (Ed.), *Sexual abuse of children. The future of children* (pp. 31–69). Los Altos, CA: David and Lucielle Packard Foundation.

Friedrich, W. N., Fisher, J., Broughton, D., Houston, M., & Shafran, C. R. (1998). Normative sexual behavior in children: A contemporary sample. *Pediatrics, 101,* e9.

Hammerschlag, M. R., & Guillén, C. D. (2010). Medical and legal implications of testing for sexually transmitted infections in children. *Clinical Microbiology Reviews, 23*(3), 493–506.

McCann, J., Voris, J., Simon, M., & Wells, R. (1989). Perianal findings in prepubertal children selected for nonabuse: A descriptive study. *Child Abuse and Neglect, 13,* 179–193.

McCann, J., Wells, R., Simon, M., & Voris, J. (1990). Genital findings in prepubertal girls selected for nonabuse: A descriptive study. *Pediatrics, 86*(3), 428–439.

O'Leary, P., Coohey, C., & Easton, S. D. (2010). The effect of severe child sexual abuse and disclosure on mental health during adulthood. *Journal of Child Sex Abuse, 19*(3), 275–289.

U.S. Department of Health and Human Services, Administration for Children and Families. (2010). *Child maltreatment 2008.* Washington, DC: Author.

Whaitiri, S., & Kelly, P. (2010, June 3). Genital gonorrhoea in children: Determining the source and mode of infection. *Archives of Disease in Childhood, 19*(3), 307–310.

Wonderlich, S. A., Ross, D., Crosby, R. D., Mitchell, J. E., Thompson, K., Smyth … Jones-Paxton, M. (2001). Sexual trauma and personality. *Journal of Personality Disorders, 15*(6), 496–504.

Wurtele, S. K., & Miller-Perrin, C. L. (1992). *Understanding child sexual abuse.* Lincoln: University of Nebraska Press.

SUGGESTED FURTHER READING

Cantón-Cortés, D., & Cantón, J. (2010, June 1). Coping with child sexual abuse among college students and post-traumatic stress disorder: The role of continuity of abuse and relationship with the perpetrator. *Child Abuse and Neglect, 34*(7), 496–506.

Jones, D. J., Runyan, D. K., Lewis, T., Litrownik, A. J., Black, M. M., Wiley, T., ... Nagin, D. S. (2010). Trajectories of childhood sexual abuse and early adolescent HIV/AIDS risk behaviors: The role of other maltreatment, witnessed violence, and child gender. *Journal of Clinical Child and Adolescent Psychology, 39*(5), 667–680.

Lalor, K., & McElvaney, R. (2010, August 2). Child sexual abuse, links to later sexual exploitation/high-risk sexual behavior, and prevention/treatment programs. *Trauma Violence Abuse, 11,* 159–177.

Reese-Weber, M., & Smith, D. M. (2010). Outcomes of child sexual abuse as predictors of later sexual victimization. *Journal of Interpersonal Violence, 26*(9), 1884–1905.

Scribano, P. V., Hornor, G., Rhoda, D., Curran, S., & Stevens, J. (2010). Multi-informant assessment of anxiety regarding ano-genital examinations for suspected child sexual abuse (CSA). *Child Abuse and Neglect, 34*(8), 602–609.

Taylor, J. E., & Harvey, S. T. (2010). A meta-analysis of the effects of psychotherapy with adults sexually abused in childhood. *Clinical Psychology Reviews, 30*(6), 749–767.

Turner, H. A., Finkelhor, D., Ormrod, R., & Hamby, S. L. (2010). Infant victimization in a nationally representative sample. *Pediatrics, 126*(1), 44–52.

Vrabel, K. R., Hoffart, A., Rø, O., Martinsen, E. W., & Rosenvinge, J. H. (2010). Co-occurrence of avoidant personality disorder and child sexual abuse predicts poor outcome in long-standing eating disorder. *Journal of Abnormal Psychology, 119*(3), 623–629.

Walsh, K., Rassafiani, M., Mathews, B., Farrell, A., & Butler, D. (2010). Teachers' attitudes toward reporting child sexual abuse: Problems with existing research leading to new scale development. *Journal of Child Sex Abuse, 19*(3), 310–336.

Yampolsky, L., Lev-Wiesel, R., & Ben-Zion, I. Z. (2010). Child sexual abuse: Is it a risk factor for pregnancy? *Journal of Advanced Nursing, 66*(9), 2025–2037.

CHAPTER 10

Crimes Against the Elderly

Tracey Creegan Hammer and Rita M. Hammer

Abuse of elders, very often of a criminal nature, is rapidly becoming a problem of significant proportions in the United States, particularly as the number of individuals experiencing increased longevity grows. A contributing variable that affects the rise in abusive or criminal behaviors toward this vulnerable group is that while individuals may be living longer, independent control of their physical, psychological, or financial state does not always accompany the extended life span. Government statistics estimate that between 1 million and 2 million older citizens are mistreated in some way, either physically through direct injury or neglect, psychologically through harassment or intimidation, or financially through direct theft or exploitation of resources (National Center on Elder Abuse, 2005). This chapter will organize information about this issue according to the types of abuse, the scope of the problem, legal protection for vulnerable elders, profile of the abusers, the profile of the abused, venues of abuse, and intervention.

CHAPTER FOCUS

» Types of Elder Abuse
» Scope of the Problem
» Legal Protection

» The Abusers and the Abused
» The Role of the Forensic Nurse
» The Consequences of Abuse

KEY TERMS

» abuse
» fiduciary
» guardianship
» mistreatment
» neglect

» ombudsman
» power of attorney
» protective services

Types of Abuse

Definitions of elder **abuse**, neglect, and exploitation are defined by state laws and thus vary considerably from state to state. The original descriptions of elder abuse emanated from the federal government as guidelines through the Older Americans Act first enacted in 2006 (Older Americans Act, 2006). In general, elder abuse is considered the intentional infliction of harm or the creation of a situation that could result in harm upon a vulnerable elder, frequently by someone entrusted with the care and welfare of the elder. The types of abuse are physical, including sexual abuse, emotional abuse, financial exploitation, abandonment, neglect, and self-neglect (NCEA, 2007).

Physical Abuse

Physical abuse is any act of physical violence that results in pain, injury, or impairment of the victim. Thus, in addition to direct assaults such as hitting, shoving, burning, kicking, etc., the unwarranted forceful use of physical or chemical restraints, forced feedings, inappropriate medication administration, and physical punishment are included. Assessment of elders for signs of physical abuse can be difficult since the elderly are prone to falls, bumps, and other mishaps that could leave them with suspicious physical signs. In addition to obvious signs that could give rise to suspicion such as bruises, fractures, wounds, welts, etc., the forensic nurse should be cognizant of more subtle signs such as absent or broken eyeglasses or dentures, fearful behavior by the victim, an unwillingness by a caretaker to allow the elder to be interviewed alone, and of course statements by the elder indicating that physical abuse had taken place.

Sexual Abuse

Sexual abuse of an elder is the nonconsensual sexual contact of any kind with an elder as well as sexual contact with an elder considered incapable of consent (NCEA, 2007). Elders are more subject to trauma during an assault because of the fragility of tissues resulting from estrogen loss that occurs with aging. There is little data available regarding the sexual abuse of the elderly—even less than the data associated with general physical abuse. Elders are frequently too weak and frail to fight off advances or assaults and then are frequently too ashamed or frightened to report the assault. In other situations, they are simply unable to communicate what happened to them. Sexual assault of individuals over the age of 65 is less frequently reported than that of those under the age of 65. It has been shown that healthcare professionals are not as predisposed to suspect sexual abuse in the elderly as in younger people and thus miss important cues (Burgess, Hanrahan, & Baker, 2005). In addition, shame and embarrassment on the part of the victim may make an elderly person more reluctant to report sexual abuse than to report abuse in general.

Emotional or Psychological Abuse

Emotional or psychological abuse includes the intentional infliction of distress, anguish, or fear through verbal or behavioral actions directed at the victim (NCEA, 2007). These include threats, harassment, and attempts to humiliate or intimidate the elder. There is a wide range of activities that are considered abusive, such as withholding food or medication as punishment, verbal threats, isolating the victim, and humiliation in front of others. This type of abuse can be the most difficult to identify, since the resulting behavior by the elder is frequently subjective rather than objectively observed and can be easily missed during assessment procedures. As always, reports or even hints by the elder that he or she is being abused should raise an immediate red flag for the forensic nurse and warrants further investigation, especially without the suspected perpetrator present. The nurse should be particularly astute when evaluating discrepancies in the reports from the elder versus the caregiver.

Financial Exploitation

Financial exploitation includes the misuse, either inappropriately or illegally, of the elder's resources, which can include such things as cash, valuable belongings, retirement funds,

TABLE 10-1   Signs of Financial Abuse

- Frequent expensive gifts from elder to caregiver
- Elder's personal belongings, papers, credit cards missing
- Numerous unpaid bills
- A recent will when elder seems incapable of writing a will
- Caregiver's name added to a bank account
- Elder is unaware of monthly income
- Elder signs for a loan
- Frequent checks made out to Cash
- Unusual activity in bank account
- Irregularities on tax return
- Elder unaware of the reason for an appointment with a banker or attorney
- Caregiver's refusal to spend money on the elder
- Signatures on checks or legal documents that do not resemble the elder's signature

checking accounts, and signatures on documents not understood by the elder (NCEA, 2007). See **Table 10-1**. Financial exploitation can be as minor as helping one's self to food purchased for the elder or more serious, such as the appropriation of things of much greater value. Indeed there is more than one instance on record of an elder signing over his/her home and/or fortune to a trusted caregiver or companion. Another example is the inappropriate sale of financial products such as insurance or annuities to vulnerable elders (Passaro, 2006). These cases are currently handled individually since no clear regulations regarding exploitative sale of such products exists. In some states there have been recent efforts to combat financial exploitation by initiating class action suits against the perpetrators. In the past, Congress has convened hearings into deceptive practices in the magazine and sweepstakes industries that target the elderly, resulting in the loss of millions of dollars annually to this age group.

CASE STUDY 10.1

Myrtle

Myrtle was in her 90s and homebound when discovered by Adult Protective Services. Her only child made a visit from out of state and found her mother in poor condition. Jim, a distant relative in his 40s, was residing in Myrtle's home. Jim claimed to be caring for Myrtle, but the home was cluttered and dirty and the food on hand sparse. Myrtle stated that she wanted to be left alone and that her daughter was a troublemaker who was after her money. On follow-up visits, Myrtle was observed to be sitting in the same filthy robe and slippers, her hair greasy and her bed linens soiled. A guardian was appointed and attempted to arrange home care, but due to Jim's interference and Myrtle's unwillingness to cooperate, services could not be provided. On the final attempt, a visiting nurse found Jim passed out on the lawn. Further investigation revealed that Jim was obtaining narcotics in Myrtle's name and that her investments had been cashed out and her bank accounts emptied. Myrtle was moved to an assisted living facility and for the first few weeks was tearful and disoriented, crying frequently and requesting to be taken home. Eventually, Myrtle's distress abated and she began to ask about her daughter. Three months after her placement, Myrtle had no recollection of Jim and was thriving. She had become an active participant in social activities and was enjoying all that the facility had to offer. Her daughter continued to visit from out of state, enjoying access that Jim had discouraged. Myrtle spent the next several years in good health and could not recall ever having been skeptical of her daughter's intentions. Jim was never heard from again. The significant monies that disappeared while Jim was living with Myrtle were not able to be recovered, and Myrtle was left with tax liabilities, interest, and penalties to pay.

Neglect

Neglect of an elder is the intentional refusal or failure of a caregiver to fulfill the obligations or duties for an elder in his or her care (NCEA, 2007). Such things as failure to seek medical attention when indicated (assuming the caretaker has the ability to recognize the indication), failure to provide adequate food, clothing, and shelter and failure to assist with or provide medications needed by the elder constitute neglect. Often these situations go unnoticed for extended periods until such time as another individual has cause to enter into the elder's environment for some reason. Unfortunately by the time this occurs the elder may have suffered irreparable harm.

Abandonment

The desertion of an elder by someone responsible for his or her care is called abandonment (NCEA, 2007). The caregiver could be a family member with whom the elder resides or a nonfamily member hired to care for the elder. Leaving a totally dependent elder alone for even a short period of time could place him/her in danger and thus can be considered abandonment. A caregiver, hired through an agency to care for an elder, who either leaves early or fails to arrive on schedule without notice can be charged with abandonment.

Self-Neglect

Self-neglect is behavior by an elder that threatens his or her health, well-being, or life. The self-inflicted neglect can include many of the behaviors described as intentional neglect by a caretaker. The elder may not maintain adequate hygiene, nutrition, sleep, or even basic safety measures to protect against injury or possible death. Some elders refuse assistance even when they are well aware of their deficiencies of care. These are difficult situations that raise ethical questions related to an individual's right to self-determination and freedom. Frequently the elder is in some degree of mental and physical decline and may need referral to Adult Protective Services (APS).

The Scope of the Problem

The numbers of elder abuse cases reported are undoubtedly an underestimate of the extent of the problem since there is no nationally recognized standard by which to gauge, report, and compile data on actual cases. It is thus difficult to accurately assess the scope of the problem and consequently to address it as vigorously and adequately as the issue merits. The lack of standardization for even defining the problem places increased importance on nurses to view each and every encounter with a vulnerable senior through a forensic lens. Lack of agreement and standardization further creates a major impediment to the recognition and reporting of abuse and inhibits the research aimed at implementing appropriate interventions to address the problem. A systematic review of multiple databases of studies on elder abuse confirms that although one in four vulnerable elders is at risk for abuse, a very small percentage of cases are actually reported (Cooper, Selwood, & Livingston, 2008). Among the many reasons for underreporting cited by these investigators is an easily corrected one. Elders and caregivers are not routinely asked about abuse, and if they were, more cases would be detected. Other reasons include the victim's fear of reprisal, shame, or an unwillingness to accuse a caretaker, who is frequently also a relative. A reversal or diminution of the underreporting phenomenon might allow for increased recognition of when and under what circumstances this population is at risk for or is actually being abused. Studies suggest that physical abuse is the form of abuse least frequently reported, while psychological abuse is the most frequently reported, with financial abuse next. Other studies cite neglect as the most frequently observed type of abuse followed by psychological abuse and then financial exploitation, with physical and sexual abuse occurring the least frequently (Cohen, Levin, Gagin, & Gideon, 2007). In 1998, Congress mandated a study to more accurately estimate the size and scope of the problem (National Center on Elder Abuse, 1998). This study, a random sampling of 20 counties and utilizing information on cases from the APS agencies, as well as interviews within the venues where elders are found, estimated that 449,924 persons ages 60 and older living in domestic settings were abused, neglected, or exploited in the United States in the year of the report. Of the total number, only 70,942 cases were reported to APS. Thus for every reported case, 378,982 went unreported (National Center on Elder Abuse, 1998). This underreporting did not include the numbers of elders residing in private homes who may not have been able to venture out into the community venues where the other elders were interviewed. Thus it can be assumed, that indeed, many other community-dwelling elders may be subject to underreported abuse.

Legal Protection

The legal system operates in two significant ways to protect the elderly. All 50 states within the United States have laws that protect the elderly from **mistreatment**, and healthcare providers in most states are governed by mandatory reporting laws for confirmed cases of abuse as well (Brody, Acker, & Logan, 2001). However there is no specific federal statute that targets the prevention of mistreatment of the elderly as there exists for victims of child abuse and domestic violence (Sellas & Krouse, 2009). A **protective services** system for the elderly was established in 1974 under Title XX of the Social Security Act. These services operate on the state level, and various degrees of service may be mandated by each of the 50 states and the District of Columbia. In addition, 43 states have mandatory reporting laws for suspected cases of abuse. Thus forensic nurses must research and identify the various specific provisions of individual clinical practice within their state since these can be quite different from state to state. The laws provide the framework within which healthcare professionals can report suspected cases of abuse without fear of adverse consequences. Yet the reporting of such incidents remains low considering the estimates of its occurrence. In a survey of primary care physicians, it was found that this group initiated only 2% of the reports of elder abuse despite having frequent contact with their patients—an average of five times per year (Kennedy, 2005)—and despite a long-standing recommendation by the American Medical Association that physicians routinely question elders about abuse or neglect (AMA, 1992). Reasons cited by the physicians included lack of awareness of the regulations and procedures regarding reporting, insufficient evidence to support an allegation, subtle signs, denial by the patient, and a lack of knowledge of how to access available community resources (Kennedy). Other reasons for underreporting include the inability of some victims to communicate, the presence of mental illness or dementia, non-English speaking elders, and infrequency of contact with the healthcare community by some elders. Nurses and social workers are the most frequent reporters. As mandated reporters, nurses are guaranteed immunity from liability for reports rendered in good faith. Every report will initiate an investigation into the accusation by the appropriate social service agency charged with enforcing the laws protecting elders from abuse. Failure to report may result in criminal or civil charges against the nurse and can also precipitate malpractice procedures (Brent, 2001). In some circumstances the abuse involves criminal activity and the issues around lack of standardization and reporting impacts these situations as well. The ability to pursue civil and criminal charges against perpetrators of elder abuse is also hampered by a lack of resources to conduct the research needed to address all aspects of the problem.

CASE STUDY 10.2

Gertrude

Gertrude was 83 years old when a pattern of being brought to the hospital by her daughters with dehydration and low blood sugar prompted a report to Adult Protective Services. APS found Gertrude's home to be in deplorable condition. Her daughters, in their 50s, appeared to have a hoarding disorder. After APS arranged for some clearing of clutter and the daughters agreed to enroll Gertrude in adult day care, the case was closed, only to be reported again the following year. When APS revisited, the home was in worse condition than before. Many rooms were impassable, and a leaking refrigerator was causing rot and slippery floors. Again, APS arranged to clear clutter. Gertrude's daughters stated that they were caring for Gertrude as best they could, cooking breakfast every morning, sending her to day care when she was willing to go, and fixing dinner every night. A guardian was appointed for Gertrude, and home care sought, but services could not be provided due to the condition of the home. Gertrude's daughters resisted any further cleaning or clearing of clutter, insisting that Gertrude wanted to hold onto every item. Gertrude herself said very little, but knew that she did not want to go to a nursing home. After several more trips to the hospital, however, Gertrude was placed in a nursing facility. Later, it was discovered that most of the kitchen appliances and the bathtub were not operational—though the daughters had reported cooking and bathing—and Gertrude's bed was infested with insects burrowed into the underside of her mattress. Gertrude had been complaining about being bitten, but her daughters thought that she had been imagining it. Gertrude's condition improved in the nursing facility. A month after placement, when asked about going home, she responded that it might be better if she stayed in the nursing home. Her daughters insisted that she desperately wanted to return home, but Gertrude never conveyed that desire to anyone else involved in her case.

Guardianship

In the event that an elder is deemed to lack the mental capacity to conduct his or her affairs in a safe and timely manner, a guardian may be appointed by the courts to manage the elder's personal, medical, and/or financial affairs. The guardian may be made responsible for such things as paying bills, managing real property, managing investments, arranging medical care, arranging home health care, and arranging placement in assisted living or skilled nursing facilities. A guardian may be needed in situations where there are not family members or friends available to provide informal assistance, in situations where family members want to assist but are unable to agree on a plan of action, and in situations where family members or friends are found to be assisting but the assistance being provided is either inadequate or exploitative. Although laws vary from state to state, generally almost any interested party may petition the courts to request the appointment of a guardian. Frequently, it is hospital and nursing home caseworkers (social workers or nurses) who initiate **guardianship** proceedings, in connection with ensuring safe discharge plans or gaining approval or consent for courses of treatment for the elder.

Power of Attorney

A **power of attorney** is an authorization to act on behalf of another person that may be granted by any adult who has mental capacity at the time of making the designation and who is acting freely and of his or her own volition and not under any undue influence or duress. An elder may wish to designate a trusted family member or friend as a power of attorney either because he or she requires immediate assistance with managing his or her affairs or because he or she wants to be prepared in the event that such assistance is required in the future. Powers of attorney may be limited or general in nature and may be designated so as to take effect immediately or at a certain time in the future. In the context of the elderly, powers of attorney are more likely to be broad and unlimited in duration, but will automatically terminate upon death. If a power of attorney states that it will remain effective after the grantor becomes incapacitated, it is called a durable power of attorney. Depending upon the jurisdiction and manner in which a power of attorney is to be used, the authority to make healthcare decisions may be included—encompassing the authority to make decisions regarding life support if necessary—or a more specific grant of authority, such as a designation of healthcare representative or agent, may be required or preferred. Unlike the actions of a guardian, which are overseen by a court, the actions of a person acting under a power of attorney or healthcare designation are undertaken entirely in private, and are not overseen by any authority. Therefore, powers of attorney are easily abused, and the ongoing trustworthiness and reliability of the person granted a power of attorney is of enormous importance.

Elder Abuse in Nursing Homes

Sad as it may seem to contemplate, elder abuse does occur within settings designed to provide competent, safe, respectful care for residents under the direction and supervision of healthcare professionals. Estimates of the numbers of residents residing in licensed nursing homes includes 1.6 million, with another 1 million in residential care facilities such as group homes, adult congregate living facilities, assisted living facilities, and rest homes (Cooper et al., 2008). Because these residents suffer from various chronic illnesses as well as in some cases developmental disabilities, they are particularly vulnerable. Further, between 40% and 60% of these residents have some degree of cognitive impairment such as Alzheimer's disease or other forms of dementia. In addition, only 12–13% of the residents have spouses residing with them and many have no close relative nearby to act as advocates for them.

As is the case of abuse of elders in private settings, the estimates of numbers of abused elders residing in residential care facilities is grossly underreported, for many of the same reasons. However, anecdotal evidence and informal studies suggest that the problem is widespread but no systematic study of prevalence has been conducted (Lauman, Leitsch, & Waite, 2008).

Elder abuse in institutional settings has been the target of congressional and federal inquiries for many years resulting in some positive actions aimed at addressing the issue. The Institute of Medicine produced guidelines for preventing elder abuse in institutional settings, the Joint Commission on the Accreditation of Healthcare Organizations developed standards for identification and management of elder abuse in medical facilities, and the Department of Health and Human Services created the Elder Abuse Task Force, which not only addresses issues of identification, treatment, and prevention of abuse, but also stipulates a plan for national research and data collection (Aravanis et al., 1993). In 1991 a National Institute on Elder Abuse was established through the Administration on Aging. The Patient Protection and Affordable Care Act of 2010 provides two new measures that will help to protect the elderly from criminal acts of abuse. The Elder Justice Act focuses on the development of measures designed to intervene and prosecute cases of abuse and exploitation. The Patient Safety Abuse Prevention Act focuses on protecting residents of nursing homes including mandating criminal background checks for those seeking to work in long-term care facilities (Alford, 2011).

Types of abuse observed in nursing homes include physical abuse such as excessive use of physical restraints, pushing, shoving, slapping, pinching, or kicking. Verbal and psychological abuse such as yelling, swearing, or insulting the resident occurs along with verbal threats to withhold food or to restrict activity. Isolation of the resident, lack of allowance of adequate time for eating or assistance with meals, refusal to answer calls for assistance, removing or turning off the resident's call light, failure to remove the resident from soiled clothing, refusal to toilet the resident or to ambulate him or her as prescribed along with the denial of physical therapeutic necessities such as range of motion exercises contributes to the abusive existence that some residents must endure. The very fact of their admittance to an extended care facility suggests that they may be even less able to defend themselves than elders being cared for at home. Abusive caretakers often do not understand the behavioral aspects of impaired residents nor do they have a grasp of the range of limitations imposed upon residents because of the aging process. Thus, occasionally a caretaker will become angry at a resident, believing that problematic behavior exhibited by the resident is intentional, in some cases mean spirited. Consequently the caretaker might view his or her own unacceptable behavior as justifiable retaliation (see **Table 10-2**). This often leads to a cycle of abusive care, other staff members taking their cues from one another, and thus branding the resident and increasing the degree of vulnerability. There are many strategies that can be employed in institutional settings aimed at reducing mistreatment at the hands of staff members. Some of these strategies relate to the staff themselves but others call for involvement of the administration, family members, and utilization of volunteers within the facility. (see **Table 10-3**). Agencies that provide information about institutional abuse

TABLE 10-2   Risk Factors for the Potential Abuse of Elders in Institutional Settings

- Unsympathetic or negative attitudes by staff
- Chronic staffing problems
- Lack of administrative oversight
- Staff burnout
- Stressful working conditions
- Inadequate preparation of staff regarding the phenomenon of aging
- Insufficient recognition of staff for their work
- Signatures on checks or legal documents that do not resemble the elder's signature

TABLE 10-3   Protective Factors for Residents in Institutional Settings

- Effective monitoring systems in place
- Clear and enforceable institutional policies and procedures for care of residents
- Systematic education regarding elder abuse for employees
- Clear understanding by administration on the correct use of durable power of attorney
- Encouragement of family involvement in care of resident
- Noticeable presence of volunteers, recreational personnel, and social workers
- Careful screening of personnel prior to employment
- Recognition of staff for their contributions to a safe and caring environment
- System for promoting pride and respect for the work of the staff

and neglect include state licensure and certification agencies, state Medicare and Medicaid fraud and abuse agencies, long-term care **ombudsman** programs (established under the Older Americans Act), state protective services programs, and nurse aid registries.

The Abusers

Family Members

It is well recognized that the most frequent perpetrator of abuse against the elderly is more than likely someone entrusted with the care of the victim, and this often turns out to be a family member. Almost one third of the abusers are the victims' spouses (Koenig & DeGuerre, 2005). The reasons for the abusive actions of the perpetrator are many and varied. The abuser may be the primary caregiver and may be stressed beyond her ability to cope not only with the care of the victim but often with outside pressures and stresses that diminish her ability to act patiently and empathically with the elder in her care. In some cases there is a history of social, mental, and/or legal problems that includes substance abuse and other dysfunctional behaviors. In other situations financial pressures cause the abuser to exploit the elder in the belief that the victim is not cognizant of the abuse or exploitation. At other times the abuser and the abused are mutually aware of the abusive behaviors but the abused feels helpless to protest and reluctant to confide in an individual who might be in a position to intervene. These situations can pose considerable difficulty to identify and prosecute because the victim may be confused or unable to remember the underlying facts; may be reluctant to report the incident or to cooperate with an investigation because she or he is too ashamed of what occurred; may desire to treat the abuse

TABLE 10-4   Risk Factors for the Potential to Abuse

- Current diagnosis of mental illness
- Current abuse of alcohol or other substance
- High levels of general hostility or anger
- Poor or inadequate preparation for caregiving responsibilities
- Inadequate coping skills
- High financial and emotional dependence upon a vulnerable elder
- Lack of social or community support for caregiver responsibilities
- Compounding personal, marital, or financial pressures
- History of strained relationship with the elder

as a family matter; or, out of compassion and grief, might not want to see the relative, especially if it is a child, prosecuted and punished. In other cases the victim is intimidated by the family member and fears retaliation if he or she speaks up. Often the elder victim is alone with a caregiver and susceptible to financial crimes without even knowing that they have been committed. In other cases, the caregiver is quite blatant about the financial abuse, which can involve large sums of money but more frequently involves only a small fixed income of the elder.

There are some theories that seek to explain the dynamics that cause a perpetrator to abuse a victim (see **Table 10-4**). One holds that violence toward elders is related to family violence and is learned behavior that arises from the perpetrator having witnessed the behavior or having been a victim himself of family violence, indeed sometimes at the hands of the very victim he is abusing. A second theory describes a psychopathology present in the perpetrator that may be compounded by alcoholism or other substance dependence and severe emotional or mental health problems. Others describe a sense of resentment that arises if the perpetrator is dependent on the victim for some reason such as lack of financial resources or homelessness. This resentment, when coupled with other factors, may give rise to abusive behaviors (Laumann et al., 2008). Stress, in addition to that created by being cast in the role of caretaker, such as economic problems, marital problems, or additional health issues, may all act in concert to predispose the perpetrator to abusive actions. Given the complexity of the issue of elder abuse, no one theory can explain the behavior of the abuser or of the abused. A unifying theoretical model through which testing of concepts and constructs could be effected is a current goal of researchers in the field.

CASE STUDY 10.3

Dot

After a brief hospitalization, Dot, in her 80s, was referred to a visiting nurse association for follow-up care. Dot was weak and confined to bed, and her sister, Helen, in whose home she lived, was caring for her. The visiting nurse observed Helen to be inappropriate during caregiving. Helen would yank Dot by the hair in order to lift her head or change her position, and would yell at her and leave her unattended for lengthy periods of time. Dot was nonverbal due to dementia. Helen denied being inappropriate with Dot and stated that she loved her sister more than anything in the world.

A guardian was appointed for Dot for the limited purpose of finding her a nursing home placement. When a nursing home was located, Helen became extremely agitated, began to yell and scream, and attempted to block ambulance drivers from transporting Dot to the facility. Helen called for emergency assistance from police. The responding officers convinced Helen to permit Dot to be transported to the nursing home, informing her that she would be arrested if she tried to interfere. In the months after Dot's placement, Helen was extremely stressed, crying each day and begging for Dot to be returned home. Helen expressed her inability to carry on without Dot, saying that she missed her sister and had no reason to live with Dot gone. Helen was encouraged to visit the nursing home frequently, and a bus pass was obtained for her to make transportation easier. Two years after Dot's placement, Dot was in good physical health but remained nonverbal. Helen, however, had experienced a significant decline in her physical and mental health, and continued to talk about how upset she was that Dot had been removed from her home.

Nonfamily Caregivers

In the case of nonfamily caregivers, the reasons for abuse are more sinister since the abuser has no emotional history involving the victim that may be fueling feelings of anger and frustration. These individuals are motivated essentially by either greed, economic desperation, or similar psychopathology that describes the family abuser but minus the dysfunctional family relationship with the victim. Caregiver abusers can be professional healthcare workers such as home healthcare aides, physicians, nursing home certified nursing assistants, nurses, administrators, and support staff. The majority of documented cases of abuse occurring outside of the realm of family caregivers are committed by nursing assistants. Institutionalized elders are frequently victims of theft and physical abuse, which may include withholding food or privileges, unlawful restraint, neglect, and sexual assault.

Fiduciaries

Fiduciaries such as attorneys, notaries, accountants, stockbrokers, real estate brokers, guardians, conservators, investment advisers, and people holding powers of attorney are often in a unique opportunistic situation to use their positions of trust to benefit themselves.

Con Artists

Con artists swindle the elderly through fraudulent door-to-door, mail, and telemarketing schemes frequently resulting in the depletion of the elder's life savings. An alarming number of elderly Americans are being conned out of their savings by a variety of swindles ranging from insurance scams, annuities, identity theft, and many different bogus investment schemes. It is estimated that one in five Americans over the age of 65 has been the victim of a financial scam through inappropriate financial investments (Leondis, 2010).

The Abused

It is important to remember that the majority of perpetrators of elder abuse are male while the majority of victims are female who in some way are dependent on the perpetrator

(Moynihan & Hammer, 2002). See **Table 10-5**. This dependency creates a situation of perceived powerlessness that serves to discourage the elder from disclosing any information relevant to mistreatment at the hands of a caregiver. The elder may fear reprisal from the perpetrator, be reluctant to level accusations against a friend or family member or simply may be too ashamed and humiliated to implicate an individual whom they should be able to trust. In the case of spousal abuse, the victim may have suffered abuse at the spouse's hand over the course of many years and thus has no frame of reference to recognize escalation of the abusive behavior. Since the majority of cases of elder abuse occur in private residences, it is easy to understand why many of the cases go unreported. If there are no witnesses to the abuse, it becomes easier to hide. Because the principal caregiver is most frequently the principal abuser, it is easy to see why the elder is at risk and frequently becomes a victim without recourse. The elderly comprise one of the most vulnerable populations that the forensic nurse will encounter. The degree of frailty, isolation, cognitive and physical impairment, and dependence dictates the likelihood that an elder will be mistreated. If the mistreatment is occurring in an institutionalized setting, fear of reprisal or escalated mistreatment may cause the elder to remain silent. Of other concern is the fact that the institutionalized elder may be unable either physically or cognitively to understand and report what is happening to him or her. Some of the important dynamics contributing to the underreporting (and thus the undertreatment) of elder abuse include denial, reluctance to disclose, traditional reliance on self to solve problems, the perception of available services or the lack of supportive services, language and cultural barriers, and the notion of suffering in silence versus revealing family shame.

The Role of the Forensic Nurse

Assessment

Assessment is an area in which the forensic nurse is uniquely and unquestionably invaluable. The assessment of vulnerable elders conducted through a forensic lens can more accurately identify cases in which the risk factors or index of suspicion is high. The forensic nurse may be instrumental in identifying isolated instances of abuse in private homes or upon presentation of an elder in emergency departments, systemic problems in group residential settings, and in communities. Identification of needed action both immediate and preemptive, involving research and education in collaboration with other agencies such as law enforcement, adult protective services, social services, other family members, and community support resources is the ideal approach. Assessment of the elder for signs of physical abuse should be implemented with each encounter of the elder with the

TABLE 10-5   Risk Factors for the Potential to Be Abused

- Age 80 years or older
- Physically or cognitively impaired
- Dependency on the caregiver
- Related to the caregiver
- Cared for within a private home
- History of living with an abusive spouse
- Absence of close family member living nearby
- Low income
- Low educational level
- History of a strained relationship with the caregiver

healthcare system. Elders should be assessed for any irregular signs of injury such as patterned bruising, fractures both recent and older unidentified, signs of malnutrition, anxious withdrawn behavior, markings that might indicate defensive wounds, all the while keeping in mind the tendency for elders to display injuries requiring only minimal trauma to produce, such as those arising from increased capillary fragility, common bumps or mishaps in the home and the tendency for bones to break more easily. There are several assessment instruments with varying degrees of reliability and validity testing done that are available for screening in different settings. One such tool is the Elder Assessment Interview, a Likert-type scale that includes 41 items in 7 sections that include abuse, neglect, financial exploitation, and abandonment (Fulmer, 2004). The instrument is easy to administer although no actual score is recorded. Thus the clinician should take action if the elder shows any evidence of abuse without an adequate explanation such that an index of suspicion is raised in the assessor or if the elder reports being abused. Another such tool with good reliability and validity is the Indicators of Abuse Screen (Reis & Nahmiash, 1998). This tool is completed by trained professionals and takes considerable time since a preliminary extensive assessment is conducted prior to the administration of the tool itself. The study consists of 29 abuse indicators that include the caregiver and the care recipient. The 29 items are organized into the following three categories:

1. Caregiver intrapersonal problems/issues (e.g., mental health, behavioral, and alcohol or other substance abuse difficulties)
2. Caregiver interpersonal problems (e.g., marital and family conflict and poor relationships generally with the care receiver, etc.)
3. Care receiver social support shortages and past abuse (Reis & Nahmiash)

Various healthcare institutions utilize their own assessment tools, but much work is needed to establish the validity and reliability of these instruments since there is lack of standardization in descriptions. Appropriate proven interventions are sorely needed.

Sexual Assault

A report of possible sexual assault encompasses not only intercourse but also other forms of nonconsensual sexual acts including touching or fondling, forced exposure of the victim or voluntary exposure of the perpetrator, sexually explicit conversation including threats, among other acts. The majority of sexual assault incidents involving the elderly take place in the elder's home by an assailant unknown to the victim (Burgess et al., 2005). In the case of reported sexual abuse, assessment should be conducted by a sexual assault forensic examiner or a geriatric forensic nurse examiner. Appropriate evidence should be collected according to established forensic protocols and the chain of evidence maintained.

Despite the difficulty of conducting a rape examination on an elderly client, it is critical to obtain vaginal, rectal, and pharyngeal specimens. In addition to the inspection that would normally be carried out for suspected physical abuse, careful inspection of external genitalia, perineum, and thighs for any signs of trauma that might indicate assault should be done. Tests for sexually transmitted disease should be conducted and appropriate antibiotics administered in the light of positive findings or prophylactically if the perpetrator is known to be infected. (See Chapter 18 for a more detailed discussion of care for victims of sexual assault.)

A victim advocate should be assigned to the elder in addition to healthcare personnel caring for the elder in the hospital and follow-up in the community or residential living arrangement. Carefully crafted questions should be used keeping in mind the possible reluctance of the victim to describe the attack because of embarrassment, shame, guilt, fear, and the shock that frequently accompanies such an incident. A specific assessment instrument, the Comprehensive Sexual Assault Assessment Tool, was developed by a team of experts convened in 2001 supported by a grant from the Department of Justice, with the objective of standardizing the collection of data about the victim and the offender in cases of reported sexual abuse (Burgess). The instrument was first developed for general use and then adapted for use specifically with elder victims. Several barriers were identified in the course of the study that acted to impede the identification and investigation of elder sexual abuse, including among others the delay in the reporting and collection of evidence, psychological response of the victim, and the relationship of the victim to the offender (Burgess). The final instrument that resulted from the study targeting elders is the Comprehensive Sexual Assault Assessment Tool-Elder (Burgess, 2006). These instruments are in wide use today and are used in the programs preparing nurses to become certified as sexual assault forensic examiners.

It should be noted that elder victims of sexual abuse generally have longer recuperative periods following an assault than younger adults. In part, this relates to longer periods required to heal from physical injuries that accompany the sexual assault in addition to the severe emotional trauma that lingers for all victims. Thus the elder may require longer periods of follow-up and more frequent contacts than a more resilient younger adult who can recover faster from physical injuries.

The Interview

One of the most significant strategies that should be employed with every elder encounter is the interview. Elders should be questioned by the healthcare practitioner with each visit. This technique has been shown to yield positive results even in the absence of overt physical or psychological evidence of possible abuse. Both the caregiver and the recipient should be interviewed together and separately, observing for any discrepancies in the narrative. Some suggestions for the process of the interview are included in **Table 10-6**. **Table 10-7** poses some questions that could be useful during the interview. A positive answer to any of the questions requires careful follow-up and elaboration taking into consideration the emotional and cognitive abilities of the individual elder.

Documentation

Documentation of suspected elder abuse must be thorough, substantive, and accurate as such documentation could be used as evidence should civil or criminal legal proceedings result. Use of language such as *victim*, *abuser*, or any other wording that implies that the clinician may have reached a conclusion regarding the guilt of the caregiver could negate the usefulness of the evidence in court (Sheridan & Nash, 2007). Verbatim statements of the client and the caregiver recorded by the clinician as well as careful documentation of suspected injuries including photographs are the most useful. The chain of evidence must also be maintained.

Referral

Following treatment, reports of abuse are generally given to APS, but in some jurisdictions reports are to be handled initially by law enforcement. However, APS caseworkers

TABLE 10-6   The Interview Process

- Keep the questions simple and direct.
- Allow the elder sufficient time to respond.
- Observe for signs that specific questions elicit guarded responses.
- Avoid questions that might imply legal ramifications as the elder may be fearful to implicate the abuser if it is believed that legal action might result.
- Include references to specific behaviors that might constitute abuse but that the elder might not conceive of such as "Do you ever feel that you are being scolded unnecessarily?" or "Do you ever feel frightened when you are left alone?" looking to ascertain if the elder is left for long periods of time without supervision. "Have you ever noticed that you are missing anything around the house?" can elicit information about possible financial exploitation.
- Allow for separate interviews of the elder and the caregiver.

TABLE 10-7   Suggested Interview Questions*

- Have you ever felt afraid?
- If so, of whom are you afraid?
- Has anyone ever taken things from you without your consent?
- Has anyone ever touched you without your consent?
- Have you ever been threatened by anyone?
- Do you feel you are able to get help when you need it?
- Do you feel safe in your current home (surroundings)?
- What would make you feel safer in your home (surroundings)?

* Depending upon the answers, each question would be expanded.

are often the first to either identify or receive a report of suspected or substantiated elder abuse (see **Table 10-8**). In any instance, the APS acts as a liaison between law enforcement and other agencies charged with providing services to elders at risk of actual or future abuse. APS determines the need for further action or provision of services either in the home or supervised facility, including the assignment of an alternative caregiver if indicated. APS acts in various capacities including the arrangement of economic and legal support, the provision of home health assistance, housekeeping help, temporary shelter, assistance with medication administration, food procurement and referrals and provision of information to law enforcement agencies. Home visits are essential as are investigations of residential facilities dependent upon the venue in which the abuse occurred. In some cases, the caregiver may be in need of supportive services, such as psychological support, economic aid, or respite care that may allow him or her to continue in the caregiver role relative to the victim. It is important to remember that the services of protective services are voluntary and the elder can choose to accept or decline any assistance. In extreme cases, APS may have to intervene to provide legal interventions such as restraint orders, emergency removal from the home, or guardianship.

Consequences of Elder Abuse

Few studies have examined the long-term effects of morbidity and mortality on abused elders. In one such study, almost 3,000 elders were tracked over a 13-year period following

TABLE 10-8 Events Involved in a Call to Adult Protective Services*

- A potentially abusive situation surfaces.
- A call is placed to the hotline or directly to APS.
- A priority is assigned.
- If it is an emergency, medical personnel and law enforcement are called.
- The report is forwarded to local authorities.
- A local investigation begins.
- APS calls someone who knows the victim.
- APS conducts a visit of the victim's home.
- A worker evaluates the information gathered, discusses the case with a supervisor as necessary, and decides if the elder person needs protective services.
- If abuse is confirmed, the case is referred to the appropriate authorities.
- If abuse is unconfirmed, the case is closed and the elder person is referred to other community resources as indicated.

* It is important to note that competent adults have the right to refuse help from adult protective services. In some states, competent adults may refuse an investigation as well.

Source: Adapted from National Center on Elder Abuse (2001, April). Elder Abuse Awareness Kit. Retrieved from http://www.ncea.aoa.gov/NCEAroot/Main_Site/pdf/basics/speakers.pdf

reports of their abuse to a local adult abuse agency (Lachs, Williams, O'Brien, Pillemer, & Charleson, 1998). The reports utilized to identify the study participants covered a 9-year period within one agency in one U.S. city. These elders were compared with a group of elders who reportedly were not abused during the same time period. Of the elders in the group who were not abused, 40% were still living at the time of the survey, compared to 9% of the abused elders (Lachs et al.). Even after adjusting the figures to account for possible factors that might affect the results, the disparity is alarming. The researchers also pose the interesting observation that simply being exposed to the interventions provided by the involved agencies could place the elder in a situation of additional stress, perhaps leading to increased risk of death. A more recent study, aimed at comparing reports of elder abuse with all-cause mortality among community-dwelling elders, demonstrated an increased risk of mortality and seems to confirm these earlier findings, bringing further urgency to the need to develop more effective strategies for dealing with this growing problem (Dong et al., 2009). Another study found that older abused women suffer from overall poorer mental health than those not abused (Mouton, Rodabough, Rovi, Brzyski, & Katerndahl, 2010). It also found that verbal abuse alone was more damaging, in terms of subsequent depression, loss of optimism for living, and other indicators of weakening mental stability than physical abuse alone. The study was based on information from 94,000 women who were part of a large Women's Health Initiative study (Mouton et al.).

Summary

Elder abuse is a complex problem, and thus any efforts at intervention must be undertaken within the context of a multidisciplinary model. Of critical concern is the lack of standardization of terms that define the problem, and that, in turn, affects data collection. Thus efforts to propose and test interventions through rigorous research are hampered. Studies are needed to support such actions as are needed to provide education, treatment, and prevention. Intervention teams to address elder abuse should include representation from local and state social services agencies, nursing, medicine, public health, police, and various nonprofit agencies with an interest in community-dwelling elders as well as those living in institutions within the community. The unique interrelationship between the abused and the abuser—often the caregiver and/or family member—will continue to hamper efforts to report and deal with the various types of crimes against the elderly. Support for the recognition of the criminal nature of much of the observed and documented abuse has increased over time as many endorse the creation of misdemeanor and felony statutes and prison sentences for punishment of abusers (Morgan, Johnson, & Sigler, 2006).

 ## QUESTIONS FOR DISCUSSION

1. What can the forensic nurse do to ensure the identification of elder abuse in the emergency department?
2. What are the legal protections in place to ensure the safety of elders?
3. What action should be taken if the forensic nurse suspects the abuse of elderly clients residing in extended care facilities?
4. What role does the forensic nurse play in the protection of community-dwelling elders?
5. What elements should be included in the assessment of an elder suspected of being the victim of sexual assault?
6. What responsibility does the forensic nurse have in relation to identified elder abusers?

REFERENCES

Alford, D. M. (2011). The Elder Justice Act. *Journal of Gerontology Nursing*. Retrieved from http://www.ncbi.nlm.nih.gov/pubmet/21667887

American Medical Association. (1992). *Diagnostic and treatment guidelines on elder abuse and neglect*. Chicago, IL: AMA.

Aravanis, S. C., Adelman, R. D., Breckman, R., Fulmer, T., Holder, E., Lachs, M., ... Sanders, A. B. (1993). Diagnostic and treatment guidelines on elder abuse and neglect. *Archives of Family Medicine, 2*(2), 371–378. Retrieved from www.archfammed.com

Brent, N. J. (2001). *Nurses and the law: A guide to principles and applications* (2nd ed). New York, NY: W. B. Saunders.

Brody, D., Acker, J., & Logan, W. (2001). *Criminal law*. Gaithersburg, MD: Aspen.

Burgess, A. W. (2006). *Elderly victims of sexual abuse and their offenders*. Report to the U.S. Department of Justice. Retrieved from http://www.ncjrs.gov/pdffiles1/nij/grants/216550.pdf

Burgess, A. W., Hanrahan, N. P., & Baker, T. (2005). Forensic markers in elder female sexual abuse cases. *Clinical Geriatric Medicine, 21*(2), 399–412.

Cohen, M., Levin, S. H., Gagin, R., & Gideon, F. (2007). Elder abuse: Disparities between older people's disclosure of abuse, evident signs of abuse, and high risk of abuse. *Journal of the American Geriatric Society, 55*(8), 1224–1230.

Cooper, C., Selwood, A., & Livingston, G. (2008). The prevalence of elder abuse and neglect: A systematic review. *Age and Ageing, 37*, 151–160.

Dong, X., Simon, M., Mendes de Leon, C., Fulmer, T., Beck, T., Hebert, H., ... Evans, D. (2009). Elder self-neglect and abuse and mortality risk in a community-dwelling population. *JAMA, 302*(5), 517–526.

Fulmer, T. (2004). Elder abuse and neglect assessment. *Dermatology Nursing, 16*(5), 473–474.

Kennedy, R. D. (2005). Elder abuse and neglect: The experience, knowledge, and attitudes of primary care physicians. *Family Medicine, 37*(7), 481–485.

Koenig, R. J., & DeGuerre, C. R. (2005). The legal and governmental response to domestic elder abuse. *Clinical Geriatric Medicine, 21*(2), 383–396.

Lachs, M. S., Williams, C. S., O'Brien, S., Pillemer, K. A., & Charleson, M. E. (1998). The mortality of elder mistreatment *JAMA, 280*(5), 428–432.

Laumann, E., Leitsch, S., & Waite, L. (2008). Elder mistreatment in the United States: Prevalence estimates from a nationally representative study. *Journal of Gerontology: Social Sciences, 63B*(4), 8248–8254.

Leondis, A. (2010). Financial abuse victimizes 1 in 5 elderly. *Bloomberg Business Week.* Retrieved from http://www.businessweek.com/print/investor/content/iu/2010/n:20100715210670.htm

Morgan, E., Johnson, I., & Sigler, R. (2006). Public definitions and endorsement of the criminalization of elder abuse. *Journal of Criminal Justice, 34*(3), 275–283.

Mouton, C., Rodabough, R., Rovi, S., Brzyski, R., & Katerndahl, D. (2010). Psychosocial effects of physical and verbal abuse in postmenopausal women. *Annals of Family Medicine, 8,* 206–213.

Moynihan, B., & Hammer, R. (2002). Elder abuse: Is it safe to grow old in America? *Forensic Nurse, 1.*

National Center on Elder Abuse. (1998). *Elder abuse prevalence and incidence.* Final report. Washington, DC: American Public Health Services Association.

National Center on Elder Abuse. (2001, April). Elder abuse awareness kit. Retrieved from http://www.ncea.aoa.gov/NCEAroot/Main_Site/pdf/basics/speakers.pdf

National Center on Elder Abuse. (2005). *Elder abuse prevalence and incidence.* Fact sheet. Retrieved from http://www.ncea.aoa.gov/NCEARoot/Main_Site/pdf/publication/FinalStatistics050331.pdf

Older Americans Act. (2006). Administration on Aging. Retrieved from http://www.aoa.gov/AoAroot/AoA_Programs/OAA/index.aspx

Passaro, G. (2006). Claims of exploitation of the elderly in the sale of financial products. *Florida Bar Journal, 80*(8) 81–87.

Reis, M., & Nahmiash, D. (1998). Validation of the indicators of abuse screen. *The Gerontologist, 34*(4), 471–480.

Sellas, M., & Krouse, L. (2009). Elder abuse. Retrieved from http://emedicine.medscape.com/article/805727-print

Sheridan, D. J., & Nash, K. R. (2007). Acute injury patterns of intimate partner violence. *Trauma Violence Abuse, 8*(3), 282–289.

Youth Exposure to Violence, Terrorism, and Sudden Traumatic Death

Paul T. Clements and Joseph T. DeRanieri

Forensic nurses can actively provide support and guidance for youth exposed to interpersonal violence, crime, terrorism, and sudden traumatic death. This chapter explores methods for increased awareness and enhanced assessment, and suggestions for intervention by forensic nurses across levels of prevention, referral, and treatment.

 ## CHAPTER FOCUS

» Youth and Traumatic Exposure
» Scope of the Problem
» Exposure to Violence
» Terrorism
» Implication of Youth Exposure to Violence
» Impact of Exposure to Violence for Youth
» Posttraumatic Stress Disorder

» Chaotic Aftermath
» Forensic Nursing Intervention
» Primary Prevention
» Secondary Prevention
» Tertiary Prevention
» Helpful Hints for Intervention
» Talking With Preteen Youth
» Talking With Teenaged Youth

KEY TERMS

» PTSD
» terrorism

» violence
» youth

Introduction

It is conceivable that **violence** and crime occur in all countries and across all cultures. Violence occurs in homes, workplaces, and places where we least expect it to happen. "People from all walks of life are subjected to many forms of violence. Some are victimized by strangers and others by family members and intimate partners. [Sometimes] it is difficult to predict when and where it will occur" (Meadows, 2001, p. vii). It is also difficult to predict the impact that exposure to interpersonal violence, crime, terrorism or sudden traumatic death can have on youth (DeRanieri, Clements, Clarke, Kuhn, & Manno, 2004). The possible sequelae of fear, grief, and intrapsychic pain are personal reactions based on individual development and beliefs and mitigated by family system and culture. These same sequelae create responses that can be potentially disruptive to the ongoing emotional, behavioral, and interpersonal development and related tasks of everyday life (Clements et al., 2003).

Youth are at particular risk for traumatic effects because they do not have an established identity and their available repertoire of coping behaviors is limited (Stevenson, 1996). Exposure to violence can leave youth with disturbing thoughts and images, numerous unanswered questions, and extreme changes in the family structure and function, and this ultimately results in the necessity of relearning the world as a potentially dangerous place (Attig, 2001; DeRanieri, Clements, & Henry, 2002). Exposure to violence can also simultaneously confound multiple developmental tasks and contribute to increased rates of depression, incapacitating anxiety, intrapsychic distress, and isolation from peers and school. Subsequent attempts at coping and adaptation are frequently complicated and can result in affective and behavioral changes including chronic depression; substance abuse; suicidal ideations, gestures, or attempts; and the potential to commit acts of aggression and interpersonal violence on others (American Psychiatric Association, 2000; Vigil & Clements, 2003).

Youth and Traumatic Exposure

During the past 3 decades, studies of youth exposure to various forms of violence and other disasters have significantly contributed to our understanding of the mental health effects in youth. (Buka, Stichick, Birdwhistle, & Earls, 2001). Such studies include Terr's (1983) work on the Chowchilla kidnapping involving an entire school bus of summer students over a 27-hour ordeal. This study was seen as groundbreaking because it was one of the first studies to involve primary interviews of traumatized youth versus obtaining descriptions of symptoms via parent interview. Prior to 1980, the assessment of youth-related trauma responses was primarily accomplished through clinical case examination and review of case records. Clinicians often reported case observations and parent or teacher reports of youth reaction to the traumatic event. Following Terr's utilization of primary interviews and examination, studies evolved to include interviews with youth exposed to violence and disasters (Eth & Pynoos, 1985; Garbarino, Dubrow, Kostelny, & Pardo, 1992; Garbarino, Kostelny, & Dubrow, 1991; Greenberg, 1994; Greenberg & Keane, 1997; Jones, Ribbe, & Cunningham, 1994; Monaco & Gaier, 1987; Terr et al., 1999). It became clear that interviewing youth directly can be an effective method of assessing their experiences and responses to the event.

Additional foundational studies include Green's (1985) work with youth traumatized by physical abuse, Eth and Pynoos's (1985) work with youth witnessing a parental death or abuse, and Lyons's (1987) work, which found that some youth who witnessed even a single violent event reported symptoms of diminished concentration in school, sleep disturbances, flashbacks, disordered interpersonal attachment behavior, increased startle response, and hypervigilance. The information gleaned from these studies has identified behavioral states of distress in traumatized youth, including depression, dissociation, aggression, and substance abuse. These disruptions may include displays of avoidance of anything suggestive of the traumatic event, as well as withdrawal from family and peers and a general decrease in activity level following the event. Additionally, agitation; aggressive behaviors toward peers, siblings, and family pets; irritability and emotional outbursts; fights at school; verbal hostility to parents; and other acts of defiance may be noted (Clements & Burgess, 2002;

O'Campo, Rao, Carlson-Gielen, Royalty, & Wilson, 2000; Osofsky, Wewers, Hann, & Fick, 1993; Rollins, 1997).

An ongoing primary issue is the helplessness of youth at having to watch or listen to the sights and sounds surrounding a violent act and being unprotected from the full emotional impact of the violence (Clements & Benasutti, 2003). Buka and colleagues' (2001) review of empirical work on the distribution, determinants, and consequences of youth witnessing of community violence indicates that males, ethnic minorities, and urban residents are at increased risk for witnessing violence and have higher rates of posttraumatic stress disorder (PTSD).

Scope of the Problem

As a public health problem, youth exposure to myriad forms of violence is not just manifest in witnessing a traumatic event or dealing with the injury or death of a victim; it is additionally an influencing factor in the ongoing formulation and formalization of a developing personality structure, intrapsychic interpretation of the surrounding environment, and attempts at effective coping and adaptation in the everyday stress found in contemporary society. Such exposure to violence is an especially unique and painful burden for youth to bear because it can violate the very basic tenets of trust in the world, social appropriateness, fairness, and basic beliefs surrounding the sanctity of life (Vigil & Clements, 2003). The impact of violence crosses all cultures, races, and both genders, resulting in youth who must interpret meaning, identify coping mechanisms, and confront realistic fear for the integrity of their minds and bodies (Ruchkin et al., 2005).

Youth exposure to violence typically includes seeing or hearing about behavioral acts that have underpinnings of power and control, and which are often exerted by an adult for some form of personal gain and often brutality (Clements & Benasutti, 2003). The Federal Bureau of Investigation Uniform Crime Reports (UCR) (FBI, 2009) provides a nationwide view of crime based on the submission of statistics by law enforcement agencies throughout the country. UCR provides insight into the nature of the barometer of violence in the United States. To best depict total crime data and to provide the most meaningful information, the UCR program collects data on only known offenses and persons arrested by police departments. The selected offenses monitored by the FBI UCR are: (1) murder and nonnegligent manslaughter, (2) forcible rape, (3) robbery, (4) aggravated assault, (5) burglary, (6) larceny-theft, (7) motor vehicle theft, and (8) arson. These are serious crimes by nature and/or volume. Additionally, in the nationwide attempt to assess, prevent, and intervene relative to violence, the Centers for Disease Control and Prevention (CDC, 2010), the U.S. surgeon general (Satcher, 2001), and *Healthy People 2020* (U.S. Department of Health and Human Services, 2010) have all declared violence and violence-related deaths to be a significant public health problem in the United States. Confronting violence in the current millennium is also presented as a significant healthcare issue by the American Medical Association (AMA, 2003), the American Nurses Association (ANA, 2001), and the International Association of Forensic Nurses (IAFN, 2011). This nationwide monitoring and promotion of strategies for prevention and intervention supports the need for increased awareness and understanding as it relates to assessment of exposed youth.

Exposure to Violence

In cities around the United States, youth are exposed to violence and crime in their neighborhoods and inside their homes; they are witnessing street fights, gang activity, domestic violence, child abuse, drug activity, shootings, stabbings, and other assaults. In our society, over 60% of youth were exposed to violence in the past year (2009), with 1 in 10 children being injured in an assault (CDC, 2009). More than 1 in 4 children witnessed a violent act and more than 1 in 10 saw a family member as a victim of assault. Numerous victimizations were common with 38.7% of children experiencing at least two direct victimizations in the past year and more than 1 in 10 (10.9 percent) were victims of at least 10 events (CDC).

Today, children are more likely to experience violence than adults. A study conducted in 2005 revealedthat young adults between the ages of 12 and 17 were twice as likely as the total population to become victims of violence (Baum, 2005).

Exposure to violence can be categorized as direct or indirect. Direct exposure requires a physical proximity that permits experiencing the violence via visual or auditory means or both. Indirect exposure indicates learning of the violence via verbal accounts of family or friends or from the news media. Indirect exposure precludes being present with the victim at the time of the event, finding the victim alive but mortally wounded, or witnessing the actual death.

Coping and adaptation have been shown to be related to cognitive development and degree of exposure and to differ with age. Younger youth have a more restricted range of coping skills than older ones, and therefore may have less flexibility and adaptation to traumatic events (Krell & Sherman, 1997; Schwarzwald, Weisenberg, Solomon, & Waysman, 1994). One study of 326 children from areas struck by Scud missiles in the Gulf War found that younger elementary school children (6th graders) were affected more than adolescents (Schwarzwald et al.). Additionally, a study by North, Smith, and Spitznagel (1994) showed that the degree of exposure and location in proximity to a mass shooting at a playground predicted the intensity of PTSD symptoms 14 months after the event.

Terrorism

The September 11, 2001, terrorist attacks resulted in more deaths than any battle on American soil, exceeding the two most devastating battles in American history—Antietam, during the Civil War, which, until 2001, was the battle with the greatest loss of life in our history, and the attack on Pearl Harbor (Clements, 2001; DeRanieri et al., 2004). Today's youth have never experienced war-time America because all incursions or defensive responses have been deployed on foreign soil. The Oklahoma City bombing and the September 11th attacks have contributed toward understanding the impact and effects of **terrorism** on contemporary American youth (DeWolfe, 2000; Hopkins & Starr, 2002; Pfefferbaum et al., 1999, 2000). For youth, now faced with understanding ongoing changes in and interpretations of the terror alert colors and the imminent threat of more terrorist acts, this can be a very uncertain and anxiety-provoking time (DeRanieri et al., 2004; U.S. Department of Homeland Security, 2004). Youth look to adults for reassurance and to explain the chaos that is happening in the world (Clements, 2001; DeRanieri et al., 2004).

Although the intrapsychic impact on youth of the September 11, 2001, attacks are not yet clear, findings from the Oklahoma City bombing indicate that youth who lost a friend or relative were more likely to report immediate symptoms of PTSD than nonbereaved youth. Trauma-related arousal and fear were evidenced within 7 weeks after the bombing and were noted to be significant predictors of a diagnosis of PTSD (Pfefferbaum et al., 1999). Two years after the bombing, 16% of youth who lived approximately 100 miles away from Oklahoma City reported significant PTSD symptoms related to the event (Pfefferbaum et al., 2000). This is an important finding because these youth were not directly exposed to the trauma of the bombing and were not related to people who had been killed or injured. PTSD symptomology was also predicted by the amount of media exposure and indirect interpersonal exposure (such as having a friend who knew someone who was killed or injured). Based on this research from Oklahoma City, it is predicted that PTSD may develop in children exposed to media coverage or who had a friend or family member who was killed or injured (Pfefferbaum et al., 2000).

Implication of Youth Exposure to Violence

Violence never occurs in a positive light. It is often sudden and unexpected and is still traumatic even when anticipated within a cycle of repetitive abuse. Violence is the purposeful infliction of pain and suffering on one person by another; it is an act of human design. The victim may suffer for hours in severe emotional or physical trauma, or he or she may die. Regardless of the mode, manner, and timing of the violence, for youth, the pain and suffering begins with exposure to the act or the results and subsequent attempts to understand such violation (Rynearson, 1995; Rynearson & McCreery, 1993). Clearly, after such exposure, a diagnosis of posttraumatic stress disorder must be considered, particularly when manifested by significantly disruptive emotional and behavioral symptoms in exposed youth (American Psychiatric Association, 2000).

For youth, exposure to violence can be particularly traumatic in light of the expected developmental tasks and inherent challenges. These include functioning with general lack of autonomy, ongoing development of a strong identification with the permanence of family and friends, and evolving attempts to understand societal norms of behavior, especially describing and defining actions within the context of right and wrong. Violence directly confounds and violates all of these developmental issues in one traumatic event. This can create highly problematic intrapsychic conflicts for exposed youth, who may subsequently express and display trauma-related symptoms and behaviors.

Developmental tasks, including moral reasoning, peer relationships, and interaction with the environment and culture expand remarkably during youth, particularly as youth move from the protection of family, neighborhood, and friends to the wider world (Clunn, 1991). Youth is a decisive period for relationships with others. Problem solving and interpretation of events and situations are based on perceptions (Erickson & Coles, 2000; Piaget, 1969, 1977; Wong, Hockenberry-Eaton, Winkelstein, Schwartz, & Wilson, 2000). Significant value is placed upon maintenance of the family unit, which includes obeying the rules, showing respect for authority, and maintaining the social order by demonstrating correct behavior (Kohlberg, 1966, 1975, 1979).

As youth develop a firm sense of stereotypical male or female behaviors, exposure to violence may create confusion about what are deemed to be appropriate gender roles. As a result in this period of development, one can anticipate a decrease in the objectivity of youth to be able to evaluate behaviors that are right or wrong. Youth also continue to explore and understand the moral tenets of truthfulness and honesty (Erickson, 1993; Freud, 1923; Gilligan, 1983; Piaget, 1977; Stoudemire, 1998).

Youth explore how to compete and cooperate with others; it is a critical time frame for learning the rules (Erickson, 1993). Youth learn how to control their instinctual impulses while dealing with their environment, particularly as they move toward functioning in a more autonomous fashion. Youth who have difficulty completing these developmental tasks may eventually demonstrate difficulty with impulse control and will exhibit a diminished capacity to sublimate their energies into task completion (Erickson; Marcus, 1997).

During formulation and formalization of a moral code and understanding the rules of family and society, the overt violation created by violence and sudden traumatic death can present a significant threat to the normal path of growth and development. It can confound a youth's ability to understand societal norms of interpersonal safety and respect for value of life. The critical foundation for personal mastery can be disrupted and can lead to confusion and misunderstanding about appropriate personal and interpersonal roles and expectations (Eth & Pynoos, 1985; Stevenson, 1996; Sunderland, 1995; Terr, 1991).

Impact of Youth Exposure to Violence

The effects of violence are not limited to the target and the offender. Family members and friends are also affected by the trauma of exposure, whether they are an eyewitness or traumatized from learning about the details of the violent act. Each violent event creates a uniquely complex set of issues for youth, including siblings, friends, neighbors, or acquaintances.

Older youth (typically greater than age 8) understand that death is irreversible and permanent. Therefore, violence activates fears and concerns regarding their own vulnerability and inability to take responsibility for themselves. Furthermore, these youth may feel multidirectional anger, which may be directed at the victim, related to feeling abandoned, and caused by the great pain and sorrow that has accompanied the traumatic event. Youth may also feel angry with themselves for not preventing the event (Clements & Burgess, 2002). There is also confusion and virtual violation of the senses accompanied by attempts to comprehend that one human could purposefully violate the life of another human, especially when that loved one was their family member. Youth may express their pain and trauma via anger, by becoming withdrawn or depressed, or by developing physical symptoms (Burgess et al., 1995; Rando, 1996; Redmund, 1996).

Posttraumatic Stress Disorder

In the aftermath of violence, youth are at significant risk to develop PTSD with accompanying symptoms that are both disturbing and disruptive to their daily routines and that can impact the trajectory of their growth and development.

According to the fourth edition, text revision of the *Diagnostic and Statistical Manual of Mental Disorders* (DSM-IV-TR), posttraumatic stress disorder (**PTSD**) (diagnostic code 309.81) refers to the cluster of symptoms that characteristically occurs after an extremely disturbing life event outside the range of human experience (APA, 2000). Although early literature linked the development of PTSD to brain injury, it is now generally accepted that the etiology is psychogenic, and the condition is classified along the continuum of anxiety disorders; it is perhaps the most extreme state of anxiety that may be experienced.

A diagnosis of PTSD requires a clear implication that the traumatic event would provoke a significant stress response in most individuals (APA, 2000). Currently, the DSM-IV-TR sets forth the following two criteria that must be met for a diagnosis of PTSD: (1)

the person experienced, witnessed, or was confronted with an event or events that involved actual or threatened death or serious injury, or a threat to the physical integrity of self or others; and (2) the person's response involved intense fear, helplessness, or horror.

Determining a diagnosis of PTSD requires significant intervention. The DSM-IV-TR requires 1 month of diagnostic-related traumatic symptomatology to make a diagnosis of PTSD. Unfortunately, youth may not be diagnosed in a timely manner because parents and caregivers may not seek assessment and intervention until the youth is demonstrating maladaptive behaviors or physiological symptoms. It is noteworthy that the DSM-IV-TR acknowledges that these symptoms and behaviors may be manifested differently in youth based upon developmental age and expected tasks and behaviors. These might include agitation, disorganization, and behavioral displays that are reminiscent or symbolic of the traumatic event.

Chaotic Aftermath

The social barometer of the United States has changed drastically during the last decade. Acts of violence have increased in frequency and have become increasingly interpersonal in nature (FBI, 2003). Such acts are often compounded by the typical dynamic of premeditation or intent of one human to cause harm to another.

Trauma and related behaviors created by violence are intertwined, and the surviving family members may seek assistance within the healthcare system for youth with emergent symptoms such as sleep pattern disturbances, dietary disruption, or significant avoidant or aggressive behavior patterns. They may also seek help from or be referred to mental health agencies.

Numerous factors related to violence can complicate the normal process for adaptive coping, including the absence of affective response (numbing or dissociation that results in a showing of no emotion), an unwillingness to speak about the violence (avoidance), expression of only positive or negative feelings about the perpetrator or victim, new or increased behaviors of aggression and destructive outbursts, persistent blame or guilt, anxiety and hypervigilance, prolonged dysfunction in school, parentification manifested by increased caregiving to adults and siblings, accident proneness, stealing or other illegal acts, and signs of addictive behavior (use of illicit drugs, excessive consumption of alcohol, and dietary alterations) (Vigil & Clements, 2003).

Within the first hours after traumatic events, a youth may crystallize an altered and restricted view of his or her personal future that will require treatment to reduce the symptom intensity and to potentially integrate the event into the youth's life history (Attig, 2001). Factors complicating the normal adaptive coping process for exposed youth include the lack of anticipation of the trauma, feelings of horror, thoughts of preventing the event as well as anger, guilt, self-blame, and shattered assumptions about the world within which they live (Clements & Burgess, 2002).

Forensic Nursing Intervention

Forensic nursing intervention with exposed youth requires sensitive and accurate assessment. Many youth may be fearful to share information regarding violence, therefore, forensic nurses must approach the assessment interview with a nonreactive and overtly nonjudgmental stance. Although youth may be asked to describe the violent events that have occurred, it is also critical for nurses to assess family strengths and use these to instill some facet of hope for the surviving youth (Clements & Benasutti, 2003).

Congruent with standard nursing assessment, forensic nursing assessment and intervention should revolve around primary, secondary, and tertiary levels of prevention when working with youth exposed to violence. It is important for each family member who has been exposed to violence to understand that he or she will need to approach adaptive coping as both an individual and a member of the family unit. It is typical for youth to attempt to suppress or hide their feelings for fear of upsetting their parents while simultaneously parents or other adults will avoid talking about the violence to avoid upsetting the youth. It is important for each family member to express individual thoughts and feelings in their own way and at their own rate, which in turn will help the family with adaptive coping and problem solving as a unit.

Primary Prevention

Congruent with the mission, scope of practice, and current goals set forth by *Healthy People 2020*, the American Medical Association, the American Nursing Association, and the International Association of Forensic Nurses, primary prevention relative to decreasing or preventing youth exposure to violence is of overarching significance. To prevent families from becoming violent or being exposed to high-risk situations for violence, forensic nurses must find opportunities to promote nonviolence in families and society at large. Forensic nurses can assess and promote primary prevention by assessing levels of family stress, communication and problem-solving abilities, psychological stress and abuse, other stress, and the degree of psychosocial nurturance provided by the family or support system.

Secondary Prevention

Secondary prevention involves early identification and intervention that prevents any reoccurrence of exposure to violence. Exposure to violence that involves youth requires a report to state child protective service agencies. Families at risk for violence can significantly benefit from referral and collaboration with available mental health agencies, school counselors, parenting workshops, and anger management seminars.

Tertiary Prevention

Tertiary intervention is necessary when exposure is ongoing and apparently unavoidable. When imminent risk for danger to self, others, or property are noted, immediate intervention must occur. Depending on the nature of the risk (disclosure of ongoing abuse, threats of harm, evidence of previous or current injury, etc.), numerous agencies (police, child protective services, etc.) may require reporting and immediate referral for additional assessment, and intervention may be needed (emergency room, primary care provider, crisis intervention agency, mental health assessment services, etc.).

Helpful Hints for Intervention

Families can be very complex, and the relationships within them are typically numerous, different, and sometimes complicated. Thinking about families as a mobile can be a helpful metaphor for assessment and intervention. Many families hang a mobile above their child's crib or just outside on the porch, and they will typically be able to identify with how gentle breezes cause it to spin and move. Families, in essence, are very similar to these mobiles. They come in all different shapes and sizes, the pieces move at different speeds and in various relations and distances from the others, and yet the common struts and wires hold the pieces together as one unit. Typically the gentle breezes of life keep the mobile moving and changing, adding to the excitement, adventure, and beauty of the family. Even when the harsh winds of life's storms blow, some of the pieces may clink and collide, but the mobile remains together and eventually returns to peaceful motion. However, even the most beautiful mobile can be changed if one of its pieces is damaged or destroyed. Exposure to violence creates such damage or destruction. Violence can damage or take away one or more pieces of the mobile, leaving just an open space, yet with a strut still connected to the rest of the mobile—a constant reminder of the damaged or missing piece.

It is important that each piece of the mobile—that is to say, each family member—takes care of himself or herself while also understanding that the family will grieve together as a whole family. The following are helpful hints for exposed youth and their families:

» Youth are often overwhelmed with emotions (anxiety, fear, anger, guilt), as well as practical matters (school, peers, family function, and structure). This is often related to the frequently asked question, "Is it normal to be feeling this way?" Because concentration and comprehension may be impaired at this stressful time, forensic nurses should provide information about resources and educational information in writing or printed form when possible. This will allow future access and referral to the information as needed.

» Many youth struggle with feelings of guilt for not having been able to prevent the violence or the sudden traumatic death. Some youth may blame themselves, believing that the violence was somehow their fault, or some form of cosmic retribution for being bad or having done something wrong. Other youth may have witnessed the event and begin to second-guess whether the event could have been prevented by grabbing the gun or otherwise intervening in unrealistic and unsafe manners. The forensic nurse can set a platform for adaptive coping and promote reduction of such guilt feelings by reminding the youth that it was not his or her fault, that any such attempts at intervention would have likely resulted in injury or other severe forms of harm, and that at times, adults make poor decisions (i.e., violent acts) that are not the responsibility of the youth to correct.

» Shock, numbness, and disbelief or overt denial are typical reactions to violent events, so a helpful first step is to encourage other family members to talk through their thoughts and feelings. Talking about the event can help validate what has occurred and can facilitate reinvesting in life. Emphasize that telling the story is a helpful way for families to begin adaptation and coping. If family members become upset and cry or get angry, this is all a normal part of the process.

» It is normal for trauma response patterns to vary among family members, even as they respond together as a unit. Trauma responses are not wrong or bad. For example, all boys do not need to cry to be effectively grieving, yet many people believe that not crying during the grief process is unacceptable behavior. Just because some people simply do not allow themselves to show emotion or other behaviors in the presence of others does not mean that they are not coping effectively. This will be mitigated by personality, culture, age, and personal style during coping and adaptation. The forensic nurse who has concerns about a certain behavior, or lack thereof, should inquire further about the individual's and the family's usual coping skills and behaviors. This will clarify the situation and help the forensic nurse promote adaptive coping or identify potentially maladaptive coping approaches that require additional assessment or intervention. Finally, the use of drugs, alcohol, and violence are not a normal part of the adaptive coping process, and anyone displaying such behavior should be referred immediately for additional assessment and possible intervention.

Talking with Preteen Youth

When talking with preteen youth, forensic nurses should remember the importance of getting down to their level, both developmentally and physically. With smaller youth, getting on the floor with them as they draw or play will provide eye contact and a sense of importance to the discussion at hand. With larger youth, sitting at a table provides a level field for communication. It is just as important to remember the expected developmental tasks and behaviors of youth. Maximize a youth's ability to explore and understand through play and fantasy (Clements, 2001; Clements & Benasutti, 2003; Clements, Benasutti, & Henry, 2001). For example, drawings or doll play can facilitate exploration and discussion of concerns and confusion. If the forensic nurse asks a youth to draw a picture of what he or she thinks happened during the violent event or to use dolls to demonstrate the events, it can provide significant insight into his perceptions and fears. Remember, any drawing or doll play is not right or wrong or good or bad, but rather a simple reflection of what the child is thinking and feeling. Avoid trying to psychoanalyze the drawing or the role play, but instead, ask the youth, "So . . . tell me what's happening in the drawing," or "So what is that doll doing now?" This can provide helpful information regarding fears or concerns that the youth may have (Clements, 2001; Clements & Benasutti, 2003; Clements et al., 2001; Clements, Benesutti, & Henry, in press).

Remember that youth have varying levels of understanding regarding violence, injury, and death. Some youth may express thoughts and understanding of violence in terms of fantasy and other related belief systems. Other youth may realize that violence is wrong and that the threat of injury and death are real. This can result in more disruption in adaptive coping and in anxiety related to the realization of their vulnerability to such violence and injury.

Talking with Teenaged Youth

Teenaged youth clearly understand the pain and suffering involved with violence. As they are struggling with the task of becoming independent in preparation for adulthood, they may also be aware of the risks and fears associated with the potential for more violence. It is important to discuss the violence with teenaged youth while making sure that normal developmental tasks and behaviors are simultaneously promoted (Clements, 2001). Actually, forensic nurses can use these normal teen behaviors to enhance processing of this information. For example, a teenaged youth's most important peer group is not his or her family, but other teenaged youth. One way to promote conversation and exploration might be to ask a teen, "Have you talked with your friends about this? What is everyone saying and thinking?" This will send a message to the teenaged youth that the forensic nurse acknowledges and understands that talking about this with friends is important, and at the same time the forensic nurse is also concerned about the traumatic events (Clements).

Teenaged youth need to continue other on-task developmental behaviors, such as going to the mall, going to the movies, and hanging out at the playground with friends. These are all behaviors that are still as normal as they were before the violence started. If parents have anxiety about keeping closer tabs on their teenaged youth, they can discuss this with the youth and perhaps negotiate some helpful and not too intrusive activities, such as an extra check-in call home. When parents explain to teenaged youth that this is not in response to an increased lack of trust but is a way of increasing communication and ensuring safety, most teenagers, if approached in a realistic and proactive way, may grumble a little, but ultimately understand and agree (Clements, 2001).

Summary

It is not unusual for youth to be upset after exposure to violent or traumatic acts. Traumatic responses never feel good but are often a typical part of the process of understanding and coping. It is important for forensic nurses to help promote and teach adaptive methods of coping because these are often reflective of the way in which youth will handle fear, guilt, and intrapsychic pain as they enter adulthood.

QUESTIONS FOR DISCUSSION

1. Why are youth at significant risk for developmental disruption after exposure to violence, terrorism, or sudden traumatic death?
2. Identify and discuss the implications of exposure to violence on youth and their family.
3. Identify how trauma can contribute to maladaptive coping and developmental disruption in youth.
4. Identify and discuss the roles the forensic nurse can take in educating youth and their families regarding trauma and adaptive coping.
5. Identify several different approaches that may be taken when working with youth of varying developmental levels or age groups.

REFERENCES

American Medical Association. (2011). Youth Violence Prevention Training and Outreach Guide. Retrieved from http://www.ama-assn.org/ama/pub/physician-resources/public-health/promoting-healthy-lifestyles/violence-prevention/youth-violence-prevention-training-outreach-guide.page

American Nurses Association. (2001). *American Nurses Association demands stricter violence protections for health care workers: Murder of Florida psychiatric nurse prompts profession's call to action.* Press Release (Nursing World, Released April 18, 2000).

American Psychiatric Association. (2000). *Diagnostic and statistical manual of mental disorders* (4th ed., text rev.). Washington, DC: Author.

Attig, T. (2001). Relearning the world: Always complicated, sometimes more than others. In G. Cox, R. Bendiksen, & R. Stevenson (Eds.), *Complicated grieving and bereavement: Understanding and treating people experiencing loss* (pp. 7–22). Amityville, NY: Baywood.

Baum, K. (2005). Juvenile Victimization and Offending, 1993–2003. Washington, DC: U.S. Department of Justice, Office of Justice Programs, Bureau of Justice Statistics.

Buka, S., Stichick, T., Birdwhistle, I., & Earls, F. (2001). Youth exposure to violence: Prevalence, risks and consequences. *American Journal of Orthopsychiatry, 71*(3), 298–310.

Centers for Disease Control and Prevention (2009). Children's exposure to violence: A comprehensive national study. *Juvenile Justice Bulletin.* Retrieved from http://www.ncjrs.gov/pdffiles1/ojjdp/227744.pdf

Clements, P. T. (2001). Terrorism in America: How do we tell the children? *The Journal of Psychosocial Nursing, 39*(11), 8–10.

Clements, P. T., & Benasutti, K. M. (2003). Mental health aspects of child survivors of abuse and neglect. In E. R. Giardino & A. P. Giardino (Eds.), *Nursing approach to the evaluation of child maltreatment* (pp. 306–329). St. Louis, MO: G.W. Medical.

Clements, P. T., Benasutti, K. M., & Henry, G. C. (2001). Drawing from experience: Utilizing drawings to facilitate communication and understanding with children exposed to sudden traumatic deaths. *The Journal of Psychosocial Nursing, 39*(12), 12–20.

Clements, P. T., Benasutti, K. M., & Henry, G. C. (in press). Drawings in abuse cases. In R. Alexander & A. P. Giardino (Eds.), *Child maltreatment* (3rd ed., pp. 129–155). St. Louis, MO: G.W. Medical.

Clements, P. T., Vigil, G. J., Manno, M. S., Henry, G. C., Wilks, J., Das, S., ... Foster, W. (2003). Cultural considerations of loss, grief & bereavement. *Journal of Psychosocial Nursing, 41*(7), 18–26.

DeRanieri, J. T., Clements, P. T., Clarke, K., Kuhn, D. W., & Manno, M. S. (2004). War, terrorism and children. *Journal of School Nursing, 20*(2), 17–23.

DeRanieri, J. T., Clements, P. T., & Henry, G. C. (2002). When catastrophe happens: Assessment and intervention after sudden traumatic deaths. *The Journal of Psychosocial Nursing, 40*(4), 30–37.

DeWolfe, D. J. (2000). *Field manual for mental health and human services workers in major disasters.* Washington, DC: National Mental Health Services Knowledge Exchange Network. Available at http://www.mentalhealth.samhsa.gov/ publications/all pubs/ADM90-537/fmrisk.asp

Erickson, E. H. (1993). *Childhood and society.* New York, NY: W.W. Norton.

Erickson, E. H., & Coles, R. (2000). *Erik Erickson reader.* New York, NY: W.W. Norton.

Eth, S., & Pynoos, R. (1985). Interaction of trauma and grief in childhood. In S. Eth & R. Pynoos (Eds.), *Post-traumatic stress disorder in children* (pp. 232–260). Washington, DC: American Psychiatric Press.

Federal Bureau of Investigation. (2009). *Crime in the United States—2003. Uniform crime reports.* Retrieved from http://www2.fbi.gov/ucr/cius2009/index.html

Freud, S. (1923). The ego and the id. *Standard Edition, 7,* 3–66.

Garbarino, J., Dubrow, N., Kostelny, K., & Pardo, C. (1992). *Children in danger: Coping with the consequences of community violence.* San Francisco, CA: Jossey-Bass.

Garbarino, J., Kostelny, K., & Dubrow, N. (1991). What children can tell us about living in danger. *American Psychologist, 36,* 376–383.

Gilligan, C. (1983). In a different voice: Psychological theory and women's development. Cambridge, MA: Harvard University Press.

Green, A. (1985). Children traumatized by physical abuse. In S. Eth & R. Pynoos (Eds.), *Post-traumatic stress disorder in children* (pp. 85–107). Washington, DC: American Psychiatric Press.

Greenberg, H. (1994). Responses of children and adolescents to a fire in their homes. *Child and Adolescent Social Work Journal, 11*(6), 475–492.

Greenberg, H., & Keane, A. (1997). A social work perspective of childhood trauma after a residential fire. *Social Work in Education, 19*(1), 11–22.

Hopkins, G., & Starr, L. (2002). *September 11: Lessons and resources for classroom teachers.* Retrieved from http://www.education-world.com/a_lesson/lesson244.shtml

International Association of Forensic Nurses. (2011). About IAFN. Retrieved from http://www.iafn.org/displaycommon.cfm?an=3

Jones, R., Ribbe, D., & Cunningham, P. (1994). Psychosocial correlates of fire disaster among children and adolescents. *Journal of Traumatic Stress, 7*(1), 117–122.

Kohlberg, L. (1966). A cognitive developmental analysis of children's sex-role concepts and attitudes. In E. MacCoby (Ed.), *The development of sex differences.* Stanford, CA: Stanford University Press.

Kohlberg, L. (1975). The cognitive-developmental approach to moral education. *Phi Delta Kappan, 56,* 670–677.

Kohlberg, L. (Ed.). (1979). *Meaning and measurement of moral development.* Worcester, MA: Clark University Press.

Krell, R., & Sherman, M. (Eds.). (1997). *Medical and psychological effects of concentration camps on Holocaust survivors.* New Brunswick: The State University of New Jersey.

Lyons, J. (1987). Post-traumatic stress disorder in children and adolescents: A review of the literature. In S. Chess & A. Thomas (Eds.), *Annual progress in child psychiatry and development* (pp. 451–457). New York, NY: Brunner Mazel.

Marcus, P. (1997). Personality disorders. In A. Burgess (Ed.), *Psychiatric nursing: Promoting mental health* (pp. 441–460). Stamford, CT: Appleton & Lange.

Meadows, R. J. (2001). *Understanding violence and victimization* (2nd ed.). Upper Saddle River, NJ: Prentice Hall.

Monaco, N., & Gaier, E. (1987). Developmental level and children's responses to the explosion of the space shuttle *Challenger. Early Childhood Research Quarterly, 2,* 83–95.

North, C., Smith, E., & Spitznagel, E. (1994). Posttraumatic stress disorder in survivors of a mass shooting. *American Journal of Psychiatry, 151,* 82–88.

O'Campo, P., Rao, R., Carlson-Gielen, A., Royalty, W., & Wilson, M. (2000). Injury-producing events among children in low-income communities: The role of community characteristics. *Journal of Urban Health, 77*(1), 34–49.

Osofsky, J. D., Wewers, S., Hann, D. M., & Fick, A. C. (1993). Chronic community violence: What is happening to our children? *Psychiatry, 56,* 36–45.

Pfefferbaum, B., Nixon, S., Tucker, P., Tivis, R., Moore, V., Gurwitch, R., ... Geis, H. K. (1999). Posttraumatic stress response in bereaved children after Oklahoma City bombing. *Journal of the American Academy of Child and Adolescent Psychiatry, 38,* 1372–1379.

Pfefferbaum, B., Seale, T., McDonald, N., Brandt, E., Rainwater, S., Maynard, B., ... Miller, P. D. (2000). Posttraumatic stress two years after the Oklahoma City bombing in youths geographically distant from the explosion. *Psychiatry, 63,* 358–370.

Piaget, J. (1969). *The theory of stages in cognitive development.* New York, NY: McGraw-Hill.

Piaget, J. (1977). *The development of thought.* New York, NY: Viking Press.

Rollins, J. (1997). Minimizing the impact of community violence on child witnesses. *Critical Care Nursing Clinics of North America, 9*(2), 211–219.

Ruchkin, V., Schwab-Stone, M., Jones, S., Cicchetti, D., Koposov, R., & Vermeiren, R. (2005). Is posttraumatic stress in youth a culture-bound phenomenon? A comparison of symptom trends in selected U.S. and Russian communities. *American Journal of Psychiatry, 162,* 538–544.

Rynearson, E. K. (1995). Bereavement after homicide: A comparison of treatment seekers and refusers. *British Journal of Psychiatry, 166,* 507–510.

Rynearson, E. K., & McCreery, J. M. (1993). Bereavement after homicide: A synergism of trauma and loss. *American Journal of Psychiatry, 150,* 258–261.

Satcher, D. (2001). *Youth violence: A report of the surgeon general. Report on community forums— Youth violence and public health.* Retrieved from http://www.surgeongeneral.gov/library/ youthviolence/forums.asp

Schwarzwald, J., Weisenberg, M., Solomon, Z., & Waysman, M. (1994). Stress reactions of school-aged children to the bombardment of SCUD missiles: A 1-year follow-up. *Journal of Traumatic Stress, 7*(4), 657–667.

Stevenson, R. (1996). The response of schools and teachers. In K. Doka (Ed.), *Living with grief after sudden loss: Suicide, homicide, accident, heart attack, stroke* (pp. 201–214). Washington, DC: Hospice Foundation of America.

Stoudemire, A. (1998). *Human behavior: An introduction for medical students* (3rd ed.). Philadelphia, PA: Lippincott Williams & Wilkins.

Sunderland, R. (1995). *Helping children cope with grief: A teachers guide. Picking up the pieces* (2nd ed.). Fort Collins, CO: Services Corporation International.

Terr, L. C. (1983). Chowchilla revisited: The effects of psychic trauma four years after a school-bus kidnapping. *American Journal of Psychiatry, 140,* 1543–1550.

Terr, L. C. (1991). Childhood traumas: An outline and overview. *American Journal of Psychiatry, 148*(1), 10–20.

Terr, L. C., Bloch, D. A., Michel, B. A., Shi, H., Reinhardt, J. A., & Metayer, S. (1999). Children's symptoms in the wake of *Challenger:* A field study of distant-traumatic effects and an outline of related conditions. *American Journal of Psychiatry, 156*(10), 1536–1544.

U.S. Department of Health and Human Services. (2010). *Healthy People 2020. Injury and violence prevention.* Retrieved from http://healthypeople.gov/2020/topicsobjectives2020/overview.aspx?topicid=24

U.S. Department of Homeland Security. (2004). *Threats & protection advisory system. Homeland security advisory system: Understanding the homeland security advisory system.* Retrieved from http://www.dhs.gov/dhspublic/display?theme29

Vigil, G. J., & Clements, P. T. (2003). Child and adolescent homicide survivors: Complicated grief and altered worldviews. *Journal of Psychosocial Nursing and Mental Health Services, 41*(1), 30–39.

Wong, D. L. L., Hockenberry-Eaton, M., Winkelstein, M. L., Schwartz, P., & Wilson, D. (2000). *Essentials of pediatric nursing* (6th ed.). St. Louis, MO: Elsevier Science.

SUGGESTED FURTHER READING

Aizer, A. (2008). *Neighborhood violence and urban youth.* Cambridge, MA: National Bureau of Economic Research.

Centers for Disease Control and Prevention. (2010). *Understanding youth violence.* Fact sheet. Retrieved from http://www.cdc.gov/ViolencePrevention/youthviolence

Dowd, N. E. (2006). *Handbook of children, culture, and violence.* Thousand Oaks, CA: Sage.

Englander, E. K. (2007). *Understanding violence.* Mahwah, NJ: Lawrence Erlbaum.

Kent State University, Institute for the Study and Prevention of Violence. (2003). *Current perspectives on violence prevention.* Kent, OH: Institute for the Study and Prevention of Violence, Kent State University.

Lawton, S. A. (2008). *Abuse and violence information for teens: Health tips about the causes and consequences of abusive and violent behavior; including facts about the types of abuse and violence, the warning signs of abusive and violent behavior, health concerns of victims, and getting help and staying safe.* Detroit, MI: Omnigraphics.

Steinberg, L. (2001). Youth violence: Do parents and families matter? *National Institute of Justice Journal.* Retrieved from http://www.ncjrs.gov/pdffiles1/jr000243f.pdf

United States National Institute of Justice. (1996). *Assessing the exposure of urban youth to violence: A summary of a pilot study from the Project on Human Development in Chicago Neighborhoods.* Washington, DC: U.S. Dept. of Justice, Office of Justice Programs, National Institute of Justice.

CHAPTER 12

Posttraumatic Stress Disorder: An Overview of Theory, Treatment, and Forensic Practice Considerations

Edwin F. Renaud

Posttraumatic stress disorder (PTSD) is an area of significant concern for practitioners in the forensic setting. Forensic nurses may come into contact with traumatized individuals such as rape victims, abused children, and victims of domestic violence. They may also come into contact with offenders who have backgrounds characterized by exposure to violence, neglect, and other severe stressors, the effects of which may go unrecognized due to the patients' criminal behavior. Understanding the nature and origins of PTSD permits the forensic nurse to provide the best care possible to this challenging population.

CHAPTER FOCUS

» Defining Trauma and Posttraumatic Stress Disorder

» Risk and Resiliency to Posttraumatic Stress Disorder

» The Effects of Single-incident Trauma Versus Chronic Trauma

» Treatment and Intervention With Traumatized Patients

KEY TERMS

» acute stress disorder
» avoidance symptoms
» cortisol
» hyperarousal
» posttraumatic stress disorder (PTSD)

» protective factor
» reexperiencing symptoms
» risk factor
» stress response
» trauma

Introduction

Considerable gains have been made in the basic science, theory, and treatment of posttraumatic stress disorder since the early 1980s. As our understanding of PTSD has improved, mental health providers have begun to consider the impact of traumatic experience on different clinical populations. The forensic population has been no exception.

The organized study of PTSD owes much of its impetus to research on combat veterans. Psychiatric casualties have become an increasingly well-documented aspect of warfare, with modern accounts dating back to the American Civil War (Dean, 1999). Many people are familiar with the term *shell shock*, which was used to describe the psychological effects of combat during World War I. The underlying belief behind the term *shell shock* was that the concussive force of exploding artillery rounds produced intracranial injury, which resulted in changes in mood and behavior. During and after World War II, psychiatric casualties commanded greater attention as thousands of returning servicemen were diagnosed with psychological conditions related to combat.

The 1980s saw renewed interest in the study of the psychological effects of combat, stimulated in large part by demands from Vietnam veterans who felt that existing mental health professionals did not adequately understand or address their needs. The study of trauma and its psychological and behavioral effects became a priority for the Department of Veterans Affairs and other federal agencies. The next 20 years yielded a considerably better understanding of the definition, theory, and treatment of PTSD. However, as interest in the study of combat-related trauma grew, it also became clear that combat veterans were not the only population that suffered from trauma-related psychopathology.

As the study of trauma attracted wider attention within the clinical and academic communities, researchers began to look at the experiences of abuse and neglect survivors, victims of crime, and people who had experienced accidents. This led to a greater recognition that psychological trauma was not restricted to combat veterans and was not limited to single episode or short-term stressors. Indeed, some of the most important contributions to our understanding of PTSD come from the study of adaptation to chronic stress.

More recently, researchers have focused on the stress-related morbidity of police, fire fighters, rescue personnel, and recovery workers assigned to deal with the aftermath of natural disasters or terrorist attacks. One area of special interest could be described as preventative trauma research, concerning efforts to predict who may be more vulnerable to suffering traumatic reactions to stress (Roy-Byrne et al., 2004), providing treatment to those who have just undergone stressful events (van Emmerick, Kamphuis, Hulsbocsch, & Emmelkamp, 2002), and understanding more about those individuals who seem resistant to high amounts of stress (Morgan et al., 2002). As the threat of terrorism becomes part of our ongoing collective experience, interest in this branch of the trauma literature is likely to grow.

Defining Trauma

Practitioners tend to use the terms **trauma** and **posttraumatic stress disorder (PTSD)** interchangeably. However, a trauma is an experience, and not necessarily the same experience for different people; posttraumatic stress disorder is a diagnosis. There is considerable variability among individuals in their vulnerability to being traumatized and further difference among traumatized people as to the specific profile of their symptoms. However, there are broad commonalities to the types of symptoms seen in patients with PTSD. These symptoms fall into three clusters.

The first cluster of symptoms is referred to as **reexperiencing symptoms**. This group of symptoms consists of nightmares, flashbacks, and other unwanted intrusions of the traumatic event into mental awareness. These symptoms may range from persistent, intrusive thoughts to full-blown hallucinations. Reexperiencing symptoms is not limited to conscious memory. It may involve symbolic reminders or reenactments of the traumatic event in dreams or behavior patterns.

The second cluster of PTSD symptoms is known as **avoidance symptoms**. These symptoms consist of feelings, thoughts, or actions meant to diminish contact with people, situations, or other cues that might remind the patient of the traumatic event. Avoidance symptoms can range from an aversion to watching war movies to marked social withdrawal. Because traumatic events often involve the actions of other people, feelings of social estrangement and a reduced capacity for emotional expression are included in this symptom cluster. Avoidance may be more difficult to observe or elicit from the patient if he or she is more passive and involved in staying out of sight. Avoidance is sometimes regarded by the patient as an adaptation rather than a symptom of PTSD.

The most severe manifestations of avoidance symptom are dissociation and derealization. Derealization (sometimes referred to as depersonalization) occurs when the patient experiences events she is participating in as if she were watching them or is otherwise psychologically detached from the events around her. The patient remains aware of herself in the context of the environment, but that awareness has a quality of being an observer rather than a participant. Dissociation is a step beyond derealization in which the patient experiences himself or herself as being completely disconnected from events, often not having any moment-to-moment awareness of the surroundings while in the dissociative state. Dissociation and derealization symptoms tend to occur episodically, usually under conditions of heightened stress, anxiety, or emotional intensity.

The last cluster of PTSD symptoms is **hyperarousal**. Of all the symptoms of PTSD, hyperarousal is often the most obvious and the most likely to attract attention (positive and negative) from family members, coworkers, and the social environment of the patient. These symptoms include difficulty sleeping, increased irritability, and a globally exaggerated autonomic and subjective response to environmental danger signals. Hyperarousal is characterized by hypervigilance (being chronically on alert for potential sources of danger), claustrophobia, and sensitivity to loud noises. Hyperarousal symptoms are a basic alteration in the perceptual experience of patients with PTSD. They often manifest as heightened sensitivity to potential sources of danger and a bias towards interpreting neutral environmental stimuli as dangerous. This can result in disproportionately aggressive or fearful responses to one's environment, a tendency for interpersonal suspicion and mistrust, and substance abuse in an attempt to diminish the heightened states of fear and anger. Hyperarousal symptoms represent an erosion of the mind's capacity to filter out extraneous information, resulting in an overflow of stimuli that can overwhelm the patient. The aggression, substance abuse, and interpersonal chaos noted in the personal lives of PTSD patients often have their roots in the patients' struggle to cope with the hyperarousal symptoms.

The *Diagnostic and Statistical Manual of Psychiatric Disorders* (DSM) definition of trauma is descriptive. As with psychiatric diagnosis in general, the DSM-IV (DSM, TR, 4th edition) definition of trauma does not point to a specific disease process or identify a pathway between organ dysfunction and symptoms. This creates a degree of ambiguity about the meaning of trauma. Having an experience that meets the DSM-IV-TR (DSM-IV, text revision [APA, 2000]) definition of trauma (criterion A) is not a guarantee of being traumatized. It is the experience of symptoms after the stressful event rather than the experience itself that qualifies one for the diagnosis of PTSD. The next logical question might be, what makes a trauma different from a stressful experience that would be diagnosed as **Acute Stress Disorder** (ASD)?

The key difference between PTSD and ASD is the timeframe for the onset and resolution of symptoms. The diagnosis of ASD sets a limit of 1 month for the onset of symptoms, whereas the PTSD diagnosis lists no such time frame for symptom onset. Also the PTSD diagnosis states that symptoms must be present for more than 1 month whereas the ASD diagnosis states that symptoms must resolve within 1 month. The timeline for ASD leaves a 2-month window for the onset and resolution of trauma-related symptoms. After the 2-month window the appropriate diagnosis is PTSD. *When a person undergoes a stressful experience that is so severe that it overwhelms his or her psychological capacity to cope, the result is trauma.* This definition, translated through different theoretical languages, is seen repeatedly throughout the trauma literature. All the theoretical models of PTSD discussed in this chapter, whether rooted in a breakdown of psychic structures, cognitive schemas, or functional neurobiology, speak to a breakdown of the mind's capacities to organize experience and the emotions that go with it, under conditions of extreme stress.

Theories of Posttraumatic Stress Disorder

It is beyond the scope of this chapter to review and discuss the myriad theories developed to describe and understand the dynamics of PTSD. Treatment interventions are driven by the utilization of a specific theory that is researched and effective in a specific population. Such theories include psychoanalytic theories, which includes cognitive behavioral theory. The biological theory has focused on the **stress response** hormones and the effect on the hypothalamic/pituitary/adrenal system of the brain. One hormone of particular interest is **cortisol** and its role in the body's stress response.

Cortisol is a steroid hormone secreted by the adrenal glands and serves various functions within the body, among them regulation of immune functions, blood pressure, glucose metabolism, insulin regulation, and the body's flight or fight response to sudden acute stress. However, in the face of severe traumatic stress, levels of cortisol may actually become depressed (Delahanty 2011). Immediately following a traumatic event, there is a significantly decreased activity within the hypothalamic-pituitary-adrenal axis leading to a corresponding decrease in cortisol. This decrease can be correlated with victims who later develop the cluster of symptoms associated with PTSD. Thus the measurement of cortisol immediately following a traumatic incident could be used as a marker for risk of subsequent development of the disorder. One psychbiological treatment strategy for PTSD aims to return cortisol levels to normal ranges as soon after the precipitating event as possible (Feldner, Monson, & Friedman, 2007).

Biological Consequences of PTSD

Researchers have identified areas of the brain that may be associated with PTSD. One observation is that people with PTSD may experience a reduction in the brain's capacity to translate traumatic memory into language that could have major implications for understanding traumatic memory.

Memory Formation and Trauma

The role of memory in PTSD has been an area of special interest for trauma researchers, because PTSD can be thought of as a disorder of remembered experience. Reexperiencing, avoidance, and hyperarousal symptoms are all contingent upon the retention of information associated with the traumatic event. Bessle van der Kolk has studied changes in memory storage and retrieval in persons suffering with PTSD. His model of traumatic memory is a useful framework for understanding the effect of stressful experience on memory and points to a biological model of psychological trauma surprisingly similar to those put forth in the psychological literature.

Coping strength is an individual trait that is subject to a considerable number of environmental and endogenous factors. What is traumatic for one person may not be traumatic for another. Individual coping may also vary depending on the type of stressor encountered. An individual may be more resilient to the stress associated with an automobile accident than an assault, for example. Although there is a great deal of individual difference in what may be traumatizing, certain risk factors have been shown to make one more vulnerable or resistant to the development of PTSD.

Vulnerability and Resilience to PTSD

One of the most puzzling questions about PTSD is why some people go on to develop the disorder after a stressful event and others do not. The National Comorbidity Survey, a study of the incidence of mental illness in the U.S. population, found that more than 50% of women and 60% of men in the general population experience a stressful event that meets the DSM definition of trauma at some point in their lives (Kessler, Sonnega, Bromet, Hughes, & Nelson, 1995). Yet the lifetime prevalence of PTSD in the general population is roughly 8%. Using the most conservative estimates, this data indicates that fewer than 20% of people who experience a stressor great enough to meet the definition of trauma go on to have symptoms of PTSD. What makes some people more vulnerable to becoming traumatized than others? What allows most people to survive stressful events without being traumatized?

The term **risk factor** is often used to describe preexisting characteristics that make a person more vulnerable to developing a particular disorder. The term **protective factor** refers to qualities that predate the onset of a disorder and diminish the likelihood of developing pathology. Because of the highly individual nature of vulnerability to being traumatized, researchers have shown interest in the risk and protective factors associated with the development of PTSD. One of the findings of this research is that risk factors and protective factors appear to be at work both before and after the traumatizing stressor.

There have been two major efforts to systematically review the findings of the trauma literature and identify the most common risk factors and protective factors for PTSD. Brewin, Andrews, and Valentine (2000) conducted a meta-analysis (an analysis of multiple research reports to look for commonalities in the literature) of 77 studies on the risk factors and protective factors for the development of PTSD. They found that the most powerful risk factors for developing PTSD that were present before the traumatic event were childhood abuse, a personal history of psychiatric illness, and a family history of psychiatric illness. The risk factors that most strongly predicted the development of PTSD after a traumatic event were a lack of social support, the severity of the trauma itself, and the occurrence of subsequent stressful events. Another meta-analysis of 68 studies conducted by Ozer, Best, Lipsey, and Weiss (2003) found generally similar results; specifically, they found that prior trauma history, prior psychological adjustment, and family psychiatric history were important pretrauma risk factors for developing PTSD. Consistent with earlier findings, perceived threat of death during the traumatic event (an aspect of trauma severity) and posttrauma social support played an important role in the risk for developing

PTSD after the trauma. Ozer and her colleagues also found that the experience of dissociative symptoms and the intensity of emotions experienced by the victim in the immediate wake of the trauma were also predictive of later development of PTSD.

The Subjective Versus the Objective Meaning of a Stressor

The National Comorbidity Survey found that being raped was more likely to lead to developing PTSD than any other stressor, for both sexes (Kessler et al., 1995). Other traumas that were found to be more likely to produce PTSD were combat exposure, physical abuse, and being threatened with a weapon. Although it is crucial to recognize the individual nature of coping, we should not ignore the evidence that certain experiences are characteristically more difficult to cope with and are more likely to result in developing PTSD. Another factor that plays a significant role in the development of PTSD is the cumulative effect of stressors over time. Later stressors are themselves a risk factor for developing PTSD after an initial trauma. This suggests that the effects of stress can be cumulative over time. Several studies have shown that there is a dose–effect relationship between stress and the likelihood of developing PTSD. This effect has been demonstrated with torture victims (Mollica, 1998), combat veterans (Zaidi & Foy, 1994), and victims of child abuse (Edwards, Holden, Felitti, & Anda, 2003).

Certain individual qualities have been found to have a positive influence on the effects of severe stress. Active coping, sociability, and internal locus of control have been associated with better outcomes for those exposed to trauma. A study of 10 Vietnam veterans who had survived heavy combat without developing PTSD (Hendin & Haas, 1984) revealed that they shared the ability to communicate with others, an ability to solicit and use social support, and an active, internalized sense of responsibility for their own destiny. This suggests that these characteristics contribute to resiliency from trauma.

Discussing what constitutes a risk factor versus a protective factor for PTSD forces us to take a look at the nature of trauma and hold competing, seemingly contradictory ideas in mind. On the one hand, experiences like rape seem more likely to produce PTSD, and certain aspects of personal history seem to make a person more vulnerable. On the other hand, there is no evidence that any single stressful event will automatically result in the development of PTSD, and there appear to be aspects of social support and later stress over time that affect the risk for developing PTSD. No formula, algorithm, or recipe exists to determine who will go on to develop PTSD. What the literature on risk and protective factors tells us is that adaptation to trauma is complex, ongoing, and individual. Although it is important to understand that the development of PTSD is not random and that certain conditions make its occurrence more likely, having a risk factor does not mean one will develop the disorder. Many patients with one or more risk factors for PTSD (or any other illness for that matter) do not go on to develop the disorder. Understanding risk factors helps identify vulnerable populations and target interventions to those patients who are most likely to require them. By identifying risk factors and protective factors, we can better target interventions to those populations at greater risk for developing PTSD and identify aspects of functioning that promote greater adaptation to trauma over time.

The Perpetration of Violence as a Risk Factor for PTSD

Most of the risk factors discussed thus far have had to do with being victimized or otherwise impacted by external sources of stress. One of the complexities of working with a forensic population is that one is confronted with patients who may have been both victims and victimizers. The literature on the psychological effects of committing violence is small in comparison to that on being the victim of violence. Committing acts of violence has been shown to have a negative impact on later psychological functioning and increases vulnerability to the development of PTSD. Much of the research on the commission of violence has been conducted on combat veterans who committed atrocities and has focused on subsequent violent behavior (Beckham, Feldman, Kirby, Hertzberg, & Moore, 1998). The bulk of the evidence suggests that the commission of atrocities is predictive of increased violent behavior later. Other studies on the effects of committing acts of violence (Yehuda, Southwick, & Giller, 1992) have been concerned with the effect of committing atrocities on later PTSD symptoms. Their findings suggest that the committing of atrocities worsens PTSD symptoms.

There is also a small but notable body of literature about the posttraumatic effects of violence committed by civilians. MacNair (2002) presents evidence that both police officers who are involved in the fatal shootings of suspects and criminals who commit violent crimes are at greater risk for developing PTSD. Using a relatively large sample of convicted felons (1,140), Collins and Bailey (1990) found that as many as 15% of felons who were impulsively violent without any secondary goal (*expressive violence* in Collins and Bailey's terms) experienced PTSD symptoms after their crime. Other researchers have found that murderers whose violence was more reactive in nature were more likely to be traumatized by the act itself (Pollock, 1999). This body of evidence suggests that violence committed based on fear or in a reactive emotional way poses a greater risk for the later development of PTSD. **Table 12-1** lists the risk and protective factors for developing PTSD.

PTSD from Single Incidents Versus Chronic Stress

Because PTSD is the consequence of experience, we are used to thinking about trauma as a discrete event, which is somewhat misleading. From our discussion of the various risks and protective factors for the development of PSTD, we know that traumatic events come in many varieties. Some traumatic events are truly singular occurrences like a plane crash or a terrorist attack—events that the victim will most likely not experience twice. Yet these single events can have enduring impact on health and functioning. On the other hand, some traumas stem from circumstances that are hardly events at all, but are chronic conditions or characteristics of their surrounding environment. Examples would include

TABLE 12-1   Risks and Protective Factors for PTSD

Pre-trauma Risk Factors	*Post-trauma Risk Factors*
Physical abuse	Trauma severity/perceived life threat
Sexual abuse	Poor social supports/social isolation
Personal psychiatric history	Subsequent traumatic events
Family psychiatric history	Severity of acute stress symptoms
Prior trauma history	Dissociative symptoms
Pre-trauma Protective Factors	*Post-trauma Protective Factors*
Secure attachment	Positive social support
Positive social supports	Effective use of anger
Active problem solving	Internal locus of control

children growing up in conditions of violent political unrest, victims of chronic sexual abuse, or abused spouses. These patients have traumatic experiences that are qualitatively different from those traumas caused by a single event. There is good evidence to suggest that the mental health effects of these two types of trauma have important differences. Studies by Lenore Terr and Judy Herman exemplify these differences.

The Long-Term Consequences of Single-Episode Trauma

In 1976, a group of 26 children on a school bus in Chowchilla, California, were kidnapped and placed in a freight trailer that was buried in the California desert. They remained in the trailer for approximately 36 hours before venturing out and finding that they had been abandoned. The kidnappers were never found and no motive for the kidnapping has ever been determined. The abducted children ranged from 6 to 12 years of age. Lenore Terr followed the victims of this group abduction and reported her findings in the book, *Too Scared to Cry* (1990). Terr's follow-up studies give us an opportunity to understand the effects of short-term trauma on long-term psychological functioning.

In the course of her follow-up studies with the children from the Chowchilla abduction, Terr made several observations. First, there were subtle and progressive alterations of the memories of the traumatic event over time. In some cases this was the effect of misleading consensus—small distortions that through repetitions and discussion with other participants took on the legitimacy of fact. Other instances involved specific memories of the kidnapping that were either distorted or elaborated upon to the point of being factually inconsistent with known aspects of the kidnapping. Terr observed that many of the children had some degree of change in their capacity to regulate fear, anger, and interpersonal connection. Various children were observed to have grown either more irritable, hypervigilant, emotionally detached, or some combination thereof.

Finally, Terr found that the themes of the kidnapping had ways of expressing themselves throughout the child's repertoire of conscious and unconscious behaviors. Many of the children had recurrent dreams and nightmares about the kidnapping. Other children reenacted various aspects of the kidnapping, either overtly or symbolically in their play. The children who were youngest at the time of the kidnapping seemed to engage in the most nonverbal and symbolically transformed behavior over time, as if they could only work through these issues using the capacities developmentally available to them at the time of the trauma. From a single identified stressor, the kidnapping, these children exhibited variable and enduring changes in psychological functioning.

Complex PTSD

Herman describes complex PTSD as a pattern of alterations to several areas of psychosocial functioning:

» *Emotional regulation:* Emotional regulation is the capacity to reign in one's own automatic emotional responses and to comfortably experience a range of emotions between extremes of good and bad. Patients with complex PTSD have difficulty feeling a moderate or slight form of an emotion. This can lead to intense feelings of sadness, rage, or fear that are vastly out of proportion to the events surrounding them.
» *Consciousness:* As already noted, stress responses can produce changes in consciousness, including dissociation, intrusive thoughts, and difficulty with memory. Patients

with complex PTSD may present experiencing these changes in consciousness on a persisting aspect of their daily lives. This may include reexperiencing phenomena as described in the PTSD diagnosis or repeated dissociation or depersonalization experiences.

» *Self-perception:* Patients with complex PTSD can present with feelings of being inadequate, shamed, or stigmatized. These feelings of being damaged are often accompanied by feelings of being alone or being incapable of being understood.

» *Perception of the perpetrator:* Because the conditions that produce complex PTSD often involve intense interpersonal relations between the abuser and the victim, usually of a coercive sort, patients who develop complex PTSD can have an assortment of ideas about their abusers. Some patients attribute special powers to their abusers or experience their relationship with them as special in a positive way. They may be preoccupied with the abuser in various ways. The overarching principle is that the patient's concept of the perpetrator takes on meaning beyond a mere object of fear or anger.

» *Relations with others:* Patients with complex PSTD often come from backgrounds where interpersonal relationships were exploitive. With that background, intimacy, trust, and the safety of others is thrown into doubt. Patients with complex PTSD have learned through hard experience that people can be dangerous. This creates difficulty in forming and sustaining positive social relationships and social support.

» *System of meaning:* Of all the aspects of complex PTSD, the patient's system of meaning has the greatest implications for long-term growth and change for the patient. The patient's system of meaning refers to the patient's overarching set of beliefs about the present, his or her self, and the future that serves to promote or diminish hope. This includes religion or other spiritual beliefs. It also encompasses the patient's set of expectations about themselves and the future. An urban youth whose only example of power, economic security, and success is drug dealers may see no benefit to other pathways to goals, such as education or conventional employment. A battered woman who only sees worsening anger and threat by her abuser may see no benefit in trying to leave him.

The symptoms of complex PTSD are not very different from the DSM definition. The changes of affect regulation, relations with others, and consciousness are similar to avoidance symptoms. What makes these symptoms different from the PTSD definition given by the DSM is that it encompasses the developmental and interpersonal consequences of living under conditions of chronic and repeated trauma, in which PTSD symptoms become part of personality functioning. What this illustrates most clearly is that chronic stress, especially in children and adolescents, has developmental consequences that are distinct from short-term or single-episode trauma. Observing that many psychiatric patients diagnosed with major personality disorders (borderline personality disorder in particular) often present with histories of major sexual or physical abuse, Herman (1992) suggests that these patients might be more accurately described in a framework that accounts for the long-term effects of trauma as expressed in adult personality functioning. Short-term effect or single episode trauma seem to produce symptoms most consistent with the DSM-IV-TR series definition of PTSD. Long-term trauma seems to produce symptoms that create enduring changes in adaptation and the interpretation of experience, becoming incorporated into more global personality functioning.

Psychiatric Comorbidity and PTSD

Depression and anxiety are common complaints for patients with PTSD and may be their initial reason for seeking out mental health treatment instead of the trauma itself. Depression appears to make one more vulnerable to developing PTSD, and PTSD appears to make one more vulnerable to developing depression. One of the confounding issues in the diagnosis of depression and anxiety in conjunction with PTSD is that certain PTSD symptoms resemble both depression and anxiety (Davidson & Foa, 1991). Hyperarousal symptoms and reexperiencing symptoms can easily resemble other anxiety disorders. Avoidance symptoms can resemble depression. The relationship between PTSD and depression is complex (Erickson, Wolfe, King, King, & Sharkansky, 2001). The literature suggests that although depression in patients with PTSD appears to have little difference from depression in clients without PTSD, there is a slightly greater experience of self-blame and lower levels of dependency in the patients with PTSD.

Substance abuse in PTSD can be especially difficult to manage and treat. Patients suffering from PTSD and substance abuse will often describe their use as a means of dampening their PTSD symptoms and may justify their substance abuse on that basis. Central nervous system depressants such as alcohol, opiates, benzodiazepines, and hallucinogens such as marijuana are fairly common substances of choice for patients with PTSD, as they can reduce the subjective experience of hyperarousal and intrusive symptoms. However, the use of stimulants or more activating drugs like cocaine is not unheard of. Using epidemiological data, McFarlane (1998) offers compelling evidence that the relationship between substance abuse and PTSD is largely unidirectional. The notion of self-medication of psychiatric symptoms is not new in the substance abuse literature, but it seems to be particularly valid for PTSD patients.

Treatment Modalities for PTSD

Most studies have found that effective treatment for PTSD consists of combined psychosocially oriented therapy (cognitive behavioral, psychodynamic, or group psychotherapy) and medication treatment. Most of the psychosocial therapies have similar common goals—symptom reduction, the improved psychological organization of the traumatic experience, and reducing the destructive power of memories and feelings associated with the traumatic memory. Their differences lie in how they broadly conceptualize the mechanisms of trauma and by extension the steps needed to provide relief.

Pharmacotherapy

The use of medication has been found to be helpful in the treatment of PTSD. The only medication currently approved by the FDA specifically for the treatment of PTSD is sertraline (Zoloft). Because of the relatively broad symptom profile (depression, emotional numbing, withdrawal, anxiety, agitation) seen in patients with PTSD, medications are often prescribed empirically to treat specific target symptoms. Although guidelines are available (Alarcon, Glover, Boyer, & Baleen, 2000; Francis, 2003), most practice seen in the community tends to be driven by symptom considerations. (An excellent overview of the pharmacological treatment of PTSD can be found in Friedman [2001].) Certain drug classes are more commonly used for the treatment of PTSD.

Research and the development of newer medications have resulted in more effective management of the often incapacitating symptoms of PTSD. We have not listed any specific medications since striving for effective management results in frequent modifications of medication regimens. Antidepressants and anxiolytics/benzodiazepines continue to provide relief in certain individuals suffering from PTSD.

The Care and Assessment of Patients with PTSD in the Forensic Setting

Assessment in the forensic setting has different areas of emphasis than those in traditional clinical settings. If the nurse is caring for the victim of a crime, evidence collection and ascertaining details of the crime take on greater importance than they would in a more conventional clinical encounter. If the nurse is caring for an inmate or an alleged perpetrator of a crime, questions of malingering, violence potential, and state of mind may take on greater importance. Caring for patients with PTSD in the forensic setting makes special demands of the nurse—demands that change with the type of patient for whom the nurse is caring.

Interviewing Techniques

The following guidelines can assist in the interviewing and assessment of trauma victims.

1. *Approach the topic of the trauma with respect and patience.* Patients will often be reluctant to talk about their traumatic experiences with strangers, even healthcare professionals. Practitioners working with trauma victims should establish a rapport before proceeding into the details of the trauma. This could consist of obtaining more general background history first, or providing other forms of care prior to the interview. It is often helpful to clearly frame questions about the trauma within the helping context (e.g., "I need to ask you some questions about what happened so I can know how to help you."). Do not demand, cajole, or otherwise coerce the victim to talk about the trauma, or to talk about the trauma more than he or she feels ready to at the time. Forcing emotional displays from the patient or demanding that patients confront or deal with their trauma in a manner of our choosing rather than theirs has no proven benefit and is poor treatment. This may include accepting the patient's limited ability to remember the details of the trauma or their being unwilling to talk about it. All the following recommendations should be taken with that caveat in mind.

2. *Start with open-ended general questions and follow with more specific and detailed questions.* Begin asking about the traumatic experience using open-ended questions. This allows the patient some obvious control of the interview and is less threatening. It is also more natural to ask about specific details of the trauma against the backdrop of the general information the patient provides. Depending on the rapport and comfort level with the patient, you may choose to ask more detailed questions as the story unfolds or after the patient has completed his or her account. As the patient gives you an account of the trauma, note areas or details that you wish to know more about and go back to. What questions come to mind? You may find that the patient answers your questions as he or she continues to describe the event, but you should

keep a mental note of your questions just in case. When the patient has completed the account, you can go back to those areas to fill in the gaps.

3. *Follow the patient's lead whenever possible.* Listen for clues the patient gives you about important aspects of his or her trauma during the interview. If a particular place, person, time, or situation keeps coming up in the patient's narrative but is not addressed, ask about it. Observe and note changes in the patient's emotional expression over the course of the account. Conspicuously intense or absent emotion are signals that the material being described is especially troubling to the patient, and this may be a sign to slow down or offer additional support. Sometimes the interview will ebb and flow, as the patient will need to move away from the topic of the trauma for a few minutes before returning to it. Patients will sometimes do this as a way of regrouping before moving forward with the account, so this should generally not be discouraged. Because of the emotional intensity of the material, the patient may require time to process a question or think about how to respond. This can lead to moments of silence during the interview. Unless the patient is visibly becoming somnolent or appears to be dissociating, resist the impulse to break the silence or probe further until the patient responds on his or her own.

4. *When possible, help the patient give words to his or her feelings.* Trauma occurs when coping is overwhelmed. As we have already discussed, one of the changes observed in the brains of patients with PTSD is that the part of the brain responsible for language operates differently in the context of trauma reminders. Words and language are powerful tools for organizing experience. One of the most subjectively disturbing problems trauma victims describe is their difficulty giving words to their emotions and their experience. This can create circumstances where the patient has torturous feelings of fear, sadness, and rage to which he or she cannot give voice. As the victim describes the aftermath of the trauma, you should also ask about his or her feelings as well as the facts of the trauma.

Without imposing your words on the victim's experience, it is often helpful to work with the patient to find his or her own words for the actual events and the feelings associated with the trauma. This helps the patient create an internal account of the trauma and his or her feelings, which can be communicated to others. This, in turn, helps the victim organize the experience in his or her own mind and speaks to the fundamental breakdown that distinguishes stress from trauma. By giving language to the facts and feelings of the trauma, those words can become the currency that the patient exchanges for the help and support of others.

Specific Patient Populations

Forensic nurses will be called upon to provide care for patients suffering from a wide variety of trauma under equally variable circumstances. To attempt to cover every possible type of trauma is beyond the scope of this chapter. However, the forensic nurse may encounter certain situations more regularly than others. The following section identifies the more common forensic patient populations seen in practice; however, this is by no means complete. The victims of violent crimes and terrorism, as well as victims of domestic events, fires, and weather-related trauma are also forensic patients. Any patient who is the victim of a violent or traumatic event may be a forensic patient.

Caring for Prison Inmates

Prison inmates present a set of unique challenges to the forensic nurse. The confinement, the closed social network of the patient population, and the involuntary nature of treatment can make the care of this patient population daunting. Yet the prison population also has a high concentration of individuals with PTSD compared to the general population. A study by Powell, Holt, and Fondacaro (1997) found that the incidence of PTSD in the inmate population in a rural state prison system was 33%, which is more than double the incidence found in large population studies outside of prison.

Inmates are at heightened risk for traumatic experiences while being incarcerated. Between 16% and 22% of male inmates are raped while in prison (Struckman-Johnson, Struckman-Johnson, Rucker, Bumby, & Donaldson, 1995, 1996). Reviewing the literature on inmate violence, Drummond (2000) summarizes several factors that make a prisoner more vulnerable to being raped. Those risk factors include youth, small physical size or weakness, having a mental illness or developmental disability, lack of street sense, lack of gang affiliation, known homosexuality, being a sex offender, being suspected of informing on other inmates, being disliked by staff, and having a history of being sexually assaulted. Very little controlled research has been conducted on the scope of inmate violence, and no official figures for prison rape are currently maintained on any large scale, so it is impossible to precisely quantify the extent of the problem. However, the problem of prison rape has attracted sufficient notice that the Prison Rape Elimination Act of 2003 was signed into law. This measure was enacted to more comprehensively study the problem of prison rape and to provide a basis for ongoing intervention and policy making.

Inmates struggling with PTSD may be reluctant to acknowledge or discuss their issues for several reasons. Acknowledging being traumatized involves an admission of vulnerability. The risk of being perceived as weak by other inmates is an important consideration in an environment where the image of strength plays such an important role in safety and daily living conditions. This may be particularly true of inmates whose trauma involved being the recipient of abuse, which may cast the patient in a weak or vulnerable light. Another consideration is that PTSD symptoms like hypervigilance and hyperarousal are adaptive in circumstances where aggression plays a pervasive role in social relations.

Despite the obstacles, there is considerable value to providing treatment to inmates with PTSD. Patients with PTSD can experience significant difficulty with substance abuse and anger management. Often these problems contributed to the behaviors that brought the inmate into contact with the criminal justice system in the first place. In addition to addressing the trauma, it is important to address other conditions that contribute to behavior that leads the patient to be in the criminal justice system. Inmates with PTSD may have substance abuse and anger management problems that can aggravate (or be aggravated by) the effects of PTSD. Group treatment can be helpful because it normalizes the experience among the group members, reduces the need for defensive aggression, and builds a support system.

Professional Practice Considerations

Feelings Toward the Patient

Forensic patients of any kind can provoke strong feelings in the professionals responsible for their care, and nurses are no exception. Healthcare professionals are often drawn to the field because of their concern for others. Working with forensic patients can pose a challenge because they often come to the forensic setting having been the victim of or having engaged in behaviors that are harmful, exploitative, or destructive. A feeling of sympathy and compassion for victims is natural, as is anger, revulsion, and fear for patients who may have committed terrible acts. Awareness and acceptance of one's own feelings for the patient, negative or positive, are essential to maintaining a professional helping stance.

Denial of one's own feelings for the patient can lead to unconscious and subtle forms of interaction with the patient that often cause substandard care and make care more difficult to provide. If one's feelings for the patient are negative, the patient will often sense that he or she is being treated badly. If one's feelings for the patient are positive, objective assessment becomes more difficult, and boundary violations are more likely to occur. It is better to acknowledge one's own feelings for a patient and talk about them with colleagues than to enact those feelings on the unit floor or in the office. Keeping in mind one's role within the larger system and the right of all patients to good care are important in maintaining perspective in working with this challenging population.

Understanding the Role of Trauma Is Not Equivalent to Sympathizing With Criminal Behavior

Working with victims of trauma in a forensic setting can evoke contradictory feelings. On the one hand, you may be working with someone who has been accused of committing terrible acts, yet who may also have been the victim of terrible acts himself. It can be a struggle to reconcile feelings of empathy for a person who has known terrible suffering with feelings of fear and revulsion for the same person who may have inflicted terrible suffering on others. When working with inmates or the alleged perpetrator of a crime, it is important to remember that understanding the contributions of traumatic experience to the patient's criminal acts is not equivalent to condoning antisocial behavior.

Mental illness does not justify a criminal act. The courts consider the role of mental illness in determining the level of culpability and the severity of the punishment for the accused. The necessary conditions for criminal responsibility in the U.S. criminal justice system are the commission of a criminal act and the presence of criminal intent. Although the performance of a criminal act may be comparatively easy to establish, mental illness calls criminal intent, and thus criminal responsibility, into question.

One of the most important tasks any forensic healthcare professional performs is translating an understanding of healthcare concepts, issues, and processes to the interdisciplinary forensic team. This is a complex skill that is part teaching, part reframing, and part diplomacy. The criminal justice system is organized around the protection of society through the adjudication and punishment of crimes, whereas healthcare provision is organized around the care and benefit of the patient. When working with trauma survivors or victims of crime, these value sets are broadly aligned, even when the professional becomes a source of information to help make the case. In investigative or correctional settings, where the survivor or victim may also be a perpetrator, these values may come into conflict. These patients are the bad guys, after all. This is a fundamental difference in orientation and is a predictable source of tension for the nurse practicing in the forensic setting.

Healthcare professionals provide assessment, care, and treatment. Judges and juries decide the role of mental illness in determining guilt or innocence of a crime. Our role as healthcare professionals is to provide good assessment and good care to our patients, and when obliged provide information to other members of the forensic team (lawyers, judges, juries) to facilitate their work in adjudicating these matters. Fulfilling that role requires that our care be provided in a professional manner and that our assessments are fair, objective, and reliable. By doing so, we allow the other participants in the process (colleagues, lawyers, judges, juries) to make arguments, decisions, and judgments with the best information possible.

Summary

Posttraumatic stress disorder is a topic of substantial interest to the field of mental health, the legal system, and society at large. The conditions that create trauma, the interventions that reduce its likelihood, and the treatment of those who suffer from it have broad social implications. It is indisputable in the face of the available empirical data that some people's feelings, thoughts, and behavior are dramatically and negatively altered by the experience of overwhelming stress. The conditions that breed trauma have considerable social components. Violence, substance abuse, and neglect all qualify as large social problems that government and mental health establishments have had mixed results in combating. These issues are also part and parcel of the work the criminal justice system and the forensic sciences engage in every day.

Although mental illnesses such as bipolar disorder and schizophrenia enjoy strong evidence for biologically based etiology and have clear symptom profiles, PTSD is by its nature an acquired mental illness that can have a variable presentation resembling other conditions. The study of trauma brings into bold relief the forensic and legal questions posed by mental illness in general. How do we know another person's mind? To what extent can the hardships of the past explain our present behavior? To what extent do those hardships diminish culpability for our actions? How do we understand the person we are treating now in terms of her past?

Nurses who practice in a forensic setting will encounter patients who have experienced the unimaginable. Sometimes they will be victims; sometimes they will be perpetrators. Too often they will have been both at different times. Patients with PTSD present unique challenges and demand treatment that is mindful of its complexities. Although general information such as that provided in this chapter is a point of departure, it is not a substitute for learning from the patient. Understanding patients with PTSD requires that we stand with them, be they sinner or saint, and bear witness to the darkest aspects of human experience. It is provocative work that demands courage. Working with traumatized patients requires a willingness to help give voice to the unspeakable and to withstand rage from the patient and within ourselves; it also requires the capacity for hope in the face of despair. By doing these things we help the patient begin to make sense of their past experience, define themselves in the present, and develop meaning for the future.

QUESTIONS FOR DISCUSSION

1. What events in your own life have challenged your coping?
2. What strengths and supports can you point to in your own life that have helped you in times of crisis?
3. Is there any similarity between society's response to large national tragedies like the September 11, 2001 attacks and individual responses to trauma?
4. How is a stressful event different from a trauma?
5. Why do some people develop PTSD and others do not?

REFERENCES

Alarcon, D., Glover, S., Boyer, B., & Baleen, R. (2000). Proposing an algorithm for the pharmacological management of posttraumatic stress disorder. *Annals of Clinical Psychiatry, 12*(4), 239–246.

American Psychiatric Association. (2000). *Diagnostic and statistical manual of psychiatric disorders* (4th ed., text revision). Washington, DC: American Psychiatric Press.

Beckham, J., Feldman, M., Kirby, A., Hertzberg, M., & Moore, S. (1998). Interpersonal violence and its correlates in Vietnam veterans with chronic posttraumatic stress disorder. *Journal of Clinical Psychology, 53*(8), 859–867.

Brewin, C., Andrews, B., & Valentine, J. (2000). Meta-analysis of risk factors for post-traumatic stress disorder in trauma exposed adults. *Journal of Consulting and Clinical Psychology, 68*(5), 748–766.

Collins, J., & Bailey, S. (1990). Traumatic stress disorder and violent behavior. *Journal of Traumatic Stress, 3,* 203–220.

Davidson, J., & Foa, E. (1991). Diagnostic issues in posttraumatic stress disorder: Considerations for the DSM-IV. *Journal of Abnormal Psychology, 100,* 346–355.

Dean, E. (1999). *Shook over hell: Post-traumatic stress disorder, Vietnam and the Civil War.* Cambridge, MA: Harvard University Press.

Delahanty, D. L. (2011). Toward the predeployment detection of risk for PTSD. Washington DC: American Psychiatric Association.

Drummond, R. (2000). Inmate sexual assault: The plague that persists. *The Prison Journal, 80*(4), 407–414.

Edwards, V., Holden, G., Felitti, V., & Anda, R. (2003). Relationship between multiple forms of childhood maltreatment and adult mental health in community respondents: Results from the Adverse Childhood Experiences study. *American Journal of Psychiatry, 160*(8), 1453–1460.

Erickson, D., Wolfe, J., King, D., King, L., & Sharkansky, E. (2001). Posttraumatic stress disorder and depression symptomatology in a sample of Gulf War veterans: A prospective analysis. *Journal of Consulting and Clinical Psychology, 69*(1), 41–49.

Feldner, M. T., Monson, C. M., & Friedman, M. J. (2007). A critical analysis of approaches to targeted PTSD prevention: Current status and theoretically derived future directions. *Behavior Modification, 31*(1), 80–116.

Francis, J. (2003). Effective treatments for PTSD: Practice guidelines from the International Society for Traumatic Stress Studies. *Bulletin of the Menninger Clinic, 67*(4), 370–379.

Friedman, M. (2001). Allostatic versus empirical perspectives on pharmacotherapy for PTSD. In J. Wilson, M. Friedman, & J. Lindy (Eds.), *Treating psychological trauma and PTSD* (pp. 94–124). New York, NY: Guilford.

Hendin, H., & Haas, A. P. (1984). *Wounds of war: The psychological aftermath of the Vietnam War.* New York, NY: Basic Books.

Herman, J. (1992). *Trauma and recovery.* New York, NY: Basic Books.

Kessler, R., Sonnega, A., Bromet, E., Hughes, M., & Nelson, C. (1995). Posttraumatic stress disorder in the National Comorbidity Survey. *Archives of General Psychiatry, 52,* 1048–1060.

MacNair, R. (2002). *Perpetration-induced traumatic stress: The psychological consequences of killing.* Westport, CT: Praeger.

McFarlane, A. (1998). Epidemiological evidence about the relationship between PTSD and alcohol abuse: The nature of the association. *Addictive Behavior, 23,* 813–825.

Mollica, R. F. (1998). The dose effect relationship between torture and psychiatric symptoms in Vietnamese ex-political detainees and a comparison group. *The Journal of Nervous and Mental Disease, 186*(9), 543–553.

Morgan, A., Wang, S., Southwick, S., Rassmusson, A., Hazlett, G., & Hauger, R. (2002). Plasma neuropeptide-Y concentrations in humans exposed to highly intense and uncontrollable stress. *Biological Psychiatry, 47,* 902–909.

Ozer, E., Best, S., Lipsey, T., & Weiss, D. (2003). Predictors of posttraumatic stress disorder and symptoms in adults: A meta-analysis. *Psychological Bulletin, 129*(1), 52–73.

Pollock, P. (1999). When the killer suffers: Post-traumatic stress reactions following homicide. *Legal and Criminological Psychology, 4,* 185–202.

Powell, T., Holt, J., & Fondacaro, K. (1997). The prevalence of mental illness among inmates in a rural state. *Journal of Law and Human Behavior, 21,* 427–438.

Roy-Byrne, P., Russo, J., Michelson, E., Zatzick, D., Pitman, R., & Berliner, L. (2004). Risk factors and outcomes in ambulatory assault victims presenting to the acute emergency department setting: Implications for secondary prevention studies in PTSD. *Depression and Anxiety, 19*(2), 77–84.

Struckman-Johnson, C. J., Struckman-Johnson, D. L., Rucker, L., Bumby, K., & Donaldson, S. (1995). *A survey of inmate and staff perspectives on prisoner sexual assault.* Paper presented at the annual meeting of the midwestern Psychological Association, Chicago, IL.

Struckman-Johnson, C. J., Struckman-Johnson, D. L., Rucker, L., Bumby, K., & Donaldson, S. (1996). Sexual coercion reported by men and women in prison. *Journal of Sex Research, 33*(1), 67–76.

Terr, L. (1990). *Too scared to cry: Psychic trauma in childhood.* Grand Rapids, MI: Harper & Row.

van Emmerick, A., Kamphuis, J., Hulsbocsch, A., & Emmelkamp, P. (2002). Single session debriefing after psychological trauma: A meta-analysis. *Lancet, 360*(9335), 766–771.

Yehuda, R., Southwick, S., & Giller, E. (1992). Exposure to atrocities and severity of chronic posttraumatic stress disorder in Vietnam combat veterans. *American Journal of Psychiatry, 149,* 333–336.

Zaidi, L., & Foy, D. (1994). Childhood abuse experiences and combat-related PTSD. *Journal of Traumatic Stress, 7*(1), 33–42.

SUGGESTED FURTHER READING

Blaustein, M. (2010). *Treating traumatic stress in children and adolescents: How to foster resilience through attachment, self-regulation, and competency.* New York, NY: Guilford Press.

Fernando, S. (2010). *Mental health, race and culture.* New York, NY: Palgrave Macmillan.

Ford, J. D. (2009). *Posttraumatic stress disorder: Science and professional dimensions.* Burlington, MA: Elsevier Academic Press.

National Center for PTSD website. http://www.ncptsd.va.gov

National Institute for Mental Health (NIH) website. http://www.nimh.nih.gov/health/topics/post-traumatic-stress-disorder-ptsd/index.shtml

Paulson, D. S. (2010). *Haunted by combat: Understanding PTSD in war veterans.* Lanham, MD: Rowman & Littlefield.

Schiraldi, G. R. (2009). *The post-traumatic stress disorder sourcebook.* Lincolnwood, IL: Lowell Hill.

Williams, M. B., & Sommer, J. F. (2002). *Simple and complex post-traumatic stress disorder: Strategies for comprehensive treatment in clinical practice.* Binghampton, NY: Psychology Press.

CHAPTER 13

Death Investigation

Edward T. McDonough

Death investigation is an essential service that involves a focus on the identification of the deceased, determination of the physical condition of the body at an investigative scene, documentation of injuries, gathering and reporting of evidence, estimation of time of death, functioning as a liaison to families, and provision of the final certification as to the cause and manner of death. Increasingly in many jurisdictions, the death investigator is a nonphysician employed by the medical examiner's office. As a representative of this office, the nonphysician death investigator plays a vital role in contributing to the ultimate findings of the medical examiner as to the cause and manner of death, performing many of the duties previously associated with the medical examiner. The death investigator is an evolving role that requires excellent observational, perception, and communication skills. A preexisting knowledge of medical conditions is a most desirable additional asset. Although death investigators traditionally have varied educational backgrounds, the requisite skills make the forensic nurse an ideal candidate to fulfill this role.

CHAPTER FOCUS

- » History of Death Investigation
- » Cause of Death
- » Identifying the Deceased
- » Clinical Forensic Medicine
- » Time of Death and Postmortem Changes

- » Human Decomposition
- » Identification of Human Remains
- » Guns and Gunshot Wounds
- » Blunt-Force Trauma
- » Asphyxia

KEY TERMS

- » abrasion
- » algor mortis
- » autolysis
- » cause of death
- » contusions
- » coroner
- » degloving
- » desiccated
- » forensic entomologist
- » forensic pathologist
- » fracture
- » homicide
- » laceration

- » livor mortis
- » maceration
- » manner of death
- » medical examiner
- » mummification
- » natural death
- » nosologist
- » proximate event
- » putrefaction
- » rigor mortis
- » saponification
- » suicide
- » toxicology

There is no single uniform death investigation system in the United States. There are at least 50 major jurisdictions, not including the District of Columbia, Puerto Rico, Guam, and all the subjurisdictions such as counties and cities. Further, statutes, law enforcement, and the attendant support structures that evolve around them are all locally generated. The 10th Amendment to the U.S. Constitution allows for these individual jurisdictions to exist and operate independently, but it also creates inherent inequity and variation. There is often not a right way or a wrong way to investigate any particular death, but a city way and a country way; that is, population centers have greater resources and larger revenue streams available to the governing body, and therefore can offer more services to the citizens than a region with fewer resources. This includes death investigation services. The methods applied to investigating various categories of deaths are well defined, but lack of available local resources may, out of necessity, modify the extent to which particular deaths are scrutinized. For example, a large metropolitan medical examiner's office with sufficient staffing, laboratory facilities, and capabilities may examine firsthand every deceased individual who comes under its jurisdiction. In contrast, some small rural counties may have no medical facilities and a limited budget for outsourcing only a few autopsy examinations annually.

History of Death Investigation

There are many historic seeds, some thousands of years old, which ultimately germinated into the modern practice of death investigation. Identification of a particular death as a suicide was important to early communities who believed that if suicide was not recognized and stopped, the community would be destroyed by the action of the evil spirits thought to be responsible. The counterpart to this community action is seen in the modern epidemiologic approach used to identify and combat infectious diseases (Hanzlick, R.L. 1996).

Some examples of historic medicolegal seeds follow. One is Hammurabi's Code, which was inscribed on stone in approximately 2000 BC and is perhaps the oldest written code of law. When Julius Caesar was assassinated in 44 BC, a Roman medical doctor named Antistius examined the body and noted and reported the presence of 23 wounds. It was his opinion that one stab wound to the chest was the lethal injury. In 1192, when Richard the Lionhearted was kidnapped and held for ransom by Leopold of Austria, the English treasury was unable to cover the ransom. This led to the development of a strategy to make use of corpses as a novel source of income. The title of *crowner* was given to those who acquired custody of a dead criminal's possessions turning them over to the English treasury, thus enriching the royal assets. The word **coroner** (crowner) was originally mentioned in 925 in the Chart of Privileges. In 1194, the duties of the coroner in England were formally delineated. The local justices provided that three knights and one clerk were elected in every county as keepers of the pleas of the crown. This coroner position dictated administrative and investigative responsibilities often carried out with the assistance of the local sheriff. One of these duties included holding inquests over the deceased to ascertain the nature of the wounds and provide for the arrest of any individual deemed responsible for their infliction (Hanzlick, 1997b).

In 1250, a Chinese treatise, *Hsi Yuan Lu*, was produced, covering such topics as blunt and sharp force injury, drowning, and deaths by fire. This writing addressed questions about whether a person was alive or dead when he went into the water or prior to the fire.

The settlers in early America brought with them the English coroner system. In 1637, records in Maryland discuss the actions of the coroner/sheriff holding inquests. The first recorded autopsy examination was done in 1647 in Massachusetts regarding a case where an individual was killed by a tree limb. Autopsy examinations were still incredibly rare events, but their usefulness was identified in this early time period.

The earliest mention of physicians collaborating with the coroner was in 1860 in Maryland, when the Code of Public General Laws authorized the coroner or his jury to require the attendance of a physician in the investigation of cases of violent death. Shortly after that, the legislature authorized the governor to appoint a physician as a sole coroner in Baltimore. In 1877, Maryland adopted a statewide system requiring that a physician known as a **medical examiner** supplant the coroner. The examiner's responsibilities primarily lie in the investigation of violent deaths. In 1890, a Baltimore city ordinance authorized the board of health to appoint two physicians with the title of medical examiner and assign them the duty of performing all autopsies requested by the coroner or the state's attorney of the city of Baltimore.

In 1915, New York City adopted a law eliminating the coroner's office and creating a medical examiner system. The medical examiner was authorized to investigate deaths resulting from criminal violence, suicide, sudden unexpected deaths, deaths that were not attended by medical personnel, or the deaths of imprisoned persons. Dr. Charles Norris was the first chief medical examiner and was given the authority to perform autopsies according to his particular judgment. This established the first essentials of a competent medical examiner system that would investigate a broad spectrum of cases with the authority to perform an autopsy when the public interest demanded it.

In 1939, the first statewide medical examiner system was established in Maryland. The medical examiner system, as developed in New York City and throughout Maryland, requires the medical examiner to be a physician. For the most part, this eliminates the death investigator having to be tied to a political party and having to campaign periodically for the office. Running for an elected office might be seen to compromise, to some degree, a coroner's true independence by creating a need to avoid alienating one or more segments of the electorate, such as law enforcement, criminal and civil lawyers, funeral directors, and other potential special interest constituencies, including families. However, many elected coroner positions throughout the United States require that the coroner be a physician (Dillon, 1999).

Death Investigator Roles

A coroner is an elected or appointed official who may or may not have any medical training, much less subspecialty training in forensic pathology; however, there are many excellent nonphysician death investigators. One advantage to the classic coroner system is the ability to hold minitrials known as inquests. In an inquest, witnesses can be examined under oath to document and certify evidence associated with a particular deceased in a formal setting.

A medical examiner is, by definition, a physician. However, the mere fact that the medical examiner is a physician does not in any way guarantee that this person has any training or experience in the field of death investigation. His or her inherent knowledge of medicine, dealing with patients and grieving relatives, and understanding of physiology and pharmacology does, however, give him or her a significant advantage over a lay nonphysician coroner responsible for investigating death.

A forensic pathologist is a physician who has trained in pathology, either in a 3-year anatomic pathology program or a combined 4-year anatomic and clinical pathology program, who then goes on to subspecialty training in an approved medical examiner's office, ultimately sitting for the Forensic Pathology board examination. It is not uncommon for a forensic pathologist to be triple board certified (holding anatomic, clinical, and forensic certificates) in pathology.

The Role of the Medical Examiner

A medical examiner's office may cover an entire state or a single county. Some state systems, such as in Massachusetts and North Carolina, have regional offices apart from the main headquarters because of the geography and large distances that need to be covered. County systems often also contract with surrounding smaller county coroners to perform necessary medicolegal autopsy examinations. A chief medical examiner, who is statutorily responsible for administering the agency, performing the death investigations, keeping records, and providing **toxicology** services, usually heads such an office. The chief medical examiner may be directly appointed by the governor or appointed by an intermediary body. The office may be a part of a larger state or county agency, such as the health department or the attorney general's office. The duties of the chief medical examiner and his office are dictated by state or county statute, which usually allow the chief medical examiner or his designee to perform investigations and autopsy examinations at their professional discretion.

The purpose of any death investigation system, however it is constructed, is according to statute—to determine the cause and the manner of an individual's death that comes under its jurisdiction. The criteria for which types of deaths must come to the attention of a death investigator were set forth by the New York City Medical Examiner's Office decades ago. Although minor variations occur between jurisdictions, the broad criteria allow a wide net to be cast and therefore decrease the chances of a case that should have been investigated being missed. The generally recognized criteria include deaths caused by trauma (blunt, sharp, chemical, or electrical trauma), suicide, accident, or homicide; deaths that are suspicious, impact public health, are in the workplace, or are unattended by medical or hospital personnel; and remains that are to be cremated or buried at sea. Other types of deaths falling within the death investigator's purview include people dying with no physician to sign the death certificate.

The Investigation

Initial Scene Observations

The investigation begins when a particular death, meeting the criteria for investigation, is reported to the administrative arm of the death investigation system. Ideally, if the deceased is still at the death scene, the investigator should be dispatched to the scene to gather information and evidence, not to determine that the individual is indeed dead. No state statutes indicate that a physician must pronounce a person dead. The statutes do indicate that a physician must certify the death (i.e., sign a death certificate), usually within 24 hours of becoming aware of it. In the field, a person is presumed/declared dead when responsible parties decline to institute emergency procedures and/or transportation to a medical facility. Conditions such as drug or alcohol intoxication and hypothermia can mimic somatic death, and there are cases reported where an apparently dead person awakened. To avoid these situations, medical control for emergency service personnel should include the documentation of lack of cardiac activity prior to the presumption of an individual's death.

At the scene, it is important to establish whether the decedent has been moved or is in the same position as initially discovered. Basic questions can then be ascertained from the police, witnesses, or family members who are also at the scene. How and why was the decedent discovered? What is the identity of the individual? When was the person last reliably known to be alive? What happened just prior to the decedent's collapse, if known? What was his condition/behavior in the 24 to 48 hours prior to his death? What are his or her known medical conditions? The investigator then should make observations about the nature of the environment in which the victim lived. Is it tidy, cluttered, or dirty? Is there anything out of order? What is the temperature of the environment (or what was the temperature of the environment when the first responder arrived?) What is the decedent wearing? What is the position of the body?

The investigator should then examine the remains for personal possessions, evidence of identification, and other clues as to his or her medical condition, such as medical alert bracelets, medications, or medical devices such as insulin pumps or pacemakers. The investigator should also observe any injuries to the body. It is unwise to try to perform a detailed examination under suboptimal conditions such as cramped space, poor lighting, or with inadequate equipment and assistance. If the person who responds to the scene is not the coroner or medical examiner or the person ultimately responsible for the autopsy examination and/or the death certification, his or her initial findings should be communicated to the autopsy pathologist. This can now be done by telephone, with video conferencing, or with digital imaging via email or the Internet.

If a crime is suspected, the investigator responding to the scene should correlate further activities with law enforcement and/or evidence technicians so that any potential evidence associated with the body is identified and collected at the scene or preserved in such a manner that it will not be damaged or destroyed prior to subsequent collection in the autopsy room. The processing of the body at the scene is optimal if permission is given by the investigator and/or the forensic pathologist he or she represents. The utilization of alternate light sources for the identification and collection of hairs, fibers, and body fluids is done most efficiently prior to wrapping, manipulating, and transporting a body to the medical examiner's laboratory. This should always be done with the full knowledge of the investigator or the responsible coroner or medical examiner, so that any artifacts associated with the identification and collection of evidence left on the body would be known to the pathologist and correctly interpreted. An example of a technique that would create such an artifact would be forming a tent around the body and fumigating the remains with cyanoacrylate (such as Super Glue) for the detection, with alternate light sources, of fingerprints.

It is also important for the investigator to search the scene, with the knowledge and permission of law enforcement, for medications. A prescription vial label contains a tremendous amount of valuable information including the name of the decedent, the pharmacy where the prescription was filled, the name of the prescribing physician, what was prescribed, the quantity, the instructions, and the date of prescription. This one item is often an invaluable tool with which to start the medical investigation and/or suggest a possible suicide.

Removal of the Body

The appropriate packaging of the remains and the subsequent removal from the scene to the autopsy facility should also be well coordinated. This can be an extremely difficult job depending on location; it might involve simply moving the decedent from a death bed in a hospital or nursing home facility to the funeral cart or transport gurney, or it could be removing someone from an outdoor location that is potentially dangerous or near the top of a multistory building with no elevator. The state of the remains might be recently deceased, badly decomposed and insect infested, or skeletonized. The investigator's observations should be reduced to a written report, transmitted to the forensic pathologist, and kept on file. The accessibility of these reports by outside parties varies from jurisdiction to jurisdiction.

Determination of Death

An investigation into the death of an individual cannot be initiated until a person has actually died. Up until about 1990, the concept of brain death had not been generally accepted. Even after the Harvard criteria were established, lawyers in particular were extremely uncomfortable with the thought of removing a normally beating heart from an individual presumed to be brain dead in order to donate it to a recipient. In fact, in one case, criminal defense attorneys attempted to charge the transplant surgeon with the death of an individual who had been declared brain dead as a result of a gunshot wound to the head, and whose family wanted to donate the heart. The attempt was not successful.

Somatic death has, by necessity, been the standard for determining the ultimate demise of a human being. This implies the objective determination that the heart and lungs are no longer functioning. This is done initially by palpation and then subsequently with the utilization of the stethoscope. There are two absolute criteria that any person, regardless of his or her training or background, can use to determine, even from some distance, that a human being is deceased—decapitation and skeletonization. All other bodies fall somewhere on the spectrum of clearly alive to probably dead.

With the development of the respirator, it became possible to supply oxygen with mechanical assistance to the subcranial organs. There are two common mimickers of somatic death, in which the mechanical detection of a heartbeat and/or respiration is difficult, if not impossible: hypothermia, particularly from immersion, and intoxication with respiratory depressants such as alcohol, benzodiazepines, and opiates. The utilization of an electrocardiogram machine and/or field defibrillator should be able to demonstrate that the individual is not deceased, and appropriate resuscitation measures can be instituted.

Organ Transplantation

The ability to prolong life through mechanical respiration allowed for the advancement of organ transplantation. The heart, lungs, kidneys, and liver can remain oxygenated and perfused for later donation, providing life-saving outcomes throughout the country and the world.

Organ and tissue procurement organizations are, by default, required to interact frequently with members of the medical examiner and coroner systems. It is not an uncommon scenario to encounter an individual with significant head injury or a spontaneous natural disease process such as a ruptured berry aneurysm, where significant trauma and anoxic encephalopathy and brain swelling ultimately lead to brain death. These types of cases come under the jurisdiction of the medical examiner and/or coroner. Most physicians are fully cognizant of the benefits of organ and tissue transplantation. The diagnosis of brain death includes clinical demonstration of loss of the cranial nerves and reflexes such as the corneal reflex, the gag reflex, and the caloric reflexes. Further, there should be laboratory demonstration that when the patient is removed from the respirator, no spontaneous respirations are evident, as demonstrated by an increasing partial pressure of carbon dioxide in the blood. Alternative tests such as repeated electroencephalograms or radioactive tagged red cell cerebral blood flow studies are also extremely useful in equivocal cases.

The forensic nurse death investigator, in particular, has the opportunity to act as a liaison between the medical examiner/coroner and the tissue bank, to facilitate the investigation and the determination of the circumstances surrounding the trauma or natural disease processes causing the brain death, to lead the recovery of the organs and tissue by the transplantation team, and to arrange for the examination of the body by the pathologist in the operating room, if necessary. After brain and somatic death have occurred, the medical examiner or coroner can also facilitate recovery of additional tissues, such as corneas, heart valves, skin, bones, and veins, for processing and subsequent transplantation. These tissues are at least life enhancing, if not lifesaving. The importance of collaboration between the medical examiner, coroner, death investigator, and organ and tissue coordinators cannot be overstated.

Cause and Manner of Death

The Death Certificate

The primary goal of any death investigation is to allow the medical examiner or coroner to have enough information based on the background data collection to correlate it with the autopsy findings in order to certify a cause and manner of an individual's death. The sole legal requirement to sign a death certificate is to be a licensed physician in the jurisdiction where the body was found dead. This occasionally causes some confusion and difficulties in border towns where an event took place in one jurisdiction and the body has been transported to the closest medical facility or if the body was surreptitiously disposed of in another jurisdiction. The result is a situation in which the certifier may be a significant distance from where the actual event took place, occasionally requiring cross-jurisdictional testimony in criminal and civil actions.

The death certificate itself is modeled after a World Health Organization document that includes basic demographic information, an opinion statement regarding the cause of death, and an area to describe the events surrounding the death if it is not natural. There are numerous variations from jurisdiction to jurisdiction based on the types of data that each region wishes to collect. The death certificate is a public document that can be obtained by anyone in a town hall or registry of vital statistics for a small fee, a necessary practice for genealogists (Messite & Stellman, 1990).

The art of signing a death certificate is usually not taught in medical schools, leaving the casual certifier somewhat bewildered. It is not uncommon for a cause of death to be listed as cardiorespiratory arrest. This merely indicates that the person's heart and lungs have stopped, which is already evident because the document that is being signed is a death certificate. Theoretically, cardiorespiratory arrest could be put on every death certificate, because that is the final common pathway for all living beings. This practice is often a way of avoiding providing an opinion based on the clinical information present. In some cases this clinical information is understandably extremely limited, thus causing the certifier to fear legal retribution if the opinion is later proven to be incorrect. However, it should be noted that the death certificate clearly states that the indicated cause of death is an opinion. A professional may render an opinion based on the available information with absolutely no fear of legal consequences. Frequently, amended death certificates, updated regarding the cause or because of correction of clerical errors, can be issued, especially if further data regarding the cause of death comes to light from an autopsy, toxicology, other laboratory tests, or historical information. This information may come days, months, or decades after the initial certification.

A signed death certificate is needed for disposition of the remains according to the family's wishes. Bodies cannot be buried or cremated without it. Causes of death such as pending further studies, pending laboratory tests, or pending investigation are all perfectly legitimate statements to record as the initial cause of death. This preliminary death certificate, containing the other demographic data such as the individual's name, the date and time of death, and pronouncement, is perfectly legitimate and will allow the funeral home to carry out its duties.

Cause of Death

The **cause of death** is defined as that injury or disease process, whether brief or prolonged, that initiates the pathophysiologic downward spiral ultimately ending in death. This means that the certifier, whether a private physician, a medical examiner, or a coroner, should ask him- or herself the question, "What started it all?" In legal terms this concept is known as the **proximate event**. The cause of death box on a death certificate (**Figure 13-1**) usually has three or four lines labeled A, B, C, and D, separated in fine print by the phrase *due to or as a result of*. This ultimately allows for a cause of death statement. For example: "Cardiac tamponade *due to* ruptured left ventricle *due to* subacute myocardial infarction *due to* ischemic heart disease" is a pathophysiologic, accurate cause of death statement. Often, simple one-line cause-of-death statements also can be completely accurate, such as "ischemic heart disease" or "atherosclerotic cardiovascular disease" (Hanzlick, 1997).

Certifications for **natural death** are sometimes more difficult than for traumatic deaths because the person may have multiple comorbid disease processes resulting in chronic individual or multiple organ failures such that the final physiologic event may not be witnessed nor readily evident. However, if it is clearly a natural death, with no evidence of trauma, either chemical or physical, a reasonable cause of death statement can still be crafted.

Traumatic deaths are also often easier to certify because it is not uncommon for a person to succumb to the trauma shortly after it is inflicted. "Gunshot wound of the chest," "Craniocerebral blunt-force trauma," and "Heroin toxicity" are all readily apparent by autopsy, toxicology, and investigative data correlation. If there is significant survival in a treatment facility, then the proximate event may be forgotten by the clinicians over time. A common example would be injuries sustained in a motor vehicle accident requiring the person to be hospitalized. Death may ensue from the subsequent effects of the injury, the healing process, and any complications that stem from either. A typical accurate cause of death statement may be, "Sepsis *due to* pneumonia *due to* blunt-force trauma of the chest."

The death investigator may find the proximate event at the beginning of the chart in the emergency department or ambulance notes that tell what initially happened to the deceased person, such as a fall, assault, or motor vehicle accident. If the person was

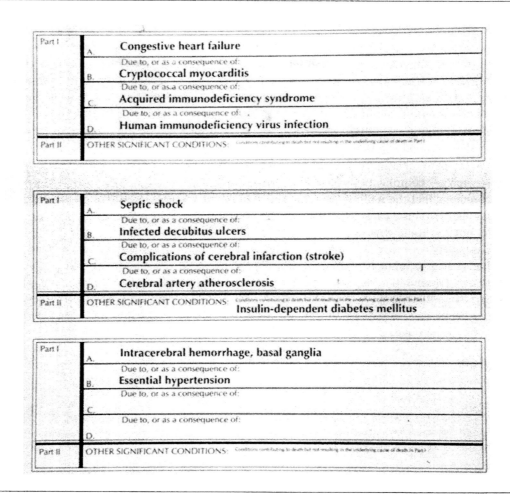

Figure 13-1 Examples of cause of death statements.

transferred from another facility, then the emergency department records from the first facility should be sought. Discussions with the paramedics or emergency medical technicians who initially transported the person, as well as the police officers who investigated the initial event, may also help to accurately identify the proximate cause of death. In cases of delayed deaths, blood samples should be sought and recovered from admission so that toxicology can be performed to help provide data as to the presenting state of the individual prior to the initiation of advanced life support and intensive care treatment.

Manner of Death

The other important aspect of signing a death certificate that is often mandated is the **manner of death**. The manner of death is defined as the circumstances that surround the cause of death. If an accurate cause of death statement indicates "gunshot wound to the chest" or "multiple blunt force injuries," this does not in any way elucidate the circumstances that surround them. Usually there are only five choices that can be certified: natural, accident, homicide, suicide, and undetermined. Medical examiners and coroners frequently have to certify natural causes of death and therefore, but not *exclusively,* the *manner of death* would be natural. Rare exceptions include cases in 2001 in which some 22 individuals were infected and 5 died as a result of inhalation of anthrax (National Academies Press, 2011). Anthrax is a naturally occurring organism causing a natural disease process; however, the circumstances surrounding contraction of this disease process were clearly intentional and assaultive in nature, leading to a homicide manner of death. The argument has also been made for homicide by heart attack, in which an assailant threatens the victim with a gun and the victim has a cardiac arrhythmia due to the immediate stress of the situation and dies. These are uncommon but documented scenarios.

Usually, medical examiners certify death with a simple one-line phrase indicating the proximate event, or if there is some significant survival between the event and the death, a phrase such as "complications of . . ." or "sequelae of . . ." are adequate. Some pathologists and clinicians feel the need to indicate the significant features of the autopsy report and clinical history on the cause of death statement. If it is sequenced correctly this is not inaccurate, but it is somewhat unnecessary.

Nosologists who work within a strict framework code the individual statements on the death certificate. What is placed on a death certificate may or may not be coded as the certifier had intended, either on paper or in their thought processes. An accidental manner of death is applied to situations where the cause is due to unintended events. These may include reactions to drugs, alcohol, blunt or sharp force, or seminatural situations such as an anaphylactic reaction to a bee sting, peanut butter, or radiologic dyes.

Homicide

Homicide is defined simply as death at the hands of another individual. It does not imply the true intent of one person to kill another, such as an assassination, but encompasses a wide range of scenarios. For example, the justified shooting of an individual by a police officer is classified as a homicide, even after internal affairs conducts a criminal investigation and the officer is found to be completely within his or her rights and responsibilities to have fired and fatally wounded the individual. The classification of homicide is often used inconsistently—one jurisdiction may call a hit and run fatality of a pedestrian by a person driving a motor vehicle a homicide, whereas another may classify it as an accident if the vehicle was not used as a weapon. Similarly, a death caused by a small child playing with a firearm may be called a homicide in one jurisdiction and an accident in another.

Suicide

A **suicide** usually indicates that the injuries have been caused intentionally by the individual to bring about his or her death. The classic scenario of Russian roulette frequently initiates debate as to whether this is a suicide or an accident. Modification of the word *intentionally* with the concept of volition, indicating a voluntary act that leads to one's death, may help clarify the debate, or at least allow consistency among forensic specialists.

Accident

For the manner of death to be certified as accident, the circumstances surrounding the death must be outside of the control of any individual. The most common accident is a motor vehicle death, unless it is determined that the vehicle was being used as a weapon. Other more subtle accidents include deaths from bee stings or unforeseen complications of a surgical procedure.

The determination of the manner of death by a coroner or medical examiner often has no effect on how other organizations interested in that particular death will act. The certification of the death as an accident does not in any way prevent or inhibit the district attorney from filing any range of charges against the person who inflicted the fatal injuries. Also, insurance companies do not automatically accept an accidental manner of death as having fulfilled the particular definition of *accident* in the death benefit policy for the deceased individual.

In other parts of the world, death investigation systems may require that the medical certifier not indicate a manner of death. This is often done by the legal authorities who correlate the medical findings with the laws of that country.

Identification

The importance of accurately identifying the deceased is paramount for obvious reasons, as exemplified by the fact that the name is the very first box to be completed on the death certificate. The family will want to have the correct remains returned to them as soon as possible for burial or cremation (**Figure 13-2**). The identification process is crucial in situations of homicide where the presentation in court must satisfy the legal standards that the deceased individual is who the prosecutors say he or she is.

Clinical Forensic Nursing

The forensic nurse has an important role in an emergency room, operating room, or walk-in clinic—to identify and document injuries in nondeceased patients. As with any type of investigation, appropriate and persistent interviewing is crucial for correlating the injuries with the event. A diagram, 35-mm photography, Polaroid photographs, and digital imaging, with and without rulers, are all valuable for documenting injuries. Also, photographic or digital documentation of injuries should be done over time, either on a daily or every other day basis for a week to 10 days. This is to show the development and possible distribution

Pa. woman mistakenly identified as victim in fatal car accident

HARRISBURG, Pa. (AP) — Funeral arrangements were being made and relatives mourned for Denise Dieter, a 23-year-old law student identified by her stepfather and grandfather as the victim of a car accident.

But as the family gathered in her father's home near Philadelphia on Sept. 15, Dieter walked into her apartment in Harrisburg. Her startled roommate said, "You'd better call your dad."

The crash the day before had obliterated the female victim's face. She had striking similarities to Dieter, who was supposed to have been in the car en route to a picnic but had changed her mind at the last minute.

The victim, Cindy Bowers, was the same height and weight as Dieter. They had the same hair color and were wearing identical hair barrettes. They both had double-pierced ears, were wearing the same earrings and had similar key rings.

"It was really bizarre and weird," Dieter said in a telephone interview.

Ms. Dieter said that when she walked into her Harrisburg apartment that Sunday, her roommate, Jackie Rodriguez, became hysterical and could only blurt out for Ms. Dieter to call her father.

"I thought somebody in my family died," Dieter said.

When Ms. Dieter called her father's home, her stepmother, Patti Dieter, answered.

"I said, 'Hey Patti, What's up?'" Dieter recalled. "She was stunned. She said, 'Denise, they're planning your funeral. Where the hell are you?'

"My father grabbed the phone, he was hysterical. He kept saying, 'Oh my God, oh my God, oh my God.' At this point, I knew they thought I was dead."

Dieter, a second-year student at Widener Law School's Harrisburg campus, had been invited to a picnic to hobnob with lawyers.

"I called and said I wasn't going," she said. "I don't know why."

Figure 13-2   Media report of mistaken identity.

of injuries, as well as the aging process and the possibility of identifying a pattern within the injuries that was not initially readily apparent. This identification and documentation is important in the event of a subsequent trial, because the victim cannot demonstrate to the jury the nature of the injuries if they have already healed. Utilization of alternate light sources for the identification, preservation, and collection of evidence can also be done by the forensic nurse.

Utilizing this particular area of forensic nursing expertise beyond direct patient care is somewhat problematic because the only true constituency for this service would be prosecutors. A clinical forensic nurse could be an extension of the medical examiner's office and ideally would be available 24 hours a day for consultation in emergency room and operating room settings. In the age of the Health Insurance Portability and Accountability Act of 1996, the patient, victim, or even perpetrator's permission would be needed to perform this service, or the nurse would need access to a search warrant. The exam would have to be done in a timely fashion because debridement and cleaning of wounds may destroy intimate trace evidence, and treatment and time delay may modify the ability to document the injury in its native state.

Forensic nurses have also made inroads into professionalizing the rape examination by developing the sexual assault nurse examiner program (IAFN, 1999). This has developed into an extremely important and valuable service that the nurse can provide, including giving comfort to the victim, explaining in detail the medical procedures and potential complications, and examining the victim for the purpose of documenting injuries and collecting trace evidence. Demonstrating the advantage of using the skills of a forensic nurse to prosecutors and possibly plaintiffs' attorneys will be a long but potentially rewarding journey in the area of forensic nursing (**see Color Plate 1**).

Time of Death and Postmortem Changes

There is *no* scientific method for determining the exact time of death outside of a monitored medical setting or an eyewitness. Beyond these modalities, there is nothing about the changes that occur to a human body after death that will in any way be entirely accurate. Only a range should be given based on numerous factors. (Saferstein, 2010). When the death investigator is asked to give an opinion about the time of death or the time since death, the investigator should establish the two limiting points: when the person was last reliably known to be alive and when the person was found dead. The point at which the person was found dead is relatively easily determined, but the point at which the person was last reliably known to be alive is not that easy. Interviews with family, friends, and coworkers are of course a place to start. The investigator can review personal computers for activity at some particular clock time, such as was done in the investigation into the death of Washington, D.C.-intern Chandra Levy in 2001. Answering machine messages and telephone records are also useful. It is important to recognize that the reliability of any information, particularly regarding when somebody was last known to be alive, must be verified. Witnesses may intentionally mislead the investigator or the witness may be incompetent, due to chemical impairment or brain disease. The time frame that is developed can be a range of minutes, hours, days, weeks, months, or years. Multiple interviews over time may identify witnesses or situations that provide additional information relevant to the times and dates when the person was last seen, thus narrowing the time frame. Even if the time period between last reliably known alive and found dead is a matter of minutes, that is the limit of accuracy.

The three classic pillars used for time of death estimations based solely on examination of the body are rigor mortis, livor mortis, and algor mortis. These are chemical and physical changes that all deceased individuals undergo, but there is such individual and environmental variability and lack of established testing criteria that they can be utilized only in the face of appropriate investigative information.

Rigor Mortis

Rigor mortis, or rigidity, is a chemical process within the skeletal muscle cells that causes the cross-linking of the actin and myosin fibers in the muscle cells due to decreased oxygen, lack of adenosine triphosphate production, and the postmortem leakage of calcium from the sarcoplasmic reticulum. This process is manifested by the progressive stiffening of muscles. Rigidity develops in all muscle cells simultaneously at the time of death with the loss of adenosine triphosphate production, although it may be detected in smaller muscle groups before larger ones. These changes, in general, come on over approximately 12 hours, will peak through 24 hours, and will begin to wane through the next 12 hours. This chemical process is accelerated by heat and retarded by cold. In warm environments, rigidity can come on more quickly and start to disappear more quickly. There is also instantaneous rigor called cadaveric spasm. The theory behind this process is the rapid premortem loss of muscular adenosine triphosphate caused by intensive muscular activity, such as a tonic-clonic seizure, a foot chase, or struggling during drowning. There are numerous reports of an individual holding some object in his or her hand in full rigor, which would not be possible if the death were not instantaneous.

There is no test for rigidity. It is strictly a qualitative assessment as to the distribution and quantity of the muscle stiffness. The investigator can attempt to manipulate the major joints, particularly the jaw, elbows, and knees, to assess the rigidity. The communication of the quality of the rigor should be descriptive, such as "the jaw is freely moveable, the elbow joint cannot be extended even with great effort, and the knee joint rigidity is easily broken." These types of descriptive phrases are more valuable to the reader than such words as *full rigor* or *partial rigor*.

The most important aspect of rigor mortis is the documentation that it is appropriate for the position in which the deceased is found. It is impossible to die, pass out after a night of alcohol, or fall asleep with one's arm straight up in the air perpendicular to the floor (**see Color Plate 2**). If the deceased individual is found in this position, one knows immediately that the body has been moved after the person has been dead long enough for rigidity to form in another position. Often that original position can be easily re-created. The determination that the deceased has been moved is important for police investigators because it indicates an altered death scene. This may have occurred innocently by a first responder, a layperson, emergency medical personnel, or the police.

Livor Mortis

The second postmortem change is **livor mortis**, or lividity. This is a chemical process that occurs after the heart stops beating and circulation through the arteries and veins can no longer be accomplished. The lack of circulation allows for the blood, particularly in the veins where the vessels are elastic and capillaries have little vascular integrity, to settle and collect in the dependent portion of the body in line with gravity (**see Color Plate 3**). If the deceased is lying on his or her back, the livor would accumulate over the posterior aspect of the body. Lividity can come on relatively quickly, depending on the integrity of the cardiovascular system. An elderly person with heart disease may already have compromised circulation, and lividity may even be evident in the perimortem period. In a healthy individual, lividity would be detectable in the first couple of hours.

The intravascular blood is liquid, and when pressure is applied to the dependent portion of the body, the blood can be squeezed out of the capillary bed and the skin will blanch. After approximately 6 hours the blood will begin to coagulate, and if the skin is compressed and it does not blanch, the livor is said to be fixed. If the position of the body is then changed, a small amount of livor may be detectable in the new dependent portion, but most of it will remain in the original dependent position. Blanched areas in the livor, where the weight of the body compresses the skin and the dermal capillaries are commonly seen over the buttocks, the elbows, and the region of the shoulder blades. It may also be notable in areas of the body that are compressed with clothing, particularly elastic in waistbands or underwear, or objects on which the person might be lying (**see Color Plate 4**).

Using lividity to determine time of death is fraught with tremendous error and must be correlated with the information as to when the person was last reliably known to be alive. Similar to rigidity, lividity is useful in assessing whether the person has been moved after death. An altered death scene is assumed if the person is lying face down and all the livor is noted on his or her back.

Algor Mortis

Algor mortis is a physical process that uses the physical concept of temperature equilibrium. Mammals and birds are homeotherms, which means they generate their own heat. The maintenance of a relatively constant body temperature is important for maximum operation of enzyme systems that have evolved over hundreds of thousands of years. This is in contradistinction to cold-blooded animals that require an external source of heat to elevate their body temperatures and cellular enzyme systems to an efficient mode. After death, the human body will cool and ultimately equilibrate to the environmental temperature. Knight (1995) indicated up to eight models by which measuring body temperature in the early postmortem period might be useful for an estimation of the postmortem interval. Numerous variables must be taken into account: the weight and relative body mass of the individual, the amount of clothing the person is wearing, the humidity of the environment, the temperature of the environment, the temperature of the surface that the deceased is lying on, wind speed, and the body temperature that the person had prior to death. Some of these, such as height and weight, can be measured and incorporated into a nomogram.

One of the models, called the rule of thumb model, states that the human body in the early postmortem period will cool off 1.5 to 2°F per hour (**Figure 13-3**). Therefore, a postmortem core (rectal) temperature of 90°F would suggest that the person has been dead approximately 6 hours. Once again, because of the numerous variables, only a range should be given, and it should ultimately be correlated with other investigative information. Many death investigation jurisdictions do not even utilize postmortem core body temperatures, and this is often a theoretical discussion.

Entomology

The most scientific estimate of the postmortem interval is achieved through forensic entomology. An entomologist specializes in the study of insects and their life cycles (**Figure 13-4**). Shortly after a death occurs, insects such as the fly are able to detect chemical

Temperature-Based Models

Eight Different Models

#1 "Rule of Thumb"

$$\text{P.M.I. (hours)} = \frac{98.6 - \text{rectal temp (F)}}{1.5}$$

Figure 13-3 Estimating time of death from temperature.

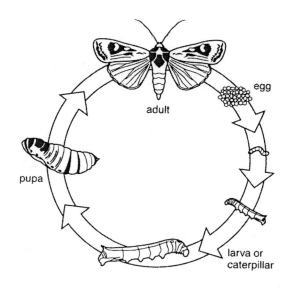

Figure 13-4 Estimating time of death from an insect life cycle.

molecules that attract them to the remains. The flies will search for a source of liquid food, which is primarily at the natural body openings that are exposed, including the mouth, nose, eyes, ears, and potentially the creases in the neck where fluids might accumulate. If there is a suitable source of food, the flies will then breed, and the female will lay hundreds of eggs. These eggs will ultimately hatch into larvae (maggots), which have teeth and will feed on the tissue in the region of their hatching. Bodies that are colonized by flies and other insects will rapidly be consumed, usually starting with the soft tissues of the head and working downward into the chest and abdominal cavities and then ultimately toward the extremities. Ultimately, if the conditions are suitable, complete skeletonization can be accomplished.

Samples of both live and dead insect larvae, as well as adult species, can and should be taken as evidence, preserved in the appropriate media, and sent to a **forensic entomologist** for evaluation. Information such as where the samples were taken, the general location of the remains (indoors, woods, open parking lot, near a body of water, etc.), and the range of environmental temperatures surrounding the 2- to 3-week period when the remains may have been exposed will greatly enhance the interpretation of the insect evidence.

Bioenvironmental evidence is useful because species of flies grow at a certain rate, and the size of the larvae can be calculated and an estimated minimum postmortem interval can be generated. Remember, this is a minimum postmortem interval and not an exact time of death. There is no way to calculate, other than by history, when exactly the remains had opportunity to be colonized. If the remains were indoors or in an enclosed space for several days prior to being deposited in a site where insects would have access to them, then that would not be known simply by the insect examination (Byrd & Castner, 2001).

Identifying, preserving, and collecting insect evidence, whether it consists of the common fly larvae, beetles, wasps, or bees, can help the consulting forensic entomologist recreate the micro and macro bioenvironmental scene. An opinion can then be offered as to what the minimal postmortem interval is, based on the evidence of insect attraction, reproduction, and maturation. The death investigator should provide as much background information as possible to the entomologist for the most accurate estimation. This should include the location of the remains (e.g., house, car trunk, forest, beach) as well as temperature variations from the closest measuring station to where the remains were located.

The anatomic site of insect collection is also important. The deceased quickly attracts flies, which, requiring liquid for feeding, go to natural body openings, such as the nose, mouth, eyes, and ears, as mentioned earlier. Therefore, these are the locations where eggs are laid and the insect larvae will hatch. Insect larval activity at other atypical areas such as hands, extremities, or torso indicate an alternate, more attractive source of liquid fuel, such as blood from a wound. Photographic and written reports as to the distribution of the insect larvae will be helpful not only in determining the postmortem interval, but also for the possible identification of morbid or fatal injuries. Bioenvironmental evidence may be beneath the body in the soil or around the body in the vegetation. This is particularly true of flying adult insects that may also give information about the microenvironmental activity; these should also be collected and appropriately preserved for evaluation.

It is also useful to collect all evident insect species, whether they are associated intimately with the remains, are under the remains, or are flying around the remains. The concept of succession indicates that various types of insects will be attracted to the remains at various stages during this type of decomposition process. Certain species are attracted to the fresh remains, other species are attracted to partly decayed remains, and other species such as beetles are attracted to the decomposers. Some species will actually feed on the insect larvae. Exploring the soil around the remains may also help identify species that have started their final development and have formed pupa casings or are feeding off of the liquid decomposition fluid beneath the body. Collecting a wide variety of specimens will ensure the best information given by the consultant.

The forensic entomologist will use the various combinations of the collected insects associated with the remains to help accurately determine the postmortem interval. Forensic entomologists Dr. Wayne Lord of the FBI and Dr. Lee Goff of Chaminade University in Hawaii point out that, "if you know the players on the field, then you can tell what inning the game is in" (Goff, 2000, p. 487).

Other Aids to Determining Time of Death

Although there is no scientific method to determine the time of death, the correlation between when the deceased was last reliably known to be alive, when he or she was found deceased, the other environmental and investigative information such as mail or newspaper deliveries, computer analysis, and witness statements, in conjunction with the early postmortem changes and modalities such as forensic entomology can be very useful in narrowing down the time of death. This is not necessary in all deaths, but for deaths where it is necessary to confirm or deny an alibi, this information would be crucial.

Human Decomposition

Autolysis

After death, unless the normal pattern of decay of a deceased entity is inhibited by such processes as freezing or chemical alteration such as embalming, the cells in the tissues will naturally break down. After death, the lack of oxygen to the cells causes the earliest form of postmortem decomposition called **autolysis**. Autolysis is Greek for "breakdown of self," and is simply due to the lack of oxygen. This is more evident in cells with large quantities of enzymes, such as those within the pancreas and the adrenal glands. Autolytic changes such as softening and loss of histologic structure are evident several hours after death. The most dramatic example of postmortem autolysis is the intrauterine death of a fetus that is retained for 1 to 2 days, if the demise is not infection related. The fetus will begin to macerate, with development of skin slip; loss of subtle, then more obvious, anatomic features; darkening of the skin that is homogeneous and diffuse; and ultimately loss of anatomic detail and darkening of the internal organs. The most typical etiology of this type of intrauterine death with **maceration** (autolysis) would be a compromised umbilical cord causing a decreased flow of oxygen to the fetus.

Skin Slip

Skin slip is an autolytic process in which the intercellular bridges, or connections, begin to break down and one layer of skin will literally slip off of or away from the layer beneath with a small amount of applied pressure. This can be seen 24 to 48 hours after death. It can occur even more quickly in situations such as carbon monoxide poisoning, because the toxicity of the gas causes rapid cellular death, and it can occur quickly where there are focal or environmental elevations of temperature. Skin slip is common in areas where there might be pressure, such as the upper back where the shoulder blades protrude, the buttocks, or the hips. This normal postmortem autolytic change can be quite dramatic. A deceased person who appears to be fairly well preserved at a scene may have dramatic evidence of skin slip when ultimately examined in the autopsy room due to the multiple manipulations of the body during the transport from the scene to the autopsy facility.

The presence of skin slip can be useful to the medical examiner. When the cellular connections break down on the hands due to immersion or the process of decay, the thick palmar skin can literally be removed intact as a glove. This is known as **degloving**. This "glove" can then be placed over the gloved hand of the examiner, and fingerprints and even palm prints of good quality can be created and be useful for identification purposes when facial feature distortion may preclude visual identification.

Putrefaction

The next, and most dramatic, aspect of decomposition is due to a process called **putrefaction**. This process is a bacterial-mediated progressive form of decay that occurs through the interaction of bacteria with all plant and animal material. This process is seen frequently in the home when milk, vegetables, or other foods begin to spoil and are no longer edible.

Both the external and internal surfaces of the body are extensively colonized by bacteria, which are held in check by the normal human immunological systems. After death, when these systems are no longer functioning, the bacteria will break through their normal constraints and utilize the tissues as a culture medium. Because of the high concentration of bacteria in the intestinal tract, particularly in the colon or large intestine, the putrefactive process is visually observed in the right lower quadrant of the abdomen as a greenish discoloration of the skin. This represents the region of the cecum and the progressive and unrelenting growth of bacteria utilizing the wall of the colon as an area of growth. In moderate temperatures, this is evident approximately 24 hours after death.

Because putrefaction is a bacterial process, it is extremely sensitive to temperature. Just as food is able to be preserved in the freezer nearly indefinitely or in the refrigerator for at least days, if not weeks, a body in a cold environment may not show evidence of putrefaction for a prolonged period of time. However, even in a morgue refrigerator, bodies will eventually decay because cold will only slow down and not kill the bacteria. This is the reason why embalming is important—the tissues are modified chemically so that the bacteria cannot act upon them, and the remains will be preserved in the short term for whatever funeral arrangements the family has made.

This putrefactive decaying process can be very rapid in warm environments. The bacteria will continue to grow, causing breakdown of the tissues similar to that seen in autolysis where there is loss of subtle and then more dramatic anatomic features, darkening of the skin associated with skin slip and bloating of the eyelids, lips, abdomen, penis, and scrotum. This is due to the production of gas by the bacteria. This gas can be foul smelling and is often the reason why deceased individuals are eventually discovered. As these gases continue to be produced they can force the liquefying tissues out of the natural body openings (the nose, mouth, and anus). This process is called purging, and it can be quite dramatic, particularly if the deceased is face down. It is often initially believed to be related to trauma and must be correlated with the scene and circumstances surrounding the death. It can have a dark purple-red-black color and may be pooling around the head. The bacteria will continue to cause the tissues to decay over a period of weeks.

Mummification

The putrefactive process is in competition with other processes such as **mummification**. This is not related to the mummification used by Egyptians caring for deceased rulers, where the tissues were actually removed from the body and the remains were wrapped and preserved chemically. Mummification refers simply to the dehydration of tissue. As the putrefactive process continues, the external surfaces of the body may begin to dry out, particularly in a warm, dry environment, to the point where either all of the skin or certain portions of the skin surface, whether it is the face, chest, abdomen, or extremities, will become leathery and so hardened that they cannot be cut with a scalpel. Mummification is often seen in the fingertips and hands where little bacterial activity occurs. This makes the process of fingerprinting the body difficult, if not impossible. The friction ridges may be visible, but because of the wrinkling and the lack of pliability, they cannot be recorded by usual fingerprint techniques. The processes of autolysis, putrefaction, and mummification are often competing, depending on the macro and micro environments.

Saponification

Another postmortem change, **saponification**, is dependent upon a wet environment. This process results in the hydrolysis of the subcutaneous adipose tissue into a waxy type material (sometimes called grave wax or adipocere) that is akin to soap. Wherever subcutaneous fat is located, this process can occur. This process can take weeks to months depending on the environment in which the remains are located. Often the internal structures that are encased by this waxy shell are fairly well preserved and easy to autopsy.

Vegetation Changes

Bioenvironmental evidence, which involves the local vegetation, may give indications and clues that a decaying body is either located at a particular place or was located there. Broken vegetation or discolored leaves from the gases produced by the bacteria and emitted from the decaying remains may give the first visual signs that there has been a disturbance or alteration in an area. Denser growth provided by the nitrogen nutrients from the decaying remains may also provide evidence that remains have been buried at a particular location. Because of this accelerated growth in the vegetation, infrared photography, particularly from an elevated platform such as a helicopter or unmanned fixed-wing drone, may assist in identifying a clandestine grave. Broken plant material should be collected, as well as any plant life that is intimately associated with the remains. These might include mosses growing on bones or individual plants that have grown through bones. The plants, including the roots, should be collected, wrapped in newspaper, and placed in a dry place in preparation for submitting to a botanist who understands the local vegetation. Photographs of the location are also crucial. This will assist the botanist in understanding the bioenvironmental locale.

Soil Samples

The soil samples in and around a suspected clandestine grave can also be useful. Decompositional proteins and fatty acids will leech into the soil, which can then be analyzed. Also, the disruption of the stratification of the soil will prove that there has been a disturbance in that area, whether remains are recovered or not. It is always important to remember that controls and providing as much information as possible to the consulting forensic scientist will yield the best analysis.

Anthropologic Evidence

Consultation with a forensic anthropologist, both at the death scene and in the autopsy facility, is crucial to the operation of any death investigation system. It is not uncommon for bones to be discovered in a variety of situations such as a family pet bringing one to the house, private or public digging for renovation or construction purposes, or discovery in fill dirt. The forensic anthropologist has to immediately be able to answer the simple question, "Are these bony remains human?" If this question can be answered in the negative, then there is no concern for police officials and nothing further need be done, although it is wise to not return the bony remains to the discovering or presenting authority, because the same bone may end up having to be reevaluated in the near future when it is rediscovered in a second site. If the question is answered in the affirmative, it then needs to be determined, probably by the anthropologist, whether the remains are historic or recent.

The discovery of historic human remains (defined as remains that are old enough that any assailant would no longer still be alive, e.g., 100 years) is not uncommon. Throughout New England and the Eastern Seaboard are numerous undocumented colonial and Native American gravesites. These are frequently discovered serendipitously. It is important to know that if the remains are identified as Native American, then all efforts must be made by the local authorities and any state archaeology group to return the remains to the tribes that were known to have been located historically in that region.

If the remains are identified as human and recent, then it is likely that they have been buried in a criminal-related manner (Forensic Timeline, 2002). It is then imperative that a forensic anthropologist have access to the remains to determine the age at death, the ancestral background (Asian, African, or European), and sex. If the remains are determined to be prepubescent, the determination of age to within 6 months to 1 year is relatively easy because the eruption of teeth and the growth of individual bones and the fusion of epiphyses (growth plates) is fairly constant. It would be impossible by morphology alone to determine the sex of the individual and also difficult to identify the ancestry.

The age of an adult can be determined to a range of approximately 5 years based on bone morphology, epiphyseal and cranial suture closure, and wear on the face of the pubic symphysis. The intact skeleton also makes it very easy to determine the sex primarily by examination of the morphology of the pelvis. The female pelvis is designed for childbirth and has a significantly different shape than the male pelvis. The nature of the muscles also shows smaller and more gracile areas of muscle attachment due to the lack of testosterone, which creates larger muscles, and therefore more robust muscle attachments to bone. Ancestral determinations are more difficult, particularly as interracial marriages and progeny are produced. Stature can be estimated from multiple measurements of the long bones.

The forensic anthropologist is also invaluable in identifying deformities of the skeletal structures that may have been caused by natural disease processes, which would help identify the individual through medical history and/or suggest a cause of death. The identification of subtle blunt and sharp force trauma, including gunshot wounds and their directionality, is also information that the consultant can provide to the forensic pathologist, the death investigators, and law enforcement. The identification of human remains that are completely skeletonized is always an interesting challenge.

Identification of Human Remains

In some instances, positive identification of a deceased individual may not occur until years after the death because of various circumstances occurring at the time or new information that surfaces long after his/her demise. In other situations time is a crucial factor and the immediate certain identification of the body is critical. Such cases involve a suspicious death, the death of a world leader, a celebrity, or possibly an international terrorist. Some fatality events require the death investigation system to utilize multiple methods so that the correct remains are returned to the grieving families. The anguish and stress inherent in these situations is played out vividly in the media and can add to a family's distress. Examples such as the identification of the victims of the terrorist attacks on the World Trade Center, the Pentagon, and United flight 93 on September 11, 2001, and the identification of the sons of Saddam Hussein are dramatic examples of such media coverage. In the case of the death of Osama bin Laden during a Navy Seal mission carried out by the United States in Pakistan, it was necessary to utilize all available evidence very rapidly because of the intent to bury the body at sea immediately after identification. Thus multiple modalities were employed. The body was first matched to the decedent's physical appearance. He was known to be 6'4" tall and thus the body was quickly measured. Facial recognition analysis was completed on a photograph taken by the Navy Seals involved in the mission and compared to a photograph on file at CIA headquarters. This analysis demonstrated with 90–95% certainty that the body was that of Osama bin Laden (Moran, Raddatz, Schifrin, Ross, & Tapper, 2011). A full biometric analysis comparing facial and other physical characteristics was also completed. A DNA sample was transmitted to the U.S. and compared to DNA samples previously on file from multiple relatives. These results confirmed the certainty of the identification with 99.9% confidence.

The process of identification is simply a comparison of premortem data with postmortem data. This can be done circumstantially, where the premortem record is somebody's memory, compared with a postmortem personal viewing of the remains and/or a photograph of the deceased. Identification is done frequently at the medical examiner's office, hospital, or funeral home.

Fortunately, most of the people in this country are who they are purported to be, and visual identification is readily acceptable, especially because true positive identification for everyone would be too costly and time consuming. Problems with visual identification as the primary method occurs in the case of identical twins; friends or family who have not seen the deceased for some period of time; trauma that obscures or modifies the identifying features, including treatment such as bandages; and/or a healing process that includes swelling, hematoma formation, and inflammation. The most recognizable features of a person are his or her eyes and hair. Distortion of these areas complicates the visual identification process. The circumstantial identification would also include appropriate circumstances where an individual of known age, race, and sex is compared using anthropomorphic techniques with the deceased individual. For example, an elderly Caucasian male who lived alone has not been seen recently and the remains of an elderly Caucasian male are found in the burned house where he was known to reside, allowing for a circumstantial identification. These are nonscientific methods. In order to positively identify an individual, premortem data such as dental records, fingerprints, direct or indirect DNA samples, or X-rays must be sought out and recovered. There may be extremely unique features of a person such as distribution of tattoos, scars, surgical clips, or prostheses that may at least give clues as to the identity of the person during the initial stages of identification, but may also rise to the level of positive identification at some point. The scientific and statistical elimination of all other persons on the planet would be a positive identification.

The investigator, with the assistance of the investigating police department, should seek out all premortem data that is available, whether the situation involves a single individual or a mass fatality situation. These would include age, race, and sex documentation; dental records; previous X-rays (from either a clinic, a walk-in immediate medical care center, or a hospital); and previous sources of fingerprints such as arrest records, military service, civil service, pistol permits, or immigration records. The premortem data is often assembled when an individual is reported missing, especially when the circumstances suggest that the individual may have been the victim of an assault and is likely to have died. The search for premortem records if no family is readily identifiable can be difficult, but personal records; hospital, medical, or dental bills; interviews with friends; and record searches of hospital or walk-in clinics in the vicinity of the person's home or workplace will generate leads to premortem records that will be helpful in identification.

The postmortem data is available from the autopsy examination. Forensic technicians are often quite skilled in obtaining fingerprints from recently deceased individuals or even badly decomposed individuals. The process of autolysis causes the thick palmar skin to slough off the deeper layers, often intact. The sloughed skin can be placed over the gloved finger of the technician, who can take his or her time to create fingerprints (**see Color Plate 5**). **Desiccated**, mummified, or waterlogged (washerwoman) fingertips require potential rehydration and/or subcutaneous injection with various fluids to reconstitute and create usable prints. Prior to any manipulation of the fingertips, a photograph should be taken in case the friction ridges are ruined or are unusable.

It may be necessary to enlist the services of a consulting dentist to help appropriately document the jaws (**see Color Plate 6** and **Figure 13-5**). A consulting dentist is also crucial to help evaluate and interpret dental records in order to make a positive identification. A forensic anthropologist is invaluable, particularly when the remains are badly decomposed or completely skeletonized, to determine the basic age, race, and sex of the individual. Other valuable individual osseous features that might be useful for identification can be documented. Appropriate samples can be taken from the deceased for DNA typing. A simple blood sample is valuable; however, if the remains are in an advanced state of decomposition, bone marrow or teeth where cellular and nuclear material are protected against decay are valuable specimens.

When we see our spouses, children, coworkers, or friends, we are comparing the known data (i.e., our memories) with the unknown data (i.e., the person who is standing before us at that particular moment). The most identifying features of a human being are his or her face, including the eyes and eye color, and his or her hair. If an individual, such as a celebrity, wishes to become somewhat anonymous, he either goes someplace where he might not be recognized or he puts on sunglasses, a hat, and generic clothing. Technically, the process of visual identification is not a positive identification. Even parents or siblings often mistake identical twins for each other. Babies and children, before they have had a chance to develop significant individuating features such as eye color and hair color, can be confused. People who are injured, such that their features are distorted by the trauma, and if they survive, by the treatment (surgical modification, suturing, and bandaging) and/ or healing processes (edema, discoloration from bruising), also may not be readily identifiable by even the closest relative or friend. Also, postmortem changes such as putrefaction and insect infestation can destroy the features that are readily identifiable, such as the shape of the nose or facial or head hair.

The vast majority of identifications, either on live people or deceased, are done visually. Somebody looking at an injured person and declaring her name, someone witnessing an event, or a family member viewing a body at a funeral home and signing an identification form are everyday occurrences that are uncomplicated. When they are complicated, or when there is a specific need for more definitive determination such as a civil (paternity) or legal reason, a positive identification must be accomplished.

Tattoos and semipermanent features may not rise to the level of positive identification, but they may help investigators establish a strong, tentative identification. Because tattoos are handmade and are of specific numbers, at certain anatomic locations, and contain

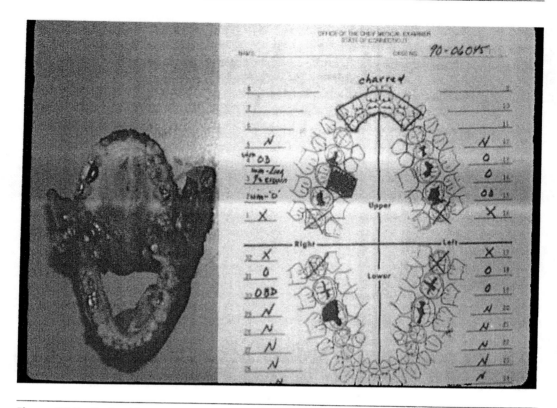

Figure 13-5 Excised jaws and charted teeth as the postmortem record.

certain details, they can be compared with an artist's tattoo log or family photographs for positive identification.

A positive identification is a statistical comparison and elimination of the possibility of anyone else on the planet being confused with the person in question. This is accomplished by (1) the determination that there is no apparent dissimilarity or discordance, and (2) the identification of multiple points of similarity. The more points of similarity, the greater statistical likelihood that one would reach a confidence level that is well beyond even the remotest chance.

The gold standard for positive identification has been fingerprint comparison. The friction ridges on the palmar surfaces of the hands, as well as the feet, are unique, even to identical twins, and for decades have been utilized in positively identifying individual human beings. The evolution of molecular biology over the last several decades, starting with simple ABO blood typing and progressing to identification of different isoenzymes within cells to the nuclear and mitochondrial extraction, even in the most minimal specimen of DNA, has and will continue to revolutionize individuation. The process of comparing pre- and postmortem dental records is also a common practice. However, this and techniques such as pre- and postmortem comparison of any X-ray can be accomplished only if a tentative identification has been done. One cannot seek out dental or medical records from their repositories without knowing who one is looking for. This is unlike comparison to large data banks such as the automated fingerprint identification system, where an unknown print can be put into the system and compared to those present in the database, and the growing development of DNA databases. The forensic nurse is invaluable in seeking, reviewing, and understanding medical and dental records and understanding where the repositories might be, such as hospitals, walk-in clinics, industrial medical offices, clinics, and private and university-based dental offices. Another unique method of either assisting or accomplishing a positive identification involves tracking down serial numbers from such items as pacemakers, breast implants, orthopedic prostheses, and hearing aids.

When a body is badly decomposed, burned beyond visual recognition, or the legal system requires a positive identification, the collection and documentation of postmortem data and the collection of premortem data may take a significant period of time as the repositories are searched. If the person is completely unidentified, the first step in identification is to consult local, state, and even national missing person registries. If no missing person reports have been filed, the remains, regardless of the cause of death, may never be identified.

Types of Injury

Blunt Trauma

Injury or damage to tissue as a result of the application of some quantity and quality of force results in what is called blunt-force trauma. The individual's tissue reaction to the magnitude and direction of force can potentially give information about the nature of the event. The force can be applied to the tissue in either of two ways: a moving object can impact the body or vice versa. Identical applications of force with the same direction and magnitude may not result in the same type of injury to different people. An important variable is the quality of the tissue of the individual to which the force is applied. A young individual who has supple, pliable skin and elastic ribs may show no external and little internal injury because the force is easily diffused throughout the tissue without overcoming the tensile or elastic strength of the tissue. In contrast, an elderly person with thin, fragile skin and osteoporosis may suffer significant injury with potentially lethal consequences from the same force that caused minor injury in the young person. Other variables include the normal cyclical interaction of the immune system, causing the same individual to react differently to the same application of force just weeks apart, based on the current capabilities of his immune system that may be affected by stress or diet. Diseases also render the tissue more or less vulnerable. Skin diseases, infection, and cancer all modify the tissues' ability to withstand the application of force.

Blunt-force trauma is the most common type of trauma seen in clinical forensic medicine or forensic pathology. Nearly every person, every day, is walking around with some evidence of blunt-force trauma, from the tiniest scratch or bruise to injury that would require intensive nursing care. The evidence of the tissues' reaction to the applied force is broken down into four categories—abrasions, contusions, lacerations, and fractures.

Abrasions

Abrasions are injuries of the skin that result in damage of various layers of the epidermis. If the force is applied tangentially, then it results in a scratch-type injury. This can be a linear injury or, if the surface is broad, it can be a very wide confluent collection of linear scratches retaining their individuality or coalescing into one large area of denuded epithelium. Close examination of the wound may find tiny, triangular-shaped tissue segments whose apical point is directed opposite to the vector of force, or pointing to the source of the force (**see Color Plate 7** and **Color Plate 8**). Also, there may be a collection of the abraded epithelium at one edge of the wound (**see Color Plate 8**). This epithelial piling also indicates the direction of force.

Even the most mundane or simple abrasion-type blunt-force injury should be documented in detail, because a history or witness statement may be confirmed or denied simply on the basis of one nonlethal, relatively minor injury. Abrasions can be superficial or deep, with the deeper ones having a much redder base and being more likely to bleed. The quantity of blood from abrasion is relatively minor compared to other types of injuries. After death, if the abrasion is exposed, it may begin to dry out. It may have a dry maroon-brown color or may even blacken. As the injury dries out, the subtleties and potentially even a pattern that it may have had in the fresh state become obscured. After death, force can still be applied to a body and cause injuries. A postmortem abrasion should have no evidence of a vital reaction such as erythema or swelling. It often has a dull yellow-tan appearance with no margin of redness. The abrasion is, by definition, the exact point of force on the skin.

Contusions

A **contusion**, or bruise, is defined simply as blood leaking into tissues after the vessels have been disrupted by the application of force. A contusion can be seen in any tissue, including the skin, brain, lungs, or liver; bone is not included because if there is enough force to break blood vessels within the bone, it will cause the fourth type of blunt trauma, a fracture. The amount of energy required to break blood vessels within the skin, in the subcutaneous tissue, or within an organ causing the leaking of red blood cells is really quite variable, depending on the quantity and quality of the force as well as the elasticity of the tissue.

A contusion or a bruise does not necessarily indicate the exact point of force. If blood vessels are broken, then the blood can dissect through the tissue planes and be affected by gravity. Individuals who survive blunt trauma and who are in a recumbent position may have significant dissection of the blood that will accumulate in the flanks or even the back. Areas where the tissues are fixed and the tissue planes have ended will also accumulate blood, such as beneath the eyes at the level of the cheekbones. Blood accumulating from a fracture at the base of the skull, behind the ear, does not indicate the point of contact. This is called Battle's sign (**see Color Plate 9**). Similarly, force applied to the head, such as a gunshot wound or other types of blunt trauma that would cause the brain to impact on the thin, delicate orbital roof causing fractures, may allow blood to dissect anteriorly into the upper and lower eyelids. There may be complete confluence of blood in the upper and lower eyelids; this is called raccoon eyes or spectacle hemorrhages (**Figure 13-6**). This can be incomplete, with only a small amount of blood seen in the medial canthus of either the right or left side. A hematoma is an actual collection of blood (the suffix -*oma* being Greek for "swelling" or "tumor"—as in lipoma, carcinoma, and sarcoma). The importance of a true hematoma is that it will take longer for the blood to resorb and heal and can actually be used as a postmortem toxicology sample, because it can be collected as a unit.

The documentation and classification of blunt-force injuries are important, but it may also be important to give an estimation of the date of an injury. Multiple injuries that appear to have been inflicted over time may lead to certain conclusions about the nature of the events. This would be important in an abusive situation, whether it be child abuse, spousal abuse, or elder abuse. The examiner should be extremely wary of rendering an opinion as to the age of a contusion or bruise solely based on its appearance and color changes (**see Color Plate 10**). The color of a bruise is based on the metabolism

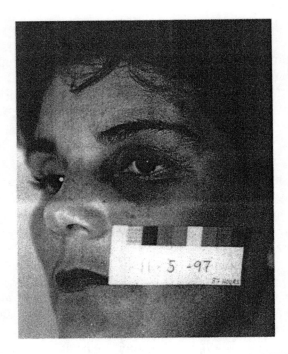

Figure 13-6 Spectacle hemorrhage (blackened/raccoon eyes).

and breakdown of the hemoglobin pigment within the red cells. The bruise appears to be initially dark purple, and then over time, as the hemoglobin breaks down, it turns a series of blue, green, brown, tan, and yellow colors. No good correlation studies provide any reasonable opinion about the age of a particular bruise based on these color changes. Bruises have numerous variables including the actual quantity of blood that constitutes the contusion and the quality of the inflammatory or healing abilities of that person. The only opinion that should be rendered is that the bruises are of various ages. This can be confirmed by a microscopic examination of the bruises to identify the quality and quantity of the inflammatory response and the breakdown of the hemoglobin. This spectrum again is quite variable and has significant overlap. In the future, identification of molecular immune mediators histologically should help clarify and increase the specificity of the timing of individual injuries.

Lacerations

A **laceration** is a tear of tissue. Once again, this can be skin or any internal organ or tissue other than bone. This injury and designation is not to be confused with a cut or incised wound. It is not infrequent to see in medical records the generic reference to "lac" when referring to any external wound noted on the body. It is important that forensic investigators are able to communicate their findings accurately and specifically because it may direct an investigation toward or away from a specific object. When sufficient force is applied to the tissue to overcome the tensile elastic strength of that entire tissue, it will tear (**Figure 13-7**). The skin should show several basic features including a marginal abrasion, tissue bridging, and possibly undermining. A marginal abrasion occurs because in the milliseconds prior to the tissue actually tearing, the skin is scraped. The dimensions and shape of the marginal abrasion may indicate the nature of the object that came in contact

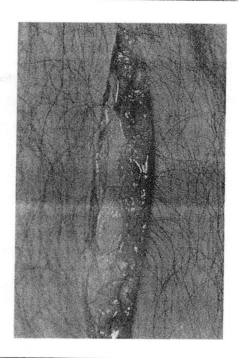

Figure 13-7 Laceration with sharp edges.

with the skin. A very narrow marginal abrasion suggests that the object had an edge to it (**see Color Plate 11**), and a wide marginal abrasion indicates that the object is broader and flatter (**see Color Plate 12**).

If the force is not sufficient to tear or destroy all of the tissue within its path, then there may be evidence of injured arteries, veins, nerves, or other elastic fibers that can be seen going from one edge of the wound to the other (**see Color Plate 13**). This is a key finding in differentiating blunt-force trauma from sharp-force trauma. An incised wound or a cut will sever these tissues and there will be no evidence of tissue bridging.

If the force is not perpendicular to the skin, then there may be more destruction beneath the skin (undermining) in the direction of the force. One might be able to do a digital or probe-type examination noting that it may be several centimeters deeper on one side than the other side. This will aid in the determination of the direction of force and should be documented. Internal organs, such as the liver and lungs, may show lacerations of the parenchyma when there is no damage to the overlying capsule. It is also not uncommon to have very little external evidence of injury but significant internal injury as the force is transmitted through the more elastic skin and subcutaneous tissue into the less resilient tissue parenchyma.

Like abrasions, lacerations indicate the exact point of force on the skin. For this reason, it is important to examine the depth of the laceration for any trace evidence that may have been deposited there. This can be collected and submitted to the police and/or crime lab for possible correlation with the object that impacted the skin. Unless there is complete perforation of the skin and subcutaneous tissue, the lacerations of internal organs should not have any trace evidence or particular pattern that would assist in determining the nature of the event. Because of their superficial nature, abrasions often do not have trace evidence associated with them.

Fractures

The final type of blunt-force trauma is a **fracture**. This is any disruption of the normal anatomy of a particular bone. There may be a minor disruption in the cortex or complete disruption of the bone with overlying laceration of the skin, called a compound fracture. A comminuted fracture is shattering of the bone into multiple pieces. A displaced fracture is one where the fractured ends are no longer in alignment. The amount of force necessary to cause a fracture is generally greater than that required to cause an abrasion, contusion, or laceration; however, there are very thin bones that are relatively easy to fracture, such as the orbital roofs and the squamous portion of the temporal bone. Also, there is great relativity in the resistance of individual bones, which can fracture depending on the moment, direction, and magnitude of the force as well as the health of the individual bone. Elderly individuals with osteoporosis or children with congenital abnormalities such as osteogenesis imperfecta are susceptible to fractures.

Pathologic fractures are those that happen spontaneously, usually with no direct application of force, due to the extensive loss of calcium such as in osteoporosis or more commonly due to the infiltration of tumor. Linear fractures, particularly of the skull, can often lead to the original point of impact as they radiate out from its center. Also, similarly to fractures in glass, fracture lines that abruptly end at another fracture line indicate that it came subsequent to the one that it meets.

Depressed skull fractures occasionally can reflect the shape of the object that caused them. Also, as the bone is depressed and then approaches its return to its original position it may "bite" tiny pieces of whatever the object may have been. Close examination of the edges of these types of wounds may yield trace evidence. Bone may also indicate directionality. The lower legs, particularly the tibia, should be examined in any case of a pedestrian struck by a motor vehicle. There may be little, if any, injury to the skin or subcutaneous or muscular tissue at the primary strike point (the point where the leading edge of the vehicle, usually the bumper, strikes the person). A triangular-shaped fracture may be seen along the shaft of the bone across its full thickness. The apex, or the point of the triangle, points in the direction of the force, unlike abrasions and lacerations where the apex of the torn tissue points in the opposite direction of the force (**see Color Plate 14**). Once again, directionality may help confirm or deny a particular piece of information that is related to the incident. If the body is badly decomposed or skeletonized, the bones must be completely cleaned and defleshed for the forensic pathologist or forensic anthropologist to examine because subtle injuries may be hidden, such as blunt- or sharp-force trauma that would help determine the cause of death.

Patterned Injury

A patterned injury is a representation of the shape of the object that caused the injury, whether an abrasion, contusion, or laceration. It is important to recognize patterns and document them because it is not uncommon for the exact shape of the object, or the object itself that impacted with the skin, to be readily and independently apparent (**see Color Plate 15** and **Color Plate 16**). Appropriate documentation by Polaroid photograph, 35-mm camera, digital imaging, drawing, and/or tracing may be useful many years later when a specific object may come to the attention of the authorities. Objects found in nature rarely have a pattern that would be reflected in an injury. Man-made objects often have a pattern, and even the simplest object such as a cylindrical pool cue or a baseball bat has several surfaces that can cause an impact. When the long portion of the shaft is impacted on the skin, these types of objects leave a patterned contusion composed of two parallel linear contusions with sparing at the center (**see Color Plate 17**). This is because when the force is perpendicular to the skin it compresses the blood vessels, forcing the blood laterally, where the increased pressure actually breaks the capillaries, causing the contusion. This is similar to the contusions seen with tire tread imprints on the skin. These are patterned contusions formed when the skin in the space between the actual treads that come in contact with the surface are forced into the grooves, leaving the pattern. The actual point of impact where the tire treads touch is without visible contusion. Patterned abrasions also may be seen in situations where the muzzle of a gun leaves the pattern of its face on the skin of a contact gunshot wound. If the force is perpendicular to the skin, the epithelium may actually be crushed instead of scraped, providing a greater opportunity to reflect the shape of the object that caused it (**see Color Plate 18**). Due to the imposition of clothing between the object and the skin, the pattern of the weave of the clothing could also be stamped into the epidermis.

Curvilinear lacerations over various surfaces of the body, particularly the head, upon closer examination may indicate a standard hammer. If the hammer impacts directly perpendicularly, there should be the suggestion of a circular abrasion or contusion with a central, possibly stellate, laceration, particularly if this involves the scalp that overlies bone. If the injury is crescent-shaped it may have fairly well demarcated edges, from the disc-shaped hammerhead to a crescent-shaped hammerhead edge (**see Color Plate 19**). A blow with a hammer may or may not cause a fractured skull and does not need to fracture the skull in order to be lethal.

Patterns, or constellations of injuries, may also be important in determining what happened to an individual or how he or she was positioned in the environment during the incident that caused blunt-force trauma. Each individual injury may not have a specific shape, but the patterns, or constellations, of the injuries, or the distributions of the injuries over the body surface may reveal what happened to the individual. An example of this would be a group of abrasions that may or may not include contusions or lacerations of the eyebrow lateral to the eye or the cheek, the tip of the nose, or the chin. This entire array, or portions of it, is typical in a fall-type pattern (**Figure 13-8**). If an individual becomes unconscious for whatever reason and is unable to protect his or her head while falling, the high points on the face will impact with the surface. This can be seen in victims of cardiac dysrhythmias who become unconscious very rapidly.

A motor vehicle driver has multiple opportunities for blunt-force trauma. An unbelted driver in a head-on collision may reveal the driver's triad—injuries to the face from the windshield, the chest from the steering wheel, and the knees from the bolster or dashboard. These injuries may be subtle and in a nondeceased individual may be reflected only in complaints of pain in those areas. Subjective focal complaints or the demonstration of point tenderness over the chest may help separate the purported driver from his or her passengers. Also, the tempered (heat-treated) glass of the side windows breaks up into small, cubelike fragments that often impact the side of the face. Having dicing-type injuries predominantly on the left side of the face is generally associated with the driver of the motor vehicle, and on the right side of the face with the passenger. It should be noted, however, that unrestrained occupants of a motor vehicle in T-bone collisions go toward the force of impact, so that a driver may have right-sided dicing-type injuries by going toward the passenger's side at the area of impact.

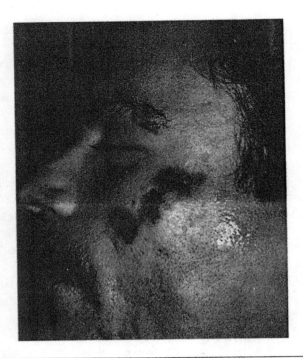

Figure 13-8   Constellation of abrasions consistent with a fall.

Pedestrians also have distributions of injuries that help identify the fact that they indeed have been struck by a motor vehicle and the relative position that they may have been in at the point of impact. Identifying the primary strike point (bumper injury) of the lower legs, whether they are anterior, lateral, or posterior is helpful. Dissecting the tibia for a possible triangular-shaped fracture would also indicate the direction of the force. If the force is enough to cause a fracture, usually only one leg shows the fracture pattern. The gait of a normal human being has the weight distributed over only one leg at a time. It is that weight-bearing leg that has enough resistance to cause the force to go through the bone, resulting in a fracture. Secondary injuries to adults happen when one is thrown upward (because he or she is struck below the center of gravity) and hits the hood of the car and/ or windshield, injuring the shoulders, chest, hips, face, and/or head. Tertiary injuries occur when the individual falls onto the surface of the roadway. It is at this point that lethal injuries often take place—the head strikes the ground and/or the weight of the body distorts the normal position of the cervical spine. Quaternary injury may then occur as the individual lying in the road is subsequently run over by another vehicle. Categorizing each abrasion, contusion, and laceration and placing it in its appropriate temporal relationship may be difficult, if not impossible; however, the general distribution of the injuries can help answer many questions. A deceased individual lying in the middle of the road with no injuries to the lower extremities, the tips of the elbows, or the hips and having bilateral anterior and posterior rib fractures, lacerations of the liver, and fractures of the pelvis indicates that the person was already lying on the ground prior to being run over, meaning that the person had not been struck while being a pedestrian. This type of correlative information may clear an individual of charges that may be brought against him.

Physical Abuse

In abuse situations, the distribution of the injuries as well as the relative age of individual injuries can be correlated with the proffered history of how these injuries took place. Injuries of various ages distributed over the back, the front, the arms and legs, and various sides of a baby's head are entirely inconsistent with a history of the baby having fallen off the changing table.

Sharp-Force Injuries

The other major type of injury is sharp-force injuries. There are only two mechanisms by which skin and internal tissues can be affected by sharp objects—cuts (incisions) and stabs (penetrations).

Incised Wounds

Cuts or incised wounds are longer than they are deep. They may be caused by any object with an edge, including paper, a knife, glass, a razor, or the lid of a can (**Figure 13-9**). Incised wounds may involve only the skin or may involve the subcutaneous tissue and even deep muscle. The depths may be the same or they may be variable throughout the course of the wound. Superficial epithelial cuts at one edge of the wound, called tails, may suggest the finishing side of the event. It is very difficult, however, to suggest a directionality to a simple incised wound. Whether the force is going from left to right or whether the perpetrator is left-handed or right-handed, or has inflicted the wound from in front or behind, is usually far too speculative to be of any true forensic value.

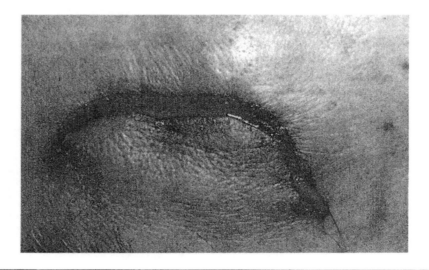

Figure 13-9   Incised wound (longer than deep).

Penetrating Wounds

A stab, or penetrating wound, is deeper than it is long. A knife, a stick, a pencil, a rod, or any object that can be thrust into the body or onto which the body can be impaled would fall under this category. Classic knife wounds can reveal significant information. Close examination of the wound may show a sharp or V-shaped edge and a blunt or squared edge (**Figure 13-10**). This reflects the cutting and noncutting edge of a single-edged blade. The vast majority of all knives are single edged. Occasionally a serrated knife upon its entry or exit from the skin may cause tiny periodic curvilinear epithelial abrasions that may be visible with a magnifying glass (**Figure 13-11**). However, the vast majority of serrated knives cause a simple stab wound with blunt and sharp edges. Two V-shaped edges or corners suggest a double-edged knife (**Figure 13-12**). The orientation of these blunt and sharp edges should be documented. One way to document them is to describe the orientation of the wound as compared to the face of a clock (e.g., "There is a sharp edge at 3:00 and a corresponding blunt edge at 9:00. The wound measures 0.75 cm in length with the blunt squared edge measuring 2 mm.").

The true nature and dimensions of the stab wounds may not be evident until the wounds are reapproximated into their previous anatomic positions. The elastic fibers will cause the wound to gape, particularly if it is vertically oriented. This is less evident if the wound is horizontally oriented, because the elastic fibers run around the body in a horizontal fashion. Wounds can be reapproximated with fingertips, clear tape, clear fingerprint lifts, or even cyanoacrylic glue (such as Super Glue). At this point, photographs and measurements can be made for documentation.

Examination of the edges of the stab wound for epithelial abrasions may also indicate the relative force of a stab wound in which the handle came into contact with the skin or forced clothing into the skin around the stab wound. The wound track should be documented by following the injury to the internal tissues beneath the skin. Documentation of whether these wounds exhibit hemorrhage is also important because stab wounds that occur after death would be bloodless.

Determining the depth of a stab wound is important, because it may help determine whether the weapon could be a 2-inch (5.08-cm) knife, a 4-inch (10.16-cm) knife, or an 8-inch (20.32-cm) knife. However, documenting the depth of the wound is fraught with great error and should be reported as a range. The very nature of the internal examination

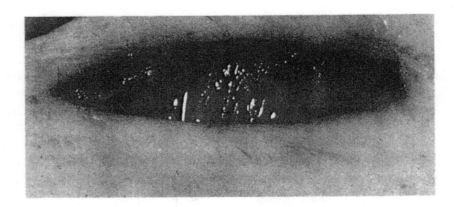

Figure 13-10 Penetrating wound inflicted by a single blade knife.

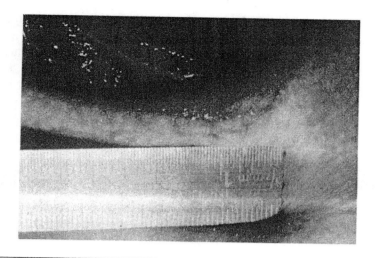

Figure 13-11   Wound inflicted by knife with a serrated blade.

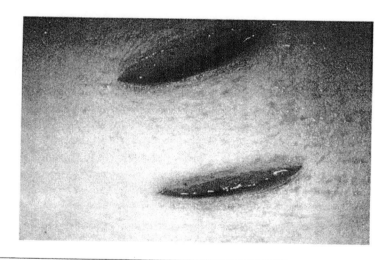

Figure 13-12   Wound inflicted by knife with a double-edged blade.

during the autopsy is a layer-by-layer, stepwise procedure. The end of the stab wound may be on the surface or within an organ. One would then have to reconstruct the dissection process, put in some sort of a probe to the deepest portion of the wound, and measure from the entrance of the skin with a ruler. However, this reconstructive process is not exact; tissues such as the lungs collapse so that the exact length within the lung as it was originally aerated would be impossible to identify, and organs are movable, particularly the heart, lungs, and intestines. Also, the abdomen, and to some degree the chest, are compressible. A 4-inch (10.16-cm) blade can easily cause a wound that is 6 inches (15.24 cm) deep. Solid, relatively movable organs such as the liver, kidneys, and to some degree the heart, provide the best chance of determining the depth of the wound.

All individuals who have suspected stab wounds should be X-rayed, because it is possible for the tip of the knife to be broken off within the body. If possible the tip should be recovered and submitted as evidence for possible physical matching to a suspected weapon.

Stab wounds that are generally perpendicular to the body surface may be more complex than a simple blunt and sharp edge. If the knife or the victim moves, which is entirely possible, then the direction that the blade enters and the direction that the blade leaves are different, forming an A- or butterfly-shaped wound of varying angles (**Figure 13-13**). Complex stab wounds may also be seen in unusually shaped areas of the body, such as the neck or the axillae, where individual cuts and then ultimately a complex stab wound may be seen as separate injuries but reflect a single event. A knife may be held in various manners and can be directed toward a target in a forehand, backhand, or thrusting motion. The knife can be directed overhand or underhand. The shape, depth, and direction of the wound cannot independently reconstruct the events that happened with regard to handedness, exact location, or relative body positions of the assailant. Penetrating injuries may be caused by weapons other than knives, such as long barbecue-type forks, screwdrivers, or other thin, natural, or man-made objects. Trace evidence such as paint, hairs, fibers, or parts of the object that caused the injury may be present within the wound tract. The wound should be explored carefully to identify trace evidence. A Phillips head or flat head screwdriver often shows patterned injuries. The flat head screwdriver has a blunt edge and the Phillips head injuries have cross or star-shaped regular linear abrasions extending from the center of the wound.

When there is sharp-force injury, it is important to also examine and document other injuries that may be evident on the hands or forearms. Cuts or even other stab wounds in these areas are commonly referred to as defense wounds, implying that the victim was conscious and able to fight back during the attack. These do not in and of themselves guarantee that the deceased person was alive and conscious, but if he wasn't, that would imply that the assailant caused injuries to these parts of the body intentionally. The identification of individual wounds, particularly in the extremities, may require them to be probed because they may represent direction of force through entry and exit wounds. It may be difficult, if not impossible, to identify the direction of these wounds unless there is an abrasion around one of them. It is certainly possible that defense wounds can be located on the

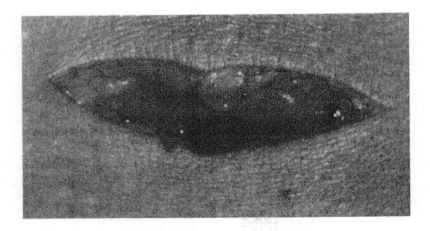

Figure 13-13 Butterfly-shaped stab wound.

lower extremities because people can defend themselves by kicking. Defense wounds also may be either blunt- or sharp-force injuries.

Guns and Gunshot Wounds
The Projectile

A lead ball traveling at several hundred feet or meters per second has significantly more energy, and therefore causes more tissue damage, than another propelled object such as one launched from a slingshot. The key to tissue damage is the translation of the energy supplied by the moving object, as represented by KE½MV2, where KE is kinetic energy, M is equal to mass (or weight of the bullet), and V is velocity. Note that if the mass of the bullet is doubled, the kinetic energy is also doubled. However, if the velocity or speed of the bullet is doubled, then the kinetic energy is quadrupled. It is the speed of the bullet that translates into tissue damage. The speed is determined by the quantity of gunpowder that is available to propel the bullet down the barrel of the gun (DiMaio, 1999).

A cartridge or round (**Figure 13-14**) is a brass cylinder with a closed base that has a hollowed out area for a disc-shaped primer cap to be installed. The gunpowder granules are then placed loosely into the cartridge case and the bullet is placed in the end and crimped, so that it will not fall out. The primer cap contains materials that are high explosives, which are then sent through a small hole called a vent in the cartridge case base that will ignite the gunpowder, producing a tremendous amount of gas that expands, forcing the bullet out of the cartridge case and down the barrel.

The handling of a recovered bullet, whether from a scene or from tissue, should be done with great care. The barrel of the gun contains grooves cut into the tube in a slight spiral pattern. These grooves help the bullet to dig in and, because of the spiral, impart spin on the bullet. Spinning the bullet along its long axis vastly increases its ability to fly straight, and therefore increases the accuracy of the weapon. This is similar to a baseball that is thrown toward home plate by the pitcher with no spin on it (a knuckle ball). It is notoriously inaccurate, and left to the vagaries of wind and humidity for its ultimate destination. In order to throw a baseball straight a spin must be imparted to it. The machined markings on the

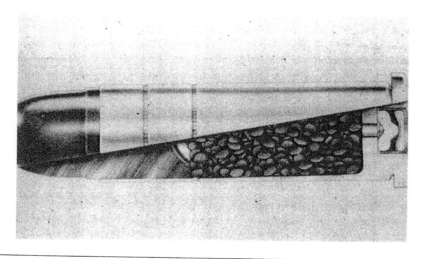

Figure 13-14 Anatomy of a cartridge or round.

inside of the barrel of the gun have a high point (the true internal diameter) called the land and a low point that has been carved out as the groove. The high point will impart a groove, which looks like a slightly angled rectangular impression, into the side of the bullet and/or bullet jacket. The number of high points and the direction of the spiral indicate the general characteristics of the barrel of the gun, for example a right or left twist and five or six lands. The individual characteristics of the machined barrel will leave tiny microscopic striations on the bullet or jacket (**Figure 13-15**). Test firing a questioned gun and comparing with a bullet recovered from a body or a scene will, using a stereoscopic microscope, essentially be able to match not only the general class characteristics, but also the individual characteristics of that bullet, similar to a fingerprint. These characteristics can change over time to some degree as the barrel of the gun handles other debris from bullets, gunpowder, and other environmental effects. Rough handling or inappropriate packaging can alter these useful striations. It is often the practice to inscribe a number or initials onto the nose or the base of the bullet for identification or chain of custody purposes; however, appropriate packaging and chain of custody receipts should obviate any problems.

Analysis of Evidence

Gunshot wounds are merely a compilation and subset of blunt-force trauma. However, their importance and implications require them to be analyzed in a different fashion in order for the forensic investigator to come up with useful opinions and conclusions (DiMaio & DiMaio, 2001). When a bullet that is spinning along its long axis impacts the skin, the skin will be indented while the bullet is spinning and forcing its way through the skin prior to overcoming its elasticity. This causes an area of abrasion that ultimately surrounds the circular defect (laceration) caused by the bullet in the skin. This abrasion collar or marginal abrasion around the central defect is the classic feature of an entry gunshot wound (**see Color Plate 20**). Depending on its kinetic energy, the bullet will then travel through tissue, causing lacerations, contusions of tissues, and fractures of any bone that it may impact. The

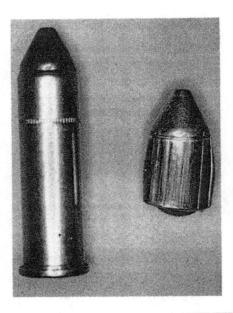

Figure 13-15 Intact round (L) and fired bullet (R) with barrel markings.

bullet may continue through the body and force its way out of the body, stretching the skin from inside toward out, ultimately causing it to tear, and the bullet continues on its way. This wound is irregular in shape, generally larger than the accompanying entrance wound, and with no marginal abrasion of the skin around the tear. These tears can be stellate or linear and of various sizes. The exit wound may have an abrasion around it if it is shored or supported. As the skin protrudes from the pressure of the bullet going from inside toward the outside, the skin may be forced up against a hard object, such as elastic clothing, a wall, a chair, or the ground. This abrasion may be very similar to that seen around the entry gunshot wound, but more typically because of the nature of the object that it impacts, flat and broad, has a wide, irregular, marginal abrasion that is dissimilar to the classic entry gunshot wound abrasion collar. Occasionally the exit wound can look very similar to the entry wound, and it can be difficult to tell which is which.

One of the important analyses to be performed on any gunshot wound is the observation and documentation of any gunshot residue. What comes out of the barrel of the gun is the bullet, unburned or partly burned gunpowder particles that become missiles unto themselves, and completely burned gunpowder called smoke or soot. If only the bullet impacts the skin, this would be called a distant entry gunshot wound. This range may actually be as close as 3 feet (0.91 meters). The absence of gunshot residue around the entry gunshot does not necessarily mean it is a distant gunshot wound if there is intermediary material such as clothing between the end of the barrel and the skin. Gunshot wounds with a classic circular defect, a marginal abrasion, and no visible gunshot residue on the skin surrounding the wound may be gunshot wounds of indeterminate range if it is known that there was clothing, a door, or a window between the gun and the victim based on the scene circumstances. If individual gunpowder particles have struck the skin they may embed into the skin, called powder tattooing, or impact the skin, leaving an abrasion or contusion, called powder stippling. Evidence of the entry gunshot wound with powder stippling or tattooing on the skin surrounding the wound is called a medium- or intermediate-range gunshot wound.

Individual gunpowder particles can be extracted from the epidermis and retained as evidence. Gunpowder particles come in multitudes of shapes, from true spheres to flattened spheres called flattened ball, to disc-shaped, to flakes, to cylinders. The shape and size of the gunpowder particles allow for variations in the length of time that this nitrocellulose material actually burns, producing the gases within the cartridge casing that expel the bullet. The radius from the center of the wound, or the total diameter of the distribution of these impacts on the skin, should be meticulously recorded and photographed. The radius of the stippling should be measured after the direction of the bullet and its angle to the skin have been determined. The radius or diameter may be different if viewed perpendicular to the skin, as opposed to a tangential entry gunshot wound from the side. A tangential entry gunshot wound will also not be circular; it will be ovoid in shape with an asymmetric marginal abrasion, the larger end being where the bullet first entered. Gunpowder particles generally, although with quite a bit of variation, will travel approximately 2 feet (0.61 m) and still have enough energy to impact the skin.

Evidence of an entry gunshot wound, powder particles having impacted the skin, and black material called soot surrounding the entry gunshot wound are all consistent with a close-range gunshot wound (**Figure 13-16**). The range of fire is in the area of less than 6 to 8 inches (15.24 to 20.32 cm). The soot is not very dense and will not carry very far. The diameter of the soot should also be documented, and a sample can be collected with a

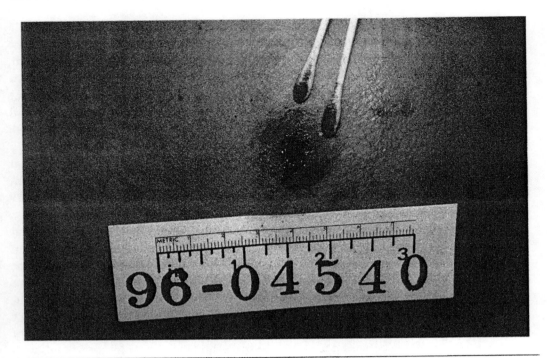

Figure 13-16   Examination of close-range gunshot wound with gunpowder residue.

cotton swab for forensic ballistic laboratory analysis. If the muzzle of the gun is in contact with the skin, there will be an entry gunshot wound that has thick accumulation of gunpowder particles and soot around its edge or within its depths, depending on how tight the contact is. As the gases penetrate the skin and expand, the skin will be stamped into the muzzle face, leaving a thin, curvilinear patterned abrasion that should mimic the shape of the face of the barrel of the gun. This is called a barrel abrasion or a muzzle stamp. This can be extremely useful in determining which gun may have caused the injury if there is a choice of more than one known gun. If the contact entry gunshot wound is over bone, commonly over the scalp in suicide situations, the tremendous gases that come out of the barrel of the gun enter between the scalp and the skull, causing a large irregular or stellate tear of the scalp. If the bullet perforates the brain and skull and exits the opposing side, it might create a relatively small wound, which flies in the face of the conventional wisdom that the entry wound is smaller than the exit wound. Identification of soot and gunpowder in the depths of the wound easily distinguishes the entry from the exit. After gentle cleaning of the wound to identify the presence of soot or gunpowder particles and the collection of any visible material, the hair surrounding the wound should be shaved so that the features of the wound can be appropriately examined and documented. The hair around the wound, regardless of how bloody or dirty it may be, should be saved for potential laboratory analysis of the gunshot residue. Even if it is not visible on the skin, the residue may have adhered to the hairs and would be helpful in estimating the range of fire. Hair around the wounds should always be shaved and never washed until after appropriate evidence collection and wound documentation has been completed.

Radiographic Studies

Any live or deceased person suspected of being a victim of a gunshot wound should have X-rays. This will help locate the bullet as evidence and at least suggest a path and, therefore, the tissue damage. Bullets generally travel in a straight line, although as they lose energy their paths may be deflected by bone. Atypical final locations of bullets can occur; if a bullet enters an artery or a vein, it can be swept either by the action of the heart or gravity into a vessel toward the heart or away from the heart and be located far away from the initial entry wound and suspected tissue path. Trying to locate such a bullet can be confounding.

In cases of multiple gunshot wounds, it may be difficult to catalog all the entries and exits and the number of bullets. The general rule of thumb is that the number of wounds plus the number of bullets equals an even number. For example, an entry wound with a bullet recovered in the chest is an even number, an entry and an exit wound is an even number, and an entry, exit, reentry, and bullet recovery is an even number. If the examination and analysis yield an odd number of wounds plus bullets, then an unaccounted for wound or a missing bullet is to blame. The exception to this rule is if a soft lead bullet comes in at a tangential angle and is split, causing a fragment of the bullet to exit and the other fragment to remain in the body. The jacket of a bullet can also be peeled off from the lead core, either by an intermediary target, clothing, or a defective unit, causing two wounds but a single bullet.

Asphyxia

Asphyxia essentially means the lack of oxygen to cells. The brain cells are the most sensitive to low oxygen states; therefore, any mechanism that results in decreased oxygen availability to the neurons would be an asphyxial death. Any situation that one could conceive that would prevent oxygen from getting into the bloodstream or blood from getting to the brain would lead to an asphyxial death.

Environmental Deficit

External environmental situations that would decrease oxygen not intimately associated with the body include an environment free of oxygen or depleted in oxygen such as an underground manhole that has been sealed for a long time, in which the normal bacterial residents have consumed the oxygen and produced carbon dioxide, or an enclosed, nonventilated space such as a vault or refrigerator. Nontoxic gases, such as natural gas or carbon dioxide, that replace oxygen in enclosed environments would also lead to an asphyxial death.

A more localized enclosed space around the body, such as a bag over the head, would rapidly deplete available oxygen. The prevention of oxygen from entering the respiratory tract, such as smothering with some object tightly sealing off the nose and the mouth or a gag forced into the mouth obstructing the posterior pharynx, which also blocks off the nasal pharyngeal passage, would also lead to asphyxia.

Compression

External prevention of respiration can be accomplished by preventing the chest from expanding. A classic scenario concerns a person working underneath a car that slips off the jack, resulting in the undercarriage resting on his chest. This would prevent the expansion of the chest cavity. Another common situation would be in a motor vehicle collision when the integrity of the passenger compartment is significantly compromised and the occupant has some materials pressing on his or her chest. This might also occur with the seat belt if the individual is in such a position that he or she can't release the seat belt, particularly if the vehicle is inverted. Another human being can also be the cause of chest compression, sometimes called traumatic asphyxia. One or more persons sitting or lying on the chest of another might inhibit that person's ability to respire.

Obstruction

Following the oxygen delivery deeper into the respiratory tract demonstrates any number of potential mechanisms whereby oxygen can be prevented from getting from the outside environment into the alveoli.

Materials such as food are not uncommon, particularly if the person's neurologic status is compromised by natural disease, such as a stroke, or chemically, such as by alcohol. Chunklike particles of food, particularly meats, the most common culprit being the hot dog, are prime candidates for this plugging mechanism. An event that would cause swelling of the upper airway, such as an allergic reaction causing edema of the vocal cords and laryngeal soft tissues or infection or trauma with subsequent hemorrhage and swelling may decrease the amount of oxygen that can flow.

Tumors eventually might close off an airway as well, although this is a much slower mechanism that should be identified long before it becomes a potential upper airway asphyxia mechanism. Conditions such as asthma could cause bronchial constriction in deep airways and subsequent death.

Chemical Asphyxia

At the cellular level, toxins such as carbon monoxide—which bonds to the hemoglobin molecule 200–400 times more avidly than oxygen itself—would cause chemical asphyxia. Cyanide is also a subcellular asphyxiant, preventing the intermitochondrial transport of oxygen.

Hanging

If oxygenated blood is prevented from reaching the brain, an asphyxial death can also occur. The most common mechanism for this would be neck compression via hanging. Oxygen can be prevented from getting into the cells of the brain either by interrupting the arterial flow or, more easily, by interrupting the bilateral venous outflow from the head, thereby disrupting the inflow of blood and oxygen transfer to the neurons. Circumferential bilateral and equal neck pressure will easily compress the veins, which require only approximately 4 pounds of pressure. The arteries, which are deeper and more elastic with thicker walls than with thin walls, require much more pressure to compress. In hanging, this occurs as the weight of the body, particularly in the unconscious state, puts relatively rapid and equal pressure on the neck, cutting off the arterial supply as well. This is why no petechial hemorrhages are seen during the ocular examination. Petechial hemorrhages are pinpoint red-purple hemorrhages caused by purely mechanical disruption of the venous flow exiting the head (**see Color Plate 21**). If there is adequate arterial flow, pressure will build up and the small delicate capillaries of the mucosal surfaces will break and be visible. These can even coalesce to be quite large, encompassing much of the sclera. They are readily apparent on the conjunctival surfaces of the globe, beneath the eyelids, and in the skin of the eyelids. Petechial hemorrhages can also be seen on the oral mucosa, although this is often not looked for and is not reflected in previous studies. People who have had their necks compressed but do not succumb may have florid petechial hemorrhages seen everywhere on the face.

Petechial hemorrhages seen in true hanging victims should be explained. The most likely reason is that a previous attempt had failed, causing damaged blood vessels that are reacting to the renewed arterial blood flow. Hanging can take place in any position. One does not have to be swinging from a tree limb. Hanging can be done fully suspended, partially suspended where the person can relieve the neck pressure at any time while conscious, in a seated position, or even lying down. As long as enough bilateral neck pressure is maintained after the person becomes unconscious to prevent blood flow, it will inhibit oxygen transfer to the brain. There should be an identifiable suspension point in the ligature furrow (**see Color Plate 22**), forming an upside down *V*.

In assault situations, a ligature can be placed around the neck. This mechanism is a process called garroting (**see Color Plate 23**). This can be done with any object and is usually accomplished from behind. A soft ligature may not leave any marks at all, whereas a narrow or patterned ligature that would reflect the shape of the object that caused it may leave specific injuries that can be identified and documented. The ligature furrow should be horizontal and circumferential around the neck. Because this occurs during a violent encounter, other injuries may also be present, such as abrasions and contusions of the face and potentially the arms. The investigator should also look for injury to the back as the perpetrator might use a knee for leverage, causing a contusion.

Manual Strangulation

Another more dramatic form of external neck compression is manual strangulation. This is a very dynamic event in which the assailant places his or her hands on or around the neck, usually involving significant struggle. During this period shearing forces occur at various levels throughout the neck structures. The hallmarks of manual strangulation include the identification of petechial hemorrhages as the veins are easily compressed but the arteries are not or are interrupted intermittently. Careful examination of the conjunctivae, the eyelids, and the oral mucosa are important in every case, particularly if the deceased is a female, if there is disruption of the clothing or she is nude, or if the scene circumstances suggest violence. Careful examination of the skin of the neck may find contusions and abrasions (**see Color Plate 24**), some of which may be small curvilinear abrasions that would represent fingernail marks. Not all fingernail abrasions are those of the assailant. During the struggle with the assailant's hands around the victim's neck, attempts to remove the hands may cause the victim to scratch him or herself. Because of the intimate nature of these types of assaults, whether they are ligature or manual strangulation, it is important to look for trace evidence. Alternate light sources are useful for foreign hairs and fibers, as well as for potential semen stains on clothing or skin.

Fingernail scrapings or the complete excision of the fingernails for potential biological material that might link the deceased to the assailant should be taken routinely, and a rape kit should be taken if the deceased is female or known to be a homosexual. This should be done even if the assault does not lead to the individual's death.

The internal examination reveals subtle, usually asymmetric, hemorrhages that may be in multiple layers of the neck structures, which should be dissected meticulously in situ for best results and appropriate interpretation. A prolonged struggle may also lead to massive internal neck hemorrhages. A delicate dissection of the hyoid bone may reveal fracture of the cornu and/or the superior horns of the thyroid cartilage. The presence of fractures in these structures is highly suggestive, if not diagnostic, of a manual strangulation because their location high and deep in the neck structures make it very difficult to apply force that would not be readily apparent from the scene, such as a motor vehicle accident or other type of drastic trauma. However, the absence of hyoid bone fractures does not rule out manual strangulation. If the victim is young, then the hyoid bone and thyroid cartilages may be quite elastic, and the hyoid bone may not have ossified and fused and therefore retained its pliability (Saferstein, 2010).

Neck compression can also be done with the arms, such as the now-discouraged police technique of the carotid sleeper, where the tip of the neck at the Adam's apple is wedged in the depths of the antecubital fossa as a person, such as a police officer or an attacker, wraps his or her arm around the victim's neck from behind. Utilizing the free arm for pressure and leverage, the upper and lower arm are squeezed onto the neck in a pincher-type motion, readily compressing the carotid arteries bilaterally and leading to rapid unconsciousness. If pressure is maintained too long, oxygen depletion, seizure, and/or cardiac dysrhythmia due to stimulation of the carotid body may lead to death. If the anterior aspect of the neck is on the forearm as it is held horizontally across the neck with pressure applied, the larynx may fracture, leading to hemorrhage and swelling and potentially an asphyxial death. This is called the bar hold, which is a very painful experience for the recipient. An inanimate object can also cause neck compression, but instances are very unusual, occurring generally in industrial situations.

Positional Asphyxia

Positional asphyxia is often discussed in police and corrections circles. Sometimes police or corrections officers have to restrain an individual who is out of control due to drugs such as phencyclidine or cocaine, or due to inherent psychoses, for the safety of himself, people surrounding him, and the officers. The necessary restraint may take four to six people, but during the struggle, pressure may be applied to the chest cavity for a prolonged period of time, causing the individual to die of traumatic asphyxia, or pressure may be applied to the neck, causing the person to die of asphyxia by neck compression. This is not a true positional asphyxia. True positional asphyxia means that the body is in a position where respiration is difficult, if not impossible. True positional asphyxias are difficult to envision and are often complicated by significant alcohol or drug consumption. A person lying on her back with her feet touching the ground while her neck, chest, and waist are bent is an example (**Figure 13-17**). Another example is an individual with a large abdomen who is handcuffed or hog-tied, causing inhibition of respiration if he is face down on a hard surface. Lying prone on a surface, such as the back of an automobile where the transmission axle hump is located, can further decrease the ability to expand the chest.

Manner of Death

All types of asphyxial deaths are traumatic except for natural disease processes such as a bacterial infection, asthma, or anaphylaxis. The traumatic mechanisms of asphyxia may

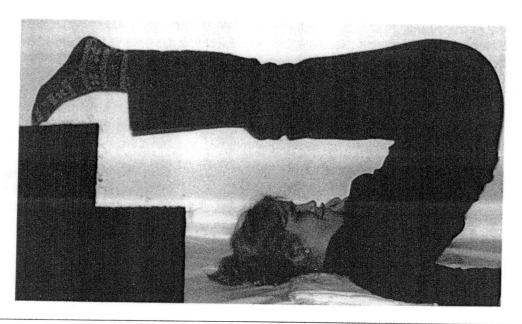

Figure 13-17   Potential positional asphyxia.

be accidental, homicidal, or suicidal. Appropriate scene investigation, including interviews with witnesses, family, and private physicians, as well as scouring the environs for a suicide note, whether written on paper, dictated, or on a home computer, should be accomplished for an appropriate manner of death determination. For example, a young male found hanging in the bedroom, although not fully suspended, may not be a suicide victim. If the genitals are exposed, pornographic material is present, and there is no previous history of suicidal ideation, attempts, or an apparent suicide message, this may fall under the category of an autoerotic asphyxia, which is an accidental death and not a suicidal death. In these particular situations, the discovery that light-headedness enhances the orgasm causes the participant to invent any one of varied and imaginative mechanisms to compress the neck. There should be an escape mechanism so that the pressure can be relieved, preventing the individual from becoming unconscious while the pressure on the neck is maintained and ultimately dying. Occasionally these escape mechanisms will fail, and the deceased can be found in sometimes very unusual situations.

Summary

In order to expand and professionalize the responsibilities of death investigation, more and more jurisdictions are utilizing nonphysician death investigators. This includes the forensic nurse and others, often with college or advanced degrees, with formal or in-house training and hands-on experience in the medical field. With these backgrounds, individuals can develop the experience required to understand the different types of deaths and how to assist the responsible physician for accurate certification.

A forensic nurse is probably the most qualified nonphysician death investigator. The advantage that the nurse death investigator possesses is medical and nursing education that results in a rapid and accurate understanding of the disease processes when reviewing medical records and obtaining pertinent history from treating physicians. The nurse also has a wide background in understanding classes and individual types of prescription medications. Nurses are also uniquely qualified to interact with family members involved in extremely stressful events, such as the violent demise of a loved one. The forensic nurse possesses expert communication skills that can be used effectively with families, loved ones, witnesses, and any other people who might impact the death investigation. Having an understanding of the collaborative nature of the death investigation role enables the nurse to become an effective team member. Even if the nurse has not had any experience in death investigation, the basic procedures, observations, and language can be learned and assimilated readily. In summary, nurses as death investigators are in a unique position to be successful and productive because of their education, experience, inherent ability to relate to people, and natural tenacity to solve problems and to pose and answer questions.

QUESTIONS FOR DISCUSSION

1. Describe the death investigation system in the area in which you reside.
2. What is the primary goal of any death investigation?
3. Describe methods one could use to identify a deceased John Doe.
4. Describe the sequence of photographs that should be taken at a death scene investigation.
5. What is the best way to determine the time of death of a deceased?
6. What is meant by the chain of custody of collected evidence?
7. What is meant by the term proximate event?
8. Describe how two bullets are compared during a ballistics test.
9. Compare the processes of putrefaction and mummification.
10. What are the responsibilities of the death investigator in relation to organ transplantation?
11. What issues might present themselves in a death investigation system that utilizes nonphysician death investigators?

REFERENCES

Byrd, J. H., & Castner, J. L. (Eds.). (2001). *Forensic entomology: The utility of arthropods in legal investigations.* Boca Raton, FL: CRC Press.

Dillon, D. (1977). *A history of criminalistics in the United States 1850–1950.* (Unpublished doctoral thesis), University of California, Berkeley.

DiMaio, V. J. M. (1999). *Gunshot wounds: Practical aspects of firearms, ballistics, and forensic techniques* (2nd ed.). Boca Raton, FL: CRC Press.

DiMaio, V. J. M., & DiMaio, D. (2001). *Forensic pathology* (2nd ed.). Boca Raton, FL: CRC Press.

Forensic Timeline. (2002). *Forensic science timeline.* Retrieved from http://www.forensicdna.com/Timeline020702.pdf

Goff, M. L. (2000). *A fly for the prosecution: How insect evidence helps solve crime.* Cambridge, MA: Harvard University Press.

Hanzlick, R. L. (1996). On the need for more expertise in death investigation (and a national office of death investigation affairs?). *Archives of Pathology & Laboratory Medicine, 120,* 782–785.

Hanzlick, R. L. (Ed.). (1997a). *Cause of death statements and certification of natural and unnatural deaths.* Northfield, IL: College of American Pathologists.

Hanzlick, R. L. (1997b). Death registration: History, methods, and legal issues. *Journal of Forensic Science, 42*(2), 265–269.

International Association of Forensic Nurses. (1999). *Scope and standards of forensic nursing practice* (3rd ed.). Washington, DC: American Nurses Publishing.

Knight, B. (Ed.). (1995). *The estimation of the time since death in the early postmortem period.* Avon, England: Edward Arnold.

Messite, J., & Stellman, S. (1990). Accuracy of death certificate completion: The need for formalized physician training. *Journal of the American Medical Association, 275,* 794–796.

Moran, T., Raddatz, M., Schifrin, N., Ross, B., & Tapper, J. (2011). TARGET: Bin Laden–The Death and Life of Public Enemy Number One. *Retrieved from* http://abcnews.go.com/Politics/target-bin-laden-death-life-osama-bin-laden/story?id=13786598&page=4

National Academies Press (2011). Review of the scientific approaches used during the FBI's investigation of the 2011 anthrax letters. Washington, DC: Author.

Saferstein, R. (2010). *Criminalistics: An introduction to forensic science* (10th ed.). Upper Saddle River, NJ: Dave Garza.

SUGGESTED FURTHER READING

Blum, D. (2010). *The poisoner's handbook: Murder and the birth of forensic science in jazz age New York.* New York, NY: Penguin Press.

Ford, J. (2006). *Forensics in American culture: Obsessed with crime.* Philadelphia, PA: Mason Crest.

Libal, A. (2006). *Fingerprints, bite marks, earprints: Human signposts.* Philadelphia, PA: Mason Crest.

Meyers, C. (2007). *Silent evidence: Firearms (forensic ballistics) and toolmarks: Cases from forensic science.* Charlotte, NC: Catawba.

Shone, R. (2008). *Corpses and skeletons: The science of forensic anthropology.* New York, NY: Rosen.

Wagner, E. J. (2006). *The science of Sherlock Holmes: From Baskerville Hall to the Valley of Fear; The real forensics behind the great detective's greatest cases.* Hoboken, NJ: Wiley.

CHAPTER 14

Evidence Collection and Documentation

Nancy B. Cabelus and Katherine Spangler

Any time two people or objects come in contact with each other, there is an exchange of physical evidence. The value of this evidence in forensic investigations may be compromised if the evidence is improperly packaged or if the reliability of the evidence cannot be shown. The forensic nurse must be aware of the proper recognition, documentation, collection, and preservation of evidence in criminal and civil investigations, such as domestic violence, motor vehicle accidents, and other situations involving physical evidence and patterns. This awareness is essential to prevent loss of critical materials and information, which can adversely affect subsequent analysis and proceedings.

CHAPTER FOCUS

» Basic Theories of Evidence
» Locard's Principle of Exchange
» The Crime Scene
» Classification of Physical Evidence
» Evidence Recognition and Collection
» Recognition of Physical Abuse

» Evidence Documentation
» Evidence Packaging
» Role of the Forensic Laboratory
» Collection of Evidence From the Deceased Patient
» Legal Considerations

KEY TERMS

» chain of custody
» cross-contamination
» documentation
» HIPAA regulations
» Locard's principle

» physical evidence
» tangible evidence
» trace evidence
» transient evidence

Introduction

Discoveries and developments in forensic science have led to changes within professional nursing practice. Because of these advances, forensic nursing is an evolving discipline that is a blend of two distinct concepts: nursing and forensic science.

The nursing profession interfaces with the law more than ever before, and in a multitude of settings. For example, there is a marked increase in the number of challenges to nursing **documentation** in both criminal and civil courts. The nurse is no longer automatically granted a high level of trust. She or he must earn that trust among colleagues and other professionals. As forensic nurses face today's challenges in treating victims and perpetrators of violent acts, they must be vigilant in recognizing changes and trends within their field of practice.

This chapter will address evidence recognition, documentation, and collection in the forensic nurse's daily practice. Standards for basic evidence collection techniques, suggested methods of documentation, and issues pertaining to patient privacy and confidentiality also will be discussed.

Basic Theories

Contemporary forensic nursing roles may be largely attributed to the vision exemplified by the earliest founders of our profession. Attention to detail and unwavering dedication were part of the foundations of nursing. Today, forensic nurses work in many contemporary roles but have built upon the nursing theories of the past. By applying critical thinking skills, forensic nurses pay special attention to fine details while never losing sight of the whole picture.

Contemporary nurses of the 21st century must acquire some knowledge in basic forensic science and the law to treat a forensic patient effectively. Forensic nurses must be aware of current statutes, legal decisions, and mandated professional obligations when treating victims and perpetrators of abuse, neglect, or interpersonal violence. Care plans and charting procedures may need to be updated to document appropriately the standards of care provided by healthcare practitioners. This documentation is always important but of even greater significance in any case that could potentially interface with a medicolegal investigation.

Locard's Principle of Exchange

Known as the father of **trace evidence**, Dr. Edmond Locard (1877–1966) was a pathologist in Lyon, France. For many years, Locard conducted scientific investigations and researched the application of analytical methods to criminal investigation. In 1910, Dr. Locard founded the first police laboratory, which was dedicated to the advancement of the forensic sciences. Forensic nurses have followed in Locard's footsteps by understanding the dynamics of trace evidence and the significance of that evidence in medicolegal investigations.

Locard's theory states that whenever there is contact between two objects, there is a mutual exchange of material between those two surfaces. This theory of evidence exchange provides a basis for linkage between the victim, the perpetrator, and the scene, as depicted in **Figure 14-1**. Locard maintained that "no one can act . . . without leaving behind numerous signs of it . . . indications of where he has been or what he has done" (Inman & Rudin, 2001, p. 44).

This evidence can lead to the conviction of an offender or, as importantly, show that the person accused is not guilty of an offense.

Profound advances have occurred in the field of forensic science since 1910, including the discovery of deoxyribonucleic acid (DNA) and its application in forensic investigations. Thus, **Locard's principle** remains as important now as it was in the early 1900s.

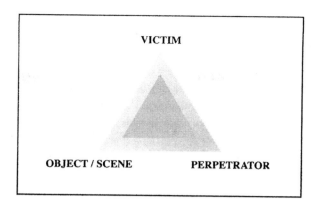

Figure 14-1 Relationship among sources of trace evidence.

Materials that have been exchanged between people or objects may be identified through application of Locard's principle; forensic advances such as DNA analysis allow for greater individualization of that exchanged evidence. (Refer to Chapter 18 for more information on DNA analysis.) Locard's theory of transfer is clearly illustrated by **Case 14-1**, involving the identification of significant transfer evidence.

CASE 14-1

Locard's Principle Linking a Victim and a Suspect

A 10-year-old girl lived in a small Midwest town with her family. She left her school at approximately 3:30 p.m. for a 20-minute walk home, but she never arrived. At 4:30 p.m., her mother became concerned and began looking for her. The mother called the homes of her daughter's friends, but to no avail. She then called the police department. A search of the neighborhood began, but the child was not found.

It was not until 3 days later that the little girl's body was discovered in a wooded area about 6 miles from the school. She was partially clothed and her body was covered with dirt and leaves. Because the ambient temperature was cool, the body was fairly well preserved. A scarf was wrapped tightly around her neck. The girl was naked from the waist down and sexual assault was suspected.

The scene was secured by police officers so that there would be no inadvertent contamination of the scene or of potential evidence. Crime scene personnel processed the scene. During a search of the crime scene, tire impressions were discovered in the moist soil and in close proximity to the body. The tire impressions were photographed and plaster casts were made in order to preserve imprint detail.

A forensic nurse representing the medical examiner's office was dispatched to the scene. The forensic nurse conducted a survey of the body, which included a written description of observations and photographic documentation. This information was provided to the forensic pathologist to assist with the examination and interpretation of the child's injuries and to corroborate findings of the autopsy.

The forensic pathologist used an ultraviolet light to perform an external examination of the victim's body. The alternate light source was used to search for further potential evidence that may have been transferred onto the victim's body or the clothing by the perpetrator. Evidence such as semen, other body fluids, chemical residues, and some fibers may fluoresce when exposed to the ultraviolet light. Fine red fibers were found on the clothing that would not have been apparent with the naked eye. Subsequent laboratory evidence of these fibers showed that they had characteristics of a carpet fiber. Samples for comparison were removed by investigators from various locations. The red fiber evidence found on the child's body ultimately linked the victim to the perpetrator; the trunk of the perpetrator's car was lined with carpet having similar red fibers.

The Crime Scene

A crime scene is the location or place where a crime occurs. The scene can be inside or outdoors. A motor vehicle, train, or aircraft can be a crime scene. In the clinical setting, the victim may be the only known crime scene, for example when a sexual assault occurs. Clinicians who treat the victim may not know where the crime occurred, but evidence on the victim's body or clothing could connect that person to the crime scene. For example, if the crime occurred in a wooded area, there may be soil or plant material on the victim's clothing or footwear that would be similar to findings at that scene. It is important for the forensic nurse to understand Locard's theory of evidence transfer and its implications. In this way, clinical findings can be interpreted while conducting an examination of the patient.

If there are multiple crime scenes within the scope of the investigation, the locations of interest may be referred to as the primary, secondary, or tertiary crime scenes. For example, in a carjacking incident, the primary crime scene would be where the carjacking occurred, and the secondary scene would be where the vehicle was recovered. In a homicide, a victim may have been abducted from one location, killed in a second place, and left in a third location. Therefore, investigators would ultimately have three crime scenes to process. The vehicle in which the victim was transported would also be considered a crime scene.

Physical evidence, when properly recognized, documented, and preserved, can provide the crucial link between the person and location or object that caused an injury. This is also true in cases of civil litigation, such as motor vehicle accidents and negligence cases. For example, a case of a failed seat belt will be greatly substantiated by identifying the presence of hair and tissue fragments in a shattered windshield, especially if those materials can be related to head injuries of the injured plaintiff.

The Forensic Nursing Role

Forensic nurses who work with evidence collection and documentation require specialized training. Because of the emphasis on forensic evidence in today's courtroom and with advances in forensic science, especially in the laboratory testing of biological evidence, nursing care plans must be modified to include policies and procedures for both the treatment of the forensic patient and the proper collection of forensic evidence. Because they are excellent communicators, forensic nurses can help to bridge the gap between law enforcement and the physician or other healthcare professionals. In addition, forensic nurses are able to provide better holistic care by applying critical thinking skills when making a nursing diagnosis. Forensic nurses may be called upon to testify in a criminal or civil courtroom because of their interaction with victims, suspects, and members of the legal community. Forensic nurses are readily accepted as credible expert witnesses because of their specialized training.

Forensic Evidence

Classification of Physical Evidence

There are many ways to classify and categorize physical evidence. Some forensic experts classify evidence according to the type of action that produced the evidence (e.g., homicide, motor vehicle accident, medical negligence); others concentrate on the type of analyses that will be required (e.g., instrumental analysis, pattern examination, radiography). For the purposes of this chapter, evidence classes that are of greatest concern to the forensic nurse are physical evidence that is identified as tangible, transient, or trace. **Tangible evidence** is touchable. It may be recognizable on sight, such as a gun, a knife, an article of clothing, or a written document. Multiple gunshot patterns, bloodstains, and other pattern evidence are included in this category. When pattern evidence is encountered, those patterns must be documented in place prior to any alteration. **Figure 14-2** shows the proper documentation of multiple gunshot pattern evidence. Note the presence of a scale and proper lighting, which assists in determining the sequence of shots and their relationship to each other on the windshield.

Physical evidence also includes so-called trace evidence, which is any material found in small quantity or size. Trace evidence cannot always be seen by the naked eye, but it may be identified with the use of a microscope or alternate light sources; for example, bite

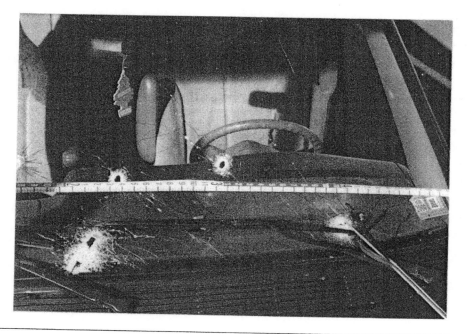

Figure 14-2 A photograph of a motor vehicle with multiple gunshot strikes to the windshield. The photograph depicts the distribution of shots and the scale allows an estimate of the distance among the shots.

Photograph courtesy of the Connecticut State Police, Central District Major Crime Squad.

mark evidence may include traces of saliva containing DNA. Although DNA is not visually apparent, the forensic nurse may recognize the significance of finding DNA evidence in a wound. If collected properly, the foreign DNA sample can potentially be linked to its source. If the nurse were to cleanse a bite mark injury prior to collecting a swabbed sample from the marking, the transferred evidence would be lost. The nurse should also note other characteristics of the bite mark such as size, shape, depth, or pattern of the mark. Use of alternate light systems often aids in locating and recognizing trace evidence.

Evidence that can be washed away, damaged, lost, or destroyed, either intentionally, accidentally, or by environmental factors, is designated **transient evidence**. Transient evidence is observed when a patient is treated with injuries having characteristics of bruising, swelling, bleeding, redness, or tenderness. The nurse should carefully document the location and description of those injuries as well as what was palpated upon examination. If possible, these kinds of injuries should also be photographed because they will no longer be visible after they have healed. Photographs of the injuries should also be taken a couple of days after they first occur. This additional documentation will demonstrate any further discoloration of the patient's skin throughout the healing process and any patterned injury that may be seen.

Transient evidence may also be detected through sense of smell, such as an odor of marijuana, alcoholic beverage, or gasoline. Again, this kind of evidence is present only temporarily. It will not be available to show to a court or jury if the case goes to trial in the future. Therefore, the importance of thorough documentation cannot be overemphasized.

Evidence Recognition and Collection

Evidence can be encountered in many situations within the forensic nursing profession. Perhaps the most common or most familiar role in which the forensic nurse must follow prescribed procedures for evidence collection is that of the sexual assault nurse or forensic examiner. Sexual assault nursing is arguably the most established forensic nursing role in the recognition and handling of physical evidence. As part of their training and education, sexual assault nurses must demonstrate proficiency in evidence collection and packaging, the ability to properly document their findings in the course of the examination, and also be able to properly initiate the **chain of custody**. Mandated collection kits or protocols have been developed in most jurisdictions to maintain the proper collection and preservation of evidence in sexual assault cases and cases of interpersonal violence. The goal is to limit the potential for challenge of the evidence at a later time.

In clinical practice, the chain of custody usually begins when a healthcare practitioner locates or obtains physical evidence. The documentation process for evidence collection and transfer is facilitated by the use of an evidence custody form. An example of a chain of custody form is shown in **Figure 14-3.** Any documentation of the evidence should include a description of what the item of evidence is, the date and time it was recovered, and from where it was recovered. A case number or identification code to be used for cross-referencing should also be noted. This initial collection information should also be written on any evidence tags. The person who receives the evidence from the nurse should sign for the evidence, initiating a paper trail that follows the transfer of evidence. A receipt should also be generated to obtain the signatures of people who have custody of the evidence. As a general rule of thumb, it is always better to write down more information than might be required if you are not sure what to include. Most evidence is presented months or years after collection, so the failure to note appropriate details could result in many hours

Case No. or ID Code No. H1234

Exhibit No.: 1

Description of item: blue T-shirt, size small, torn on right sleeve

Taken from: Kathy Smith

By whom: S. Jones RN

Date/Time: 1/2/03 4:10am

Transferred to: Off. Coffey My City P.D.

Taken from: Off. Coffey

By whom: Sgt. Bagel

Date/Time: 1/2/03 6:15 a.m.

Transferred to: State Lab

Taken from:

By whom:

Date/Time:

Transferred to:

Figure 14-3 Chain of custody form.

providing testimony. In some cases, improperly documented evidence or chain of custody may result in the judge ruling the evidence inadmissible during court proceedings.

When providing care to victims or perpetrators of interpersonal violence, the forensic nurse must be aware of what could potentially be physical evidence of a crime. The forensic nurse must consider that when treating a gunshot wound victim, guns, gunshot residue, bullets, bullet projectiles, or fragments may be present on the patient's skin, in the clothing, within applied bandages or dressings, or even on the stretcher on which the patient was transported. Law enforcement officers may arrive at the hospital to collect such evidence. Forensic nurses can better assist the investigative team by recognizing what law enforcement investigators may consider important evidence.

The forensic nurse should also keep in mind that safety is a very important concern. If weapons are found on a patient, security measures must be taken immediately to protect medical staff and other patients in the facility. Documentation of safety interventions by the nurse who secured the weapons should be noted (e.g., "Handgun, magazine, and 8 bullets turned over to hospital security department."). Because many people are not firearms experts, the nurse should not record information about the weapon that is uncertain (model number or caliber). However, the nurse should document what types of weapons were found (knives, brass knuckles, etc.). If possible, photograph the weapons as shown in **Figure 14-4.** As always, care should be taken to avoid disrupting other evidence that may be on the weapon's surface.

Victims of motor vehicle accidents, especially pedestrians struck by motor vehicles, may be covered with telling evidence at the time of physical examination. Dirt, debris, glass fragments, and paint samples frequently transfer onto the body or clothing of a victim at the point of impact or in the moments following a crash. Additionally, the forensic nurse can

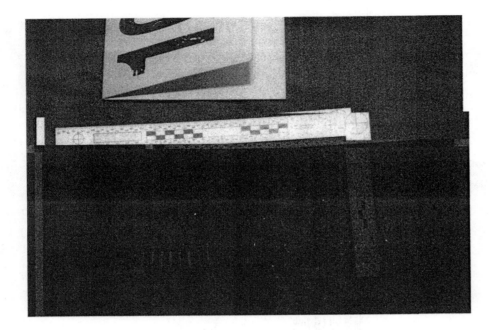

Figure 14-4 Proper photographic documentation of an unloaded, semiautomatic pistol with empty magazine and eight live rounds.

assess for evidence of the driver of the vehicle or where a passenger may have been seated in the vehicle. Types of injuries to evaluate would include abrasions caused by seat belts, shoulder harnesses, or airbags; lacerations to the face or scalp; and contusions to the chest or knees. In car vs. pedestrian accidents, especially hit-and-run incidents, patterns of injuries caused by impact with vehicle bumpers, side-view mirrors, or tires will often help investigators to match up evidence at the accident scene or to reconstruct the incident. **Figure 14-5** depicts an example of hair evidence located on the windshield of a vehicle involved in a hit-and-run accident. The victim's clothing should be carefully handled to preserve stains, rips, and tears in the fabric, as well as trace evidence such as glass, paint, dirt, or debris.

When victims or perpetrators are treated, they may have electronic devices, such as cell phones, digital planners, iPhones, and other digital equipment on their persons. These items may contain critical information for the investigation by law enforcement personnel. It is critical that the forensic nurse does not turn these digital items on for any reason. Turing on electronic devices may result in the loss of information. Such evidence should be documented and collected as other evidence.

Recognition of Physical Abuse

Victims of physical abuse, domestic violence, or child or elder abuse who seek medical treatment may present with evidence of injuries such as slap marks or grab marks from the hand of their offender, bite marks, burns, contusions, or scars. If an injury appears to have a pattern, the nurse should describe and document the pattern in the patient record. Photo documentation is very useful to support clinical findings in such cases.

The nurse could ask the patient if he or she was hurt by someone, who did this, or with what he or she was struck. If the patient is nonverbal or cannot effectively articulate this information, the nurse's job becomes more challenging and difficult. The victim might not

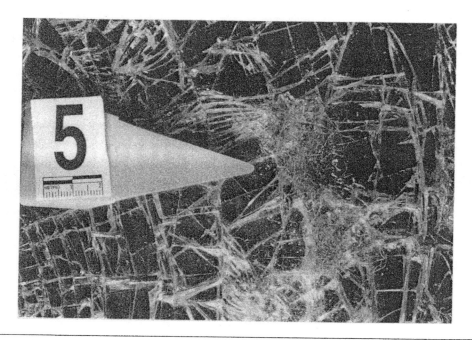

Figure 14-5   A close-up photograph of evidence identified in the search of a motor vehicle involved in an accident. Strands of hair can be seen caught within fractures of the windshield glass.

answer the nurse's questions for fear of the consequences. The forensic nurse should be aware that the evidence at hand may not be consistent with the story that is being told.

Many times, the perpetrator of abuse is related to the victim in a role such as a caretaker, a relative, or an intimate partner. Sometimes the offender will accompany the victim to the hospital and will stay with the victim during an examination to ensure that the victim does not disclose information or report the offender. Chapters 9 and 10 discuss relationships and abuse in greater detail and may provide additional guidance regarding these considerations when collecting evidence from victims of abuse.

Nurses must be familiar with mandated reporting statutes in their state. In general, nurses are mandated to report cases of abuse or neglect in children, the elderly, and the mentally retarded. Contact with the agencies that protect these populations should be made verbally and also in writing. Most agencies have required documents that must be completed by the clinician. Copies of those documents should be included with the patient record.

Collection of Physical Evidence

Crime scene investigators know what types of basic evidence collection materials are needed to process a crime scene. Such items include paper or plastic bags, paper envelopes, boxes, clean rolled paper, and containers of various sizes. Tools that are useful at the crime scene include tape rulers, a sketchbook, a compass, and a camera. It becomes automatic for the experienced crime scene investigator to arrive at the crime scene prepared to complete the lengthy and meticulous process of gathering evidence.

In the clinical setting, the caregiver may not be as readily prepared to receive a patient who could later be considered a crime scene or source of civil legal dispute. It is important to train medical staff about advances in forensic medicine so that they, too, are ready when a forensic patient is whisked through the hospital doors. In trauma centers, staff may be equipped with prepackaged cut-down sets used to insert intravenous catheters or tracheal intubation sets used to establish an airway for a trauma patient who is not breathing. Staff members should also be supplied with evidence collection kits filled with collection materials necessary to conveniently and properly preserve evidence that could link the victim to the crime scene or to the suspect.

Preservation of life is the foremost priority when treating a trauma patient. In a stressful and chaotic environment, it is easy to overlook forensic evidence that may be inadvertently destroyed or discarded. Evidence of interest to investigators could include the patient's clothing, footwear, hairs or fibers, stains, glass fragments or debris, or any noticeable patterns of injury including cuts, lacerations, abrasions, or bite marks. Prior to packaging evidence, the forensic nurse should refer to the workplace photography policy regarding seized evidence.

Evidence Packaging

In general, physical evidence should be packaged to prevent alteration of the evidence or deleterious change. Some suggestions for packaging commonly encountered physical evidence are listed here.

Clothing

If possible, the nurse should collect items of clothing and place each item into a separate paper bag to avoid **cross-contamination**. If articles of clothing are wet, they should be air dried before packaging. If this is not possible, the articles may be temporarily placed into separate plastic bags to avoid leakage or cross-contamination. Then, as soon as possible, transport the items to a place where they can be hung to dry (e.g., drying room or evidence drying cabinet). Failure to completely dry items prior to packaging could result in bacterial or mold growth, contamination, and breakdown of biological evidence. Whenever possible, clothing should not be deposited on the floor or area where there may be biological evidence, cellular material, or other trace evidence that may be transferred to the clothing.

Patterns of stains, holes, or tears in the clothing fabric should be noted. Effort must be made to preserve such patterns for forensic specialists to examine. A frequent mistake made by first responders and hospital personnel is to cut through the patient's clothing at the site of bullet holes, stab wounds, or tears in the fabric made by a penetrating object. Forensic examiners may be limited in their capability to interpret or reconstruct the incident if the evidence has been altered in such a manner. First responders may not be aware of the value of the evidence that they are destroying or discarding. Although it is acceptable to cut through clothing to enable the administration of first aid, whenever possible defects in the clothing should remain intact. Careful handling of these items by the forensic nurse can help the forensic scientist to successfully complete a laboratory examination.

Footwear

Footwear should be packaged separately from the clothing and each shoe packaged individually. Footwear from both the victim and the perpetrator may be of significance and link each to the crime scene. Soil or debris may have collected within the grooves and ridges of the soles and may match soil at the scene. Footwear sole patterns, stains, or evidence of spatter should be noted. Footprints and shoe impressions should be photographed to scale, as shown in **Figure 14-6**.

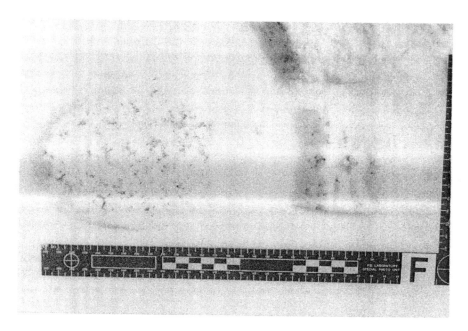

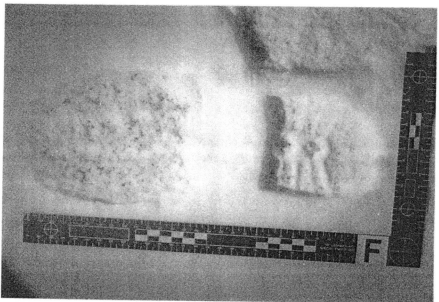

Figure 14-6 A footwear impression in snow photographed with scale using a standard flash (top) and an alternate light source (bottom). Note the additional imprint detail in the photograph taken with alternate light.

Hairs or fibers found on the victim's *body* are best preserved when carefully removed; hairs, fibers, and other trace evidence on clothing as a rule should not be removed prior to packaging the clothing. Hair and fiber evidence may be collected by area (e.g., patient's right hand or patient's left hand). When the hair or fiber is removed it should be packaged inside a paper druggist fold and then sealed in a paper envelope. Clothing should be carefully folded and placed in a clean paper bag or in paper wrapping to avoid loss of the trace materials.

Stains or Other Deposits

Dried secretions, samples of dirt, or debris should be swabbed with a sterile swab moistened with sterile water or saline. These swabs should be air dried before packaging. Some facilities use a simple rack in which swabs can dry before they are inserted into paper envelopes. Small, electric, or battery-operated dryers are sometimes used to facilitate the drying process. However, caution should be used to avoid cross-contamination with samples from other specimens or patients when using these devices. It is necessary to clean the drying apparatus after each use to avoid contamination. Also, a dryer with fans may introduce foreign, airborne particles or bacteria onto the collected sample. Avoid using heat lamps or hair dryers because these may alter the physical properties of the sample or degrade the biological material.

Bullets and Projectiles

Bullets or projectiles may contain trace evidence such as fibers, blood, or tissue. The nurse should preserve the projectile by placing it into a clean druggist fold or gauze before sealing it in a clean envelope. The surface of the projectile should be protected from rubbing against hard surfaces or other objects to preserve ballistic markings and detail.

Sharps

Sharp objects such as needles, razor blades, or knives need to be secured in such a way as to prevent injury to others and also to preserve trace evidence on the item. Plastic or glass specimen jars may be used to secure needles, razor blades, or pieces of broken glass. Knives should be secured in cardboard boxes of the appropriate size. Containers that have been designed to store these hazardous objects safely are commercially available.

Evidence collection techniques and choice of collection products can vary among jurisdictions. Training and experience will assist the nurse in determining what to collect, how it should be collected, and how much to collect. It is important for the forensic nurse to be familiar with collection and packaging guidelines specific to the laboratory where the evidence will be tested.

Function of the Forensic Laboratory

Once evidence has been collected, it is transferred to the forensic laboratory for analysis. It is important to understand what the laboratory can do when analyzing evidence, but it is also important to understand what the lab cannot do.

Many services within the forensic laboratory are available to police departments, state agencies, and, occasionally, to the private sector. Some of the services available may include, but are not limited to:

» Biological analysis is for the identification and individualization of blood and body fluids. This also includes the fields of immunology, serology, biochemistry, hematology, and molecular biology.

» Chemical analysis is used to identify accelerants that have been collected during arson investigations or other cases in which chemicals have been used in the commission of a crime.

» Fingerprint analysis is available and includes processing for identification of latent prints and fingerprint comparisons from agencies around the world.

» Firearms analysis includes the examination of guns, bullets, and bullet fragments. Tool marks are also examined and compared to tools when encountered during the investigation of a crime. This is a mark that is left when a hard surface comes into contact with a soft surface, leaving telltale marks that may identify the type of tool used.

» Document examination is the analysis of documents, whether in written form or produced by a machine, including typewriters, computers, or copiers. Characteristics of paper and ink may also be included in this process.

» Trace evidence analysis is done using a number of different modalities. It may include the use of a scanning electron microscope or gas chromatograph. The types of trace evidence that may be analyzed are enumerable and may include paint, soil, glass, minerals, fiber, hairs, and plant material.

» Controlled substances/toxicology analysis identifies drugs of abuse and chemicals that may be used in drug-facilitated sexual assaults. Alcohol or drug levels in urine, blood, or other body fluids are also analyzed in toxicology sections.

» Forensic photography utilizes specialized techniques to document and enhance information from crime scenes. Photographic documentation of a note from a crime scene is shown in **Figure 14-7.**

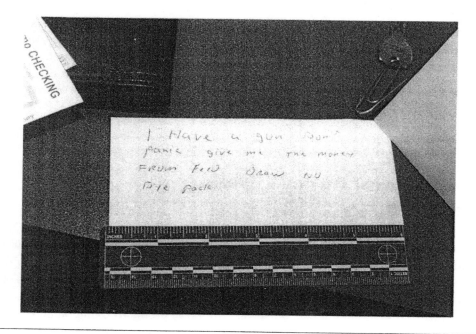

Figure 14-7   A handwritten note that was left at the scene of a bank robbery. As shown in this photograph, evidence should be documented in place prior to collection.

CASE 14-2

The Importance of the Chain of Custody

In 1973, a young woman parked her vehicle on the upper level of a public parking garage. As she exited her vehicle, she was attacked, chased by her attacker, and stabbed as she entered the descending stairwell. The woman was fatally stabbed through the chest by an unknown assailant. The attacker returned to the victim's vehicle and drove it to a lower level of the garage. While in the victim's vehicle, he noticed that his hand was bleeding and reached into the back seat of the vehicle for a box of tissues. In doing so, he left a bloody fingerprint on the box. The assailant then exited the victim's car, proceeded to his own vehicle, and drove his vehicle out of the garage. He handed his parking stub to a ticket taker and paid for parking. The ticket taker recalled having to wipe the blood from the ticket in order to read the time stamped on it. He watched as the assailant quickly drove away.

A short time later, the victim's body was discovered in the stairwell. Investigators responded to the scene and documented their findings. Items of evidence that included the victim's dress, samples from a bloody trail within the garage, blood from the vehicle, and the tissue box with the bloody fingerprint were seized.

For nearly 3 decades this case remained unsolved, until one day, when a diligent fingerprint expert entered this bloody fingerprint into the automated fingerprint identification system. The automated system identified a matching print on file, which was confirmed by the examiner. The suspect identified by the fingerprint match still lived in the area of the crime.

Evidence gathered at the scene had been tested by various laboratories over a period of several years. The defense challenged the admissibility of the evidence because of the many years and multiple handling of the evidence. However, the chain of custody had been maintained by extensive photographs of the evidence and documentation in the written records. In addition, the evidence remained securely stored at the police department and laboratory. Evidence preservation, integrity, and documentation by the investigative agency led to successful prosecution of this case that resulted in a 30-year sentence for the perpetrator.

Documentation of Physical Evidence

Written Records

Nurses who document reports of the treatment of a forensic patient and the collection of physical evidence must adhere to quality charting standards that are typically required for all medical records. Documentation standards are set by licensing statutes, nurse practice acts, the American Nurses Association, and the Joint Commission (Austin et.al., 2004). Errors made by healthcare personnel in the medicolegal documentation of a case could lead to disastrous outcomes in the courtroom. Common problems found in medical charts include the use of sloppy jargon, confusing abbreviations and statements, vague descriptions, and lack of clarity. Failure to report information as stated by the patient, omissions of interventions provided, and late entries in the record could raise legal concerns about the nurse's actions.

Nurses need to communicate the information effectively into the written record by being accurate, comprehensive, and legible. It is important to document the facts as discovered and to avoid personal opinions about the patient or the case.

When charting in the forensic patient's record, the nurse should address the patient's response to treatments given and also describe the recommended plans for follow-up care. Referrals made to protective agencies such as battered women's shelters, sexual assault counseling services, or victims' advocacy groups should be noted.

Other Documentation Methods

In addition to a written description of a patient's injuries, it is often helpful to use drawings and diagrams, sometimes referred to as body charts. For example, if a person sustained multiple stab wounds or bruises, a sketch of the injuries could better depict the location of the injuries than a written description. Rather than describing the injury as being in the upper left chest or the lower portion of the arm, a body chart better clarifies the location, size, or shape of the injury in question.

The use of photography is an excellent way to document findings of forensic evidence while either at the crime scene or treating a clinical patient who has sustained an injury. In clinical environments, it is important to have policies in place regarding use of photography to document injuries relating to trauma as well as domestic violence, sexual assault, or any means of abuse. The authors' recommended guidelines when implementing clinical photo documentation policies are outlined in **Table 14-1.** Detailed guidelines for forensic photography can be found in Appendix 2.

Case 14-3 illustrates the importance of evidence collection, documentation, and the integrity of the chain of custody. The hospitals in this case were a short distance away from each other. Hospital A did not have a forensic nurse on duty. Hospital B personnel had some training in evidence collection.

TABLE 14-1 Considerations for Clinical Photography

- Who will take the photographs? What kind of training does the photographer have?
- What kind of camera will be used? What type of film/equipment will be used?
- What will be photographed?
- Is there a written consent from the patient to be photographed? Or is the consent to photograph included in the all-inclusive consent to treat the patient?
- Who will develop/process the film and maintain the chain of custody for the film so it does not end up in the hands of a third party?
- Where do the developed photographs end up? They belong with the medical record, but is there a place to securely store them?
- If using digital photography, where are the disks that contain the medicolegal documentation stored?
- Consider confidentiality and privacy regulations. What steps are taken to ensure that HIPAA standards are maintained? If the photos are subjected to court subpoena, what is the procedure for duplication of the negatives?
- Who pays for the taking of photos and the processing of the film?

CASE 14-3

The Importance of Proper Evidence Collection and Documentation

Hospital A

A 25-year-old female who was 7 months pregnant was having a domestic dispute with her boyfriend. The boyfriend, in a fit of rage, stabbed the woman repeatedly with a knife. Neighbors heard her cries for help as she exited the apartment and ran to the parking lot. Police arrived shortly thereafter and ordered the man to drop the knife. The man refused to comply and was shot dead. The female victim was transported to a hospital with wounds to her chest and neck. She was rushed to the operating room where her baby was delivered via cesarean section. When investigators arrived at the hospital to retrieve the victim's clothing for evidence, the clothing could not be located. Neither the emergency department nor the operating room personnel knew what had happened to the clothing. After several inquiries, it was discovered that the blood-saturated clothing was put into a plastic bag and tossed into the laundry chute. There it became lodged between floors within the hospital. Comingled with hospital linens, this evidence was eventually recovered, but it was cross-contaminated by multiple sources. How would the presence of a forensic nurse on staff have affected the proper collection and preservation of this evidence?

Hospital B

The subject, an intoxicated, adult male, threatened to kill his parents with a knife. The subject's mother ran from the house and called 911. Screaming for help, she told the dispatcher that her son was going to kill her husband. When the first responding officer arrived, he ordered the man, several times, to put down the knife. The man shouted back at the officer and lunged toward him. The officer shot the man in the chest. The wounded man was transported to the local hospital and was rushed to the operating room where he died a short time later. The forensic nurse in this case preserved the clothing and potential trace evidence for police investigators, although the subject's brother was demanding to see the deceased. Detectives photographed the subject's injuries, collected gunshot residue samples, and fingerprinted the subject for the purposes of identification. Once the evidence was collected and documented, hospital staff members addressed the needs of the family. **Figure 14-8** shows the decedent's clothing as it was documented before packaging. Quick documentation with a scale in the ER assisted the investigation at a later time.

This case, as police-involved shootings often are, was scrutinized by the general public. Questions frequently arise pertaining to the justification of the shooting. Some of these questions are: Was there reasonable use of deadly force? Was the officer in fear for his life? What was the direction of the shots fired (e.g., front to back vs. back to front)? How close was the officer to the subject? Examination of physical evidence can sometimes answer questions that even eyewitnesses may have difficulty in recollecting or answering.

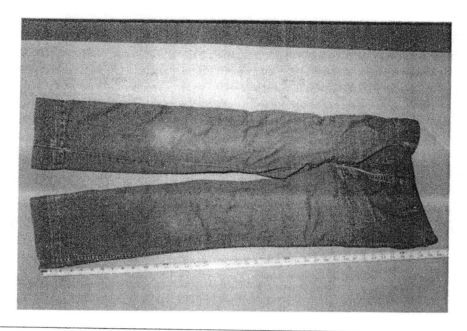

Figure 14-8   An overall view of the clothing removed from the decedent in a police-involved shooting case.

Collection of Evidence from the Deceased Patient

Identity of the Deceased

At the scene of a homicide or at a death that was not witnessed, investigators will search for evidence to attempt to obtain the identity of the deceased. This could include an attempt to locate the next of kin or a picture ID card, such as a driver's license with the name and date of birth of the victim. Investigators at the scene may check through the victim's clothing and inventory the victim's wallet, the contents of pockets in clothing, and any jewelry that the victim may be wearing. Electronic pagers and cellular telephones, frequently found on or within clothing, are also noted and secured by investigators. In some cases, none of the aforementioned items is present. In those instances, identification is made through fingerprint or dental record comparisons or through DNA sampling if known materials are available for comparison purposes.

Trace Evidence from the Decedent

If the victim appears to have been in a struggle or was shot at close range, investigators will secure paper bags over the hands of the deceased to preserve trace evidence that could potentially be destroyed or lost during transport of the body to the morgue. The body is then wrapped in a clean sheet before being placed into a body bag. Again, this is done to preserve trace evidence.

Prior to autopsy, the victim is photographed and trace evidence is collected from the body by the forensic pathologist. Once this is done, the victim can be fingerprinted.

If the victim is transported to a hospital in a resuscitative effort, preservation of trace evidence becomes very difficult. When the victim is pronounced dead, the past practice of the nurse was to provide postmortem care by cleaning up the body so that the next of kin could make identification. Forensic nurses now know that the practice of washing away trace evidence is detrimental to an investigation.

The forensic nurse can take some helpful steps that may aid investigators in the preservation of physical evidence. Important points for consideration in preserving physical evidence on the deceased follow. Once these steps are taken, the nurse may either assist family members of the decedent to make identification at the hospital or direct family to the medical examiner's office and to the investigative authorities.

1. If clothing was removed from the body, preserve, document, and package as described in this chapter.
2. Do not wash or attempt to improve the appearance of the deceased until a death investigator or forensic nurse has had an opportunity to photograph the victim and remove trace materials.
3. Bag hands to prevent loss of evidence. Gunshot residue samples or other trace samples may need to be collected as soon as possible.
4. Fingerprints may need to be obtained by investigators.
5. Keep dressings, bandages, catheters, and endotracheal tubes intact with the patient.
6. Other items of evidentiary value (weapons, drugs, documents) may need to be turned over to police or death investigators.

Evidence from Poisoning or Overdose

Sample Documentation

In cases of suspected poisoning or drug overdose, it is important for the forensic nurse investigator not only to obtain a social and medical history of the deceased, but also to record an inventory of prescription medications found at the scene. Information in a medications inventory should include:

» The name of the patient
» The name of the medication
» The dosage
» Date filled
» Number dispensed
» Number of tablets remaining in the vial
» The physician's name
» The pharmacy that dispensed the order

This information is not only helpful for determining an antidote for a surviving patient, but also assists the forensic pathologist or death investigator in the course of the autopsy and investigative inquiry should the cause of death be an issue. Medications at the scene should be documented in place prior to complete inventory of the materials, as shown in **Figure 14-9.** It is also important to note the quantity of medication remaining in the containers upon collection.

Poisons can be introduced into the body by ingestion, injection, or inhalation. The elements that may affect the body are many. The forensic nurse must maintain an

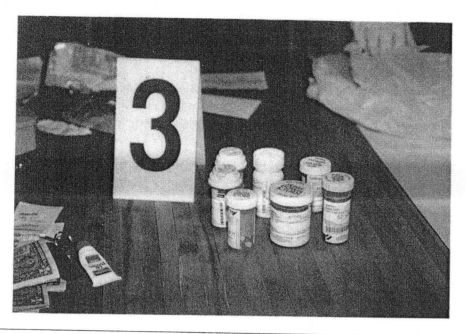

Figure 14-9   Prescription medications located at the scene of a questioned death.

objective mind-set and use critical thinking in analyzing the possibility of poisoning, whether intentional or unintentional.

Sample Collection and Analysis

Determining the element of a poisoning may be done by analyzing any or all of the following:

1. Body fluids, which include blood, gastric contents, urine, breast milk, or fluid in the eye
2. Hair, particularly head hair
3. Tissue, which includes sampling of muscle, brain, and liver

All these tissues may be tested for the identification and quantitation of chemical poison levels. If tissue is collected for testing, the sample must be handled to prevent cross-contamination with other specimens such as blood. Samples should be kept in separate containers for submission to the laboratory (Lee & Harris, 2000).

If administration of poison is intentional and results in a death, the manner of death may be ruled either a suicide or a homicide. If administration of poison is unintentional and results in a death, the manner of death would be accidental. Many deaths of accidental nature are caused by mixed drug intoxication. This means that the individual, though not intending to cause her own death, has taken a mixture of agents such as heroin, alcohol, and painkillers.

Death or injury from poisons may be exacerbated if there are underlying medical conditions such as heart disease or diabetes. Also, a person may be taking prescribed medications that may interact negatively with recreational drugs. Thus, a medical history is important in ascertaining the potential interactions of materials. In addition, when assessing a patient who may have been poisoned, the forensic nurse should understand what types of analyses may be done to detect the possible poisons.

If blood is to be analyzed, the first blood drawn should be saved prior to any other medication being administered in the effort to resuscitate the patient. The type of analysis to be done will dictate what type of tube to collect the sample in and how that tube should be treated (e.g., refrigerated or not). If the forensic nurse is unsure of the analytical process that will be required, she should consult the toxicology laboratory for detailed instructions.

Legal Considerations
Collection by Warrant, Court Order, and Consent

During the course of a criminal investigation, known biological samples, including hairs, blood, or buccal swabs, may be requested from the victim or a perpetrator by law enforcement. This collection can be accomplished legally by either written consent or applying to a judge for a search warrant or court order to obtain samples. The results of these tests are to be provided to the law enforcement agency that obtained consent with the authorization of the aforementioned documents. An overview of the legal requirements to collect evidentiary samples from suspects and victims can be found in Appendix 1.

HIPAA

There has been much confusion in the interpretation of patient confidentiality as outlined by the Health Insurance Portability and Accountability Act (HIPAA) (HIPAA, 2002). Law enforcement officers may have difficulty in obtaining information because healthcare workers do not understand what HIPAA is and what it is not. The following information should help to clarify the impact of HIPAA on the forensic nurse.

All subsets of forensic nursing practice are subject to the standards set forth by HIPAA. **HIPAA regulations** are categorized into three areas:

1. *Administrative simplification*: Regulations were implemented to create uniform standards and requirements for any health information that is transmitted electronically. This includes health information that may be faxed or e-mailed to another facility. This transfer of information impacts not only the healthcare providers who have physical control over the health information of individuals, but also any person or entity who has received this information for purposes other than providing treatment to an individual. This could include attorneys, courts, police departments, and insurance companies.
2. *Security:* Regulations are outlined for maintaining the security and integrity of medical/health information. Documentation that contains any health information and specific individualizing information must be kept safe and secure while in the possession of the receiving party. This includes protecting information from being viewed by unauthorized individuals, keeping that health information in a secure location, and preventing any possibility of unauthorized duplication.
3. *Privacy:* Regulations exist regarding how that health information may be used, as set forth by the individual whose health information is at issue.

Questions have arisen as to who would fall under the category of healthcare provider. If information is obtained for a purpose other than providing care, does that entity remain under the guidelines as set forth by the HIPAA regulation? It is the authors' opinion that any person or institution that has physical control of health information must follow the HIPAA guidelines as they pertain to privacy and security.

Nurses have always been acutely aware of the fact that confidentiality is of utmost importance when dealing with health information of the patient for whom they are caring. However, HIPAA promises more extensive monitoring of confidentiality requirements and stiffer penalties for violators than at any previous time.

Generally, the job of the forensic nurse would be easier if standard forms were utilized for the release of medical information, but HIPAA only sets guidelines. It is each entity's responsibility to follow those standards. The individual or healthcare facility must determine how to apply those standards. One hospital may accept a standard release form, while another hospital may require its own form to be signed before information can be released. These individual differences can cause the requestor some confusion and delay in obtaining important information. However, time will likely ease the difficulties encountered when preserving the confidentiality, privacy, and security of the information.

According to the Department of Health and Human Services, the implementation of the HIPAA privacy rule:

1. gives patients more control over their own health information.
2. sets boundaries on how the health information is to be released and how it is to be used.
3. establishes safeguards so that those in control of the health information are better able to provide protection of the privacy of the patient and of the patient's health information.
4. holds violators of this privacy mandate accountable with resulting civil and criminal penalties.
5. provides a balance when disclosure of health information is needed in order to protect public health.
6. allows patients the ability to make informed decisions as to the care they receive and reimbursement for the care based on how the health information is utilized.
7. advises patients how the health information is to be used and what information is released.
8. possibly limits the information that will be released to the minimum needed for disclosure yet ensure quality of care based upon that information.
9. gives the patient the right to examine the records to be released and enables him or her to get a copy of his or her own health records.
10. allows the patient to request corrections to the medical records should discrepancies be found that are inconsistent with the actual facts.
11. enables the patient to control the use and disclosure of his or her own health information (USDHHS, 2003).

HIPAA and Evidence Documentation

The use of photographs, videotapes, and digital images has become an important aspect of the forensic nursing practice. These and other methods are used frequently in the documentation process. Caution must be exercised to protect the privacy and confidentiality of the client while ensuring thorough documentation of important materials and patterns. Policies and procedures regarding security of photos, video, and digital images should be in place in any facility that intends to use them as part of their documentation protocol.

The liability issues related to photographs or videotapes of patients are of utmost importance. HIPAA Section 160.103, which relates to the issue of photo documentation, states:

> Health information means any information whether oral, recorded in any form or medium that 1. Is created or received by a health care provider, health plan, public health authority, employer, life insurer, school or university, or health care clearing house; and 2. Relates to the past, present or future, physical or mental health or condition of an individual; the provision of health care to an individual; or the past, present or future payment for the provision of health care to the individual. (HIPAA, 2002)

Thus, the federal regulations regarding other forms of evidence documentation should be followed to ensure privacy, just as one would follow the handling of other health information. The authorization form for the release of this information must contain specific information. The following information must be provided on an authorization for release of information:

» A description of the information to be disclosed or used. This includes any specific request for the release of X-rays, laboratory findings, history and physical, discharge summary, or office notes.
» The identification of the persons or class of persons authorized to make use of the information to be disclosed. The name and address of the physician from whom information is requested. The entity's address should be included in this request.
» The identification of the person or persons making the request. This includes an attorney who represents a client for whom the medical records are requested for the purpose of litigation.
» A description of the reason why the health information is requested. An example of this would be, "for the purpose of litigation."
» An expiration date must be provided on the authorization form. If health information is requested, an end date or time is required for this request. This time could be "the conclusion of the case" or may be a specific date.
» The signature of the individual whose health information is being requested and a date must be provided on the authorization form.
» If the form is signed by an individual other than the person named on the form, such as a personal representative or guardian of the person, the authority of the signer must be documented and must accompany the authorization form. For example, if the person requesting the information represents the estate of a deceased individual, then the letter of administration must accompany the request. If the individual is the guardian, then the court documents showing appointment of the guardian must accompany the request.

Other Regulations and Guidelines

In addition to the HIPAA regulations that mandate privacy issues of health information, other regulations impact both the forensic nurse and the forensic patient. For those facilities that are accredited by the Joint Commission, that organization, formerly known as the Joint Commission on the Accreditation of Healthcare Organizations (JCAHO), also provided guidelines to the forensic population (JCAHO, 2003). Specifically, JCAHO stated that the goal of the patient assessment function is to determine what kind of care is required to meet the patient's initial needs and his or her needs as they change in response to care. Further, JCAHO pointed out that it is important to provide a patient with appropriate care at the time the patient is in need of that care, and that care must be provided by a qualified individual (JCAHO, 2003). Appropriate care implies that a forensic patient must be provided care by a person who is trained to recognize and evaluate the forensic patient's needs. The process of developing and implementing a plan of care in forensic situations clearly includes the recognition and collection of evidence. Thus, only when the caregiver is trained to recognize the needs of the forensic population and act accordingly will the mandate of the Joint Commission be met.

The American Nurses Association takes this requirement a step further by describing the qualified provider. The *Scope and Standards of Forensic Nursing Practice* deals specifically with the education of the forensic nurse: "The forensic nurse acquires and maintains current knowledge in forensic nursing practice" (McHugh, Leake, IAFN, & ANA 1997, Standard III). Continuing education in the field of forensic science/forensic nursing is required to meet the changing needs of the forensic patient and to keep pace with the advances made in the field of forensic science. Forensic nurses must not only keep their knowledge current, but also integrate that knowledge in their everyday practice.

Summary

The role of the forensic nurse has evolved as the needs of the populations served have significantly changed. Caring for victims and perpetrators of interpersonal violence has led the field of forensic nursing to meet the challenges of the forensic patient by developing the ability to recognize, document, collect, and preserve evidence. Forensic nurses also must understand the importance of what may seem like insignificant minutiae to an outsider. Whether collecting bite mark evidence in a case of abuse or gathering paint and glass fragments from a victim of a motor vehicle crash, it is the forensic nurse who makes a difference in the collection and documentation of physical evidence. By providing true, holistic care to the forensic patient, Florence Nightingale's legacy—treating the whole patient and not just the injury or symptom—is being carried out within the forensic setting.

Although nurses have protected the privacy of patients as this role has evolved, the forensic nurse is a mandated reporter who frequently interfaces with members of the criminal justice system. It is the responsibility of the forensic nurse to keep abreast of the advances made in the field of forensic science and to stay informed of legal implications pertinent to forensic nursing practice and evidence collection.

    QUESTIONS FOR DISCUSSION

1. What types of evidence collection materials would be useful to store in hospital emergency departments and trauma centers?
2. Give examples of how cross-contamination of articles could occur if clinical staff is not aware of proper evidence collection procedures. How could cross-contamination of evidence be detrimental to an investigation?
3. How has HIPAA impacted the forensic nurse's role pertaining to evidence collection and documentation?
4. The newly hired nurse manager of the emergency department asks the forensic nurse specialist on staff to write an evidence collection and documentation policy for the emergency department. What agencies should the forensic nurse

consult with prior to writing the policy? What HIPAA regulations must be included? What patient consent issues should be addressed?

5. A 25-year-old male is admitted to the emergency department with a superficial gunshot wound to the leg following a gang-related altercation. It is discovered upon physical assessment that the patient is armed with a semiautomatic handgun. The police are en route to interview the patient. As the forensic nurse on duty, what steps would you take to ensure safety, document and collect evidence, and initiate the chain of custody?

REFERENCES

Austin, S., Brooke, P., Glenn, L., Guido, G., Keepnews, D., Michael, J., ... Wright, L. (2004). *Nurse's legal handbook* (5th ed.). Philadelphia, PA: Lippincott, Williams, & Wilkins.

Health Insurance Portability and Accountability Act of 1996, Public Law 104191. (Revised 2002). 45 CFR Part 160 and Subparts A and E of Part 164. Retrieved from http://www.hhs.gov/ocr/privacy/hipaa/administrative/statute/index.html

Inman, K., & Rudin, N. (2001). *Principles and practice of criminalistics.* New York, NY: CRC Press.

Joint Commission for Accreditation of Healthcare Organizations. (2003). *Hospital accreditation standards.* Oakbrook Terrace, IL: Joint Commission Resources.

Lee, H. C., & Harris, H. (2000). *Physical evidence in forensic science.* Tucson, AZ: Lawyers & Judges Publishing.

McHugh, J., Leake, D., International Association of Forensic Nurses, & American Nurses Association. (1997). *Scope and standards of forensic nursing practice.* Washington, DC: American Nurses Publishing.

U.S. Department of Health & Human Services, Office for Civil Rights. (2003). *Summary of the HIPAA privacy rule.* (OCR privacy brief). Washington, DC: Author. Retrieved from http://www.hhs.gov/ocr/hipaa

SUGGESTED FURTHER READING

DiMaio, D., & DiMaio, J. (1993). *Forensic pathology.* Boca Raton, FL: CRC Press.

Dutelle, A. (2011). *An introduction to crime scene investigation.* Sudbury, MA: Jones & Bartlett Learning.

Gaensslen, R., Harris, H., & Lee, H. (2008). *Introduction to criminalistics and forensic science.* Boston, MA: McGraw-Hill.

Nightingale, F. (1992). *Notes on nursing: What it is, and what it's not.* Philadelphia, PA: Lippincott.

Reik, T. (1945). *The unknown murderer.* New York, NY: Prentice Hall.

Saferstein, R. (2010). *Criminalistics. An introduction to forensic science* (10th ed.). Upper Saddle River, NJ: Prentice Hall.

U.S. Department of Justice. (1999). *Death investigation: A guide for the scene investigator.* Washington, DC: Author. Available at www.usdoj.gov

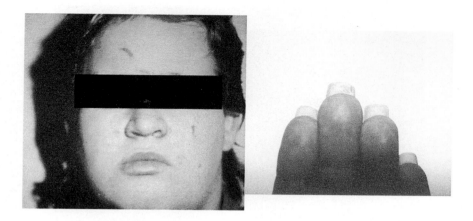

CP-1 Left: A suspect in a sexual assault homicide with scratches on his face. Right: Tissue fragments under the fingernail of the victim.

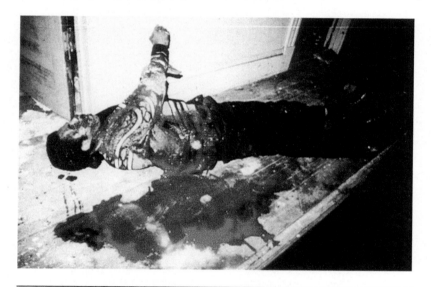

CP-2 Inappropriate rigor mortis (rigidity) for a supine position.

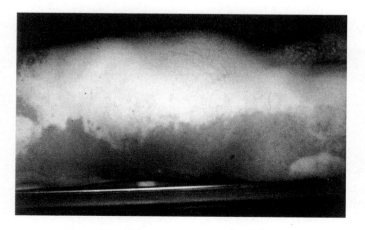

CP-3 Livor mortis evidenced by posterior pooling of blood.

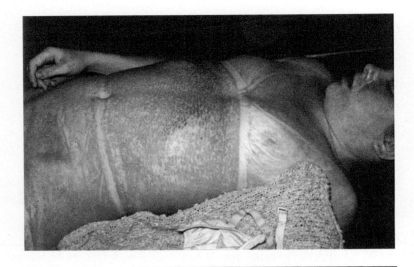

CP-4 Livor mortis showing blanching from undergarments.

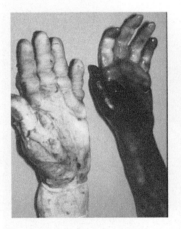 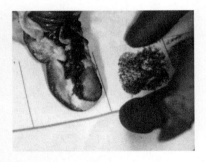

CP-5 Autolyzed glove placed on technicians hand to effectively roll fingerprints.

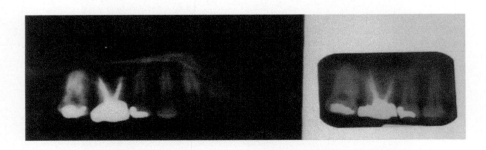

CP-6 Post- and premortem dental x-rays for comparison.

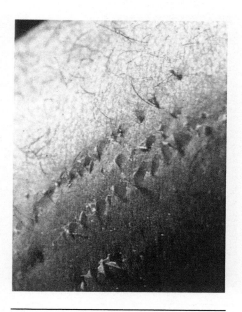

CP-7 Scrape-type abrasion with force directed top right to bottom left.

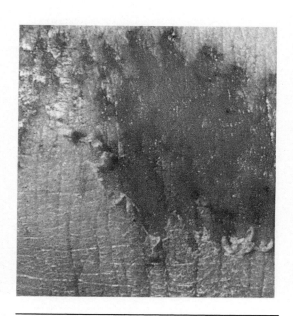

CP-8 Abrasion with piled epithelium indicating downward directionality of injury.

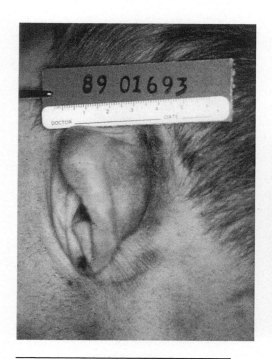

CP-9 Battles sign (blood accumulating behind the ears following a skull fracture).

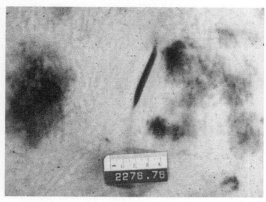

CP-10 Bruises in varying stages of resolution.

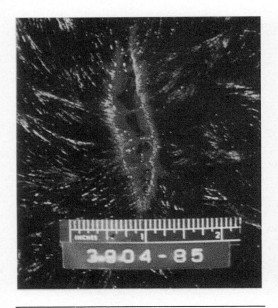

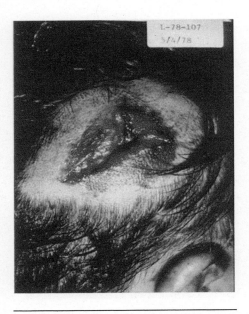

CP-11 Laceration with marginal abrasion and tissue bridging.

CP-12 Laceration with wide marginal abrasion.

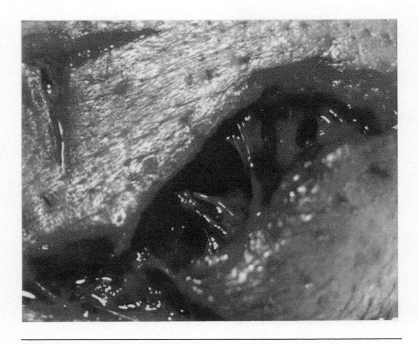

CP-13 Laceration with evidence of structures transversing the wound (tissue bridging).

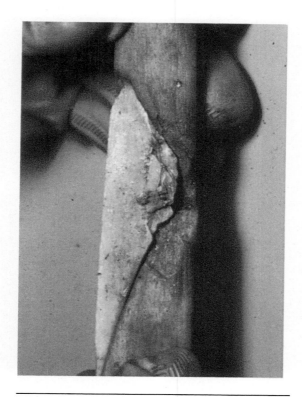

CP-14 Triangular fracture showing left to right force.

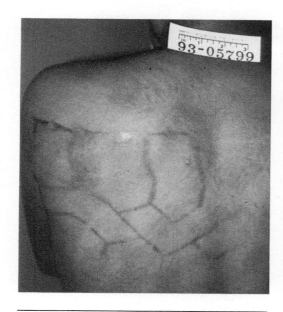

CP-15 Pattern of contusions resulting from tire treads.

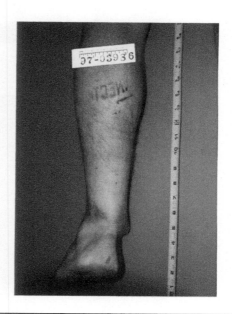

CP-16 Compression abrasion resulting from license plate imprint.

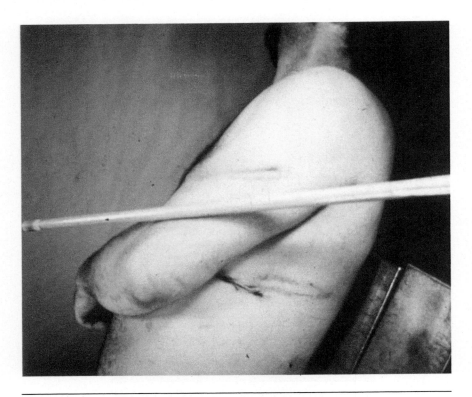

CP-17 Pool cue pattern (linear contusions with sparing at center).

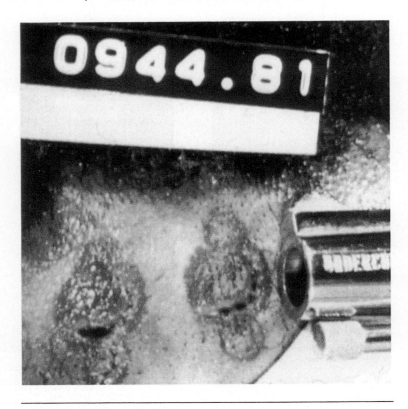

CP-18 Gun muzzle pattern.

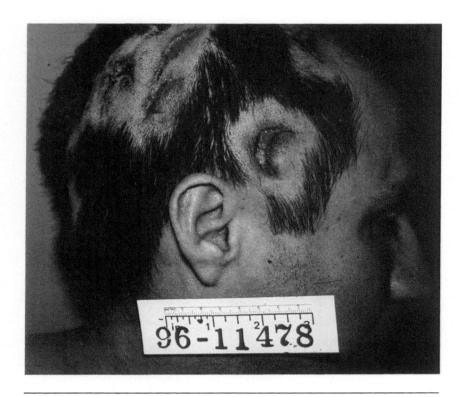

CP-19 Crescent-shaped lacerations consistent with the head of a hammer, as the head is angulated relative to the skin.

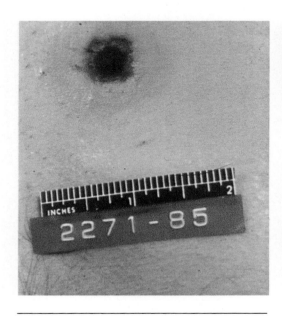

CP-20 Entry wound demonstrating marginal abrasion around the central defect.

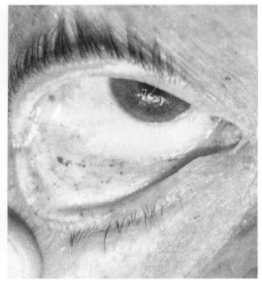

CP-21 Petechial hemorrhages resulting from interference with venous blood flow in asphyxia.

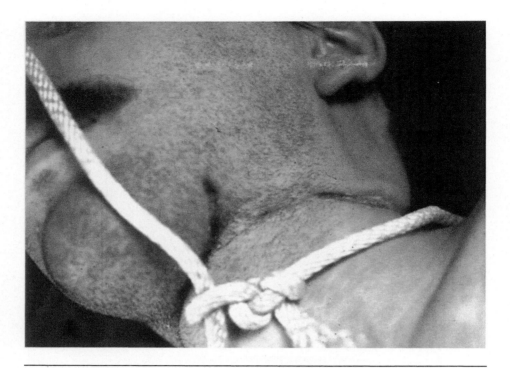

CP-22 lResults of hanging: furrow on neck resulting from suspension point in ligature.

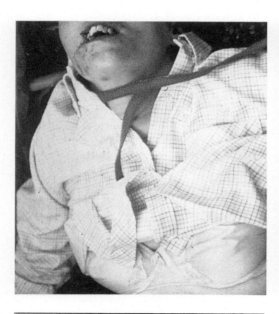

CP-23 Garroting (ligature around neck).

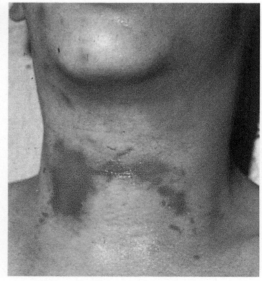

CP-24 Contusions and abrasions on neck resulting from strangulation.

CHAPTER 15

The Use of Biological Evidence and DNA Data Banks to Aid Criminal Investigations

Carll Ladd and Henry C. Lee

The development of DNA analytical methods and their application to forensic analysis have changed the face of forensic science. DNA technology has revolutionized areas such as genetic counseling, paternity testing, and criminal investigations. One of the most significant advances in criminalistics is the creation of statewide and national DNA databases that contain DNA profiles of convicted offenders. When DNA is obtained from evidence in no suspect cases, the resulting profiles can be compared to the data on file in the offender database. Thousands of cases that would have previously remained unsolved have been adjudicated due to the implementation of the DNA data banks.

CHAPTER FOCUS

» Sources of Biological Evidence
» Modes of Evidence Transfer
» Collection and Preservation of Biological Evidence
» History of Biological Evidence Examination

» Individualization of Biological Evidence by DNA Analysis
» Offender DNA Data Banks
» Challenges to DNA Admissibility

KEY TERMS

» allele
» base
» Combined DNA Index System (CODIS)
» deoxyribonucleic acid (DNA)
» DNA data bank

» frequency
» mitochondrial DNA (mtDNA)
» nucleotide
» polymerase chain reaction (PCR)
» profile

Introduction

Beginning in the 1960s, crime rates in the United States rose dramatically. As a result, the public grew increasingly concerned about the impact of crime on our society. Even before the attacks of September 11, 2001, Americans routinely identified improving public safety as a key national priority (Lee & Ladd, 1997). Crime rates, though decreasing significantly since 2001, remain unacceptably high, especially in the area of interpersonal violence. The amount of violent crime is staggering. Nationwide, almost

1 million aggravated assaults and sexual assaults are reported to the police each year. U.S. Department of Justice victimization surveys put the number even higher (U.S. Department of Justice, 2010).

During this period of heightened concern about public safety, physical evidence has become increasingly important in criminal investigations. Courts often view eyewitness accounts as unreliable or biased. Numerous studies have shown this distrust is well founded. Physical evidence, however, such as deoxyribonucleic acid (DNA) may independently and objectively link a suspect or victim to a crime or develop important investigative leads. Physical evidence may also prove invaluable for exonerating the innocent.

The natural consequence of the greater emphasis on physical evidence is increased legal scrutiny. Evidence integrity begins with the first investigator at the crime scene or with the collection of physical evidence in the emergency room. High-profile cases such as the Nicole Brown Simpson and JonBenet Ramsey homicides highlight standard challenges to the use of physical evidence in criminal investigations and suggest that scrutiny of evidence collection, preservation, and handling will continue unabated. An entire case may be jeopardized if evidence is mishandled during the initial stages of the investigation. Indeed, evidence that is not properly recognized, documented, collected, and preserved may ultimately be of no probative value. This chapter reviews the use of biological evidence, including the recognition, collection, preservation, identification, and individualization of that evidence in criminal investigations. This chapter will also examine some of the legal challenges to the collection and use of DNA evidence.

Sources of Biological Evidence

Biological evidence has been associated with numerous crimes, but is typically seen with violent crimes such as homicide, assault, sexual assault, child abuse, and hit and run accidents. Although any substance of biological origin may be useful for analysis, common sources of biological evidence submitted to forensic laboratories include:

- » Blood and bloodstains
- » Body fluid stains
- » Tissues and organs
- » Objects contacted by persons
- » Nonhuman sources

Table 15-1 lists various sources of biological evidence that are used in forensic investigations. The identification of the type or source of biological material may be as significant as any subsequent testing for genetic markers. The sources of biological evidence listed can be used to link one individual to another, to a piece of physical evidence, or to a crime scene. In addition, the evidence may substantiate or disprove an alibi or assist with crime scene reconstruction.

Biological Evidence Transfer

Although the identification of the type of evidence is the first vital step in analysis of biological samples, the method of deposit of that sample may be of equal or even greater importance in case analysis and interpretation. In general, biological evidence can be transferred by direct deposit or by secondary transfer.

TABLE 15-1   Sources of Biological Evidence

Source	Types of Materials
Body fluids	Blood, semen, saliva, urine, tears, bile, perspiration, vaginal fluid
Soft tissue	Skin, organs, hairs, fingernails
Structural tissue	Teeth, bones
Other human sources	Fecal matter, vomit
Objects contacted by persons	Lipstick, toothbrush, hairbrush, razor, cigarette butts, drinking glasses/bottles, articles of clothing
Nonhuman sources	Animal, vegetative, microbial

Blood, semen, body tissue, bone, hair, urine, saliva, and other body fluids can be transferred to an individual's body or clothing, to an object, or to a crime scene by direct deposit from the source of that sample. Once liquid biological materials are deposited, they adhere to the material on that surface, the substratum. Those deposits become stains. The exact characteristics of those stains depend on the nature of the substratum, movement before the liquid dries, and other factors. Space does not allow for an extensive discussion of the factors that will affect the general appearance of a body fluid stain. However, the forensic nurse must be aware of those characteristics of stain patterns that may be important for future analysis and should consider those characteristics when collecting and preserving biological materials.

Non-fluid evidence, such as tissue, bone, or hair, can also be transferred by direct contact with the primary source of that biological material. Because these types of biological materials often sit on top of the target surface, subsequent actions may dislodge nonliquid samples. Liquid biological material may also be associated with these nonliquid samples, such as blood on tissue or bone, resulting in a deposit with characteristics of both types of materials.

Blood, semen, tissue, hair, saliva, or urine may also be transferred to a victim, suspect, witness, object, or location through an intermediary. This process is referred to as *secondary transfer.* With secondary transfer, there is no direct contact between the original source (the donor of the biological evidence) and the final target surface. Rather, some type of contact between the first stained substratum or individual and another surface or person results in a second transfer of the biological sample. For example, seminal fluid on a rape victim's clothing may rub against a car seat, leaving some semen in the vehicle. If a second individual sits in the same location, an additional transfer of the semen may occur. Another example of secondary transfer is when a person picks up a victim's hair from the suspect's vehicle onto his jacket. The hair has now been transferred from the victim to the car and then from the car to a piece of clothing. The transfer intermediary can be a person, an object, or a scene. The secondary transfer of physical evidence may, but does not necessarily, establish a link between an individual and a specific crime.

It should be noted that the stain or pattern of deposit that results from evidence transfer may be as important as or more important than the individualization of the material itself. For example, whether semen found on a carpet is an ejaculated direct deposit or a smear-type transfer may be important in supporting the victim's description of a sexual assault.

Collection and Preservation of Biological Evidence

The ability to successfully analyze biological evidence recovered from a crime scene, person, or object depends greatly on the types of specimens collected and how they are preserved. Thus, the technique used to collect and document such evidence, the quantity and type of evidence that should be collected, the way the evidence should be handled and packaged, and how the evidence should be preserved are some of the critical issues in an investigation. Unless the evidence is properly recognized, documented, collected, packaged, and preserved, it will not meet the legal or scientific requirements for admissibility into a court of law. If the evidence is not properly documented prior to collection, its origin can be questioned. If it is improperly collected or packaged, cross-contamination may occur. Finally, if the evidence is not properly preserved, sample degradation may result. Therefore, it is extremely important to follow established procedures and use standardized techniques to collect and preserve biological evidence. An overview of sample documentation, collection, and packaging procedures for the forensic nurse may be found in Chapter 14 of this book. Many other publications discuss the collection and analysis of biological evidence in detail (Lee, Ladd, Scherczinger, & Bourke, 1998; Lee, Pagliaro, Zercie, & Maxwell, 1995).

Collection of Sexual Assault Evidence

The collection of evidence using a sexual assault kit warrants special consideration. Unlike most other crimes where typically the police collect the evidence, victims of sexual assault, domestic violence, and child abuse are examined by medical professionals in hospitals, clinics, or other centers. If no sexual assault nurse examiner/sexual assault forensic examiner program exists at the facility, critical biological evidence may be collected by medical personnel who historically have been less familiar with the forensic and legal issues pertaining to chain of custody and evidence collection. This may become an issue during DNA analysis or interpretation of DNA **profiles** obtained from the biological evidence. Most jurisdictions have developed standardized sexual assault evidence collection kits and procedures. For the successful resolution of any criminal investigation, it is essential that all medical personnel attending victims or suspects have the requisite knowledge and experience to recognize, collect, and preserve potential evidence for forensic analysis. In addition, communication and cooperation among hospital staff, police, and the forensic laboratory is extremely important.

When following standardized procedures, care must be taken to avoid collection techniques that may raise subsequent analytical issues. For example, it is useful to place the swabs in a specially designed cardboard swab collection box to ensure complete drying and minimize contamination. To minimize the recovery of skin cells from the body, collect any blood/body fluid stains as gently as possible. This can be accomplished by *lightly* swabbing the stained area. If fingernail scrapings or clippings are collected, it is important to avoid applying excessive force in this process; doing so will minimize the chance of collecting the victim's blood or skin.

After the evidence is collected, a cool, dry environment is optimal for preserving biological samples for DNA analysis. Moisture and heat can promote bacterial growth, which may seriously degrade DNA in the sample.

Statutory sexual assaults, which have been vigorously prosecuted in recent years, may also involve evidence collection by the forensic nurse. Sexual assault kits are not routinely collected in statutory or juvenile sexual assault cases because those assaults may not be reported until weeks or months after the incident. Because consent cannot be a defense in the statutory sexual assault case, if a pregnancy has occurred as a result of the rape, the product of conception is itself proof of the crime. In such cases, the samples collected are typically blood from the suspect, from the mother, and from the child or the abortus. In the event of an abortion, tissue samples should be placed in a specimen jar and submitted for forensic testing as soon as possible. It is vital that the specimen *not* be put in any preservative, such as formalin, which will seriously degrade DNA. If the pregnancy is terminated early in the first trimester, it may be necessary for a medical examiner or other trained professional to examine the sample to isolate tissue of fetal origin before collection or testing.

History of Biological Evidence Examination

Serological Testing

The identification of an individual by analyzing his or her biological material, such as blood, semen, hair, and bone, has been reported in forensic science literature since 1904 (Lee, 1982). Over the years, numerous red blood cell antigen systems, isoenzyme markers, red cell protein variants, serum protein markers (Gaensslen, 1983; Gaensslen & Lee, 1984), and human leukocyte antigens have been characterized and applied to forensic work (Lee, Gaensslen, Pagliaro, Mills, & Zercie, 1991). Historically, variation was detected by either immunological reactions, such as with the ABO blood group system and secretor status; Rh typing; human leukocyte antigen histocompatibility antigens; or the electrophoretic separation of isoenzymes and serum proteins such as phosphoglucomutase, adenosine deaminase, or group-specific component variants (Gaensslen, Desio, & Lee, 1986). Some of these, such as typing stains for ABO group antigens, were very useful methods with old samples; other markers were temperature and time sensitive and of limited forensic use. For decades, these tests were the standard techniques applied to biological samples. **Figure 15-1** is an overview of methods utilized in forensic biology for the identification and individualization of biological evidence.

DNA Testing

DNA typing procedures have become increasingly important in the fields of forensic science and forensic medicine (Lee, 1994; Lee, Ladd, Bourke, Pagliaro, & Tirnady, 1994). Several DNA typing methods have been widely implemented for forensic use. If the examiner adheres to applicable national guidelines and standards (DNA Advisory Board, 1998), DNA analysis is generally considered reliable. At this time, DNA evidence and testimony are accepted in all courts. DNA testing may assist greatly in the resolution of criminal and civil investigations.

Genetic variation can be detected by many DNA-typing techniques, including restriction fragment length polymorphism (RFLP) analysis, polymerase chain reaction (PCR), and DNA sequencing. Developments from 2001 to 2011, such as more sensitive and discriminating PCR typing methods, the felon DNA data bank, and increased federal and state funding, have greatly enhanced DNA typing in forensic casework.

The first widely publicized forensic use of DNA technology was in 1985 in the United Kingdom. Dr. Alec Jeffreys of the University of Leicester applied his newly developed

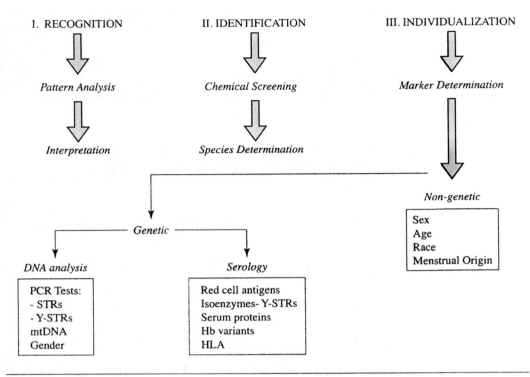

Figure 15-1 Methods used to analyze biological evidence.

DNA "fingerprinting" procedures during the investigation of a double rape-homicide case in England. DNA was first applied to casework in the United States in late 1986 in the case *Pennsylvania v. Pestinikas*. In that case, DNA was used to determine if internal organs were switched by a funeral director in an effort to confuse the issue of the cause of the victim's death. The FBI began accepting DNA cases in 1989, and widespread use of DNA testing occurred in the 1990s. Today more than 130 laboratories in the United States, both public and private, perform forensic DNA analysis. Each year, more than 40,000 DNA cases are processed by these facilities (Federal Bureau of Investigation, 2010).

The two major applications of DNA typing in forensic science are paternity testing and criminal investigation. The former application, because it deals with fresh blood samples, is relatively straightforward. However, the quality of DNA samples from criminal cases is generally unpredictable, so the latter application has been challenged more vigorously during trials and hearings (U.S. Congress, Office of Technology Assessment, 1990). Several national and international committees have been formed to address the use of DNA in criminal cases, and extensive studies have been conducted in this area (Committee on DNA Technology in Forensic Science, 1992, 1996).

Laboratory Analysis of Biological Evidence

Prior to the widespread use of DNA testing in crime laboratories, forensic serology and immunology were employed to identify the source of the biological evidence, to determine if the sample was of human origin, and then to include (or exclude) an individual as a potential source of that sample. As more forensic laboratories developed DNA capabilities over the past decade, serological methods (especially ABO blood grouping and isoenzyme typing) have been significantly scaled back or eliminated. Today, serological analysis is generally limited to identifying the type of biological evidence collected. Nevertheless, sample identification is key in supporting the elements of crimes such as sexual assault and in interpreting the results obtained from subsequent testing. After the type of biological material is identified, the evidence is individualized; that is, linked to (or excluded from) a particular person by DNA typing.

Serological Methods for Identifying Body Fluids

The process of examining items for the presence of biological evidence begins with recognizing and identifying likely materials for further testing. Various screening tests that determine if a stain could be blood, saliva, semen, and so on exist. Evidence screening saves considerable time and money by eliminating those stains that are not consistent with the body fluid of interest. The acid phosphatase test, for example, is a well-known screening test for seminal fluid. Confirmatory tests conclusively demonstrate the presence of a particular body fluid. Lastly, the body fluid is individualized by DNA.

Reddish-brown stains that may be blood are also screened prior to DNA typing. Screening tests for blood are based on the reaction of the heme component of hemoglobin with chemicals such as o-tolidine, phenolphthalein (Kastle-Mayer reagent), luminol, and tetramethylbenzidine. These tests are extremely sensitive; however, reactions with enzymes or oxidizers may result in false positives. Thus, a positive reaction with any of these reagents indicates that the sample *could* be blood. The presence of *human* blood can be determined using any immunological method that tests for human hemoglobin.

This one-step procedure is the preferred method in forensic laboratories today, because it consumes a smaller amount of sample and is extremely sensitive.

The most commonly analyzed body fluid in criminal cases is semen. As stated earlier, the common screening method for semen is the acid phosphatase test. Acid phosphatase is usually present in high levels in semen, but it can also be found in other substances such as plant matter. In addition, usually lower levels of acid phosphatase can be found in other biological samples (e.g., vaginal fluid, saliva, and fecal matter). Some forensic nurse examiners have suggested the use of acid phosphatase as a screening tool during the hospital examination. Because no confirmation of semen is possible by this test and many factors can affect the results, such analyses are best suited for laboratory testing. The presence of semen must be confirmed by identifying spermatozoa microscopically or by detecting the human seminal protein p30, also called prostate specific antigen, PSA. Recent developments in forensic science have greatly increased the sensitivity of some of these confirmatory tests.

Other enzyme and biochemistry tests may be conducted to identify biological substances such as saliva, urine, gastric fluid, and fecal matter. Microscopic examination may also be used for analysis of biological stains. For example, hairs are examined microscopically and compared to reference samples from the victim and suspect(s) and checked for the presence of hair root material. Microscopical examination of samples is often conducted to identify epithelial cells from swabs; at the present time it is not possible to identify the source of epithelial cells with techniques commonly used in forensic laboratories. Current research includes the use of RNA for the forensic identification of tissue of origin for body fluid stains. These techniques, when perfected for casework, could eliminate many of the questions about the origin of stains and cellular materials.

Individualization of Biological Evidence by DNA Analysis

The forensic application of DNA typing methods constitutes a major advancement in the examination of biological evidence and the successful investigation of many crimes. DNA is important because it is remarkably sensitive, tremendously discriminating, and stable. DNA has become a key focus in the fields of forensic science, forensic medicine, anthropology, and paternity testing. Most forensic cases involve matching the DNA profile from evidence with a sample of DNA from a known source, usually a suspect, victim or an associated sample. As seen with the identification of Osama bin Laden in May 2011, DNA analysis can confirm identity with 99.9 % accuracy, even when the DNA profile is compared to results obtained from close relatives. (McNeil & Belluck, 2011) **Figure 15-2** shows an overview of the DNA analysis of a biological sample.

The Genetics of DNA

Deoxyribonucleic acid (DNA) is the genetic or hereditary material in living cells. DNA is a polymer with individual building blocks called **nucleotides**. Each nucleotide consists of a sugar (deoxyribose), a phosphate group, and a nitrogenous base. The four different nucleotides found in DNA are classified by the corresponding **base** in the structure—adenine, guanine, cytosine, and thymine. The functional DNA molecule contains two strands of DNA bound together by complementary base pairing (hydrogen bonding) to form a double helix. Adenine always pairs with thymine, and cytosine always pairs with guanine. DNA is primarily located in the nucleus of the cells, arranged into long threadlike structures called chromosomes. Humans have 23 pairs of chromosomes. One set is inherited maternally; the other is derived paternally. The estimated 3–4 billion base pairs of DNA in the human genome encode approximately 30,000 genes on those chromosomes.

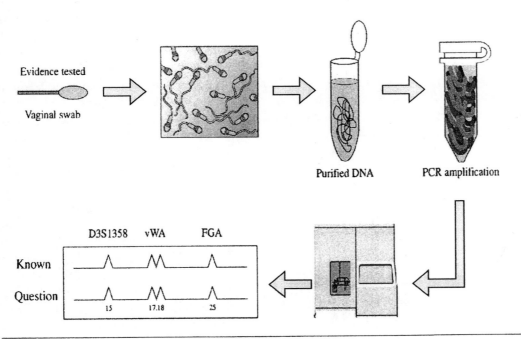

Figure 15-2 Overview of STR typing procedure.

Scientists have estimated that more than 98% of the human genome is the same or very similar in most individuals (Lander, Linton, & Birren, 2001). However, considerable genetic variation exists in the DNA of noncoding regions (which are not genes); these areas are exploited by forensic DNA typing systems.

Sources of DNA

Evidence that is suitable for DNA typing, with the exception of mitochondrial DNA (mtDNA), is limited to biological samples containing nucleated cells. Table 15-1 earlier in the chapter lists sources of those biological samples suitable for conventional DNA analysis. Note that conventional DNA typing is possible only on hairs with roots. The hair shaft does not contain nuclei and can be typed only by mtDNA analysis methods. Other types of biological evidence, such as tears, perspiration, serum, and other body fluids without cells, are not amenable to standard DNA analysis. DNA has been isolated from materials such as gastric fluids and fecal stains; however, it is difficult to obtain sufficient DNA from these sources in case samples. It should also be noted that although DNA can often be recovered from the specimens mentioned in Table 15-1, in many cases the quality and/or quantity of the sample proves inadequate for standard DNA analysis.

Four factors affect the ability to obtain DNA typing results. The first issue is sample quantity. PCR-based DNA typing methods are very sensitive, but not infinitely so. The second factor is sample degradation. For example, prolonged exposure of even a large bloodstain to the environment or to bacterial contamination can degrade the DNA and render it unsuitable for further analysis. It is important to note, however, that degradation will not change DNA profile A into profile B. The third consideration is sample purity. Although most DNA typing methods are robust, dirt, grease, some dyes in fabrics, and other materials can seriously inhibit the DNA typing process (Lee et al., 1998). The last issue is the ratio of DNA in mixtures of fluids from more than one person. DNA profiles can readily be detected with approximately equal amounts of material (e.g., 1:1 and 3:1 DNA mixtures). However, with mixture ratios such as 25:1 or 50:1, the quantity of the major DNA specimen (larger quantity) prevents the detection of the minor source (smaller quantity of DNA). This situation occurs with some vaginal swab samples where semen is detected. In such cases, the standard DNA tests detect only the victim's DNA.

Genetic Variation and Forensic DNA Typing

Two different classes of genetic variation are exploited by forensic DNA typing methods: sequence variation (single base changes) and length differences produced by variation in the number of tandem repeats. Important features of the two classes of genetic variation are illustrated in **Figure 15-3**.

DNA tests that detect length differences are currently the most common type of variation studied in forensic DNA analysis. Many well-characterized genetic regions (loci) contain sets of nucleotides (core elements) that are tandemly repeated. The number of these repeated units can vary from person to person. Certain base sequences called recognition sites flank these repeats. Specialized enzymes called restriction enzymes cut the DNA at those recognition sites that flank the repeats. This restriction endonuclease digestion results in DNA fragments ranging in size from 500 to 22,000 base pairs long. The resulting fragments are separated by agarose gel electrophoresis. This process is termed restriction fragment length polymorphism (RFLP), and is the oldest DNA typing method

Sequence and Length Variation

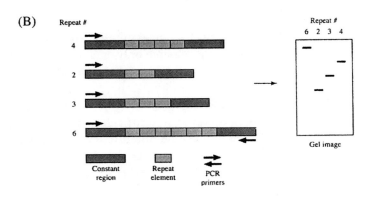

(A)   Type 1 CGATCGGAATGGC
       Type 2 CGATCGGTATGGC
       Type 3 CGATGGGAATGGC

Figure 15-3 Types of genetic variation. (A) Sequence variation. DNA variations are highlighted. Only one strand of the DNA double helix is shown. (B) Length variation. PCR primers bind to the constant regions flanking the repeats.

for both criminal and paternity cases. Conclusive results obtained from RFLP testing are highly individualizing, but the time required to obtain those data often meant that months were required to generate one case report. The most commonly used DNA testing method today (a PCR method termed STRs, discussed in the following section) omits the restriction enzyme step. Instead, small synthetic pieces of DNA, known as primers, target the site of interest and bind to DNA, flanking the repeats (see Figure 15-3B).

Polymerase Chain Reaction

The ability to amplify small segments of DNA by **polymerase chain reaction (PCR)** constitutes one of the more significant developments in molecular biology. PCR has facilitated revolutionary advances in many scientific disciplines and has proven an invaluable tool in biological research as well as in the diagnosis of genetic disorders and infectious diseases.

PCR was invented in 1985 and was subsequently adapted to forensic science. The procedure amplifies (duplicates) small segments of DNA. This process is sometimes called molecular photocopying. At the end of the amplification process, the target DNA molecule has been copied 1–10 million times.

PCR requires only trace quantities of DNA—typically, approximately 1 nanogram (ng) of human DNA is optimal for PCR, compared with 300–500 ng for RFLP typing. One ng is the amount of human DNA that typically can be obtained from a single hair root. Consequently, PCR permits DNA typing of evidence with minute samples, such as a cigarette butt containing epithelial cells. PCR generates a large quantity of product in a very short period of time, and degradation of the DNA sample is less of a concern because it amplifies small segments of DNA. The first PCR tests in widespread forensic use were DQA1, Polymarker, and D1S80. DQA1 and Polymarker **alleles** display sequence variation that was detected by a colorimetric assay. DQA1 and Polymarker DNA profiles are determined by the pattern of blue dots that develop. D1S80 typing, also called amplified fragment length polymorphism analysis, is a PCR-based DNA-typing strategy that detects length variation. D1S80 alleles contain different numbers of repeats similar to RFLP.

These three PCR systems are very sensitive; hence they permit the analysis of minute samples. However, they are much less discriminating than RFLP.

Short Tandem Repeats

The standard DNA typing method employed by the forensic community today involves the analysis of short tandem repeats (STRs). Conceptually, STR analysis can be thought of as a combination of PCR and RFLP. As with RFLP, the different STR types exhibit variation in the number of repeated core elements they contain and have tremendous discriminating power. In addition, like other PCR methods, STR typing is very sensitive. Furthermore, the use of different fluorescent dyes allows the analysis of multiple STRs in a single reaction with the aid of a laser and computer. This saves considerable time and limits sample consumption. For these reasons, STR analysis has replaced the first generation of PCR tests (Holt et al., 2002). **Figure 15-4** shows typical results obtained when multiple loci are detected using a fluorescent dye and a laser detector.

Y-chromosome STR typing constitutes an important forensic method for processing sexual assault samples. For example, sexual assault cases routinely require the testing of intimate samples that are a mixture of male and female body fluids. In some cases, as described previously, only the female profile or a predominantly female profile can be detected using standard STR systems, even when spermatozoa or semen are identified by serological or microscopic methods. This is usually due to the large amount of female cellular material in the sample collected when compared to the number of male epithelial cells or spermatozoa. A Y-chromosome STR system significantly overcomes the problems associated with a large female-to-male DNA ratio that can lead to incomplete or no amplification of the male DNA. This ability to selectively target the male contributor(s) is a substantial tool for the DNA analyst in these cases. Indeed, in sexual assaults where the semen donor is aspermic (e.g., vasectomized males), Y-STR typing may be the best approach for detecting a foreign DNA profile (a profile that does not originate from the victim). In addition, Y-STR typing may assist in evaluating mixtures by providing information regarding the number of male contributors.

Forensic DNA Analysis Case Studies

The value of DNA analysis in forensic casework is well known. The forensic nurse is well aware that a DNA profile generated from physical evidence can be used to identify a perpetrator or to exonerate the innocent. Thus, it is not necessary to discuss extensively the strength of this type of evidence. The two case studies that follow should suffice to demonstrate the impact DNA analysis has had on casework in the 21st century.

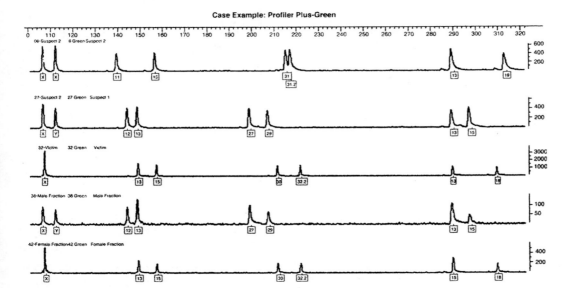

Figure 15-4   DNA typing results by STR analysis. Samples were amplified using the AmpFISTR Profiler Plus kit (Applied Biosystems). The results for the green loci (XY, D8S1178, D21S11, D18S51) are shown for a sexual assault case where a vaginal swab sample was submitted for STR analysis and comparison to known DNA profiles. A differential DNA extraction procedure was performed to separate the male and female DNA from a vaginal swab. Fluorescent DNA profiles were detected using the ABI Prism 377 DNA Sequencer (Applied Biosystems). Open boxes indicate the STR profile for each sample. The results are consistent with suspect 1 being the source of the DNA profile from the male fraction (vaginal swab, sperm DNA profile). The female fraction (vaginal swab, epithelial DNA profile) matches the victim.

CASE 15-1

A Serial Rapist

DNA was the key evidence from a young woman who was sexually assaulted by a male unknown to her. This sexual assault was similar in several elements to two other rapes that had occurred in the neighborhood. The woman was able to give a description of her assailant to law enforcement but could offer few other details about the incident. The police conducted a standard investigation and developed a suspect after consulting a number of their regular informants. The person who was the focus of the police investigation was a homeless male who roughly fit the description provided by the victim. After several hours of interrogation by detectives, the suspect confessed to all of the sexual assaults, although his version of the crime differed in some details from the actual assault. As part of their investigation, the police collected known blood and hair samples from the suspect for comparison to the biological materials in the sex assault evidence kits collected in all three cases. Laboratory scientists conducted DNA testing on vaginal swabs in the three cases. All three sperm-rich samples yielded identical DNA profiles—there was indeed a serial rapist in that city. The evidentiary profiles generated, however, did not match the person who had confessed to the crimes. Initially, detectives were sure that some error was made during the lab analysis because of the confession. The profiles generated in these cases were entered into the local and national DNA offender databases, but no match was found initially. Several months later, a sample collected from a convicted offender matched the profile generated in those three cases. The person identified by his DNA "hit" pleaded guilty to all three crimes. Certainly without DNA analysis, an innocent person who confessed for some reason to crimes he did not commit would have gone to jail for many years. At the same time a dangerous sexual predator would have been released into the community. The **DNA data bank** *provided investigative information that would not have been possible only a few years earlier.*

In another case, the search against the DNA database did not identify a suspect. After a suspect was identified by a fingerprint database search, DNA was used to corroborate the suspect identification. That case involved the investigation of an almost 30-year-old homicide.

CASE 15-2

A Cold Case Analysis

A woman was stabbed to death in a parking garage. Based on the bloodstain patterns and other evidence at the scene it was apparent that the killer had been injured during the incident. When a suspect was finally identified 25 years after the crime through a search of the automated fingerprint identification system database, the prosecutor wanted additional corroboration of this individual as the perpetrator of the murder. A few aged blood samples that had been stored in less than optimal conditions, some of which had been treated with numerous chemical reagents, were available for DNA testing. Although many other stains were originally recovered, years of serological testing reduced the number and size of material available for DNA profiling. However, DNA was extracted from some of the remaining stains and PCR analysis was conducted. STR profiles were generated from many of these samples. Although some of the bloodstains showed the presence of more than one DNA profile, the suspect was included as a possible donor to those stains. Significantly, a 13-locus match to the suspect was obtained from one of the bloodstains on a handkerchief found near the victim. The accused was convicted 29 years after the murder, and these DNA profiles were key evidence presented during the trial.

Low-Copy-Number DNA

The sensitivity of DNA typing techniques has increased significantly since the first PCR cases. Today the ability to detect small amounts of transferred DNA on surfaces and even skin means that the forensic nurse must be particularly careful in collecting and preserving biological evidence (Gill, 2001). Forensic nurses should wear masks to prevent contamination from saliva during conversations; other protective clothing may be advised depending on the setting and type of evidence that is being collected. By using various sets of DNA primers and changing the analytical protocols, profiles can be developed from just a few cells. Opponents of low-copy DNA analysis point out that this test does not identify the last person to handle the evidence, as sometimes alleged by proponents, and the actual material that is the source of the DNA is unknown (Wulff, 2006). Results obtained from low-copy testing can vary, depending on where and how the samples are taken by examiners. While some are skeptical, testimony related to low-copy testing has been allowed.

Mitochondrial DNA Typing

Mitochondrial DNA (mtDNA) typing has also been adapted for forensic purposes. Mitochondria, organelles located in the cytoplasm of the cell, have their own DNA distinct from the DNA in the nucleus. The mitochondrial genome contains 16,569 base pairs of circular DNA. Mitochondrial DNA is present in multiple copies per cell. Because of the large number of mitochondria in a single cell, forensic nurses collecting evidence and personnel conducting analyses must be careful to avoid contamination with even just a few cells. In addition, mtDNA is maternally inherited. Typically, mtDNA typing involves PCR amplification followed by direct sequencing of the DNA. Sequencing involves the determination of the exact sequence of bases composing the amplified portion of the DNA molecule.

Mitochondrial DNA testing is particularly useful with the following three types of biological evidence: old or degraded skeletal remains; human remains from mass disasters; and hair shafts that contain no intact cells and only mtDNA. An additional objective test provided by mtDNA analysis of hairs can be applied to hairs that could previously only be compared microscopically. Given its inheritance, a mtDNA profile can be compared to anyone with the same maternal lineage, which makes this testing useful for human remains analysis and search against a mtDNA database such as the national missing and unidentified persons system, NamUs. This testing, however, is not as discriminating as standard STR analysis. The procedure was first introduced in a U.S. criminal trial in the summer of 1996 (State of Tennessee v. Ware, 1999 WL 233592 [Tenn. Crim. App.]).

Interpretation of DNA Results

The objective of forensic DNA analysis is to compare the evidentiary DNA profiles to the known profiles in a case, such as that of a victim or suspect. Whenever DNA results are generated in a case, one of three basic interpretations can be made:

1. *Inclusion:* DNA markers from known source A are present in the evidentiary or questioned sample. Therefore, person A could be the source of the DNA evidence.
2. *Exclusion:* DNA markers from known source A are not present in the evidentiary or questioned sample. Therefore, person A could not be the source of the DNA evidence.
3. *Inconclusive:* No conclusion can be made as to a possible source of the DNA evidence. Results, if any are obtained, cannot be interpreted.

Using these basic criteria, the DNA analyst can address an important but limited question: Could the individual tested be the source of the biological evidence? The more challenging question of guilt or innocence is the purview of the courts.

In the event of an inclusion or DNA match (interpretation 1), person A is the source of the sample, an identical twin of person A is the source of the sample, or another person who coincidentally has the same profile as person A is the source of the sample. Hence, the analyst must provide the court with a statistical assessment of the significance of the match—how common or rare the evidentiary profile is. This typically involves calculating the random match probability, which can be thought of as the expected **frequency** of individuals in the general population who could be the source of the evidence.

Offender DNA Data Banks

One of the more significant developments in forensic science is the development and growth of offender DNA data banks. Given the high rate of recidivism associated with sexual assault, felon DNA data banks are particularly useful for solving these crimes; they also have been a valuable tool in the investigation of many other violent and property crimes. When the sexual assault victim or police are unable to identify a suspect, these types of sexual assaults are often referred to as no-suspect cases. Prior to establishing offender databases, forensic analysis of biological evidence was of little value because there was no known person other than the victim to compare with the evidence. With the creation of large offender data banks, however, it is possible to process a no-suspect case and compare the DNA profile obtained from a sample of unknown origin to a library of felon/arrestee DNA profiles. To date, data bank technology has generated more than 127,100 cold hits nationwide, leading to numerous convictions (Federal Bureau of Investigation, 2010).

All 50 states have statutes that require biological samples to be taken from convicted felons, and over 4 million felon profiles have been collected. Indeed, a majority of states now collect DNA from all felony convictions, and some even mandate the collection of DNA from all arrestees. Needless to say, this has sparked great debate about the rights of individuals not convicted of crimes, as well as the privacy rights of those whose samples are in the data banks. In 2010, all 50 states were linked to the national DNA data bank system, the **Combined DNA Index System (CODIS)**, which now contains approximately 9 million felon profiles and more than 300,000 forensic unknown profiles. This national CODIS data bank allows states to compare no-suspect profiles that have not matched state or local data banks to the profiles from all 50 states in the national repository. As greater resources are provided for processing no-suspect cases, the number of cold cases solved at both the state and national level will continue to rise.

Emerging DNA Technologies

Recently, ethnic or race-specific DNA markers have been used to provide investigative leads in several cases. By studying a set of DNA single nucleotide polymorphisms, the DNAPrint Genomics Inc. laboratory was able to assess the biogeographical ancestry of a suspect in a 10-year-old sexual assault-murder case. (DNAPrint Genomics, 2003). Since the first widely publicized case of this kind in 2003, there has been much interest in biogeographical DNA testing by citizens and law enforcement alike. (Reuters, 2008). In fact, any individual can contact these companies and have a laboratory provide an ethnic ancestry assessment. The problems associated with eyewitness accounts have been widely reported. The typing of race-specific DNA markers could point investigators in a more objective direction by providing typical, general physical information about the assailant (Wade, 2002). This information could result in considerable savings of time and resources.

This type of application of DNA typing clearly has its detractors among some scientists, privacy advocates, civil libertarians, and other individuals. They argue that there is great potential for abuse of this technology in the form of racial profiling. The interest of investigators and citizens in the origins of a person of interest, however, cannot be denied. Other scientists have been concentrating their efforts on pigmentation and eye color genes as sources for investigative leads, believing that such a focus would provide less divisive and more practical information for investigators.

Nonhuman DNA Analysis

The DNA of dogs and cats has been characterized for breeding purposes and classification. Zoos and animal protection organizations use animal DNA profiling when mating endangered species to limit harmful genes. They also have used DNA typing to determine if animals are new species or are members of a known, existing species. Nonhuman DNA has also played a significant role in several criminal cases. Cases have been reported where DNA profiling of animal hairs were used to link the suspect with the crime. In cases where there are no human hairs, analysis of animal hairs on the victim's clothing may provide significant leads or linkage to the suspect. Plant material profiles have been compared to link a suspect to the location where a body was found. Studies have also been conducted to link large caches of illegal plants, like marijuana, with each other, which can increase the charges against drug dealers. While nonhuman DNA seems to have potential as a tool to provide valuable circumstantial evidence in difficult cases, some courts have rejected the use of this testing during trial because of the lack of appropriate databases or the inability to determine the significance of a match. Even in jurisdictions where animal or plant data are not admitted in court, these nonhuman DNA tests may still provide valuable information to investigators.

Challenges to DNA Admissibility

The forensic use of DNA typing methods has played an important role in the successful resolution of many crimes. DNA is important because of its tremendous discriminating power and its stability. However, this very strength is also a prime reason that DNA tests have been challenged so vigorously in court.

Since their introduction into forensic science, DNA typing methods have been strenuously attacked in numerous protracted court battles. Initially, the general reliability of DNA typing procedures was questioned along with the statistical methods used to calculate DNA profile frequencies. In the last few years, legal challenges regarding the admissibility of DNA have shifted their focus away from the general reliability of the methods. Although most courts accept the basic methodology behind DNA analysis, some defense objections regarding DNA evidence continue to be effective. Indeed, successful challenges to the admissibility of DNA testing in court often attack the initial collection, preservation, and subsequent handling of the biological evidence. Thus, it is important for forensic nurses to be aware of the potential negative effects on DNA admissibility if physical evidence is mishandled or not documented correctly. A second type of challenge concedes that DNA typing methods are reliable *in theory*. In such a case, the defense argues that critical mistakes were made in testing that should invalidate the findings. With this strategy, typically the specific protocols and technical expertise of a particular laboratory or analyst are scrutinized.

With the sensitivity of PCR DNA typing systems, the issue of potential DNA contamination is often raised in court to challenge or minimize the significance of the DNA findings. Although contamination can occur, the greater impact may be on the prosecution. It is important to note that because multilocus DNA profiles are rare, contamination will predominantly lead to a false exclusion or an artificial mixture rather than a false inclusion. Consequently, although contamination could complicate result interpretation, it would typically not include an innocent defendant.

Summary

The importance of biological evidence has grown rapidly since 1991. Eyewitness accounts have often been viewed as unreliable or biased, and the courts have looked for more objective criteria to determine guilt or innocence. DNA analysis may *independently* and *objectively* link a suspect or victim to a scene, or it might link a victim to a scene. DNA's power as an exclusionary tool is equally noteworthy. Postconviction testing has been used to exonerate more than 130 wrongly imprisoned individuals, primarily those who were convicted based on eyewitness accounts and other less discriminating forensic procedures (Conners, Lundgeran, Miller, & McEwan, 1996). The feasibility of postconviction relief has been greatly enhanced by the latest DNA typing methods, especially STR and mtDNA analysis. Those methods are particularly sensitive, and old evidence can now be reexamined. Clearly, DNA analysis has proven an extremely powerful tool for both prosecution and defense, and the technology continues to improve rapidly. Greater use of robotics and the development of plant and animal DNA analytical tools are well under way. The number of STR cases processed each year will continue to grow. In addition, mitochondrial and Y-STR DNA typing will be utilized on a much larger scale.

It is arguable that the biggest problems in forensic DNA analysis, as in forensic science generally, involve issues of judgment, ethics, and attitude, and not inadequate technology or funding. Job performance failures prominently aired in high-profile cases such as those of Nicole Brown Simpson and JonBenet Ramsey, and exposés of laboratory problems that appear periodically in the news may have significantly eroded public confidence (Lee & Ladd, 1997). Forensic nursing is not immune to these problems, as evidenced by appellate court decisions in several states. Further discussion of the problems that may arise when a forensic nurse acts as an expert witness may be found in Chapter 20.

The greater challenge in the forensic community today is in finding ways to maintain independence and impartiality within an *intentionally* adversarial system. Effective solutions may require cultural change (Bromwich, 1997). Forensic practitioners must place greater emphasis on dispassionate and professional testimony. Forensic nurses must avoid the traps of emotion and advocacy. Furthermore, the current system built around the expert witness, discovery, and cross-examination can be very effective and deserves renewed appreciation. The forensic nursing community needs to enhance its standing in the eyes of both the public and the courts if it is to make a greater contribution as an advocate for victims of sexual assault and other personal violence. Integrity and honesty are the cornerstones of public trust. We must submit to the discipline of the results. Avoid anything that could be seen as whitewashing when questions are raised. If science is served, justice will be well served.

QUESTIONS FOR DISCUSSION

1. What steps in forensic analysis are preferred before conducting DNA analysis? How do evidence documentation, collection, and preservation affect the DNA typing process?
2. What is polymerase chain reaction? In what ways did it revolutionize clinical and forensic testing?
3. How has the development of DNA profiling affected the ability to analyze evidence such as vaginal swabs in a sexual assault case?
4. What challenges may be brought against the collection of evidence from convicted felons for inclusion in a DNA database? Explain why some state that the issues change when samples are collected from persons arrested for certain crimes.
5. Data shows that ethnic origin may be indicated from certain DNA testing. Discuss whether you think this information should be developed for investigative purposes and stored in national databases.
6. How do DNA data banks contribute to the successful resolution of many crimes?
7. How can new developments such as Y-STR typing and mtDNA analysis assist in the investigation or prosecution of sexual assault cases?

REFERENCES

Bromwich, M. R. (1997). Justice Department investigation of FBI laboratory: Executive summary, Department of Justice Office of the Inspector General. *The Criminal Law Reporter, 61,* 2017–2039.

Committee on DNA Technology in Forensic Science, National Research Council. (1992). *DNA technology in forensic science.* Washington, DC: National Academy Press.

Committee on DNA Technology in Forensic Science, National Research Council. (1996). *The evaluation of forensic DNA evidence.* Washington, DC: National Academy Press.

Conners, E., Lundgeran, T., Miller, N., & McEwan, T. (1996). *Convicted by juries, exonerated by science: Case studies in the use of DNA evidence to establish innocence after trial.* National Institute of Research Report NCJ 161258. Washington, DC: United States Department of Justice.

DNA Advisory Board. (1998). *Quality assurance standards for DNA testing laboratories.* Washington, DC: U.S. Department of Justice, Federal Bureau of Investigation.

DNAPrint Genomics, Inc. (2003, June 5). Press release.

Federal Bureau of Investigation. (2010). *CODIS-NDIS statistics.* Retrieved from www.fbi.gov/about-us/lab/codis/ndis-statistics

Gaensslen, R. E. (1983). *Sourcebook in forensic serology, immunology and biochemistry.* Washington, DC: U.S. Government Printing Office.

Gaensslen, R. E., Desio, P. J., & Lee, H. C. (1986). Genetic marker systems for the individualization of blood and body fluids in forensic serology. In G. Davies (Ed.), *Forensic science* (pp. 209–240). Washington, DC: American Chemical Society.

Gaensslen, R. E., & Lee, H. C. (1984). *Procedures and evaluation of antisera for the typing of antigens in bloodstains: Blood group antigens ABH, RH, MNSs, Kell, Duffy, Kidd, serum group antigens GmlKm.* Washington, DC: National Institute of Justice, U.S. Government Printing Office.

Gill, P. (2001). Application of low copy number DNA profiling. *Croatian Medical Journal, 42*(3), 229–232.

Holt, C. L., Buoncristiani, M., Wallin, J. M., Nguyen, T., Lazaruk, K. D., & Walsh, P. S. (2002). TWGDAM validation of AmpFlSTR PCR amplification kits for forensic DNA casework. *Journal of Forensic Sciences, 47,* 66–96.

Lander, E., Linton, L. M., & Birren, B. (2001). Initial sequencing and analysis of the human genome. *Nature, 409,* 860–921.

Lee, H. C. (1982). Identification and grouping of bloodstains. In R. Saferstein (Ed.), *Methods in forensic science* (pp. 267–337). Englewood Cliffs, NJ: Prentice Hall.

Lee, H. C. (Ed.). (1994). *Crime scene investigation*. Taoyuan, Taiwan: Central Police University Press.

Lee, H. C., Gaensslen, R. E., Pagliaro, E. M., Mills, R. J., & Zercie, K. B. (1991). *Physical evidence in criminal investigation*. Westbrook, CT: Narcotic Enforcement Officers Association.

Lee, H. C., & Ladd, C. (1997). Criminal justice: An unraveling of trust? *The Public Perspective, 8,* 6–7.

Lee, H. C., Ladd, C., Bourke, M. T., Pagliaro, E. M., & Tirnady, F. (1994). DNA typing in forensic science. *American Journal of Forensic Medicine and Pathology, 15,* 269–282.

Lee, H. C., Ladd, C., Scherczinger, C. A., & Bourke, M. T. (1998). Forensic applications of DNA typing: Collection and preservation of DNA evidence. *American Journal of Forensic Medicine and Pathology, 19,* 10–18.

Lee, H. C., Pagliaro, E. M., Zercie, K. B., & Maxwell, V. (Eds.). (1995). *Physical evidence*. Enfield, CT: Magnani and McCormick.

McNeil, D., & Belluck, P. (2011, May 3) Experts say DNA match is likely a parent or child. *The New York Times*, p. F2.

Pennsylvania v. Pestinikas (1992), 617 A. 2d 1339 (Pa. Super.).

Reuters News Service. (2008). DNAPrint genomics helps Boulder police solve 10-year-old rape/murder case using cutting edge DNA technology. Retrieved from http://www.reuters.com/article/pressRelease/idUS145130+30-Jan-2008+MW20080130

State of Tennessee v. Ware (1999), WL 233592 (Tenn. Crim. App.).

U.S. Congress, Office of Technology Assessment. (1990). *Genetic witness: Forensic uses of DNA tests*. OTA-BA-438. Washington, DC: U.S. Government Printing Office.

U.S. Department of Justice, Federal Bureau of Investigation. (2010). Uniform crime reports. Retrieved from http://www.fbi.gov/about-us/cjis/ucr/crime-in-the-u.s/2010/preliminary-annual-ucr-jan-dec-2010

Wade, N. (2002, October 1). For sale: A DNA test to measure racial mix. *New York Times*, p. 4.

Wulff, P. H. (2006). Low copy number DNA: Reality vs. jury expectations. *Silent Witness Newsletter, 10*(3). Retrieved from http://www.denverda.org/DNA_Documents/LCN%20DNA%20NDAA%20Silent%20Witness%20Article.pdf

SUGGESTED FURTHER READING

Long, H. (2008). DNA profiling: The ability to predict an image from a DNA profile. In H. Coyle (Ed.), *Nonhuman DNA typing: Theory & casework applications* (pp. 185–204). Boca Raton, FL: CRC Press.

Maguire, W., Elway, B., Bowyer, V., Graham, E., & G. Rutty. (2008). Retrieval of DNA from the faces of children 0–5 years: A technical note. *Journal of Forensic Nursing, 4*(1), 40–44.

Mayntz-Press, K., Sims, L., Hall, A., & Ballantyne, J. (2008). Y-STR profiling in extended interval postcoital cervicovaginal samples. *Journal of Forensic Sciences, 53*(2), 342–348.

Rothstein, M., & Talbott, M. (2006). The expanding use of DNA in law enforcement: What role for privacy? *The Journal of Law, Medicine & Ethics, 24*(2), 153–164.

CHAPTER 16

Computer-Assisted and Internet Crime

Monique Mattei Ferraro and Rita M. Hammer

From Facebook to the operating room, computers are ubiquitous. Every aspect of our lives is touched in some way by computers and the networks that facilitate sharing their sometimes life-saving, sometimes life-taking information. While the benefits of computers are obvious, the nefarious uses are less so. Certain populations, especially children and the elderly, are particularly vulnerable to computer-facilitated crimes. Through research, experience and opportunities to interact regularly with these victims, the forensic nurse can help identify victims of computer- and Internet-facilitated crimes and educate at-risk populations.

CHAPTER FOCUS

» Computer-assisted and Internet
  Crime Defined
» How Computers and the Internet are
  Used to Facilitate Crimes

» Focus on Internet Crimes Against Children
» Child Pornography

KEY TERMS

» *actus reus*
» child pornography
» computer
» computer-assisted crime
» denial of service
» identity theft
» Internet

» Internet-faciliated crime
» *mens rea*
» Ponzi scheme
» pyramid scheme
» spam
» unauthorized access

Introduction

There are many ways to define the term **computer**. A computer could be defined as a personal computer; however, most computer crime laws define computer more broadly than that. The definition most often used is a programmable electronic device capable of accepting and processing data. This broader definition encompasses much more than personal computers, including such items as digital cameras, fax machines, mobile telephones, and personal digital assistants. All of those items are electronic devices that accept and process data. Any of those machines may be used to commit, facilitate, or store evidence of a crime. This definition also embraces new technologies as they develop.

The **Internet** is a computer network, an association connecting computers so that they can communicate, share information, and share files. The Internet is an innovation that exposes its users to a wide variety of knowledge and opportunity and also exposes them to the potential of becoming victims of computer-assisted crime. The expertise of the forensic nurse can be utilized in relation to such Internet crimes as healthcare fraud, including illegal prescriptions and solicitation of organs, illegal sexual encounters, and child pornography.

Computer-assisted crime is any crime in which a computer is used to commit the crime or to facilitate the crime. Computer-assisted crime also includes situations where the computer contains evidence of the crime. Similarly, **Internet-facilitated crime** is crime that takes place through the Internet or where computers connected to the Internet contain evidence of the crime. The next section discusses the history of computer-assisted and Internet crimes and provides examples of the types of crimes most frequently committed.

How Offenders Use Computers and the Internet to Facilitate Crimes

Computer-facilitated crimes we see today had their beginnings before the personal computer or the World Wide Web. When computers were first used, they were huge, expensive, and delicate. An interruption of service, misuse of computer systems, or destruction of data could cost staggering amounts of money. It may be hard to imagine, but the computing power that one can store in a space the size of a dime today would take up an entire room and require around-the-clock attention 35 or 40 years ago. Even during that time, computer-associated crimes were being perpetrated.

The principal federal law governing traditional computer crimes can be found at 18 U.S.C. 1030 (2003). The federal law creates a class of protected computers, defined as any computer used by the U.S. government, by a financial institution, or in interstate commerce or communication, such as computers connected to the Internet. Most personal computers are used to access the Internet, so the federal law covers most computers. The federal law protects the computers from unauthorized access, theft, or misuse of information stored by the computer, alteration or destruction of data or equipment, and physical harm or property damage as a consequence of the unauthorized access.

Types of Computer-Assisted Crime

Unauthorized access to a computer system comes in a variety of flavors. Exceeding one's authority to access a computer or a system can be characterized as a "plain vanilla" type of computer crime. It isn't very exciting and it is fairly commonplace. In the world of violent crime, exceeding authority is similar to a crime of violence committed by a relative or friend. The attacker is known and the motivation most often stems from the relationship between the offender and the victim. Examples of exceeding authority include the help desk employee who has access to users' passwords and uses the personnel officer's user identification number and password to access confidential files that include disciplinary histories, performance evaluations, and salary information on coworkers. Another example of exceeding authority would be an individual providing a friend with her Internet access account identification and password for a single use, and that friend using the account to send spam messages advertising pornography sites.

The other type of unauthorized access—a bit more exotic—is an outright intrusion. The intrusion type of unauthorized access is similar to violent crimes committed by strangers. The offender is often unknown to the victim and the motivation is less easily identified. The attack evokes more fear because of the stranger-to-stranger and seemingly unprovoked genesis of the activity. Examples of this type of unauthorized access are also easy to find. An individual sends an e-mail with an attachment that contains a virus. An unknown recipient opens the e-mail and the file attachment that contains the virus, which installs itself on the recipient's hard drive; subsequently, the virus reveals the person's user identification and password to the sender, who then accesses the e-mail recipient's account to send e-mail or to perpetrate identity theft. This type of unauthorized access to a computer system is what many people refer to as hacking or cracking.

Another type of computer crime is a **denial of service**, which can take many different forms. Attacks might affect one system, a network, a particular business, a website, or the entire Internet. Basically, anything that an individual does to interrupt or shut down a computer or network is a denial of service. Denial of service attacks range from the very simple to the extremely complex. A simple denial of service might be that someone accessed another party's Internet account and sent a number of offensive e-mails. In response to the e-mails, several users reported the event to customer service, which shut the account down for violating the terms of service agreement. (Internet service providers usually have a terms of service agreement that forbids obscene or annoying behavior online.) A more sophisticated attack might target the internal network of a major utility, like the phone company or electric company. Hacking into the server and disrupting operations only briefly could affect service provision to all of the utility's users. The consequences of such a disruption or denial of service in the case of a utility can be life threatening. Imagine a hacking incident that causes phone service to be disrupted and at the same time there are users trying to call an ambulance or the fire department to report a fire, or a doctor is cut off while explaining a life-saving procedure to another doctor performing the procedure on the other end of the line.

Yet another vexing type of denial of service is the distributed denial of service attack, in which the attacker first breaks into other computer systems by sending out a virus or by other means. Software is installed on the victim systems. The software is later activated and used to launch the attack—the attacker sends a command to the compromised computers instructing them to begin the attack against a target. The exact method of attack varies, but often the attacker aims to overwhelm a service or website by sending too many messages or requests for it to handle. When a computer receives too many requests or is overloaded, it takes a time out, shutting down when it exceeds its capacity for processing.

Computer-assisted fraud is a primary target of the federal computer crimes law. Since the advent of e-commerce and online auctions, fraud has reached unprecedented levels. During 2002, the Internet Fraud Complaint Center received over 75,000 complaints—a 300% increase over the previous year (Internet Fraud Complaint Center, 2003). Almost half of the complaints related to online auction fraud. Most complainants lost less than $1,000.

Applying the same tactics used for thousands of years to part people from their money, fraudsters use the Internet to access millions of potential victims. The more people a fraud offender can access, the more likely that someone will participate in the scheme. The Internet has been used to further **pyramid schemes, Ponzi schemes,** sale of defective merchandise, and outright larceny. **Box 16-1** outlines the distinction between Ponzi schemes and pyramid schemes often in operation on the Internet.

> ### Box 16-1   *Ponzi schemes versus pyramid schemes.*
>
> *The Ponzi scheme is named after its creator, Charles Ponzi. In the early 1920s Ponzi promised investors that he could provide a 50% return on their money in 45 days. The promise of such a large return brought him over $15 million. He was able to pay out the first investors with money from investors coming into the scheme later. The later investors were encouraged to invest because they saw that investors received the guaranteed return. Eventually, the money ran out and the Ponzi scheme failed. The smart fraudster takes the money and runs before the jig is up.*
>
> *A pyramid scheme relies on contributors to recruit new contributors. Usually, the scheme centers around the sale of merchandise and is referred to as "multilevel marketing." It is called a pyramid scheme because there is someone at the top, then a few people under the top person, then more people under the second level, and so on, resembling a pyramid when sketched out. A new contributor or recruit gives money to the person who recruits them for training or for a "franchise" or membership as an investor. The new recruit makes money by recruiting new contributors or recruits. The people at the top make a proportion of whatever the people below them bring in. When the crop of new recruits runs out, the money stops and the scheme is over.*

It used to be that the most common type of Internet fraud was from online auctions. When online auction fraud began, law enforcement received hundreds of reports a day complaining that the merchandise paid for never came or that it didn't work or that a seller sent merchandise and did not receive payment. Fine tuning of online payment systems, rating of sellers and buyers on the auction sites and educating of the buyers and sellers has vastly reduced the incidence of auction fraud. That, however, has not put the online fraudster out of business. Where one type of fraud is discovered and reduced, another pops up and becomes more prevalent.

A popular scam that is remarkably successful is the so-called Nigerian fraud scheme. There are many different versions of the e-mail, but usually a purported high-ranking official or a doctor or lawyer from an impoverished or war-torn country sends out an appeal for someone to be kind enough to hold onto his or her money for a short period. In return for holding onto the individual's money, she or he will provide a fee—$10,000 or more—just for the seemingly simple act of allowing him or her to park some money in your account for a few days. Many people who receive these e-mails report them to law enforcement. Of course, there isn't much law enforcement can do with only the e-mail. Based on existing statutes, few jurisdictions would consider the e-mail an attempt to defraud. And often the sender of the e-mail is in another country, making it difficult or impossible to fully investigate the event. Of course, such e-mails are easily dealt with by simply pressing the Delete key. Surprisingly, some people do provide their bank account information and end up victims of theft, either directly from the person's bank account or through identity theft, which will be discussed shortly. A description of the Nigerian 4-1-9 scheme as highlighted by investigators is provided in **Figure 16-1**.

Many people approach the Internet with a reduced sense of suspicion. The same people who would never provide a Social Security number to a stranger over the phone enter it freely onto Internet forms. People send postal orders for goods purchased online. Many people send cash overseas freely, along with birthdates, addresses, and phone numbers. These factors are well known to Internet fraudsters who, like all criminals, seek to exploit

Nigerian Advance Fee Fraud "OPERATION 4-1-9"

The perpetrators of Advance Fee Fraud are often very creative and innovative. This fraud is called "4-1-9" fraud after the section of the Nigerian penal code that addresses fraud schemes. Nigerian nationals, purporting to be officials of their government or banking institutions, will fax or mail letters to individuals and businesses in the United States and other countries. The correspondence will inform the recipient that a reputable foreign company or individual is needed for the deposit of an overpayment on a procurement contract. The letter will claim that the Nigerian government overpaid anywhere from $10 to $60 million on these contracts. There is the perception that no one would enter such an obviously suspicious relationship; however, many victims have been enticed into believing they can share in such windfall profits.

Individuals are asked to provide funds to cover various fees and for personal identifiers such as Social Security numbers, bank account numbers, and other similar data. Once this information is received, the victims find that they have lost large sums of money. It is hard to pinpoint how much has been lost in these scams since many victims do not report their losses to authorities due to fear or embarrassment.

In response to this growing epidemic, the U.S. Secret Service established "Operation 4-1-9" to target Nigerian Advance Fee Fraud on an international basis. Indications are that losses attributed to Advance Fee Fraud are in the hundreds of millions of dollars annually.

Agents on temporary assignment to the American Embassy in Lagos, Nigeria, in conjunction with the Regional Security Office, supplied information in the form of investigative leads to the Federal Investigation and Intelligence Bureau (FIIB) of the Nigerian National Police. This project was designed to provide Nigerian law enforcement officials with investigative leads to enable them to enforce their own jurisdictional violations.

On July 2, 1996, officials of the FIIB, accompanied by Secret Service agents in an observer/advisor role, executed search warrants on 16 locations in Lagos that resulted in the arrests of 43 Nigerian nationals. Evidence seized included telephones and facsimile machines, government and Central Bank of Nigeria letterheads, international business directories, scam letters, and addressed envelopes and files containing correspondence from victims throughout the world.

Source: United States Secret Service (n.d.).

Figure 16-1 Nigerian advance fee fraud scheme

the weakness in their justice system to conduct their illegal transactions with virtual impunity.

Identity theft is frequently perpetrated either entirely online or is greatly facilitated by the Internet. Identity theft occurs when an individual poses as another person in order to gain goods, services, or some other benefit. Without question, identity theft has quickly become the bane of our 21st-century existence. The victim of identity theft may suffer the consequences of the crime for many years, requiring constant vigilance to correct credit and criminal history information. Many victims do not learn they have been a victim of identity theft until most of the damage has occurred—when they apply for a loan or a credit card only to learn that dozens of accounts falsely taken in their name by the offender have been maxed out. By that time, the offender is often long gone and has assumed another person's identity. A series of recent commercials have done much to provide a comical warning to the public of the serious effects of identity theft.

Identity information is everywhere for thieves to plunder. Some thieves harvest identity information through their workplace. Anyone with access to credit card information can compile it and use it to co-opt the true owner's identity. For instance, retail cashiers and wait staff deal directly with credit card information. Also, people who have access to their employer's database of customer information can harvest potential victims. Think about where your personal identifying information is stored. Usually information is in an insurance company database, your employer's human resources database, everywhere you shop, and each place you have a credit account. Personal identifying information can also be obtained by dumpster diving. Yes, people really do go through other people's garbage in search of personal identifying information. Discarded mail, such as preapproved credit card applications, bank statements, and credit card receipts, are rich sources of data that an identity thief can use to establish himself as the true owner.

Armed with another person's personal information, an identity thief can go online and pose as the victim. The Internet greatly facilitates identity theft through the anonymous nature of electronic commerce. Before e-commerce, most transactions were face-to-face. If a white, 21-year-old male presented a cashier with a platinum credit card bearing the name of a female, the cashier would likely have checked to make sure the card was not missing or stolen. Another e-commerce development is that one need not possess an actual credit card. Simply providing identifying numbers, like a Social Security number rather than a Social Security card or a credit card number rather than the actual card, is the rule rather than the exception online. When transactions are face-to-face, the card is usually required.

While shopping on the Internet, the identity thief can make a high number of purchases in amounts too little to merit immediate attention either by the vendor or the credit card company. Purchasing a little bit at one website and a little at another website, the identity thief hovers under the radar. By the time either the credit card company or the true identity owner detects the theft, the identity thief has moved on. Sometimes, identity thieves are discovered before the goods are delivered and a controlled delivery of the goods is arranged. Often, though, victims and law enforcement remain frustrated.

In addition to fraud, a host of other crimes can be facilitated by the Internet. The Internet provides greater access to victims and a resultant higher volume of completed crimes. Just as fraud schemes have enjoyed great success on the Internet, so has trafficking in narcotics. It does not require much searching to discover that one can obtain prescription drugs without the required prescription, as well as illicit narcotics, through the Internet. Using a credit card, check routing number, or cash, one may purchase any sort of drug. **Spam** (unsolicited commercial e-mail) fills Internet users' mailboxes advertising sildenafil (Viagra), diazepam (Valium), and all sorts of prescription drugs. Some vendors offer an online service through which a doctor writes a prescription, but many others simply provide the drugs upon request and payment. Narcotics also can be obtained online. Through local chat rooms, newsgroups, and e-mail, buyers order what they want, and the transaction is completed either in person or by mail. Although there are legitimate vendors, clients need to be under the care of a professional for treating a medical condition, especially if they have self-diagnosed. Evaluation relative to the ordering of a medication to treat a specific illness requires a thorough medical history, a physical examination, instructions as to adverse effects, and provision for follow-up of the condition and the response to therapy. Obtaining medication is only a part of effective management of a condition. An individual can request the name of the prescribing physician and then check on his or her credentials through the state licensing board. The same can be done for the pharmacist involved. Any difficulty encountered in this process should send up red flags for the consumer.

The Internet is also used to facilitate prostitution. Hookers have flocked to the Internet with websites and webcams that provide live sex acts. Internet users can log onto a website and, for a fee, dictate the sex action. Individuals may also arrange to use the services of the hooker. Often, a sex transaction is something that takes place after a series of e-mails or online chat to ensure that the client is not a law enforcement officer or dangerous.

Gambling is another popular criminal activity facilitated by the Internet. Although laws against gambling may have lost their influence in the wake of legalized gambling in certain cities and states, many jurisdictions prohibit gambling. Although federal law prohibits online gambling, many websites located overseas make huge sums from online gambling. Even though it is illegal, there is no evidence that the law dissuades either the providers of gambling sites or online gamblers.

Computers and Crimes Against Persons

So far, the discussion has been concentrated on traditional nonviolent computer crimes. However, the Internet also facilitates the crimes of murder, rape, robbery, assault, and child pornography. The remainder of this chapter discusses these crimes against persons in detail.

There are myriad ways to meet people on the Internet. There are dating services of all types. Some are specific to heterosexuals, others specialize in homosexual couplings, and others connect people with peculiar interests or fetishes. There are also countless chat rooms catering to every interest under the sun. Conversation in chat rooms often revolves around romance and sex. Online profiles—data entered by the Internet subscriber about him- or herself—can be accessed to find out about the people in the chat room. If a particular chat participant or profile sparks interest, individuals often instant message each other requesting further information.

People often meet people from the online world in the real world. Because of the anonymous nature of the Internet, it is impossible to guarantee that when one meets another in the real world that either person will be who he or she claims to be. Therefore, Web surfers should use a variety of methods to attempt to ensure their safety by confirming the identity of the person they intend to meet. They might request a picture, meet in a public place, talk on the phone first, and conduct a reverse directory check to confirm that the subscriber to the phone number is the same as the name the person provides. They might check the sex offender registry. All of these things can help to make a meeting with a stranger from the Internet safer; however, it is important for Web surfers to be aware that none of these measures, alone or in combination, can guarantee that the meeting or potential ensuing relationship will be safe.

Illegal Sexual Encounters and the Internet

While children continue to be the victims of unwanted sexual advances online, that number appears to be declining over time. While in 2001, Finkelhor, Mitchell, and Wolak reported that 1 in 5 study subjects under the age of 17 had been solicited on the Internet during the past year, in a replication of the study in 2006, the researchers reported that a smaller proportion of minors were solicited online and a smaller proportion were talking to strangers.

Compare Wolak, Mitchell, and Finkelhor, 2006 to Finkelhor, Mitchell, and Wolak, 2001. Whereas chatrooms were once the most common hangouts for minors using the Internet, researchers report a decline in chatroom use and an uptick in the use of social networking sites (SNS), where the nature of online victimization has changed somewhat. According to research conducted by the Crimes Against Children Research Center at the University of New Hampshire, "In fact, sex crimes with juvenile victims have declined substantially since the mid-1990s, and the proportion of such crimes committed by offenders who use the Internet to meet victims is quite small in comparison to sex crimes against children overall. Indeed, in 2006, there were an estimated 615 arrests for sex crimes involving online meetings between offenders and teenage victims, compared to 28,226 arrests for all sex crimes against teen victims in the same time frame" (Mitchell, Finkelhor, Jones, & Wolnak, 2010).

It is important to note that while law enforcement and the media often portray the relationships between child victims and online offenders as prey-predator, the actual relationships bear a more realistic resemblance to classic statutory rape scenarios (Wolak, Finkelhor, Mitchell, & Ybarra, 2008). While forming close relationships is typical adolescent behavior, the experience of forming these relationships online is a recent and potentially dangerous practice. The normal attraction of adolescents to risk taking combined with technologic proficiency in computers act in concert to create a very vulnerable population. All adolescents are at risk for involvement in this Internet activity, but some may be more inclined to carry on a virtual relationship to an actual one, occasionally with tragic consequences. Studies have shown that some adolescents are more at risk than others. Adolescents who are experiencing difficult relationships with their parents, those who have experienced prior victimization or depression, or are troubled in one way or another may be more vulnerable to online exploitation (Wolak, Mitchell, & Finkelhor, 2003). **Table 16-1** provides some additional statistics related to sexual solicitation of minors on the Internet.

Recent studies have demonstrated that overall the majority of teenaged activities involving online social networking are safer (Anderson-Butcher et al., 2010). Relatively few teens engage in inappropriate behaviors that could lead to dangerous or even tragic outcomes. While the case of Christina Long (see **Case Study 16-1**) is frightening to parents of young children and teenagers, it is not commonplace. What the millions of technologically savvy teens are doing is exactly what teens have always done except in a different venue. They discuss their day, exchange information, gossip a bit, express emotions (anger, depression, jealousy, disappointment, joy) and generally communicate with their peers much as teenagers used to do face to face after school or later at home on the telephone. However, there are occasions when these same teenagers may not use good judgment and share things in a public format that should not be shared. These things include inappropriate photographs and suggestive sexual discussions (sexting) or simply too much personal information about themselves that a stranger should not have. Sexting has become a growing problem with approximately one quarter of all teenagers having engaged in it in one form or another (FBI, 2010). A major concern is that these same teenagers see nothing wrong with it, and indeed a fair majority readily admit to sharing the sexually oriented materials with others via the Internet. Since sexting can be considered pornography under federal law, these teens could face criminal charges. Some teenagers have engaged in an activity termed *sextortion,* in which teenagers who have exposed themselves on the

TABLE 16-1   Statistics Related to Unsolicited Exposure of Youth to Sexual Images on the Internet

Based on interviews with a nationally representative sample of 1,501 youth ages 10 to 17 who use the Internet regularly

- Approximately one in five received a sexual solicitation or approach over the Internet in the last year.
- One in 33 received an aggressive sexual solicitation—a solicitor who asked to meet them somewhere; called them on the telephone; or sent them regular mail, money, or gifts.
- One in four had an unwanted exposure to pictures of naked people or people having sex in the last year.
- One in 17 was threatened or harassed.
- Approximately one-quarter of young people who reported these incidents were distressed by them.

Source: Finkelhor et al, 2000.

Internet become victims of exploitation or extortion. The photos, which are impossible to remove from the Internet, are used by others, including pornographers who threaten to expose them to family and friends unless they agree to provide or pose for more explicit pictures (Baker, 2010). Many states have passed statutes that limit the charges against teens who engage in sexting to misdemeanor charges if they have only distributed the pornographic images among other teens.

CASE STUDY 16-1

Christina Long

In 2002, a 13-year-old girl, Christina Long, from Danbury, Connecticut, became the first confirmed death in the United States at the hands of an Internet predator. There have been many since then. By all accounts, Christina was a good student, a cheerleader, and seemingly socially well adjusted despite being a child of divorced parents who was sent to live with an aunt. Unbeknownst to her aunt, Christina had a history of meeting up with individuals whom she met on the Internet. As with most teenagers, Christina's ability to navigate around various social venues online was more sophisticated than her judgment regarding safe behavior with her newfound friends. On the night of her death, Christina chatted with Saul Dos Rios, age 25, an undocumented immigrant from Brazil, and agreed to meet him at the Danbury Mall. There in his car in the parking garage, the two engaged in what was described as rough sex that culminated in the strangulation death of Christina. Her body was later found in a ravine in Greenwich, Connecticut. Dos Rios was convicted of first-degree manslaughter and second-degree sexual assault. He was sentenced to 30 years in prison all the while maintaining that the death was accidental.

Source: http://www.cbsnews.com/stories/2003/05/07/earlyshow/living/parenting/main552841.shtml

An analysis of law enforcement records from various agencies throughout the United States reveals that it is important to consider all of the sites that teenagers access, in addition to the most popular social networking sites such as Facebook, MySpace, YouTube, Xanga, Foursquare, Places, etc. It turns out that while one third of all arrests for Internet-related sex crimes against minors involved SNSs, most of the offenders began their relationships with the victims at other websites, most frequently chat rooms but also through blogs and instant messaging, although these formats lately are diminishing in popularity (Mitchell et al., 2010).

It is difficult for educators, health professionals, and parents to employ strategies aimed at keeping minors safe while not impinging upon their need for privacy and age-appropriate autonomy in their lives. While some strategies may appear appropriate and rational to parents, they may have the effect of backfiring and creating a situation of resistance or outright rebellion if perceived as intrusive by a teenager. This can lead to efforts by the teen to conceal his/her activities from the rest of the family even though the activities may actually be safe and not placing the teen in harm's way. There can be a fine line between monitoring a teen's activity and invading his/her privacy. The Children's Online Privacy Protection Act of 1998 requires that if a child is under 14 years of age, a website must have a parent's permission to collect personal information. Experts suggest one strategy that advises parents to become directly involved in the setting up of the SNEs that the minor wishes to access, allowing for transparency of the social networking activities (Silverman, 2010). This has the additional benefit of familiarizing the parents with the various aspects of the site as well as becoming an observer of the minor's postings and those of the friends on the site. Many parents are not knowledgeable about these sites and they are most certainly less knowledgeable than their child so that direct involvement with setting up the site, establishing passwords, designing the website, and the profile of the participant can be controlled and modified where indicated. Parents need to be informed as to the nature of each site, what privacy safeguards are in place, and how the teen might be able to stray from the site and invite potential danger. The parent might agree not to post anything on the site but just to be kept in the loop as to what is actually transpiring between the teen and his/her friends. Trying to relate the teenager's online behavior to real-life behavior is another strategy suggested by Silverman to help to facilitate the teen's appreciation of the potential hazards. For example, a parent could describe the similarities between a real person who might follow or stalk her and a real person who might be following her around on FourSquare. The online follower could physically materialize after learning some of her favorite haunts. In the digital age, children and teenagers are going to continue to communicate socially in a variety of new and innovative ways, and this is appropriate and beneficial to their social well-being, sense of self-worth, and to their psychosocial maturation. The challenge is to be able to keep a naturally vulnerable, inquisitive, and risk-taking population safe without alienating the members. The suggestions in the following list should be part of the safekeeping plan. The forensic nurse can act to promote the safety of children using the Internet through educational venues.

Education and Assistance for Parents
» Locate the computer in a common area where there is maximum family activity.
» Assist the children in setting up the social networking sites.
» Provide software that filters and monitors undesirable sites.
» Advise children to never provide personal information in an Internet chat room.
» Advise children to never send photographs of themselves over the Internet.

» Advise children to never arrange a meeting with someone they encountered on the Internet.

» Have children report any innocent-looking Internet link that takes the children to an inappropriate site.

» Limit the amount of time the children can spend in chat rooms or surfing that does not have an educational purpose.

» Familiarize yourself and the children with resources and mechanisms for reporting undesirable, unintended transfer to objectionable sites.

» Do not overreact to a child's inappropriate Internet activities, as it may cause him to become less open about future activities.

» Encourage children to discuss their Internet experiences openly and freely.

Education for School Personnel and Healthcare Professionals

» Be alert for behavioral changes in children that may signal an inappropriate Internet relationship, such as avoiding classmates, acting aloof, and signs of depression.

» When counseling children and adolescents, be sure to include an assessment of their Internet use along with other measures of social relationships.

» Collaborate with community members interested in the issue of Internet safety for children.

» Become actively involved in the process that seeks to address Internet safety for children through policy and legislation.

» Develop a system for evaluating Internet sites, chat rooms, and filtering software and make recommendations to school personnel.

» Conduct research aimed at understanding the impact of unwanted exposure to sexual material among children of varying ages (younger children report more distress after such exposure than older children).

» Involve children in the process of promoting safety and awareness of their responsibility for Internet standards.

» Facilitate the awareness of youth of sources of help for Internet offenses and ways to more easily report such offenses.

It is important to remember that minors and adults alike might be the victims of Internet-facilitated rape. Adults, too, should engage in safe practices while using the Internet. Because adults increasingly use the Internet to meet prospective partners, rapists increasingly use the Internet to find potential victims.

Once an offender has selected a target, he/she can monitor potential or existing victims on several levels, ranging from participating in a discussion forum and becoming familiar with the other participants, to searching the Internet for related information about an individual, to accessing a potential victim's personal computer to gain additional information. Furthermore, by giving offenders access to victims over an extended period of time (rather than just a brief encounter) the Internet enables offenders to gain control of their victims or gain their victims' trust and possibly arrange a meeting in the physical world (Casey, Ferraro, & McGrath, 2004).

Cyberbullying

Bullying is a specific form of aggressive behavior that consists of repeated, purposeful mistreatment of one individual over another involving an imbalance of power between the victim and the perpetrator. Online or electronic bullying is the same type of behavior carried out through phones and computers (Wang, Iannotti, & Nansel, 2009). Cyberbullying is an area of concern for school personnel, including forensic nurses. A study of high school students in Hawaii revealed that more than 50% reported having been the victim of cyberbullying during the previous year and that serious mental health issues followed many of the encounters (Goebert, Else, Matsu, & Chung-Do, 2010). Other statistics show that one in three school-aged children report either being a bully or having been bullied within the last year. An alarming number of recent teenage suicides have been reported to have been preceded by an episode of bullying, either physical, or, increasingly, online. Cyberbullying on college and university campuses takes place routinely, and the significance is frequently minimized as typical campus behavior among young adults. Tragic results have followed in this venue as well. It has been shown that bully-victims, whether traditional victims or cyber-victims, report significantly higher levels of depressive symptoms than their non-bullied adolescent peers (Perren, Dooley, Shaw, & Cross, 2010). Although this area is quite unsettled when it comes to the complex legal issues involved, most states have at least begun to address the issue looking for court rulings that could provide precedents for guidance going forward. Most schools and states have policies that address traditional bullying that takes place in school, but few address the issue of bullying that takes place using some form of electronic communication. Since cyberbullying generally takes place off of school campuses, it can be argued that it does not involve the school system or any of its existing rules regarding bullying that could offer a way to intervene. It can also be argued that a child has a right to feel safe in school and to not intervene if a child is being bullied does not afford the child that right. Moreover if it can be demonstrated that the school knew about the bullying, did not act to intervene, and the student suffered harm, the school could be legally charged with deliberate indifference and could thus be held liable for the student's injury/injuries. If the cyberbullying is accompanied by physical bullying, which often takes place in school or on the way home from school, school officials might feel justified in intervening regarding the physical bullying but are unclear what to do about the online incidents. This occurs despite the fact that the online attack might include threats, derogatory language, sexually explicit accusations, and generally horrific comments directed at the victim and shared for all of the child's friends and classmates to see. At times, there is confusion about whose phone or computer was actually involved. School officials do not feel that they can search a child's phone or computer, particularly because of the phenomenon of sexting, which may involve a situation of child pornography. While there is not a universally accepted interpretation regarding legally appropriate interventions, all agree that education is the key, and that programs that address the cyberbullying phenomenon and appropriate behavior in social networking sites in general must be developed. The forensic nurse can play a key role in the development of such programs particularly in school venues and in mental health settings.

Issues that need to be addressed include a comprehensive program to promote online civility in all matters related to online communication and relationships. The anonymity provided by the Internet serves to encourage an attitude of noninvolvement in the face of inappropriate behavior by others, including online harassment and bullying. Students must be encouraged to step up when they witness bullying and provide support for the victim. Parents as well as educators need to be involved in the educational process, taking advantage of every teachable moment occurring either in the home or in the school. It should also be recognized that the bully has needs that must be recognized and addressed as well. It should be stressed that while the activities of the bully must be curtailed, care should be taken to avoid humiliating him/her since it has been shown that these individuals already suffer from humiliation. It is this humiliation that fuels the desire to humiliate others through bullying. The relative newness of the phenomenon of cyberbullying is contributing to the ineffective efforts thus far to gain control of the situation and provide safety for students and other victims. The consequences for a student accused of bullying are not always clear and thus are not communicated well. One thing that does seem clear, however, is that criminalization is not an effective solution. For example, it can prove quite difficult to specifically attribute a tragic outcome such as suicide directly to the bullying, in terms of criminal charges. The student or students committing the bullying most likely do not foresee the tragic outcome. It seems more important to try to change the social culture that allows or even encourages the inappropriate behavior to begin with. Programs that include a suicide prevention component must be developed, since many victims of bullying report suicide ideation at some point during their victimization. School nurses in particular, observing individual children as well as group interactions through a forensic lens, can play a crucial role in identifying victims and proposing interventions to address this type of peer aggression.

The ability of the Internet to instantly transport any message, article or photograph to potentially millions of viewers globally presents a unique and disturbing problem, most especially for the young. At this point, there is no effective means for removing anything that is posted on the Internet, despite claims of safety and confidentiality promised by the various social networking sites. The alarming reality is that anything posted on the Internet has guaranteed immortality. Although research efforts are under way at various technical and academic institutions to develop software that will address the problem, it is far from being perfected—much less implemented (Rosen, 2010). Technically sophisticated hackers are able to compromise any social networking site creating mayhem and possible lifelong emotional devastation for risk-taking adolescents and young adults. There are well-documented cases in which foolish but understandable teenaged behavior resulted in a lifetime of misery, and in a few tragic cases, suicide resulted from the inability to face the humiliation and heartbreak experienced by a victim due to one act of inappropriate and perhaps impulsive behavior by a bully.

While the Internet facilitates online bullying, it does have the unforeseen benefit of providing a valuable forensic tool. As previously mentioned, communications that take place via the Internet remain somewhere forever. Because of that preservation of evidence that digital forensic examiners can retrieve, analyze, and document the communications that took place and can very often connect the communications to the bully.

Child Pornography

Child pornography is the scourge of the Internet. Child pornography is the graphic depiction of a minor engaged in sexual activity or in an explicit sexual pose. Child pornography is distinguished from erotica and adult pornography because the actions depicted in the images are criminal by their very nature. In the case of sex acts, the action is either statutory rape, forcible rape, or at the least a crime akin to impairing the morals of a minor or risking the injury of a minor. When the conduct depicted is a lascivious exhibition of the genitals, the act may not be a sexual assault or statutory rape, but in many jurisdictions, the soliciting of the suggestive pose by the photographer or adult is impairing the morals of a minor or risking injury to a minor. Minors are set apart from adults because they, by law and by developmental capacity, lack the ability to consent to certain conduct and obligations. For example, minors may not enter into contracts, enter into marriage, or consent to sexual activity. Along the same vein, minors may not consent to a picture being taken of criminal activity in which they are also a victim. By the same force of argument, minors whose pictures have been taken while being victimized cannot consent to allowing those pictures to be distributed.

Before the Internet, due to heavy federal and state penalties for manufacturing and distributing child pornography, it was difficult to find sources of such materials. Transactions were all conducted either hand-to-hand, as in the case of a bookstore or other purveyor, or through the mail. It was easy for police to keep the lid on bookstore trafficking of child pornography because they knew where the stores were and who worked there. All police had to do was show up and walk around the store. They could see anything in plain view that was offered for sale, and if there was evidence that the store sold child pornography, a search warrant and arrest ensued shortly thereafter. The United States Postal Service postal inspectors have a keen eye for contraband, and especially child pornography. Postal inspectors often conducted undercover stings and controlled deliveries of suspicious materials. Between the actions of local police and the postal inspectors, the physical exchange of child pornography had been slowed substantially in the United States prior to technological advances that made digital images and their rapid exchange over the Internet possible.

Digital imagery revolutionized the child pornography trade. Before digital imagery was possible, child pornography was limited to photography, film, and video. Photography and film require at least some equipment and specialized knowledge to develop the film. To mass distribute photographs, one must employ a printer; to distribute film or videotapes in large quantities, a professional processor would be needed. Getting the product to the consumer posed other logistical difficulties. Issues of advertising and the physical distribution of the material were complicated by corporeal existence of the contraband. Thus, the expense of producing child pornography made it prohibitively expensive to most people to purchase. Unfortunately, the ability to create, to store, and to traffic in child pornography in digital format has eliminated most of the traditional law enforcement and logistical barriers to mass producing and distributing that material.

Using a digital camera, one can sexually abuse a minor in the privacy of one's own home and record it as digital video or still images and instantly broadcast it to an unlimited number of recipients via the Internet. The one-time cost of the camera can be less than $50 for a small webcam. The cost of distributing the image is next to nothing. A personal computer can be purchased for less than $500. A used computer costs much less than that. An Internet connection could be $10 a month or even less with various offers.

Detection and Proof of Distribution of Child Pornography

Since 2000, federal law has mandated that Internet service providers report suspected child pornography that they detect travelling through their networks to the National Center for Missing and Exploited Children. From there, analysts review the material and refer the information to the appropriate law enforcement agency for follow-up investigation (42 U.S.C. 13032). This new practice has resulted in a tremendous increase in the number of child pornography investigations in the United States.

Law enforcement agencies also initiate investigations. One of the more successful nationwide initiatives has been use of software engineered to search peer-to-peer networks for shared known child pornography images. Once the software locates the images, investigators review the inventory of a peer-to-peer user's shared directory, viewing a sample of the files to determine if they contain child pornography. If the investigator determines that the shared files do depict child pornography, a search warrant is obtained, the computer is seized and searched and the computer user is usually arrested soon thereafter for both possession of child pornography and distribution of child pornography.

Box 16-2   Federal task force programs.

Internet Crimes Against Children Task Force Program

Since the Internet Crimes Against Children Task Force Program began in 1998, more than 288,000 state and local law enforcement officers, prosecutors and other professionals have been trained to investigate online crimes committed against children and to provide assistance to victims of those crimes. By 2010, there were 61 task forces representing more than 2000 law enforcement agencies and prosecutorial authorities. (www.ojjdp.gov)

History of Innocent Images

While investigating the disappearance of a juvenile in May 1993, FBI agents and Prince George's County, Maryland, police detectives identified two suspects who had sexually exploited numerous juveniles over a 25-year period. Investigation into the activities of the suspects determined that the adults were routinely utilizing online computers to transmit child pornography. Further investigation and discussions with experts, both within the FBI and in the private sector, revealed that the utilization of computer telecommunications was rapidly becoming one of the most prevalent techniques by which some sex offenders shared pornographic images of minors and identified and recruited children into sexually illicit relationships. Based on information developed during this investigation, the Innocent Images National Initiative was started in 1995 to address the illicit activities conducted by users of commercial and private online services and the Internet.

During the early stages of Innocent Images, a substantial amount of time was exhausted on commercial online service providers that provide numerous easily accessible chat rooms in which teenagers and preteens can meet and converse with each other. By using chat rooms, children can chat for hours with unknown individuals, often without the knowledge or approval of their parents. Investigation revealed that computer sex offenders used chat rooms to contact children. Chat rooms offer the advantage of immediate communication around the world and provide the pedophile with an anonymous means of identifying and recruiting children into sexually illicit relationships.

Sources: U.S. Department of Justice (n.d.) and Federal Bureau of Investigation (n.d.).

Today's Innocent Images

Today, the FBI's Innocent Images National Initiative focuses on individuals who indicate a willingness to travel interstate for the purpose of engaging in sexual activity with a minor and major producers and/or distributors of child pornography.

> *In addition, the Innocent Images National Initiative works to identify child victims and obtain appropriate services/assistance for them.*
>
> *Online child pornography/child sexual exploitation is the most significant cyber-crime problem confronting the FBI that involves crimes against children. Throughout the FBI, there was a 1,997% increase in the number of Innocent Images National Initiative cases opened between fiscal years 1996 and 2002, from 113 to 2,370. It is anticipated that the number of cases opened and the resources utilized to address the crime problem will continue to rise during the next several years.*
>
> *The FBI has taken the necessary steps to ensure that the Innocent Images National Initiative remains viable and productive through the use of new technology and sophisticated investigative techniques, coordination of the national investigative strategy, and a national liaison initiative with a significant number of commercial and independent online service providers. Innocent Images has been highly successful. It has proven to be a logical, efficient, and effective method to identify and investigate individuals who are using the Internet for the purpose of sexually exploiting children.*
>
> *Source:* Federal Bureau of Investigation (n.d.).

In 1996, Congress amended the child exploitation sections of the federal penal code to anticipate that virtual images—that is, digital images rendered by computer technology—would be used to depict sexually explicit images of minors. The new provisions also prohibited the depiction of individuals who appear to be minors in sexually explicit acts. These two provisions became lightning rods for free speech advocates and legitimate, adult pornographers. A group called the Free Speech Coalition sued Attorney General John Ashcroft, claiming that these elements of the law were overbroad and vague. The United States Supreme Court held in *Ashcroft v. Free Speech Coalition* that prosecutors must prove that there is an actual minor depicted in the picture and that minor must actually be sexually abused. The Court reiterated its holding in *New York v. Ferber* (1982) when it stated that the distinguishing feature that allows child pornography to be treated differently than constitutionally protected speech is that it is a visual preservation of a criminal act against a minor. There were many other features of the *Ashcroft v. Free Speech Coalition* (2002) case that are of importance, and the case is far more complex than the explanation here. Although this discussion of *Ashcroft* is a grossly simplified summary, it provides sufficient highlights of some issues relative to prosecuting a child pornography case following the *Ashcroft* decision.

Some prosecutors have interpreted *Ashcroft* to require that the state must prove beyond a reasonable doubt that the person portrayed in an image is not an adult or a computer-rendered image and that there is actual, prohibited sexual activity taking place. Thus, in order to try a child pornography case, investigators and forensic examiners often are required to prove that the person depicted in the picture actually exists and was the person depicted in the pictures. To facilitate these identifications, the NCMEC maintains a database of identified child pornography images. Investigators send images to NCMEC requesting a search of the database, and NCMEC confirms whether any of the images are of known victims. The NCMEC database has solved a small part of the problem of proving that a person depicted in an image is a minor being sexually abused. But the database cannot deal with pictures of new victims that enter the stream of trade every day.

Two thirds of offenders who were convicted of sex crimes against minors were found to be in possession of child pornography, the majority of which depicted children between the ages of 6 and 12. Many successful cases of prosecution have come about as a result of individuals reporting instances of the crime to the CyberTipline (http://www.cybertipline.com).

Forensic nurses need to be aware of the methods by which they can facilitate the reporting of such crimes. The forensic nurse can be an advocate for the protection of children through assessment, counseling, and parent and community education.

Healthcare Fraud

Individuals diagnosed with chronic illness, particularly progressive or life-threatening conditions, frequently seek information and products to treat their conditions on the Internet. Almost 100 million adults in the United States use the Internet as a resource for health information for themselves, family members, or friends (Bren, 2001). The populations most at risk for healthcare fraud are adolescents and the elderly. Adolescents regularly seek remedies for or advice about health-related issues such as weight, acne, depression, eating disorders, plastic surgery, and exercise. One might think that the elderly, a large segment of the population with chronic illness, might not be computer literate, and therefore not risk falling prey to such fraud. However, this is increasingly not the case, as even those elders who do not own their own computers often become proficient in their use through Internet classes offered at senior centers, libraries, and assisted living facilities.

Healthcare fraud is defined by the Food and Drug Administration (FDA) as the deceptive sale or advertising of products that claim to be effective against medical conditions or otherwise beneficial to health, but which have not been proven safe and effective for those purposes (FDA, n.d.). It is estimated that healthcare fraud costs Americans an estimated $30 billion per year. More ominous is the fact that these practices, in some cases, may cost individuals their lives.

There are many websites that advertise products of little or no therapeutic value. In some instances, the claims for the products are simply without proven merit. In other instances, the clients order and pay for products and then do not receive them. Clients may also illegally obtain prescription medications on the Internet, some approved but many not yet approved by the FDA. Counterfeit drugs have also found their way onto the Internet and are currently the focus of major pharmaceutical companies, Internet providers, and law enforcement seeking to curb the abuses in this market. The secondary market in which dealers buy excess inventory of drugs for resale is largely unregulated and also serves as a means of distributing counterfeit drugs. Forensic nurses should be alert to situations in which it is suspected that individuals, particularly the elderly, may be using prescription medication without proper medical oversight.

In vitro diagnostic tests are marketed freely and if used as the sole predictor of health or disease, can be potentially disastrous for vulnerable populations. Using these products, individuals may self-diagnose and self-treat themselves inappropriately and dangerously. Examples of tests available from the Internet include tests for HIV, hepatitis, drugs of abuse, and cholesterol. Physicians routinely use such tests, but only in conjunction with other standard medical practice such as physical examination, medical history, evaluation of other presenting symptomatology, additional more sophisticated in vitro diagnostic testing and so forth (CDRH, 2001). Self-diagnosis could rely on a test that yields either false-positive or false-negative results. Tests that yield quantitative data may be misinterpreted by the individual and could compromise his or her health if not followed up by a visit to a certified professional healthcare provider. Thus the advertising of products for use at home without further medical oversight is misleading at best and possibly quite dangerous for the clients using them. In addition, while some in vitro diagnostic tests are effective, many are of poor quality and some are clearly illegal—that is, they are being marketed without approval by the FDA. Others may be approved for professional use but are marketed for unapproved uses (CDRH). Potential users must be educated about the fact that all such products should first be researched and approved by the FDA.

Recently there has been increased activity involving direct-to-consumer marketing of personal genetic or genomic tests. These tests are designed to provide consumers with information regarding their likelihood of developing a wide array of diseases and conditions. These tests are marketed through print media, television, and the Internet. Since the individuals ordering these tests may not have the benefit of a healthcare professional to guide them through the report, there exists a great potential for misinterpretation, false reassurance concerning their health, and in some cases unnecessary anguish. An individual may learn that he has a gene specific for a severe medical disorder but doesn't realize that the disease is so rare that he has a 1 in 5 million chance of ever developing it. As with other types of healthcare information offered over the Internet, there exists the potential for fraudulent activities. The Genetic Information Nondiscrimination Act of 2008 (GINA), in its present form does not protect against discrimination in regard to life, disability or long-term care insurance (Steck & Eggert, 2011). Thus an individual may find him/herself unable to purchase long-term care insurance if a genetic test reveals a health problem that insurers might want to avoid. The Affordable Health Care Act seeks to address the shortcomings of GINA by not allowing insurance companies to deny an individual on the basis of a pre-existing illness but seniors seeking these tests need to be advised that they are currently not protected.

The Oncology Nursing Society has issued a position statement that includes a requirement that clients of such products or services receive pre- and posttest education, counseling, and informed consent (Oncology Nursing Society, 2010).

It is estimated that one in three clients avail themselves of some form of alternative therapy, the majority of whom do not disclose the information to their healthcare provider. Some of these therapies are fraudulent, and others, while not illegal, are purported to have beneficial effects that are clearly without scientific validation. The availability of these products on the Internet can have potentially dangerous consequences as the (illegally obtained) medications or ineffective treatments may interact adversely with those already legitimately prescribed for the client, or in other cases substitute for proven conventional medical treatments that could help. Some examples of recently prosecuted cases include a claim that St. John's wort was a safe treatment for clients with HIV or AIDS when there exists a potentially dangerous interaction with protease inhibitors used to treat the disease and the marketing of a device that claimed it could kill the agents of diseases such as cancer and Alzheimer's disease by delivering a mild electric current (Bren, 2001). While one cannot blame clients who are experiencing major illness for which there is little hope and who wish to try anything that might prolong their lives or at least relieve their suffering, the problem is that some might be forgoing proven medical therapies that could help. Although many alternative therapies are helpful or at the least, not harmful, the forensic nurse can act as an advocate to ensure that clients do not rely on products that are clearly fraudulently advertised and will not improve their state of health. Forensic nurses must be aware of these potentially dangerous websites, monitor them where feasible, and actively engage in policy making to curtail this type of healthcare fraud. Workshops and/or educational seminars held for the elderly in senior settings or for adolescents (in educational settings) should also strive to aim their program toward educating these vulnerable populations as to the dangers involved in engaging in activities related to personal health on the Internet. Observing and assessing clients through a forensic lens may alert the nurse to situations in which the clients might be being victimized and/or are compromising their health. Educating clients should include the following points:

» Always consult your healthcare provider when using any products obtained through the Internet.
» Avoid products that claim to treat a wide array of illnesses.
» Be suspicious of products that claim to be all natural, as this implies a level of safety that may not be justified.
» Avoid products that can only be obtained through one supplier.
» Obtain full information regarding the firm's name, address, and phone number.
» Do not rely on the results of any one in vitro diagnostic test without medical validation.
» Be wary of any product described in grandiose terms such as guaranteed cure.

The passage of the Affordable Care Act of 2010 has opened up a new avenue for health care scams aimed at the elderly or otherwise vulnerable populations. The HHS secretary recently warned that scammers are contacting individuals through e-mail advising them of the need for them to purchase new health insurance policies required by the act. In some cases, victims have purchased new insurance policies; in others they have provided personal information that allows the scammers to steal their identities.

In still other situations, they have been duped into providing their Medicare numbers thus allowing the scammers to submit fraudulent claims. However, the act does promise to provide new measures aimed at preventing this type of fraud that costs the citizens billions of dollars in fraudulent claims (U.S. Department of Health and Human Services, 2010).

Human Organ Transplants

Trafficking in Human Organs

Long thought to be an urban myth, trafficking in human organs for transplant has become an increasingly significant legal, moral, and ethical problem. Organ trafficking refers to the procurement of living or deceased persons or their organs involving payment or benefits to a third party for the purpose of organ transplantation. Although outlawed in virtually every country in the world, such procurement and sale of organs continues to warrant concern. This practice frequently involves the exploitation, fraud, deception, or other abuses of power over vulnerable individuals (American Society of Nephrology, 2008).

A report by the secretariat of the World Health Organization (WHO) (2003) acknowledges that while payment for human organs and tissue is illegal in most countries, there are many reports from various countries that living donors, particularly of kidneys, have received direct payment for their donation and may indeed have been exploited in the process (WHO, 2003). While it is a violation of federal law in the United States to receive or provide remuneration in exchange for a body part, Internet solicitation of organs for transplantation exists and may in some cases involve a financial transaction. One such Internet site, http://www.matchingdonors.com, claims to have over 9539 willing donors and 2092 willing donors in the altruistic paired kidney exchange program. These donors are willing to be incompatible donors meaning they will donate their kidney without a designated receiver. The first transplant of an organ from a donor solicited from this site was performed in October 2004.

Transplant Tourism

Transplant tourism describes the travel of individuals seeking an organ transplant or other medical procedures to jurisdictions where they can obtain the organ or procedure through payment, as for a commodity. Most often this activity involves travel to countries having a large segment of vulnerable individuals desperate for money. In these situations, vulnerable individuals, many not fully comprehending the ramifications of their decision, enter into a life-altering procedure for what amounts in the long term to a pittance for their donation. One such country, China, has long been known for its lucrative trade in organs, most of which are harvested from executed prisoners. In many instances, prisoners are executed for relatively minor infractions that in other countries might not even warrant a jail sentence. Since China executes more prisoners in 1 year than the entire rest of the global community combined, the organs are plentiful, fetching prices of upwards of $30,000 per organ; however, some expenses are as high as $200,000 for the transplant procedure (Glaser, 2005). Chinese officials claim that the routine harvesting and sale of organs removed from executed prisoners is not domestic policy and that the organs are donated voluntarily by the prisoners. These claims cannot be substantiated. Because the cost for the incarceration and execution of prisoners falls to the families of the prisoners, the hardship endured by the families is great. Yet it appears that in no way are their obligations for payment lessened despite the huge amounts of money paid for their relative's organs. The critical shortage of organs available for transplant in the United States continues to and will continue to encourage individuals with end-stage chronic disease to seek organs on the Internet or through other sources and subsequently engage in transplant tourism. Many ethical issues arise from this situation and are the focus of many in the medical, ethical, and scientific fields (Rhodes & Schiano, 2010).

In 2005, five doctors were arrested in South Africa and charged with illegal trading in human organs. The illegal practice of kidney transplantation involved recipients from Israel and donors from Brazil (Sidley, 2004). Israel is one country that has acted to promote the global trade in kidneys by refusing to condemn the practice. In 2006, the Jerusalem district court ordered the HMOs to pay the donors involved in living kidney transplants, essentially legalizing the practice (Bakdash & Scheper-Hughes, 2006). Their rationale included the fact that their citizens were engaging in transplant tourism by leaving the country to obtain a transplant, and they would be safer by staying in their homeland and seeking a donor who was willing to provide a kidney for reimbursement (Bakdash & Scheper-Hughes, 2006). While arguments can be made on both sides of this issue, the fact remains that procuring organs from vulnerable individuals in poor countries involves exploitation of desperate individuals who may see no other way for themselves and their families to survive. In 2008, a meeting of more than 150 representatives from around the globe met in Istanbul to develop a legal and professional framework to govern all aspects of organ transplantation, including setting up regulatory bodies to oversee and control such activities (American Society of Nephrology, 2008). At this meeting, several principles that addressed the ethical and legal implications of organ trafficking and specifically banned commercial transplantation at every level were identified (American Society of Nephrology).

Living Donors

Donations of organs by living donors involves three distinct situations. The first is the most typical and is considered a directed donation to a relative or friend, providing the donor and recipient are biocompatible. In the second type, the organ goes into the general pool to be given to the biocompatible donor at the top of the waiting list. The third type is called a directed donation and is made to a stranger with whom the donor has no previous relationship but perhaps heard of the recipient's plight through the Internet or another form of mass media (Truog, 2007).

In 2007, the National Organ Transplant Act of 1984 was amended to address the issue of organ donation from living donors unrelated to the intended recipient. This practice has gained in popularity in recent years and is greatly facilitated by Internet access to willing and compatible donors. These organ donations are of two types. The first involves a living donor who hears of the plight of an individual in need of an organ and comes forward voluntarily to offer a whole or part of one of his or her organs. These offers are generally of an altruistic nature and involve no direct compensation, although in some instances the medical expenses of the donor are paid for by the recipient.

The second type involves relatives of the individual in need of a transplant who are willing to donate all or part of an organ but are not a biologic match. These individuals are placed on a list with other potential donors and recipients in similar circumstances. Thus the incompatible relative may become the donor for an unrelated recipient while his or her relative receives an organ from another potential donor who is considered a biologic match. The Amendment to the Transplant Act addresses the issue of compensation for the living donors stating that "no valuable consideration is knowingly acquired, received, or otherwise transferred with respect to the organs" (Charlie W. Norwood Living Organ Donation Act, 2007, p. 1). It has been suggested that perhaps discussion concerning the feasibility of offering payment in the case of a living donor might be in order, following a study by researchers at the University of Pennsylvania that polled people on their interest or willingness to donate a kidney if monetary compensation was involved (Halpern et al., 2010). While one can assume that the donors in the United States participating in such organ exchanges are well informed of the risks and have undergone sufficient psychological and physical assessments to assure informed consent, the same cannot be guaranteed for donors from poorer countries who often sell their organs, most often their kidney, for money.

A recent study reported in a U.S. medical journal found no existing health consequences for living kidney donors, although the limitations of the study included the lack of long-term follow-up. However, the recipients of many of the organs have endured a higher than normal expectation of complications from the surgical procedure, and managing patients in the United States who have undergone illegal procedures in foreign countries can present ethical challenges (Rhodes & Schiano, 2010). The amendment to the National Organ Transplant Act requires that the Secretary of Health and Human Services report to the Congress on progress made toward identifying the long-term complications of living organ donation (Charlie W. Norwood Living Organ Donation Act, 2007).

In cases of living donation of organs from strangers, referred to as altruistic donors, the forensic nurse should be attuned to the possible vulnerability of the donor. In some instances the donor may be considered to be the victim, since in many cases the donor is young, in need of money, and inadequately informed as to the long-term health consequences of his or her action, which in some cases are quite serious. When a young adult surrenders a healthy kidney, for example, if illness ensues in later life, the donor might find himself or herself in need of a transplanted organ. Careful psychological screening methods must be employed prior to allowing a young, healthy adult to donate a body part to a virtual stranger, such as one met on the Internet. An index of suspicion must be employed when caring for clients in areas where organ transplantation is involved, particularly in cases where the donor may not be fully informed of the risks and consequences. When caring preoperatively for a transplant donor, forensic nurses in clinical settings may be in a position to ensure that the consent form signed by the donor is truly informed consent as required by law. Forensic nurses in the community must be knowledgeable when providing services to families and community groups about the possible implications of deviating from the prevailing medical system of organ procurement.

CASE STUDY 16-2

Illinois Fire Captain

After spending 6 years on a waiting list for a kidney transplant, an Illinois firefighter suffering from Alport's syndrome received a kidney from a stranger donor he encountered on MatchingDonors.com. He had tried unsuccessfully to seek out a biological match from among his family and friends. In the interim he was forced to undergo peritoneal dialysis at home for 12 hours each day and was forced into early retirement because of his failing health. The 56-year-old grandfather of four wrote his biography and his plea for an altruistic donor after becoming discouraged with his health and the wait time that he had spent in hopes of receiving a donor kidney from the usual route, through the United Network for Organ Sharing agency, a nonprofit agency contracted with the U.S. Department of Health. His biography caught the eye of a potential donor who wanted to provide an opportunity for this individual to spend time enjoying his grandchildren in better health. The donor proved to be a compatible match and the surgery was scheduled. Now the recipient's daughter has signed up to become a living donor to a stranger (Matching Donors.com, 2010).

The shortage of available organs for transplant and issues of fairness of distribution of such organs through the United Network for Organ Sharing have fueled dialog about the need to formulate another method of encouraging and allocating organ donations. There are estimated to be over 100,000 patients awaiting an organ transplant in the United States alone. Yet according to statistics from the United Network for Organ Sharing, only approximately one quarter that number receive transplants each year (United Network for Organ Sharing, 2011). There is increasing discussion about the idea of providing some type of reward system for those individuals and families who might consider donating organs for transplant. The ethical issues associated with such a program continue to pose a significant challenge to the idea. It remains to be seen how widespread the use of the Internet by clients in need of an organ transplant will become.

Summary

The Internet age has brought with it great benefits as well as great challenges. As with any technological breakthrough, computer technology has outpaced our ability to prepare for the unexpected, sometimes negative, consequences. Law enforcement, forensic science, and the law are in a chaotic state in the early years of the 21st century because all disciplines are trying to identify the consequences, formulate a response, and institute methods of dealing with computer-related crime. While this process of trying to make sense of things takes place, the Internet is similar to the wild, wild West—the 19th century's "www." Lawlessness rules, and it is unclear whether or when the dust will settle. Amid this turmoil the forensic nurse can provide assistance by being an educator, an advocate for the victims of Internet crime or exploitation, and an activist for appropriate, effective legislation.

QUESTIONS FOR DISCUSSSION

1. What computers do nurses use that might contain digital evidence?
2. How can nurses help to determine if a computer or the Internet was part of the crime?
3. What are the two components of a crime?
4. What is the difference between a pyramid scheme and a Ponzi scheme?
5. After reading this chapter, how would you change your Internet activities?
6. What will you recommend to others about using the Internet safely?
7. What is sexting, and how can teenagers protect themselves from unintended consequences?
8. What role does the forensic nurse play in addressing the issue of cyberbullying?

REFERENCES

42 United States Code § 13032 [2004]

American Society of Nephrology. (2008). The declaration of Istanbul on organ trafficking and transplant tourism. *Clinical Journal of the American Society of Nephroplogy, 3*, 1227–1231.

Anderson-Butcher, D., Lasseigne, A., Ball, A., Brzozowski, M., Lehnert, M., & McCormick, B. (2010). Adolescent Weblog use: Risky or protective? *Child and Adolescent Social Work, 27*(1), 63–77. DOI: 10.1007/s10560-010-0193-x

Ashcroft v. Free Speech Coalition, 122 S. Ct. 1389; 152 L. Ed. 2d 403; 2002 U.S. LEXIS 2789 (2002).

Baker, B. (2010). Online 'sextortion' of teens rising—sexual extortion—what is it and how to prevent it? Retrieved from http://news.gather.com/viewArticle.action?articleId=281474978448754

Bakdash, T., Scheper-Hughes, N. (2006). Is it ethical for patients with renal disease to purchase kidneys from the world's poor? *PLoS Med 3*(10), e349. DOI: 10.1371/journal.pmed.0030349

Bren, L. (2001). Agencies team up in war against Internet health fraud. *FDA Consumer Magazine,* 1–4. Retrieved from www.fda.gov/fdac/features/2001/501_war.html

Casey, E., Ferraro, M., & McGrath, M. (2004). Sex offenders on the Internet. In *Digital evidence and computer crime: Forensic science, computers, and the Internet* (2nd ed.). Boston, MA: Academic Press.

Center for Devices and Radiologic Health (CDRH). (2001). Buying diagnostic tests from the Internet: Buyer beware! *CDRH Consumer Information,* 1–3. Retrieved from http://www.fda.gov/

MedicalDevices/ResourcesforYou/Consumers/BuyingMedicalDevicesandDiagnosticTestsOnline/ucm142453.htm

Charlie W. Norwood Living Organ Donation Act. (2007). Global Legal Information Network. Retrieved from http://www.glin.gov

FDA Consumer Health Information (2011). FDA 101 Health Fraud Awareness. Retrieved from http://www.fda.gov/downloads/ForConsumers/ProtectYourself/HealthFraud/UCM167504.pdf

Federal Bureau of Investigation. (2010, July). Sexting. *Law Enforcement Bulletin*. Retrieved from http://www.fbi.gov/publications/leb/2010/july2010/sexting_feature.htm

Federal Bureau of Investigation. (n.d.). *Crimes against children.* Retrieved from http://www.fbi.gov/hq/cid/cac/crimesmain.htm

Finkelhor, D., Mitchell, K. J., & Wolak, J. (2001). Highlights of the youth Internet safety survey. *OJJDP Fact Sheet,* pp. 1–2. Washington, DC: U.S. Department of Justice.

Glaser, S. (2005). Formula to stop the illegal organ trade: Presumed consent laws and mandatory reporting requirements for doctors. *Human Rights Brief, 12.* Washington, DC: American University College of Law.

Goebert, D., Else, I., Matsu, C., & Chung-Do, J. (2010). The impact of cyberbullying on substance abuse and mental health in a multiethnic sample. *Journal of Maternal Child Health, 1,* 1–5. DOI: 10.1007/s10995-010-0672-x

Halpern, S. D., Raz, A., Kohn, R., Rey, M., Asch, D., & Reese, P. (2010). Regulated payments for living kidney donation: An empirical assessment of the ethical concerns. *Annals of Internal Medicine, 152,* 358–365.

Internet Fraud Complaint Center. (2003). *Welcome to IFCC.* Retrieved from www.ifccfbi.gov

Illinois fire captain will receive a life saving kidney transplant from a complete stranger he met on the Internet (2010). MatchingDonors.com

Mitchell, K. J., Finkelhor, D., Jones, L., & Wolnak, J. (2010, April 25). Use of social networking sites in online sex crimes against minors: An examination of national incidence and means of utilization. *Journal of Adolescent Health.*

National Center for Missing and Exploited Children. (n.d.). Home page. Retrieved from www.missingkids.com

New York v. Ferber, 458 U.S. 747; 102 S. Ct. 3348; 73 L. Ed. 2d 1113 (1982).

Oncology Nursing Society (2010). Position: Direct-to-consumer marketing of genetic and genomic tests. *Oncology Nursing Forum, 37*(4).

Perren, S., Dooley, J., Shaw, T. and Cross, D. (2010). Bullying in school and cyberspace: Associations with depressive symptoms in Swiss and Australian adolescents.*Child and Adolescent Psychiatry and Mental Health. 28*(4), 1–10.

Rhodes, R., & Schiano, T. (2010). Transplant tourism in China: A tale of two transplants. *American Journal of Bioethics, 10*(2), 3–11.

Rosen, J. (2010, July 25). The end of forgetting. *NYT Magazine,* pp. 30–37, 44–45.

Sidley, P. (2004). South African doctors arrested in kidney sale scandal. British Medical Journal *329,* 190.

Silverman, M. (2010, May 13). Social media parenting: Raising the digital generation. *Mashable: The Social Media Guide.* Retrieved from http://mashable.com/2010/05/13/parenting-social-media

Steck, M. B., & Eggert, J. A. (2011). The need to be aware and beware of the Genetic Information Nondiscrimination Act. *Oncology Nursing Society, 4*(15), 1–8.

Truog, R. D. (2005). The ethics of organ donation by living donors. *New England Journal of Medicine, 353*(5), 444–446.

U.S. Department of Health and Human Services. (2010). Press conference on health care fraud and the Affordable Care Act. Retrieved from http://webcache.googleusercontent.com/search?q=cache:http://hhs.gov/secretary/about/speeches/sp20100513.html&hl=en&strip=0

U.S. Department of Justice, Office of Justice Programs. (n.d.). Retrieved from www.ojp.usdoj.gov

United States Secret Service. (n.d.). *Home page.* Retrieved from www.secretservice.gov

Wang, C., Iannotti, R., Nansel, T. (2009) School bullying among adolescents in the United States: Physical, verbal, relational, and cyber. *Journal of Adolescent Health, 4*(45), 368–375.

Wolak, J., Mitchell, K., & Finkelhor, D. (2006). Online victimization of youth: Five years later. Alexandria, VA: National Center for Missing and Exploited Children.

Wolak, J., Mitchell, K. J., & Finkelhor, D. (2003). *Internet crimes against minors: The response of law enforcement* (pp. 1–14). Alexandria, VA: National Center for Missing and Exploited Children.

Wolak, J., Finkelhor, D., Mitchell, K. J., & Ybarra, M. L. (2008). Online "predators" and their victims: Myths, realities and implications for prevention and treatment. *American Psychologist, 63*(2), 111–128.

World Health Organization. (2003). *Human organ and tissue transplantation: Report by the Secretariat.* Retrieved from http://apps.who.int/gb/archive/pdf_files/EB112/eeb1125.pdf

SUGGESTED FURTHER READING

Bear, G. (2010). *School discipline and self-discipline: A practical guide to promoting prosocial student behavior.* New York, NY: Guilford.

Crone, D., Hawken, L., & Horner, R. (2010). *Responding to problem behavior in schools* (2nd ed.). New York, NY: Guilford.

Ferraro, M., & Eoghan, C. (2005). *Investigating child exploitation and pornography: The Internet, the law and forensic science.* New York, NY: Elsevier.

Varjas, K., Talley, J., Meyers, J., Parris, L., Cutts, H., & West, B. (2010). High school students' perceptions of motivations for cyberbullying: An exploratory study. *Journal of Emergency Medicine, 1*(3), 269–273.

CHAPTER 17

Hidden in Plain Sight: Modern-Day Slavery and the Rise of Human Trafficking

Barbara Moynihan and Mario Thomas Gaboury

This chapter will help readers to develop an understanding of the factors that contribute to human trafficking as it pertains to the victims and their health. As medical professionals, we have a responsibility to identify the indicators of human trafficking and provide safe and specific interventions to the victims of this tragic human rights violation.

CHAPTER FOCUS

» History of Human Trafficking
» The Magnitude of the Problem
» Victim Criteria

» Action by Healthcare Providers
» The Legal System

KEY TERMS

» Human trafficking
» The *Trafficking in Persons Report* (TIP Report)

» Trafficking Victims Protection Act

Introduction

Human trafficking is often referred to as modern-day slavery and takes many forms (United States Department of State, 2009). We will primarily focus on sex and labor trafficking in this chapter; so, we need to be alert to the presentations of those who are the victims of sex trafficking and labor trafficking, which includes child care, restaurant workers, fast food employees, and, in other areas of the world, children who are conscripted into military service of the cruelest kind and forced to engage in combat. These are the boy soldiers who have gradually been identified. Boy camel drivers are yet another population of children forced into the most horrific roles that steal both their childhood and any hope for the future. They are systematically malnourished to reduce the weight on the camel to the point of the child's starvation, and then they are discarded. Statistics are hardly accurate but do provide some information about the magnitude of these human rights violations.

According to the International Labor Organization (ILO), there are at least 12.3 million adults and children in forced labor, bonded labor, and commercial sexual servitude at any given time (ILO, 2005). It is estimated that at least 1.3 million are victims of commercial sexual servitude both nationally and internationally. According to the ILO, 56% of all forced labor victims are women and girls.

There are eight different identified types of human trafficking. These include sex slavery, slave soldiering, sex tourism, organ trafficking, skin trafficking, Internet criminal pedophilia, ritual torture, and labor slavery (Gemmell, n.d.).

It is beyond the scope of this chapter to elaborate in depth on any one of these types of human trafficking. Suffice it to say that this human rights violation is rampant, occurs in the United States, and we are often witnesses who take no action.

History of Human Trafficking

Human slavery is almost as old as humanity itself, dating back to hunter–gatherer societies. The modern-day view of human slavery and trafficking contains certain components that have surfaced in recent history. These characteristics include exploitation of a vulnerable individual for the use of labor or sex. The idea of contemporary human trafficking can be first seen with the movement against white slavery in the late 19th century. The term *white slavery* combined the movements of slavery and prostitution awareness and prevention. There is question as to whether a high number of women and girls being trafficked existed at this time, but numbers show there was a significant trade in the early 1900s, with 402 known traders of women documented in Hamburg, Germany (Kangaspunta, 2010). In the United States, an investigation in 1908 and 1909 called Importation and Harbouring of Women for Immoral Purposes, found that a large number of women were being trafficked into the United States (Kangaspunta). In 1921, the League of Nations hosted a convention including 34 nations that began to look at the issue of trafficking. The language was changed from white slavery to traffic in women and children, which in turn affected the scope and awareness of the problem, to more than white women and girls. This was the first time that the international community recognized males as victims of human trafficking. The convention's outcomes included an increase in monitoring migration as well as educating women and girls about the threat of trafficking. This conference led to an ongoing investigation and effort to understand the greater context of trafficking. Reports released in 1921 and 1932 by the League of Nations described the movement of women and girls and the methods used to sustain the trafficking industry. These tactics have not changed much and are similar to those used in the 21st century; the motivation within the industry is money. Factors that can help to prevent or reduce trafficking are knowledge, international cooperation, and the criminalization of trafficking as well as the contribution of civil society.

In 2000, *The Protocol to Prevent, Suppress, and Punish Trafficking in Persons Especially Women and Children* (also known as the Palermo Protocol) was written by the United Nations in Palermo, Italy. This was the first global, legally binding protocol, and it was adopted by 117 countries and 137 parties. This document sets forth a clear definition of trafficking with the intention of using this as a means to solidify both a national and international standard to prosecuting trafficking in persons cases (Kangaspunta, 2010).

Magnitude of the Problem

The magnitude of this crime is almost incomprehensible. Today, the monetary value of human beings is decreasing. Due to an explosion in population, it is easy and cheap to find slave labor. The price of slave labor is cheaper than traditional African slaves in the past. Many human trafficking victims become slave laborers because of debt incurred, which can be passed down from generations. Modern-day slavery has many forms, spanning all ethnic, racial, and religious backgrounds. Poverty has replaced metal chains for controlling victims of slavery and human trafficking (Gemmell, n.d.).

Factors That Contribute to Victimization

Human trafficking is a humanitarian crisis—an egregious exploitation of the innocent and vulnerable. Victims have little or no access to health care, and the health risks are overwhelming. Pregnancy, sexually transmitted diseases, injuries, and poor nutrition are only a few of the consequences of sexual servitude. Substance abuse, suicide attempts, and untreated injuries may bring a victim of trafficking to a medical facility. The nursing process involves assessment, planning, intervention, and evaluation. Assessment is a skill that nurses are experts at conducting and is key in identifying victims of trafficking. This is a population not easily identified, and few victims, if any, understand the resources possible within the medical facility. The nurse or medical provider must be able to recognize the indicators consistent with victims of trafficking as well as the skills to interview without placing the victim at further risk. Key to protecting the victim is to try to see her or him alone. This may be difficult, since the person with the victim will insist on remaining throughout the visit. There are various strategies that can be undertaken to afford the victim the opportunity to see the provider alone; however, this could put the victim at greater risk for harm once he or she leaves the facility unless the victim is hospitalized. The presenting problem or chief complaint can be mistaken for intimate partner violence and the trafficking victim, in effect, becomes invisible as such a victim.

The red flags that should raise the index of suspicion that a client is a possible victim of trafficking include not only the reason for presenting but body language. The patient is usually young, usually not proficient in speaking English, has no form of identification, is fearful, and is reluctant to answer questions if able to speak English.

The priority is, as always, assessment to determine the need for immediate medical attention. Once this need is established, then the medical care, which may include admission, surgery, or consultative services, is provided. When medical needs are not immediately available, a more in-depth assessment should be conducted. Pregnancy, sexual assault, and urinary tract infections are all potential sequelae of trafficking, as is the possibility of substance abuse—either by choice or forced in order to insure compliance with the trafficker.

Trafficking victims are hostages, taken against their will, forced to engage in unwanted, dangerous, and frightening activities. Labor trafficking can involve many hours of work, little or no time off, exposure to physical harm or disease, and no hope for rescue. This chapter focuses mainly on sex trafficking; however, it is essential that the forensic nurse be well trained in all aspects of human trafficking in order to begin to address the needs and plight of those fortunate enough to be able to seek medical care.

Health Considerations

The following conditions or findings on assessment should raise the index of suspicion that this patient is or has been a victim of trafficking:

Unmet health issues, including those listed previously, may also include injuries in various stages of healing; bruises consistent with restraint –or undiagnosed cardiac or medical conditions; depression; posttraumatic stress disorder; and substance abuse. These patients should also be screened for the risk of suicide. Other findings may include pelvic inflammatory disease, which, if untreated, can lead to serious or life-threatening conditions. Consideration should also be directed toward assessment for illegal abortions, sexually transmitted diseases, and pregnancy. All patients who are allowed to present for medical care should be screened for all of the above and appropriate laboratory studies as well as other diagnostic examinations should be performed. Since the person is usually not alone—and time is a factor, essential studies should be completed in a timely fashion in order to avoid any suspicion on the part of the person accompanying the patient, since this may result in an abrupt departure. Any and all identifying information must be obtained as soon as possible in the event that the patient is not admitted and is forced to leave prematurely.

Although the medical considerations have focused on the female victim, it is important to recognize that males are also victims of trafficking and may present differently but deserve the careful scrutiny that the female victim does as well.

Role of the Healthcare Provider: Taking Action

Historically, human trafficking has been under the radar for most healthcare providers, perhaps due to the misunderstanding related to this issue. Many believe it does not happen here. Perhaps it is not included in the curricula of nursing or medical schools. Historically, issues such as rape and domestic violence have been seen as women's issues and marginalized or seen as inevitable. Sexual assault has only recently been addressed as vigorously as it is now due to myths and misunderstanding regarding the dynamics of this violent crime. Trafficking falls into this category as well. We have begun to address and recognize the magnitude of this human rights violation and are slowly developing strategies to identify and address not only the health risks but the devastation that is created in the lives of the victims of trafficking. "The journey of a thousand miles begins with the first step" (Confucius). The following are perhaps first steps:

» Training of healthcare providers
» Multidisciplinary training
» Development of protocols
» Public awareness campaign
» Forming a task force
» Creating emergency and safe resources for the victim
» Cultural sensitivity (diversity) training
» Mental health services

Questions that are crucial in obtaining important information from a screening examination of a suspected trafficking victim include:

» Can you leave your job or situation if you choose?
» Can you move about freely?

» Have you been threatened if you tried to leave?

» Have you been physically or sexually harmed?

» Has your family been threatened?

» Has your identification been taken away?

» Where do you sleep?

» Do you have enough food to eat or water to drink?

» Are you afraid to leave?

» Are you being forced to do anything that you do not want to do? (U.S. Department of Health and Human Services, 2010)

Needless to say, these questions must only be asked if the suspected victim is alone — and you have resources to assist him or her. A healthcare provider must exhibit cultural sensitivity to the anxiety regarding not only hearing these questions but responding as well. Safety is a primary concern; if the person is returning to the situation, this could put him or her at greater risk. Ideally, a person who speaks the person's language should conduct the interview; once the door is open, the person is most vulnerable and must be protected. There are many screening tools available from various government sources, such as the U.S. Department of Health and Human Services.

Documentation

It is essential that we document any and all pertinent information about any patient that we treat — even those who leave before treatment, as long as we have at least minimal information. This is particularly true in the case of victims or suspected victims of trafficking. Not only is this important for follow-up medical treatment (if the person is able to return) but it is also important for legal issues as well as data collection regarding the incidence or magnitude of this issue. Documentation alerts the next provider and establishes directions for training and the development of resources.

International Response to Human Trafficking

Since human trafficking involves the movement of humans across borders, it is a major concern for the international community. As with other types of organized crime, the human trafficking business has gone global. The human trafficking industry has become big business, with the value of illicit human trafficking estimated at $32 billion. About $10 billion is derived from the initial sale of individuals, with the remainder representing the estimated profits from the activities or goods produced by the labor of the trafficking victims (UNODC, 2007). Markets have expanded from regional areas to encompass multiple countries.

There are many causes that enable and support the trafficking of human beings. The human trafficking phenomenon of the 20th and 21st century can be linked to certain supporting factors. The explosion of the human population, from 2 billion to almost 7 billion since 1960, linked to civil unrest, disease, natural disasters, kleptocratic governments, etc., dissolves opportunities leading to extreme vulnerability in a percentage of the population. The third factor that is necessary for slavery to exist is the absence of law and order. When corruption within the police force is prevalent, the strong can take advantage of the weak and harvest them into slavery.

For the individual who is enslaved, it is often the safety and health of her family that convinces her to take the offer of a job from a stranger who arrives in the community.

Not until she is far away and completely isolated does she realize that she has lost her free will to leave. This story is similar to what slavery has been in the past, but another new phenomenon today involves the collapse in the price of humans. Due to the population explosion, the price of humans dropped from $40,000 over the past 4,000 years to $90 on average today (Bales, 2010).

The United Nations' *Protocol to Prevent, Suppress and Punish Trafficking in Persons, Especially Women and Children*, supplementing the UN Convention against Transnational Organized Crime in November 2000, has been adopted by many countries in an effort to create laws in which to investigate, prosecute, and punish criminals involved in human trafficking.

The United Nations' Office on Drugs and Crimes (UNODC) has set forth a protocol that provides a mandate for the "increase in the level of protection and assistance provided to victims of human trafficking crimes" (UNODC, 2007, Articles 2[b], 6, 7, and 8). According to the UNODC, the protocol serves as a major source for eliminating human trafficking. The assistance provided to countries who adopt the protocol includes the following:

» Assisting the review and revision of domestic legislation concerning assistance and protection of victims
» Training criminal justice practitioners and service providers on protection of victims of trafficking in persons
» Supporting countries in the provision of physical, psychological, and social assistance to the victims, including cooperation with Non-Governmental Organizations (NGOs) and civil society
» Securing the safety of victims

Response of the Legal System

Trafficking in persons is a worldwide enterprise that is perpetrated in every country around the globe. It is perpetrated by organized criminals and also by less formalized criminal networks, as well as small groups and individuals. In its *Trafficking in Persons: Global Patterns*, the United Nations Office on Drugs and Crime (UNODC) listed 127 countries as source countries from which victims were trafficked, 95 transit countries through which victims were trafficked, and 137 destination countries where human trafficking victims end up and are exploited (UNODC, 2006b). The UNODC and U.S. Department of State (in its *Trafficking in Persons Report*, 2010) both describe various types of groups and individuals perpetrating transnational trafficking in persons ranging from groups of traffickers who are highly organized and coordinated and are illegally trafficking other goods such as drugs and weapons to those operations that are much smaller and loosely connected (UNODC, 2006b; U.S. Department of State, 2010).

Trafficking in persons seems to most typically be perpetrated in conjunction with other crimes that seriously jeopardize public safety. In their comprehensive survey of U.S. law enforcement agencies, Farrell, McDevitt, and Fahy (2008) noted that 92% of U.S law enforcement agencies report a connection between trafficking and other crimes, including kidnapping, unlawful confinement, rape, forced abortion, assault, torture, murder, prostitution, drug trafficking, document forgery, immigration violations, money laundering, tax evasion, public corruption, fraud, theft, seized documents, and extortion. Clearly, comprehensive and coordinated law enforcement and prosecutorial responses are needed. The authors also note, however, that most law enforcement agencies were not equipped to handle this issue, as of the time of their survey, in terms of available policies and procedures, training, and the establishment of officer assignments and units.

As noted previously in this chapter, traffickers target victims and achieve and maintain control over their victims through force, deception, threats, coercion, and physical violence. Although some cases of trafficking in persons begin as human smuggling cases where the victim agrees to be brought across country borders illegally, or even with victims entering a country illegally only to be forced or coerced into a trafficking situation after that point, most often traffickers transport victims across borders illegally and often by using force, guile, or deception. Trafficking victims may be kidnapped or fooled by false promises about the job that awaits them at their destination. Victims' identity documents are often confiscated.

The Trafficking Victims Protection Act and Related Law and Policy

The **Trafficking Victims Protection Act** of 2000 (TVPA) signaled a new era in law, policy, and enforcement in the United States. The TVPA provides a comprehensive and victim-oriented approach to combating trafficking in persons. There is an important focus on law enforcement and prosecution to disrupt and dismantle trafficking operations, but the victim-centered perspective contained in the law recognizes the importance of rescuing victims in the short term and providing longer-term assistance to trafficking victims, including the potential to obtain permanent resident status in the United States. Victims of human trafficking are viewed as just that—victims—and not the perpetrators of crime (as was a common misconception in the past). Victims must have suffered severe harm and also must cooperate with law enforcement and prosecution to obtain continuing presence in the United States and apply for permanent residency (Trafficking Victims Protection Reauthorization Act of 2005). Federal grant funds distributed by the Office for Victims of Crime and the Bureau of Justice Assistance, both U.S. Department of Justice agencies, and the U.S. Department of Health and Human Services provide for both coordinated task forces and related victim support and services for identified trafficking victims. Sigmon (2008) describes the underlying approach that created these coordinated and cross-disciplinary team approaches to address trafficking:

> The victim protection and assistance measures outlined in the *TVPA* address many of the special issues faced by foreign national victims of trafficking in the U.S. without proper documentation. The U.S. experience with trafficking victims has shown that their needs are unique depending upon their experience and situation, but their fundamental rights as crime victims were established in law long before the *TVPA*. The crime victims' movement in the U.S. is more than three decades old and has prompted the enactment of thousands of federal and state laws that enumerate crime victims' rights. Today crime victims' rights and services are a recognized part of the criminal justice process. Law enforcement and prosecutors' offices employ victim assistance coordinators to provide information, referrals, and assistance to crime victims. Moreover the Federal Crime Victims' Fund has provided crucial financial support (exceeding one billion dollars) for thousands of non-governmental organizations that provide direct services to victims of violent crime. This strong foundation of victims' rights contributed significantly to the creation of a victim-centered approach to combating trafficking (Sigmon, 2008, p. 250).

Major initiatives addressing this issue, particularly focused on the global level, are provided through the State Department's Office to Monitor and Combat Trafficking in Persons (the TIPS Office). The annual *Trafficking in Persons Report* (TIP Report) is a significant product of this work, along with many millions of dollars in grant funding provided to governments and nongovernmental organizations around the world.

The TIP Report assesses the status of approximately 1,450 countries and rates them on essentially a four-point scale. The report also contains country narratives that describe the particular situation in each country and discuss their contributions as a source, transit, or destination country. This assessment can either assist a country in obtaining assistance or result in the potential for sanctions against the country.

The State Department's TIP Report rates countries, including the U.S. in terms of a tier system, to quote the report:

The Tiers

Tier I

Countries whose governments fully comply with the Trafficking Victims Protection Act's (TVPA) minimum standards.

Tier 2

Countries whose governments do not fully comply with the TVPA's minimum standards, but are making significant efforts to bring themselves into compliance with those standards.

Tier 2 Watch List

Countries whose government do not fully comply with the TVPA's minimum standards, but are making significant efforts to bring themselves into compliance with those standards, AND:

(A) The absolute number of victims of severe forms of trafficking is very significant or is significantly increasing;

(B) There is a failure to provide evidence of increasing efforts to combat severe forms of trafficking in persons from the previous year; or,

(C) The determination that a country is making significant efforts to bring themselves into compliance with minimum standards was based on commitments by the country to take additional future steps over the next year.

Tier 3

Countries whose governments do not fully comply with the minimum standards and are not making significant efforts to do so (U.S. Department of State, 2010, p. 47).

The United States Department of State rated the U.S. government's performance as being in Tier 1, the highest rating, and justified this rating decision in its country description. Although not without its difficulties in terms of implementation, the U.S. government has adopted an abolitionist perspective on human trafficking, changed laws and procedures, and provided many millions of dollars in funding and technical support both domestically and globally since the TVPA was passed in 2000.

The TVPA provides a mechanism whereby identified victims can be provided with the immediate rescue assistance they need, and then, at the request of law enforcement and prosecution, provided with continuing presence in the United States while the case is being investigated and prosecuted. After this, temporary resident status can be granted, and after a 3-year waiting period, permanent residence may be applied for (with assistance

HHS Tracking Number
000000 00000

NAME OF ADULT
c/o. ADVOCATE
ADDRESS
CITY, STATE, ZIP CODE

CERTIFICATION LETTER

Dear NAME OF ADULT:

This letter confirms that you have been certified by the U.S. Department of Health and Human Services (HHS) under section 107(b) of the Trafficking Victims Protection Act of 2000. With this certification, you are eligible for benefits and services under any Federal or State program or activity funded or administered by any Federal agency to the same extent as an individual who is admitted to the United States as a refugee under section 207 of the Immigration and Nationality Act, provided you meet other eligibility criteria. Certification does not confer immigration status.

Your certification date is **MAY 25, 2002**. The benefits outlined in the previous paragraph may offer assistance for only limited time periods that start from the date of this certification. Therefore, if you with to seek assistance, it is important that you do to as soon as possible after receive of this letter.

You should present this letter when you apply for benefits or services. **Benefit-issuing agencies must** call the toll-free trafficking verification line at 1 (866) 401-5510 to verify the validity of this document and to inform HHS of the benefits for which you have applied.

You must notify ORR of your current mailing address. Please send a dated and signed letter with any changes of address to: Trafficking Program Specialist, Office of Refugee Resettlement, 5th Floor West, 570 L 'Enfant Promenade, SW, Washington, DC 20447. We will send all notices to your current mailing address and any notice mailed to your current mailing address constitutes adequate service. You may also need to share this same information with state and local benefit-issuing agencies.

Sincerely,

Director
Office of Refugee Resettlement

Figure 17-1   TK

provided by a nonprofit agency). In order to obtain services and assistance though the TVPA, the victim must be officially certified as a victim of a severe form of human trafficking. A letter such as that reproduced in **Figure 17-1** is sent to the victim to confirm this certification has been provided.

T Visas

The T visa is available for victims of severe forms of trafficking. **Table 17-1** contains the number of T-visa applications, denials, and approvals for 2005–2009, according to the U.S. Citizenship and Immigration Service, Department of Homeland Security's January 26, 2010, National Stakeholder meeting.

It is important to note in a forensic nursing context the connection between prostitution and sexual exploitation, which has been central to the United States' approach to combating human trafficking, according to Sigmon (2008).

TABLE 17-1   Number of T-Visa Applications, Denials and Approvals (2005–2009)

Fiscal Year	I-914 T Visa		I-914 T Visa (Immediate Family Members)	
	Approvals	Denials	Approvals	Denials
2005	113	321	73	21
2006	212	127	95	45
2007	287	106	257	64
2008	243	78	228	40
2009	313	77	273	54

Source: Adapted from U.S. Citizenship and Immigration Services (2010). http://www.uscis.gov/portal/site/uscis/menuitem.5af9bb95919f35e66f614176543f6d1a/?vgnextoid=74adc3531a176210VgnVCM10000008 2ca60aRCRD&vgnextchannel=994f81c52aa38210VgnVCM100000082ca60aRCRD.

The U.S. policy was expressed in a national security directive announced by the White House in early 2003: "Prostitution and related activities, which are inherently harmful and dehumanizing, contribute to the phenomenon of trafficking in persons, as does sex tourism, which is an estimated $1 billion per year business worldwide."(Office of the Press Secretary, 2003) This position is consistent with the *Protocol to Prevent, Suppress and Punish Trafficking in Persons, Especially Women and Children,* .... Article 9.5 of the *Trafficking Protocol* includes demand reduction as a key component of preventing human trafficking. It says that all party states shall adopt measures "to discourage the demand that fosters all forms of exploitation of persons, especially women and children, that leads to trafficking" (Sigmon, 2008, p. 251).

In discussing the appropriate legal framework to combat human trafficking, the TIP Report (U.S. Department of State, 2010) provides a useful distillation of the key components for good laws to combat human trafficking:

What Makes a Good Trafficking in Persons Law?
Throughout the last decade, most of the world has developed new legislation to conform with the Palermo Protocol. In so doing, many countries have looked to other countries' existing laws, model laws offered by the United Nations and other international organizations or donor governments, and advice from anti-trafficking experts in crafting legislation most appropriate for their legal systems and cultures. This diversity in contextual factors prevents the development of detailed language that would apply to all countries. Some basic principles can and should be considered as best practices in designing legislation to fight modern slavery (U.S. Department of State, 2010, p. 13).

See **Box 17-1** for an outline of what makes a good anti-trafficking law.

Box 17-1   Anti-trafficking Law

A good anti-trafficking law should include the follow:

- *A broad definition of the concept of "coercion" that covers its many manifestations in modern forms of slavery, including the threat physical, financial, or reputation harm sufficiently serious to compel a reasonable person to perform or to continue performing labor or services in order to avoid incurring that harm.*
- *A well-articulated definition of trafficking that facilitates effective law enforcement and prosecutorial responses and allows for the collection of meaningful data. The*

definition should incorporate all forms of compelled service in addition to forced prostitution. The definition should not simply criminalize the recruitment or transportation of prostituted persons. The definition should not include related but distinct crimes, such as alien smuggling or prostitution.

- *A mechanism of care provided to all suspected victims of trafficking through which they have the opportunity to access basic services- including shelter, food, medical care, psycho-social counseling, legal aid, and work authorization.*
- *Explicit immigration relief for trafficking victims, regardless of their past legal status, and relief from any legal penalties for unlawful activities committed by victim as a direct result of their trafficking.*
- *Specific protections for child victims of trafficking ensuring a responsible chain of custody and a priority placed on the best interests of the child in all decisions made in providing services to them.*
- *Explicit provisions ensuring identified victims have access to legal redress to obtain financial compensation for the trafficking crimes committed against them. In order to be meaningful, such access must be accompanied b options to obtain immigration relief. Trafficking victims should not be excluded from legal services providers who can assist with these efforts, whether NGOs or government program.</BL>*

Source: U.S. Department of State, 2010, p. 13.

Responding to Human Trafficking

Given this backdrop, there has been much progress in the area of combating human trafficking since the TVPA was passed and related international protocols were endorsed. Much of this has come in the form of collaborative responses that have teamed enforcement and victims' assistance perspectives. An excellent summary of these various efforts is contained in the annual attorney general's report to Congress on human trafficking, *Attorney General's Annual Report to Congress and Assessment of U.S. Government Activities to Combat Trafficking in Persons Fiscal Year 2009* (U.S. Department of Justice, 2010).

Major examples of this are the U.S. Department of Justice's Bureau of Justice Assistance and Office for Victims of Crime task forces that exist now in approximately 40 jurisdictions. According to the Bureau of Justice Assistance's website, by June 30, 2008, the then-42 Bureau of Justice Assistance/Office for Victims of Crime-funded task forces had identified 3,336 persons as potential victims of human trafficking and had requested either continued presence or endorsed T-visa applications for 397 of those potential victims. The task forces also trained 85,685 law enforcement officers and others in identifying the signs of human trafficking and its victims. Currently the Bureau of Justice Assistance, in coordination with Office for Victims of Crime, is funding these task forces. (See http://www.ojp. usdoj.gov/BJA/grant/httf.html.)

The map in **Figure 17-2** indicates where these task forces have been funded. A total of 42 task forces have been funded, but it appears that there were 40 task forces operating as this book was in press.

These task forces require both the law enforcement and prosecutorial side and the victims' assistance side to work together to collaborate on interventions that result in both good investigations and, when victims are identified, that immediate rescue services be

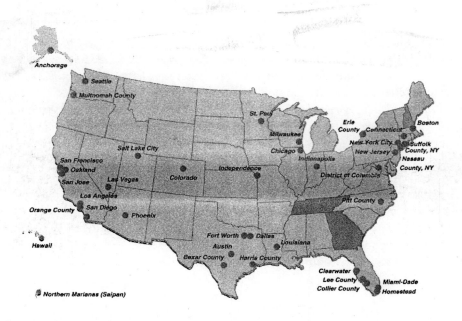

Figure 17-2 Funded task forces in the United States.

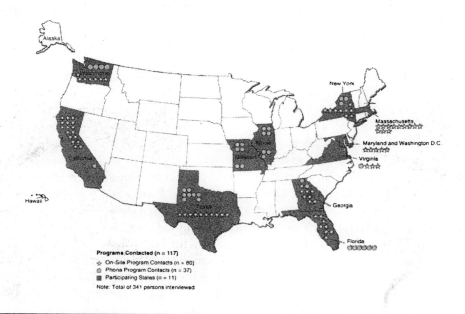

Figure 17-3 Program locations funded by the United States Department of Health and Human Services.

provided for victims when the traffickers are arrested. Moreover, longer-term victim assistance is provided through cooperating services agencies.

Another important effort is that provided with funding from the U.S. Department of Health and Human Services. The map in **Figure 17-3** indicates where many of these programs are located.

The Department of Health and Human Services also funds the National Human Trafficking Resource Center through the Polaris Project, where a hotline is housed (http://www.polarisproject.org), as well as public awareness campaigns, training, and other program activities. Other resources include the HHS Campaign to Rescue and Restore Victims of Human Trafficking (http://www.acf.hhs.gov/trafficking) and HHS's specific information for healthcare providers (http://www.acf.hhs.gov/trafficking/campaign_kits/index.html#health).

Issues in Victim Identification and Assistance

The focus of the underlying TVPA law as it is effectuated through the agencies funding these and other programs is to recognize the difficulties in identifying and serving hidden victims. As discussed previously, there are many disincentives and obstacles for trafficking victims to access services. Sigmon (2008) listed these in her experience at the State Department as follows (there is greater detail in the original article):

> (1) Trauma, (2) Fear for Their Physical Safety or the Safety of Their Loved Ones; (3) Mistrust of Those in Power and Others; (4) Fear of Being Arrested and Deported; (5) Cultural and Linguistic Barriers; (6) A Lack of Public Awareness about Trafficking; (7) A Lack of Awareness Among Allied Professionals; (8) A Lack of Training and Procedures for Identifying Trafficking Victims; (9) Difficulty Differentiating Human Smuggling from Human Trafficking; (10) Governments Often Approach Victim Assistance in a Reactive Manner; (11) Insufficient Resources to Investigate and Prosecute Traffickers and Assist Victims (p. 253–255).

Victims' vulnerabilities contribute to what the TIP Report refers to as the supply chain, where the commodity is comprised of human beings. The TIP Report provides a nice synopsis of the methods and measures that are required to break this supply chain by addressing the barriers to victims' accessing services **(Box 17-2)**.

Box 17-2   Breaking the (Supply) Chain

With the majority of modern slaves in agriculture and mining around the world, and forced labor prevalent in cotton, chocolate, steel, rubber, tin, tungsten, coltan, sugar, and seafood, it is impossible to get dressed, drive to work, talk on the phone, or eat a meal without touching products tainted by forced labor. Even reputable companies can profit from abuse when they do not protect their supply chain—whether at the level of raw materials, parts, or final products—from modern slavery.

Consumer spending and corporate investment in business are leverage points that can turn around a system that has for too long allowed traffickers and economies to operate with impunity. There is an increasing push for consumer transparency, certification, and more rigorous regulation.

Research suggests companies investing in fair labor practices and labeling their products accordingly improve conditions on the ground and drive up the demand for, and price of, their product.

A new paradigm of corporate accountability is emerging demanding companies cast their attentions beyond the places where their product are produced or processed, such as apparel factories and seafood processing shops, to places where the raw materials are collected, harvested, or mined.

Human trafficking is a crime and no level of corporate best practices can replace a government responsibility to prosecute and protect victims. Still, verifiable corporate policies prohibiting the use of forced labor through the supply chain all the way down to raw material are a critical prevention tool.

Key principles in setting supply chain standards:

- *Statements of corporate policy must incorporate truly independent verification.*
- *While remediation is important, when labor abuses rise to the level of a human trafficking offense, authorities should be notified.*
- *Government must redefine norms and set standards to create a space for companies to take the lead on combating modern slavery.*
- *Lending institutions should consider establishing whether a company has a forced labor supply chain policy as a factor for determining that company's credit rating.*

There is no way to effectively monitor a supply chain without tracing it all the way down to raw materials. Such research will lead to an understanding of supply and demand factors used to encourage greater protections of the workers whose labor contributes to downstream profits.

Modern slavery exists in diverse areas, including manufacturing, harvesting of raw materials, and the market for commercial sexual activities so often aimed at the business traveler. In this environment, companies should stuff and source their supply chains in a manner decreasing the demand traffickers so often satisfy through violence. To that end, companies should adopt policies that commit to:

- *Taking accountability for all that labor in the supply chain all the way down to raw material, with a pledge to monitor compliance, remediate noncompliance, and verify those actions by an independent third party;*
- *Honoring the role and voice of the worker as the best check on abuse;*
- *Publicly disclosing mechanisms for providing independent, unannounced, and thorough audits;*
- *Providing effective whistleblower and complaint procedure;*
- *Providing clear guidelines for security procedures throughout the supply chains to ensure that security forces are not used to intimidate, hold, or abuse workers;*
- *Regularly updating shareholders and stakeholders on creation, maintenance, and implementation of their related policies;*
- *Guaranteeing all workers mobility by strictly forbidding any confiscation of official documents;*
- *Committing to providing restitution for victims and other forms of remediation;*
- *Complying with trafficking related local laws and international standards for confronting human trafficking and protecting victim; and,*
- *Holding employees accountable for any violation or exploitative conduct contributing to trafficking in persons.*

Source: U.S. Department of State, TIP Report, 2010, p. 30.

Law Enforcement and Prosecutorial Responses

The passage and reauthorization of the TVPA and the related foundational international conventions and protocols have engendered a significant amount of law enforcement and prosecutorial activity each year. In general, investigations, arrests, and prosecutions are increasing in the United States and worldwide. For example, in the *Attorney General's Annual Report to Congress and Assessment of U.S. Government Activities to Combat Trafficking in Persons Fiscal Year 2009* (U.S. Department of Justice, 2010), federal law enforcement and prosecutorial efforts were summarized as follows and as in **Table 17-2**:

> During FY 2009, ICE initiated 566 cases with a nexus to human trafficking, a substantial increase over FY 2008. These investigations led to 388 criminal arrests, more than double the number of arrests from the previous fiscal year, resulting in 148 indictments and 165 convictions (p. 44).

Internationally, the State Department's TIP Report summarized international law enforcement and prosecutorial efforts in this way:

> The Trafficking Victims Protection Reauthorization Act (TVPRA) of 2003 added to the original law a new requirement that foreign governments provide the Department of State with data on trafficking investigations, prosecutions, convictions, and sentences in order to be considered in full compliance with the TVPA's minimum standards for the elimination of trafficking (Tier I). The 2004 TIP Report collected this data for the first time. The 2007 TIP Report showed for the first time a breakout of the number of total prosecutions and convictions that related to labor trafficking... (U.S. Department of State, 2010, p. 45).

The numbers of total prosecutions and convictions related to labor trafficking are shown in parentheses in **Table 17-3**.

TABLE 17-2   Attorney General's Annual Report to Congress and Assessment of U.S. Government Activities to Combat Trafficking in Persons Fiscal Year 2009

Fiscal Year	Investigations	Arrests	Indictments	Convictions
2005	274	101	58	10
2006	299	184	130	102
2007	348	164	107	91
2008	432	189	126	126
2009	566	388	148	165

Source: U.S. Department of Justice, July 2010, http://www.justice.gov/ag/annualreports/tr2009/agreport humantrafficking2009.pdf

TABLE 17-3   Global Law Enforcement Data on Trafficking Prosecutions and Convictions (Numbers in Parentheses indicate prosecutions and convictions related to labor trafficking)

Year	Prosecutions	Convictions	Victims Identified	New or Amended Legislation
2004	6,885	3,026		39
2005	6,593	4,766		41
2006	5,808	3,160		21
2007	5,655 (490)	3,427 (326)		28
2008	5,212 (312)	2,983 (104)	30,961	26
2009	5,606 (432)	4,166 (335)	49,105	33

Despite these significant efforts, the TIP Report also noted many obstacles and issues that hinder our progress in combating trafficking in persons and summarized these in a list **(Box 17-3).**

Box 17-3   10 Troubling Government Practices

1. *Complicity of law enforcement officials in trafficking offenses.*
2. *Legal and administrative penalties imposed on trafficking victims as a direct result of their enslavement, including, but not limited to, penalties for engaging in prostitution or immigration offenses.*
3. *Guest worker programs giving sponsors or employers inordinate power over migrant workers' legal status and basic freedoms and denying victims any ability to make a complaint.*
4. *Lack of meaningful legal alternatives to the involuntary repatriation of victims.*
5. *Trade policies and agreements/regimes that fail to safeguard against forced labor exploitation, particularly when involving states that have a poor record of addressing labor exploitation.*
6. *Barrier to citizenship. Without birth certificates, national identification cards, or other identity documents, stateless persons and some indigenous groups are vulnerable to being trafficked.*
7. *Bilateral labor agreement between source and destination governments that allow employers to confiscate/withhold travel documents and allow summary deportation of workers without trafficking victim protections.*
8. *Lack of education available to women, girls, and other populations, which blocks them from mainstream economic advancement and leaves them vulnerable to trafficking.*
9. *Internal migration controls. When populations within a country can move within the country's borders only with special permission, they often turn to the underground economy, where traffickers flourish.*
10. *Clumsily conceived antitrafficking activities, such as wholesale raids of worksites or brothel districts without initial investigation to determine whether trafficking is occurring, or of the suspension of emigration or immigration or other activities (in the name of fighting trafficking) for an entire country or nationality.*

Source: U.S. Department of State 2010 (31) p. 31.

Summary

In this chapter we have attempted to identify and address the crisis of Human Trafficking. This egregious violation of Human Rights has been "under the radar" in this country until recently. As healthcare providers we may be the only hope of rescue for these unfortunate victims. Identification may be difficult; however, the indicators that may raise one's index of suspicion have been carefully outlined, and the legal resources identified. Cultural and language barriers are formidable obstacles to overcome, and further, there are challenges due to the fear and mistrust of the victim. The tools and resources described will enhance assessment and perhaps freedom from slavery.

QUESTIONS FOR DISCUSSSION

1. What is human trafficking?
2. Why does it occur?
3. How serious is this problem?
4. What are the forms of human trafficking?
5. How can the victim be identified
6. Once identified, what is the next step?
7. What resources are available?
8. What are the cultural constraints that may deter disclosure?

REFERENCES

Bales, K. (Speaker). (2010, March). How to combat modern slavery: Ideas worth spreading [video]. TED. Retrieved from http://www.ted.com/talks/kevin_bales_how_to_combat_modern_slavery .html

Farrell, A., McDevitt, J., & Fahy, S. (2008). Understanding and improving law enforcement responses: Responses to human trafficking. Washington, DC: Institute on Race and Justice.

Gemmell, N. (n.d.). Human trafficking: The effects of modern day slavery on the global economy. Retrieved from: http://www8.georgetown.edu/centers/cndls/applications/postertool/index .cfm?fuseaction=poster.display&posterID=1752

International Labor Offices. (2005). A global alliance against forced labor. Report I (B) International Labor Office, Geneva. Retrieved from http://www.ilo.org/wcmsp5/groups/public/@ed_norm/@ declaration/documents/publication/wcms_081882.pdf

International Convention for the Suppression of the Traffic in Women and Children, 1921.

Kangaspunta, K. (2010, November 14). A short history of trafficking in persons. Freedom From Fear Magazine. Retrieved from http://www.freedomfromfearmagazine.org/index.php?option=com_ content&view=article&id=99:a-short-history-of-trafficking-in-persons&catid=37:issue-1&Itemid=159

Office of the Press Secretary. (2003). Trafficking in persons national security presidential directive. The White House.

Sigmon, N. J. (2008). Combating modern-day slavery: Issues in identifying and assisting victims of human trafficking worldwide. Journal of Victim and Offenders, 3, 245–257.

Trafficking Victims Protection Act of 2000. Div A of Public Law No. 106–386 § 108, as amended.

Trafficking Victims Protection Reauthorization Act of 2005. PL 109–164.

United Nations. (2000). Protocol to prevent, suppress and punish trafficking in persons, especially women and children, supplementing the United Nations. Convention against Transnational Organized Crime. Retrieved from http://www.unodc.org/documents/treaties/UNTOC/ Publications/TOC%20Convention/TOCebook-e.pdf

United Nations Office on Drugs and Crime. (2006a). Toolkit to combat trafficking in persons. New York, NY: Author.

United Nations Office on Drugs and Crime. (2006b). Trafficking in persons: Global patterns. Vienna, Austria: Vienna International Centre.

United Nations Office on Drugs and Crime. (2007, March). UNODC perspectives No. 3—The global initiative to fight human trafficking. Retrieved from http://www.unodc.org/newsletter/en/ perspectives/no03/page009.html

U.S. Citizenship and Immigration Services. (2010). USCIS National Stakeholder meeting. Retrieved from http://www.uscis.gov/portal/site/uscis/menuitem.5af9bb95919f35e66f614176543f6d1a/?vgnex toid=74adc3531a176210VgnVCM100000082ca60aRCRD&vgnextchannel=994f81c52aa38210Vgn VCM100000082ca60aRCRD

U.S. Department of Health and Human Services. (2010). Look beneath the surface: Role of health care providers in identifying and helping victims of human trafficking. Administration for Children and Families. Rescue and Restore Campaign tool kits. Available at: http://www.acf.hhs.gov/trafficking/campaign_kits/index.html

U.S. Department of Justice. (2010, July). *Attorney general's annual report to Congress and assessment of U.S. government activities to combat trafficking in persons fiscal year 2009.* Retrieved from http://www.justice.gov/ag/annualreports/tr2009/agreporthumantrafficking2009.pdf.

U.S. Department of State. (2009, June). *Trafficking in persons report.* Washington, DC.

U.S. Department of State (2010). *Trafficking in persons report.* Washington, DC: Foreign Policy Association.

SUGGESTED FURTHER READING

Bales, K. (2005). *Understanding global slavery: A reader.* Los Angeles: University of California Press.

Bales, K., & Soodlater, R. (2009). *The slave next door.* Los Angeles: University of California Press.

Cullen-Dupont, K. (2009). *Global issues: Human trafficking.* New York, NY: Infobase Publishing.

Fernando, B. (2005). *In contempt of fate.* Merrimack, MA: BeaRo Publishing.

Kristof, N., & WuDunn, S. (2009). *Half the sky.* New York, NY: Alfred A. Knopf.

U.S. Department of Justice (2007). *Trafficking in persons: A guide for non-governmental organizations.* Washington, DC: Civil Rights Division.

CHAPTER 18

Sexual Assault Intervention and the Forensic Examination

Patricia LaMonica and Elaine M. Pagliaro

Sexual assault is one of the most frequently committed crimes in the United States and has the highest annual victims' costs, estimated at $127 billion per year. Although sexual assault most frequently happens to females, males may also be sexually assaulted. The role of the sexual assault forensic examiner is multifaceted and encompasses a wide array of client needs following a sexual assault, such as providing medical and/or nursing care to the client while performing forensic procedures that include objective documentation, which may be utilized in a legal setting at a future date. By providing expert care and information to the client throughout the exam, the forensic examiner allows opportunities for the client to make informed decisions about his or her care, and thus begin the healing process.

CHAPTER FOCUS

» Definitions and Laws
» Effects of Sexual Assault on Victims
» Special Circumstances and Concerns
» Sexual Assault Forensic Evidence Collection

» Drug-facilitated Sexual Assault
» Medical/Legal Examination of Sexual Assault Victims

KEY TERMS

» colposcope
» drug-facilitated sexual assault (DFSA)
» forensic evidence
» prophylaxis
» rape

» rape trauma syndrome
» sexual assault
» sexual assault crisis service (SACS)
» sexual assault response team
» TEARS

Introduction

Sexual assault is one of the most frequently committed crimes in the United States and has the highest annual victims' costs, estimated at $127 billion per year (U.S. Department of Justice [DOJ], 1994). It has been estimated that as many as one in every three women and one in every five men is at risk of being sexually assaulted at some point during their lifetime (Federal Bureau of Investigation [FBI], 2009). That abuse is often perpetrated by close family members, friends, or adults in positions of authority. Various studies have shown that approximately 60–80% of assailants are known to their victims. Riggs, Houry, Long, Markovchick, and Feldhaus (2000) studied the cases of 1,076 sexual assault victims and found that 61% of the victims knew their assailants. Statistics also indicate that *date rape* (assault by a known social acquaintance) occurs to approximately one out of every six college women. One of the most startling aspects of sex crimes is how many are unreported. According to recent Justice Department statistics, only 55% of rapes and sexual assaults were reported to law enforcement officials (U.S. DOJ, 2010). When sexually abused children in grades 5 through 12 were questioned, 48% of the boys and 29% of the girls did not tell about their abuse, not even to a friend or sibling (Commonwealth Fund Survey of the Health of Adolescent Girls, 1998). Common reasons given by victims for not reporting these crimes include guilt, self-blame, the belief that the abuse is a private or personal matter, and that they fear reprisal from the assailant.

Sexual assault is a violent crime most frequently perpetrated against women (Aiken, 1993). That violence is not committed for sexual gratification, but rather is usually a sexual expression of aggression. Often the focus of a sexual assault involves power and control for the assailant (Burgess & Holmstrom, 1974). Further discussion of the relationship between violence and sexual assault may be found in Chapter 9. The effects of sexual violence on victims and their families or significant others can be devastating. All are impacted in some way—psychologically or physically—and these effects can last a lifetime.

CASE STUDY 18-1

Carol

As a freshman at a state university, Carol was sometimes overwhelmed. She did not have many friends in her dorm, so she was particularly pleased when two of the students across the hall invited her to their party. The girls were juniors and seemed very popular. Carol waited until there seemed to be a good crowd and went across the hall. After a while she felt a little woozy, even though she had only consumed two beers. Michael, a boy from the second floor, offered to help her back to her room. He had been really nice during the first few weeks of school so Carol was happy to have his help. Michael walked Carol back to her room, closed the door, and proceeded to help her to the bed. When Carol protested Michael assured her it was fine. At the bed, he pushed Carol down and proceeded to pull at her clothing. Carol tried to protest, but felt dizzy and couldn't seem to get any strength behind her protests. Several hours later Carol awoke with her pants off and her shirt pulled up. She remembered nothing after getting back to the room. When Carol's roommate came in at 2:00 a.m. she urged Carol to go to the hospital for an exam. It took several hours, but finally Carol agreed to go to the clinic, where the nurse talked to Carol about the incident. Eventually, Carol agreed to an exam. Even though several hours had passed, the nurse took samples for a toxicology test in addition to other samples in the evidence kit.

Because Carol sought medical assistance, the lab was able to obtain sufficient evidence from the kit to show the presence of semen. When Michael was accused of raping Carol, he claimed Carol consented to, in fact initiated, sex after they left the party. The nurse's complete documentation of Carol's condition, her bruises, and statements about the incident were key in the case prosecution, especially since the toxicology findings were negative.

The Sexual Assault Forensic Examiner

The role of the sexual assault forensic examiner (SAFE) is multifaceted and encompasses a wide array of patient needs after a sexual assault. Often the examiner meets multiple needs of the patient simultaneously, providing medical and/or nursing care to the patient while performing forensic procedures along with objective documentation that may be utilized in a legal setting at a future date. Patients may seek assistance by entering the system with the chief complaint of rape or sexual assault, or at times, the sexual assault examiner may discover that the patient has been sexually assaulted through assessment findings, when the patient has entered the system for an entirely different reason. Clients may also enter the healthcare system as a result of victim conduct or through referrals from other sources, such as ruling out child abuse that may include sexual assault. Thus, it is essential that assessments of those clients be holistic in nature, such that the client is able to disclose when a sexual assault has occurred.

The role of the sexual assault forensic examiner as described by the International Association of Forensic Nurses (IAFN) addresses the comprehensive needs of the patient (IAFN, 1996). The practice includes assessment, evaluation, diagnosis, and implementation of comprehensive care designed to restore and promote the bio/psycho/social health of the client, which is the primary focus of the examiner. As part of this process, the forensic examination may consist of the following:

1. Obtaining the history of the assault
2. Providing crisis intervention
3. Obtaining the history of the patient's pertinent health issues
4. Performing a physical exam and assessment with a focus on inspection and evaluation of the forensic evidence of the body
5. Collecting forensic evidence
6. Treating and/or referring the client for subsequent medical treatment
7. Documenting all findings objectively
8. Interacting with clients in an objective and neutral manner that promotes informed decisions related to the available treatment options and the collection of forensic evidence

The forensic examiner is uniquely qualified to fulfill these requirements for a comprehensive examination. Studies have shown that when evidence is collected by trained sexual assault forensic examiners, it is more likely to have been collected thoroughly and properly and maintained appropriately (Sievers, 2003).

Definitions

An understanding of the legal definitions of rape and sexual assault and of the physical and psychological effects of sexual assault on the client are essential if the sexual assault forensic examiner is going to meet the immediate and long-term complex needs of the client. Both the definition and legal implications of rape or sexual assault vary from state to state. Historically the term **rape** has been used primarily to connote the sexual assault of a female by a male (other than her husband), usually involving vaginal penetration by the assailant's penis. Rape is currently considered forced sexual intercourse that includes both psychological coercion and physical force. Forced *sexual intercourse may involve vaginal,* anal, or oral penetration by a body part such as a penis or finger, or by a foreign object such as a bottle. More recently the term **sexual assault** has been used interchangeably with the term *rape* and refers to both male and female victims of any age. Sexual assault is often defined as any type of sexual activity or act performed without a person's consent. *Consent* is considered a cooperative act of free will and can be granted only when a person is able to provide consent. In most circumstances, an adult of a statutorily specified age who is of sound mind may provide consent. By law, depending on the state the assault occurred in, people may not be considered capable of providing consent due to their age (minors), cognitive impairment (such as being under the influence of a drug or alcohol), or disability (such as being comatose). Sexual assault includes a wide range of victimizations, distinct from rape or attempted rape. These crimes include completed or attempted attacks generally involving unwanted sexual contact between the victim and offender. Sexual assaults may or may not involve force and include such acts as grabbing or fondling. Additionally, there are common informal subclassifications of rape or sexual assault that include the following:

» *Acquaintance rape:* Unwanted sexual contact or activity performed by someone known by the victim (accounting for 75–85% of sexual assaults)
» *Date rape:* Unwanted sexual contact or activity performed by someone with whom the victim is in a dating relationship
» *Drug-facilitated rape:* The use of drugs, both legal and illegal, by a potential rapist who sedates the victim prior to unwanted sexual contact or activity
» *Incest:* Sexual contact or activity performed by someone who is related to the victim
» *Statutory rape:* Sexual contact or activity performed with a minor (age determined by law) by someone who is older by a specific number of years (age determined by law)
» *Spousal or partner rape:* Unwanted sexual contact or activity with one's spouse or partner

Each sexual assault classification is defined by statute and differs slightly from state to state. For example, the definition of statutory rape may vary in the age of the victim or number of years' difference between the perpetrator and the victim.

Effects on Victims of Sexual Assault

The effects of sexual assault can be devastating to its victims and victims' families in a multitude of ways, and its consequences may produce both physical and emotional sequelae. Those close to the victim of sexual assault can also experience feelings of rage, helplessness, and vulnerability, and may also benefit from intervention. Not all victims will present with physical injury or obvious signs of trauma. It is essential for the forensic examiner to be aware of the potential psychological effects of sexual assault, which can be far-reaching but may not be immediately evident. Individual emotional styles of clients lead to different reactions to the stress of sexual assault. Other factors affecting responses of the client include age, coping skills, culture, gender, and support systems (Ledray, 1990).

In 1974, Burgess and Holmstrom studied the emotional effects of sexual assault on victims. The cluster of emotions or emotional responses that are specific to the extreme stress surrounding sexual assault was designated **rape trauma syndrome** by these authors. This response is very similar to posttraumatic stress disorder, which is experienced by victims who are exposed to other types of extreme stressors, such as war. Rape trauma syndrome can be divided into two phases—the acute phase and the reorganizational phase (Burgess

& Holmstrom, 1974). The acute phase may occur immediately or within a short period of time following the assault. During the acute phase the victim experiences a period of disorganization. The victim's observable reaction may vary from no apparent response to being completely out of control. The specific response depends on the emotional style of the client and other influences. Although the victim is dealing with the immediate trauma of the sexual assault, he or she may also experience a variety of somatic symptoms, such as gastrointestinal problems, genitourinary problems, difficulty sleeping, or hypervigilance. According to Burgess and Holmstrom, victims also experience a wide gamut of feelings. The range of responses can include fear, guilt, humiliation, embarrassment, and self-blame. Fear of physical violence including death was the primary feeling described.

The second stage of rape trauma syndrome includes a period of reorganization. It is during this period that the victim attempts to gain mastery of the event. These attempts may include changing address, changing telephone numbers, leaving school or a job, or changing/ending relationships. It is important to note that some victims of sexual assault, for a variety of reasons, may be at high risk for depression, suicide, or inappropriate/dangerous behaviors during this time. The process of coping with the assault may begin at various times for each individual.

Understanding the potential effects of sexual assault on clients should enhance the forensic examiner's ability to communicate with them. This understanding can be beneficial to both the client and his or her intimate circle. Because of his or her unique training and experience, the forensic examiner can provide the client and others with educational and anticipatory guidance. Interactions that the examiner has with the client may positively impact the recovery phase of the client and others because it enables those individuals to regain hope for the future and a return to the previous level of functioning or better. Not all clients will agree to further intervention in an attempt to regain control.

Special Circumstances and Concerns

Sexual assault is a crime that affects all socioeconomic, cultural, ethnic, and religious groups. These differences may affect the manner in which the client responds to the assault and to the subsequent forensic and medical examinations. When the sexual assault forensic examiner is aware of the effect these parameters may have on the client and his or her perception of the process, modifications in language or actions should be made to make the client more comfortable with the forensic examiner and the examination process. Several circumstances that should involve special consideration include the age of the client (children, the elderly, and adolescents), any client disability, the client's gender, and the sexual orientation of the client.

Age is a critical consideration when dealing with a client who has been sexually assaulted. The client's age may affect his or her ability to describe the incident, relate symptoms, and understand the examination process as it proceeds. In addition, age will likely impact the client's response to the assault as well as the legal implications of that attack. Elderly clients often experience extreme humiliation, shock, and disbelief similar to that of other victims of sexual assault. In addition, the elderly may be acutely aware of their vulnerability and mortality as a result of the assault (Commission on the Standardization of the Collection of Evidence in Sexual Assault Investigations, 2010). Elderly victims of sexual assault may also experience more extreme physical injuries because they generally are physically more fragile or may be suffering from age-related conditions. Some studies support that postmenopausal women who have been sexually assaulted sustain more genital trauma than younger victims (Ramin, Satin, Stone, & Wendel, 1992). The recovery process for the elderly can be lengthier than for other victims due to their lack of resilience. Additionally, they may experience feelings of loss of independence and self-reliance or experience overwhelming shame and guilt (Girardin, Faugno, Senski, Slaughter, & Whelan, 2002). Recovery is dependent on nurturing and sensitive, appropriate interventions by significant others with counseling geared toward the needs of the older client. The older client also may require more frequent medical follow-up. Most states currently have mandatory reporting for the abuse of the elderly, including sexual assault.

The special needs of children who are victims of sexual assault are well documented. Although it is difficult to obtain true figures of the rate of child sexual assault, most authorities agree that there is widespread underreporting. Additionally, research shows that exposure as a child to sexual behaviors may be linked to early onset of sexual activity and increased sexual vulnerability in adolescence, including an increased risk for sexual revictimization (Fergusson, Horwood, & Lynskey, 1997). A study by Fergusson and colleagues demonstrated a higher rate of teenage pregnancy, early onset of sexual activity, unprotected intercourse, and sexually transmitted diseases in women who reported childhood sexual assault as compared to women who were not assaulted as children.

Many children are abused in various ways over long periods of time. As a result, the collection of **forensic evidence** may not be possible at the time of the exam, especially in cases where the child is under 12 years of age. Most jurisdictions have detailed guidelines for the pediatric physical examination, and the forensic examiner should always proceed according to those guidelines. In general, however, additional support personnel including parent or guardian, child advocates, or other professionals should assist the SAFE, when appropriate, to obtain the child's medical history (Adams, Harper, Knudson & Revilla, 1994; New Hampshire Sexual Assault Protocol Revision Committee, 1998; State of Connecticut Supplemental Guidelines, 1998). Because statistics have shown that the offender is often a family member or close acquaintance whom the child trusts, the examiner should interview the child away from any potential offender. Children require special interview techniques to obtain clear, objective history, so the interview should be performed by a specially trained interviewer whenever possible. Additionally, specialized equipment may be needed for the physical examination.

As with all other clients, the sexual assault forensic examiner should take the time necessary to explain procedures to the child victim and to reassure the child as much as possible during the examination. It may be helpful to the examiner to utilize a developmental staging tool such as the Tanner Scale, which stages out female and male reproductive development to assist with further medical treatment and care.

Female adolescents are especially at risk for vaginal injury and for acquiring a sexually transmitted infection (STI) because they may be physiologically more susceptible, depending upon their developmental stage.

Special concerns also exist regarding clients with physical, mental, or communicative disabilities. These people may have limited cognition or difficulties that impair their perceptual abilities. These difficulties may cause clients to be frightened, unsure of exactly what occurred during the assault, or unable to understand that they have been a victim of a crime (American College of Emergency Physicians, 1999; Commission, 2010). As with the pediatric population, assaults within this population may go undetected for a long period of time because the offender is often a family member or a caretaker (Haddix-Hill, 1997). If speech or other communication appears to be difficult, the SAFE should make every opportunity to obtain the proper assistance in the form of an interpreter or electronic communication device. Most protocols recommend that victims with disabilities and their circle of support be given the highest priority. Extra time must be taken with the disabled client to communicate effectively during the examination process and to understand the questions or concerns of the client. Ideally, the interviewer has received specialized training regarding interviewing techniques in order to obtain a clear and objective history of the assault. The examiner may need to assist the patient in assuming the necessary positions for complete forensic collection and medical examination. Reporting of sexual abuse of disabled persons is mandated in every state.

Gays and lesbians comprise another population that requires special considerations. As with other victims of sexual assault, there is often a resistance to report the sexual assault due to a fear of judgment by the police but also due to potential rejection from the gay community. Contrary to common public opinion, both gays and lesbians are more frequently assaulted by heterosexual males. The exam process is similar to that for heterosexual victims; however, the forensic examiner should be sensitive to their special needs, and counseling is best done by someone from the gay community whenever possible.

Many experts believe that sexual assaults of males are among the least reported of any group (U.S. Department of Justice, Bureau of Justice Statistics, 2010). Men commit most of the sexual assaults of boys, male adolescents, and adult men. It is not uncommon for the male victim to have multiple assailants and to have a high degree of nongenital trauma. In fact, males often seek medical attention for physical injuries and initially only disclose the physical assault. An awareness of this fact allows the forensic examiner to investigate further whether the male was sexually assaulted.

Male victims demonstrate the same responses to sexual assault as discussed previously. The male victim will have additional concerns about his inability to protect himself and his maleness, and may feel less masculine (Girardin et al., 2002). The extent to which male victims attempt to control their environment after a sexual assault may cause them to be less communicative during the medical examination and the collection of forensic evidence. Men may be less willing to discuss in detail the types of abuse they have suffered, which makes it more difficult to obtain appropriate forensic samples and to provide the necessary health care. The male victim may be embarrassed or concerned that the examiner or the police will question his masculinity. Sensitivity to these concerns on the part of the forensic examiner can often help to obtain an objective and clear history and may lead to obtaining appropriate forensic evidence.

The Forensic Examination

It is critical that the forensic examiner maintain an objective and neutral approach during the examination and subsequent interaction with the client. Initial contact should occur in an environment that is both private and comfortable for the client. Adequate time for explanations of care and forensic procedures is critical; clients should not be rushed through the exam. The client should understand all that is about to occur and be given the opportunity to refuse those procedures with which he or she does not feel comfortable. Knowing that exams can be refused meets some of the client's need to assume some control of the situation after the assault and also provides education to allow the client to make informed decisions about care (Hampton, 1995).

Initial Considerations

Prior to starting the examination, the sexual assault forensic examiner should bring the client into a private location and establish a rapport with the client utilizing a neutral and objective approach. Whenever possible, clients should be interviewed alone at some point to avoid inadvertently being questioned in the presence of the offender, as in the case of a child. Also, prior to starting the exam, the assistance of the local **sexual assault crisis service (SACS)** should be offered. Its services are invaluable to both the client and the examiner. For the client, the SACS counselor can become a long-term connection to counseling and legal advocacy. SACS often serves as a lifeline for any needed future assistance. Generally, its services are free of charge and available 24 hours a day, 7 days a week. The SACS counselor assists the forensic examiner by providing support to the client during the physical examination and the evidence collection process. This allows the examiner to focus on the actual exam, evidence collection, and documentation. Should the client choose not to have a SACS counselor present at the time of examination, local SACS information should be provided to the client at discharge so that the client has the option of calling at a later date. In addition, if the client wishes to have another person present during the examination, those wishes should be respected. It may take some time to establish rapport with the client and to provide the desired people for support during the process. However, the forensic examiner will be able to conduct a more thorough examination and to provide better care for the client if the necessary time is spent prior to initiating the actual examination process.

The SAFE should begin by explaining what she is planning to do and allow the client to control the speed of the exam and participate by selecting the order of the exam, whenever possible. The client always maintains the right to refuse any part or parts of the exam, and this should be explained to the client before any action is taken and prior to each step in the process, thus allowing the client to make informed decisions. The examination must be done in a nonhurried way and allow opportunity for explanations and education by the SAFE. In addition, the client must have ample opportunity to ask questions throughout the examination. The client should also be told that he or she may stop the exam at any time.

The examiner should obtain a detailed history of the assault from the client, documenting on the medical record or other examination documentation form (see **Figure 18-1**). The SAFE should quote the client's own words as much as possible. This history should include all events surrounding the assault, where the sexual assault occurred, and when it occurred. A critical factor in sexual assault prosecution is often consistency between the assessment findings and the history of the sexual assault as related by the patient. Thus, no detail provided by the client should be omitted from the history, no matter how insignificant it may initially appear. The examiner should also obtain a health history from the client that includes current medical problems and a listing of medications that the client is taking, including when the client last took the medications. During the initial stages of the exam, the SAFE should determine if the client wishes to report the assault to the police, if he or she has not already done so. The examiner should be familiar with the mandatory reporting requirements independent of the client's consent. If the SAFE is required by statute to report the sexual assault to law enforcement, this fact and the reasons for the report should be explained to the client. These laws vary from state to state. However, one law that appears to be consistent throughout the United States requires that sexual assaults of a minor be reported to the police. Reporting may also be mandated with other populations, such as mentally handicapped persons, elders, and victims of assaults that include the use of a firearm.

STATE OF CONNECTICUT
SEXUAL ASSAULT MEDICAL REPORT
(Additional writing space provided in Section 9, if needed.)   CG819e-112a

HEALTH CARE FACILITY: _____

1. CHIEF COMPLAINT: _____

A. Date and Time of Arrival _____
                                 Month   Day   Year   Time

B. Date and Time of Assault _____
                                 Month   Day   Year   Time

2. MEDICAL HISTORY AS RELATED BY PATIENT:

A. History of Assault: _____

_____

_____

_____

_____

_____

_____

_____

_____

_____

_____

B. Nature of Sexual Assault:

	Contact By	Penetration By	Ejaculation
	Penis Hand Oral Other Unsure	Penis Hand Oral Other Unsure	Yes No Unsure
Mouth:	☐ ☐ ☐ ☐ ☐	☐ ☐ ☐ ☐ ☐	☐ ☐ ☐
Breasts:	☐ ☐ ☐ ☐ ☐	☐ ☐ ☐ ☐ ☐	☐ ☐ ☐
Vagina:	☐ ☐ ☐ ☐ ☐	☐ ☐ ☐ ☐ ☐	☐ ☐ ☐
Penis:	☐ ☐ ☐ ☐ ☐	☐ ☐ ☐ ☐ ☐	☐ ☐ ☐
Anus/Rectum:	☐ ☐ ☐ ☐ ☐	☐ ☐ ☐ ☐ ☐	☐ ☐ ☐
Other:	☐ ☐ ☐ ☐ ☐	☐ ☐ ☐ ☐ ☐	☐ ☐ ☐

(specify): _____

C. Between the assault and present has the patient: ☐ douched

☐ wiped/washed off   ☐ rinsed mouth   ☐ defecated

☐ bathed/showered   ☐ brushed teeth   ☐ vomited

☐ changed clothes   ☐ ate or drank   ☐ urinated

(specify): _____

D. Nature of Physical Assault (specify, e.g., struck, bit, choked, etc.):

_____

_____

_____

_____

_____

PATIENT STAMP (If handwritten, record name, unit number and birth date.)

E. Did assailant: Use lubricant?   ☐ Yes ☐ No ☐ Unsure
              Use condom?   ☐ Yes ☐ No ☐ Unsure
              Insert foreign object(s)? ☐ Yes ☐ No ☐ Unsure

(specify): _____

                                                    Yes No Unsure
F. Was the patient menstruating at the time of assault?.... ☐ ☐ ☐

If yes, is tampon present? .... ☐ ☐ ☐

G. Any additional physical injuries? .... ☐ ☐ ☐

If yes, describe: _____

_____

If yes, any bleeding? .... ☐ ☐ ☐

H. Any injuries to assailant resulting in bleeding? ...... ☐ ☐ ☐

If yes, describe: _____

_____

3. PAST MEDICAL HISTORY:

A. Any sexual intercourse in the last 72 hours? .... ☐ ☐ ☐
If yes, type: ☐ Vaginal ☐ Anal ☐ Oral ☐ Other
If yes, date:_____ time:_____
Was condom used? .... ☐ ☐ ☐

B. Is contraception used? .... ☐ ☐ ☐
If yes, type:_____
C. Last menstrual period: _____
Is the patient pregnant? .... ☐ ☐ ☐
If yes, duration of pregnancy:_____

D. Additional medical history: _____

_____

_____

_____

_____

_____

Sections 1, 2 & 3 completed by _____

Figure 18-1   Victim interview and initial examination documentation sheet.

Although some clients access the system immediately following a sexual assault, many victims of sexual assault initially experience a sense of disbelief or shock, which delays access to any form of assistance. Often the victim will not go directly to a hospital or police department, but will shower or bathe or tell a friend or family member of the assault. The timing of an official report is critical because it will determine if a sexual assault evidence kit should be used. In general, forensic evidence collection is most useful within 72 hours of the sexual assault. After 72 hours, most of the physical evidence useful to confirm the crime or identify the assailant has been lost, especially if the client has showered or bathed.

Adult patients may refuse forensic evidence collection with a sex crimes kit for a variety of reasons. These reasons include fear of retaliation by the perpetrator, embarrassment, and cultural influences, as mentioned previously. Depending upon the state in which the assault occurred, a sexual assault evidence kit may be used only if the assault is reported to law enforcement. Other states, however, allow for the collection and storage of the evidence for the statute of limitations, allowing the client to revisit the decision not to make an official complaint. Those states provide an option of allowing a patient to have forensic evidence collected using a sex crimes kit that can be entered anonymously for a period of time; the client can then take more time to make a decision concerning the filing of an official complaint. In these delayed reporting situations, the evidence will be given a specific code and then transported to the police or laboratory to maintain the appropriate chain of custody. This holding procedure benefits those patients who are ambivalent about the legal aspects of the assault. The forensic examiner should help the client make informed decisions about reporting the crime by providing information about the use of the evidence and related matters. Clients should also be informed of the potential loss of some types of forensic evidence due to delays in collection. It is important to keep in mind, however, that even if a forensic evidence collection kit is not used, the medical record of the client may provide evidence of the assault through the accurate documentation of the assessment findings.

Collection of Forensic Specimens

Before beginning the physical assessment, all equipment that the examiner needs for the examination should be available in the room. The ideal situation is to collect forensic evidence simultaneously with the medical specimens during the physical assessment. Usually, the examiner should perform any procedures for medical management of the patient after forensic and medical specimens are collected. All forensic evidence collected should remain in full view of the examiner and never be left unattended, to maintain an intact chain of evidence.

If the patient chooses to have forensic evidence collected, a sex crimes kit may be used. Kits vary from state to state depending on what types of analyses are recommended by the forensic laboratory of that jurisdiction. **Figure 18-2** shows a typical sexual assault evidence collection kit. Most kits are designed to provide the examiner with the materials to collect and preserve samples in an appropriate manner. These kits also allow for flexibility in specimen collection, based on the client's wishes and the history of the sexual assault. The examiner should assure that the kit is fully sealed and has not been opened prior to being used. Before opening the examination materials, the SAFE should put on latex or nitrile gloves. The examiner should remain gloved during the examination, changing into new gloves as necessary to avoid contamination of the forensic specimens. Some examiners use an alternate light source or an ultraviolet Wood's lamp, if this is the only light source

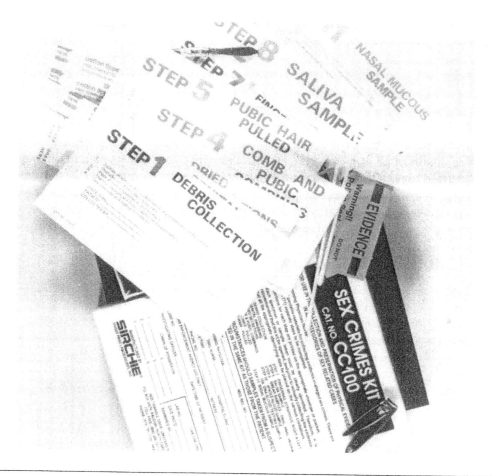

Figure 18-2   Typical sexual assault evidence collection kit and contents.

available, to perform a cursory inspection of the client's body. Body fluids such as semen appear fluorescent in that light and may provide the examiner with an additional site for forensic specimen collection.

The following paragraphs outline a suggested sequence for the examination of the client and the collection of forensic evidence using a standardized sex crimes kit. Many variations in these procedures exist, although the Department of Justice (2004) has supported the formulation of national guidelines for the collection of sexual assault evidence. Often the examination is performed from the least invasive to most invasive procedure, or from external to internal examinations. Forensic evidence collected during this examination includes materials used as standards for comparison, samples used to prove that a sexual assault occurred, and specimens that may be linked to the perpetrator(s) of the crime. Those items that may be included in the forensic evidence collection include the following: blood from the client; fingernail scrapings/cuttings; hair from the client's head; oral swabs and smears; dried secretions found on parts of the body other than the genital area; pubic hair combings; pubic hair of the client; genital swabbing; vaginal swabs and smears; anal swabs and smear; and any other physical evidence that may be evident, such as a condom, tampon, or debris on the patient.

Fingernail scrapings and cuttings may provide trace materials or tissue/blood samples of the perpetrator. If the forensic laboratory conducts hair analyses, hair from both the head and pubic area are used in comparison to other hairs collected as evidence, such as in the pubic combings. Oral, anal, and vaginal swabs and smears are collected to identify seminal fluid or spermatozoa; if semen is found, DNA analysis may be conducted on those samples. Similarly, dried secretions collected from other parts of the victim's body, such as from bite marks, may be used to identify the perpetrator.

The forensic examiner may be able to obtain only an incomplete history of the sexual assault as the client may not recall portions of the assault or may be too embarrassed to provide details of all aspects of the assault. For example, older women often may be too embarrassed to relate that the assault included oral penetration. Therefore, it is important that the sexual assault forensic examiner perform a thorough physical assessment to identify any injuries and collect all significant forensic specimens, even if not indicated by the history at the time of the initial examination.

Steps in Evidence Collection

The following steps for sample collection are presented in a common sequence, based on the recommendations of several states. The exact order in which samples will be collected from the client will depend on the type of evidence, the guidelines of the locality in which the examination takes place, the physical and emotional condition of the client, and any particular requirements based on the assault history. Any procedures used by the sexual assault forensic examiner should be flexible enough to satisfy the legal requirements for evidence admissibility and the forensic requirements for evidentiary analysis while addressing the concerns and health needs of the client during the examination.

1. ***Clothing.*** The first step in the examination is usually the collection of clothing. Before the client undresses, the examiner should determine if the client is still wearing the clothing that he or she had on during the sexual assault. If the client has not changed clothing, these items should certainly become part of the evidence collected with the client's consent. In addition, even if the client has changed clothing since the assault, the forensic examiner may choose to collect the underpants if there was a vaginal or anal assault or if the victim did not bathe prior to changing clothes.

   Before the client undresses, the examiner should place a paper sheet from the sex crimes kit on the floor. The client should stand on this paper while he or she removes each item of clothing. Standing on the paper will catch any debris, such as fibers or vegetation, that may fall off the clothing during the disrobing process. As each item of clothing is removed, it is placed in a separate paper bag. Each bag is sealed and clearly marked with the contents, the patient's name, the date and time of collection, and the examiner's name. In general, the examiner should not remove any substances from the clothing prior to packaging. The location of material or the pattern of deposits may be significant forensic information that can be used during analysis or during the trial. Rather, when necessary, the forensic examiner should assist the client while he or she is taking off clothing to prevent loss of these types of physical evidence. Only if there is danger of evidence being lost or destroyed when the client disrobes should the examiner remove and package appropriately any loose materials. If the foreign material is removed from an item of clothing, the examiner should note in detail the location and amount of that sample.

When collecting clothing from a male victim, the forensic examiner should take every precaution to prevent contamination of any body fluids with those that may have originated from the client. For example, the underwear of a male victim may contain semen from the client that should be kept away from areas that may represent seminal deposits of the assailant; paper between the folds of the clothing may help to prevent this cross-contamination.

After all of the clothing is removed, the paper on which the client is standing should be carefully folded, so evidence is not lost or contaminated, and it should be properly packaged.

Clothing should be packaged in folded paper or paper bags. Paper bags are preferable to plastic bags or containers because plastic promotes mold and bacterial growth that can cause deterioration of the evidence. Any wet items of clothing should be air dried whenever possible prior to packaging. If items are soaked with blood or body fluids and they cannot be air dried, those items may be placed temporarily in a plastic bag; however, if this occurs, the examiner should turn over the evidence as soon as possible to law enforcement for further drying or transport to the forensic laboratory. If a wet item has been placed in plastic, the SAFE should draw attention to this fact by placing prominent stickers or notations on the outer packaging. A liquid biohazard or wet designation alerts the police or the laboratory that special handling of this type of evidence is required.

2. ***Known Specimens for DNA Comparison.*** Collection of known blood specimens is often the next step in the examination process. Collection of blood at this time provides the opportunity to process specimens and to obtain results that are required for medical treatment before the end of the examination. Blood specimens needed for forensic DNA analysis should also be collected at this time. DNA testing protocols recommend the use of a purple-cap tube containing ethylenediaminetetraacetic acid (EDTA) to collect blood. Client-identifying information should be placed on the blood tube, along with the name of the person collecting the sample, the date, and the time.

Because only a small amount of sample is required for DNA analysis utilizing current standard procedures, some states collect buccal swab samples as standards for DNA analysis instead of blood samples. If buccal swabs are used, the known DNA standard from the client must be collected so that there is no possibility of contamination by other swabs or fluids from the kit or persons at the time of collection. Buccal swabs for DNA standards should be collected after all other evidence has been collected from the oral cavity, and the victim should rinse thoroughly with distilled water prior to sampling the buccal epithelial cells.

3. ***Debris and Foreign Material.*** Examination of the client often reveals the presence of blood, semen, or saliva on the body in various locations. These body fluids are the most common secretions deposited by the assailant, although urine and feces may also be encountered. When these foreign materials are observed, the sexual assault examiner should collect each foreign sample using a sterile swab. The swab should be moistened with a minimum of sterile water for collection and allowed to air dry before packaging. In addition to body fluid deposits, debris and other materials that can be associated with the scene of an assault or with the perpetrator of the crime may be noted. This debris may include vegetative material, fibers, soil, hairs, or other types of trace material. For example, in one case, after a woman was sexually

assaulted in a vehicle, fine metal shavings were collected from her hair by the SAFE. When a suspect was identified, both his car and his garage work area contained metal shavings determined to be of the same composition and appearance. Traditionally, examiners used an ultraviolet Wood's lamp to examine the client for evidence of these materials. Other alternate light sources are now available at a relatively low cost and have been shown to be more effective in identifying body fluids or small samples of fibers or other trace evidence that should be collected.

Bite mark evidence is one of the more common situations in which foreign body fluids, usually saliva, may be found. Bite marks are seen on clients who are the victims of sexual assault and other violent crimes. When bite mark evidence is recognized, it is important that the evidence in this area be processed prior to cleaning the wound. After appropriate photographic and written documentation of the bite mark are completed, the saliva should be collected. It is important to use a minimal amount of sterile water on the swab when collecting from this area. The bite mark should be gently swabbed, rotating the swab and applying light pressure during collection; the SAFE should concentrate on areas along the inner arch of the bite mark. Use of too much force when swabbing bite marks may result in a sample that contains too little foreign material in relation to the amount of client cells, often leading to an inconclusive DNA profiling result.

4. *Fingernail Scrapings and Clippings.* Fingernails may be important specimens, especially if they contain biological material such as tissue or trace evidence from the assailant or crime scene. Factors that will determine whether fingernail scrapings should be taken include the amount of time since the assault, whether the client has bathed or washed his or her hands since the assault, and the history of the incident. Some protocols advise taking scrapings and clippings even if the client has no specific memory of scratching the perpetrator. The forensic examiner should obtain the client's permission before clipping fingernails.

5. *Known Hairs From the Client.* If the forensic laboratory conducts microscopic hair analysis, known head and pubic hairs should be collected from the client at the time of the examination. This step is usually carried out after pubic combings are collected from the client. The pubic combings will be examined at the laboratory to determine if any hair evidence was transferred from the assailant during the incident. The recommended method of hair collection differs among jurisdictions. These various methods reflect some of the different philosophies among **sexual assault response teams**, sexual assault counselors, and laboratories. Some procedures recommend that no hairs be collected at the time of the examination; those protocols often state that known hairs can be collected at a later date if foreign hairs are identified in the other evidence. Scientifically, this is the least desirable situation because of the physical and microscopic differences that can occur in the hairs, even over a short period of time. It is important to collect contemporaneous hair samples for analysis because of the effect that time, diet, stress, physiological or physical conditions, and other factors can have on the morphological characteristics of hairs.

After conducting hair comparisons, scientists are only able to determine whether a hair is similar and could have originated from an individual, dissimilar to hairs from an individual, or whether the comparison is inconclusive. Microscopic hair comparisons do not serve as a positive means of individualization. Because of the limitations of this type of analysis, some experts recommend that only combed hairs be obtained as standards and that pulled hairs be collected at a later date, only when necessary. Those forensic nurse examiners believe that the potential for pain that pulling hairs may cause the patient outweighs the limited evidentiary value of pulled hair specimens. However, opponents of obtaining only combed hairs point out that there is no way to associate definitively the source of those hairs in a combing—a comb will collect telogen (about to be shed) hairs from the client as well as any loose hairs transferred from the assailant during the incident. A mixture of hairs may be present in the combing that can present difficulty during legal proceedings. If, during laboratory examination, the hairs are found to be microscopically dissimilar to the victim, the laboratory should conduct mitochondrial DNA analysis for comparison to the suspect in a case. Clearly, there is a need to associate or exclude questioned hairs in a forensic sample.

One compromise, which allows the collection of an identifiable standard while preventing any further trauma to the client, is to cut known hairs at the skin line. This method provides the entire length of the hair for microscopic examination but employs a painless collection process. Another approach is to have the patient pull his or her own head or pubic hairs. This method often reduces the client's embarrassment and the trauma of collection. Hairs should be cut or pulled as standards from various areas of a particular location to obtain a random sample of hairs that represent the various types of hair in the region. For example, hairs should be collected from the top, back, front, and sides of the client's head. The total number of hairs recommended varies, but ranges from 20 to 100 total hairs. The sexual assault forensic examiner should follow the specific recommendations of the state protocols or the healthcare facility or state when collecting hair samples.

6. *Swabs and Smears.* It is important to take swabs from each body orifice to collect evidence of penetration in the sexual assault. When collecting samples, the sexual assault forensic examiner should take every precaution to prevent contamination of the swabs with other samples or secretions. It is usually recommended that swabs and smears from the mouth, vagina/penis, and anus be collected, even if the client does not relate during the examination that such contact took place. However, as stated previously, if the client insists that he or she does not want a sample collected, that refusal should be honored. Swabbing of the mouth, vagina, and/or anus and the smears made from those swabs will be checked for the presence of spermatozoa or seminal fluid. If identified, DNA analysis can be conducted in an effort to individualize the source of that semen. If no semen is identified, condom lubricants may be detectable on the swabs. Penile swabbing of the male victim may reveal the presence of saliva on the penis that could indicate oral–genital contact. In some cases, such as the statutory sexual assault of a boy, the penile swabbing may be checked for the presence of vaginal epithelial cells and a female DNA profile.

Sterile swabs should be moistened with a minimum of sterile distilled water before swabbing the area being examined. Since swabs may be tested for the presence of condom lubricants and trace material, the forensic examiner should wear only nonlubricated, powder-free gloves during the swab collection process. Subsequently, the swabs are used to make a smear on a glass slide that will be examined for spermatozoa at the laboratory. The swabs and smears should be air dried before packaging.

The following swabs should be collected:

- Oral swabs should be collected using at least two swabs. Particular care should be taken to swab those areas in the mouth where material, including semen, may become lodged, such as between the gums and lips and in the pockets around teeth.
- Vaginal swabs should be collected without diluting the secretions or aspirating the area. Collection of vaginal swabs should take place after external genital swabs and pubic combings are collected.
- Penile swabs should be collected using light pressure. All outer areas of the penis and scrotum should be swabbed.
- Anal/rectal swabs may be moistened with a small amount of sterile water to reduce the discomfort to the client during swabbing. Whenever possible, avoid heavy deposits of fecal matter on the swab or smear.

7. *Pubic Hair Combings.* Contact between two people will result in the exchange of various materials, depending on the extent and type of contact. During a sexual assault, contact may result in the transfer of hairs, fibers, and other trace materials from the assailant, as well as materials from the crime scene. Combing the pubic area provides for the collection of these trace materials for identification and comparison at the laboratory. The sexual assault examiner should comb the area using a clean comb after placing a specimen envelope or paper under the buttocks. This location for the collection envelope or paper will prevent the loss of trace materials during the combing process. If any clumps of material are noted adhered to the hairs or if there are apparent deposits of semen or other liquid, the SAFE should ask the patient if the hairs in this area can be cut for collection. If the client does not agree to have the hairs cut, the forensic examiner should swab the deposits prior to combing the area.

8. *Genital Swabbing.* The exterior genital area should be sampled using a slightly moistened swab. When swabbing any visible secretions in this area, ensure that all the swab surfaces are exposed to the sample by turning the swab during collection. If the client is female, the vulva and inner thighs should be swabbed, even if no secretions are visible. If the client is male, the SAFE should use one swab to collect samples from the glans and shaft of the penis, a second swab for the base of the penis and the testicles, and a third swab for the thighs.

9. *Additional Evidence, as Noted.* At times there may be additional materials, such as a condom or tampon, that may provide valuable information about the perpetrator or provide evidence of a crime. When such evidence is encountered, that evidence should be collected, appropriately packaged, and included in the sexual assault evidence kit.

Drug-Facilitated Sexual Assault

Since the end of the 1990s information concerning **drug-facilitated sexual assault (DFSA)** has become readily available to the public. Many popular magazines, television shows, and news programs have provided good background on the problem and various ways that potential victims of DFSA can protect themselves. In spite of this awareness, the problem persists, especially among young adult females, and many clients express the fear that they have been the victims of DFSA. Drugs are frequently mixed with alcohol or other beverages to incapacitate the victim. Once the victim recovers from the initial effects of the drug, it may be difficult for her or him to recall the event or any details concerning the assailant. According to Welner (2001), the modus operandi of perpetrators who employ drugs to incapacitate or otherwise affect a chosen victim has four components: means, setting, opportunity, and a plan to avoid arrest and prosecution. As this list implies, there is no one drug, one type of perpetrator, or one situation in which DFSA occurs. Various types of drugs are used, depending on the social setting, access to different drugs by the perpetrator, and the relationship between the victim and the assailant (more opportunities to use a drug will arise when there is a preexisting relationship). Although no one particular group appears to be at risk, studies indicate that there may have been an increased incidence of drug-facilitated sexual assaults among college and university students in the late 1990s (Fisher, Cullen, & Turner, 2000).

A study by ElSohly in 1999 showed the presence of various types of drugs in the urine of more than 2,000 victims who believed they had been drugged prior to a sexual assault. More than 20 different chemical substances were identified in those urine samples, but the most prevalent drug detected was alcohol (ethanol); approximately 40% of the samples tested were positive for this compound. Other common drugs identified in those urine specimens were marijuana, 18%; cocaine, 8%; gamma hydroxybutyrate (GHB), 3%; and flunitrazepam (Rohypnol) 0.3%. Remarkably, tests in more than one third of the urine samples (37%) failed to reveal the presence of *any* drug. However, it should be noted that many of the drugs used in DFSA are quickly metabolized and remain detectable for relatively short periods of time in the blood and urine. If the client delays reporting a DFSA, evidence of the drug may be irretrievably lost.

The identification of alcohol as the most common drug in these urine samples should not be a surprising fact. Alcohol is a legal substance that is readily available and acceptable in most social environments. Alcohol is common at many social gatherings and at parties on campuses around the country. In fact, much of the social contact of university students revolves around alcohol or takes place where alcohol is served. The symptoms of intoxication are well known and include a reduction in inhibitions, decreased motor coordination, reduced ability to think logically, and increased response time. This is the perfect drug for an assailant who can induce his victim to consume a sufficient amount of alcohol to achieve the desired effects.

Symptoms of the use of flunitrazepam and gamma hydroxybutyrate are similar to each other and may last several days. They include drowsiness, lightheadedness, dizziness, fatigue, decreased blood pressure, and memory loss. It should be noted that GBL (gamma butyrolactone), the chemical precursor to gamma hydroxybutyrate, is available in many legal, commercial products, but it is not approved for human consumption (LeBeau, 1999).

Collection of Evidence in Drug-Facilitated Sexual Assault Investigations

In general, the sexual assault forensic examiner should not collect samples for forensic toxicology screening unless the client exhibits symptoms or a history that indicates DFSA or if it is medically indicated. The collection of DFSA evidence should be considered if:

» the patient or companion states that the client was or may have been drugged.
» the client suspects drug involvement because there is no recollection of the event.

» in the opinion of the examiner, the client's medical condition appears to warrant screening for optimal care (i.e., he or she exhibits symptoms consistent with the presence of a drug).

» the amount of time since the alleged incident does not exceed the recommended time for collection. In general, if ingestion was within 72 hours, the collection of toxicology samples is indicated.

Even if these criteria are met, the SAFE should collect a blood or urine sample for forensic toxicology testing only with informed consent from the client. Informed consent requires that the forensic examiner discuss the following information with the client:

» The effects of time since the incident on the ability to detect and identify any drugs that may have been used
» The inability to predict the success of the toxicology analysis
» The fact that toxicology testing is not limited to well-known date rape drugs, but will detect the presence of many other drugs, including legal and controlled substances that the client may have voluntarily ingested
» The negative impact on the criminal investigation of the refusal to undergo testing

Before any evidentiary samples for toxicology testing are collected it is important to thoroughly advise the client of these factors. It is usually a good idea to involve a sexual assault crisis counselor during these discussions. Because of the potential implications and impact of toxicology testing for forensic purposes, most protocols require the client to sign a separate consent form prior to the collection of toxicology samples. **Figure 18-3** shows a typical consent form for toxicology evidence collection.

Collection Procedures

The specific requirements in each state or county may vary, as outlined in the guidelines for toxicology collection established by the healthcare facility in conjunction with the local forensic toxicology laboratory and law enforcement organizations. Guidelines commonly recommend the collection of both urine and blood samples if ingestion occurred within the last 48 hours. If ingestion occurred between 48 and 72 hours prior to the collection, only urine should be collected. Collection of samples for toxicology after 72 hours is not recommended in most circumstances (LeBeau, 1999).

Blood samples should be collected in gray-top vacuum tubes using sterile procedures. Gray-top tubes contain sodium fluoride, a preservative, and potassium oxalate, an anticoagulant. Approximately 10–20 milliliters of blood should be collected. Failure to use a blood tube with the correct preservative may lead to false negative results upon testing. It should be noted that the blood tubes used for DNA testing that are present in the standard sexual assault evidence collection kits contain EDTA and are unsuitable for toxicological analysis. Thus, if there is no standard DFSA kit at the healthcare facility, the sexual assault examiner should obtain the proper tubes from hospital stock.

Urine is collected in a sterile urine collection vessel. Approximately 30–50 milliliters of midstream urine is recommended for toxicology testing. The urine vessel should be placed in a plastic bag that is sealed in a tamper-evident manner.

After the blood and the urine samples are collected, each should be labeled with the client's name and control number, along with the initials of the person collecting the sample, and date and time of collection.

CONSENT FOR TOXICOLOGY SCREEN
CGS19a-112a

PATIENT STAMP (If handwritten, record name, unit number and birth date.)

To Examining Clinician:

Please review information in this form with patient, allowing ample time to discuss any questions the patient may have. It is important that the patient understand all segments of this form prior to signing it. If patient chooses to consent to toxicology screen:

(1) Have patient sign and date the form in the space(s) indicated
(2) Provide your signature and date in the space(s) indicated
(3) Place and maintain this form in patient's medical record

To Patient:

Please read and review all information in this form with the clinician prior to signing it. Please discuss any questions you may have to ensure that you understand all of the information presented. If you choose to consent to toxicology screen, provide your signature and date in the space(s) indicated.

I consent to and authorize the collection of urine and/or blood samples for the purpose of detecting the presence of drugs or other substances that may have caused sedation and/or amnesia in the context of a sexual assault.

I understand that any samples must be obtained within 72 hours of ingestion.

I understand that the toxicology screen may detect any substances, medications or drugs (both legal and illegal) that may be in my system from the weeks prior to the sexual assault.

I understand that the results of the toxicology screen may be very important for the possible arrest and prosecution of the offender.

I have discussed toxicology screen with the clinician and have had an opportunity to ask questions and discuss concerns.

_____   _____
Signature of Patient   Date/Time

_____   _____
Signature of Clinician   Date/Time

Figure 18-3 Specialized consent form for collection of drug-facilitated sexual assault evidence.

Toxicology samples should be appropriately labeled as biohazardous materials and forwarded immediately to the appropriate laboratory for testing. Most healthcare facilities do not have the appropriate equipment or procedures in place for testing of some drugs commonly seen in DFSA investigations. More importantly, the necessary chain of custody must be maintained for the results of the testing to be admitted during a trial; hospitals and other healthcare facilities usually are not equipped to meet the legal requirements for chain of custody and admissibility of toxicology evidence.

Perpetrator Evidence Collection

At times, it is necessary to collect specimens from alleged perpetrators accused of sexual assault. Some states provide a suspect evidence collection kit that is similar to the sex crimes kit used for victims. The evidence often includes the collection of blood, hairs, fingernail scrapings, or other samples for comparison and standards for DNA analysis. Depending on how soon after the assault the perpetrator is apprehended, additional specimens may be collected, such as clothing or swabs, which can be used to search for materials transferred from the victim at the time of the assault. Suspect evidence is collected in a manner similar to that of evidence collected from victims. Documentation should be concise and clear. Because of the rights of the accused, suspect evidence collection takes place only after appropriate consent from the suspect or a search warrant is obtained by law enforcement officers. Proper protocols for the collection and preservation of evidence and proper chain of custody are vital with this evidence. At times, the attorney representing the accused may also request assistance when biological samples are required for defense purposes. The forensic examiner should follow the same type of collection and documentation protocols required when assisting police with evidence collection.

The Physical Examination

Clients entering the healthcare system should be initially examined and treated for life-threatening injuries. It is not uncommon for clients to appear uninjured or to present with minor injuries, such as abrasions or bruises. The physical examination and collection of specimens for medical treatment ideally should be performed at the same time as the forensic examination and collection of forensic evidence.

The forensic examiner will begin the physical examination with a general body survey of the patient. If no critical injury or condition requires immediate attention, the physical examination then proceeds from the least invasive assessment, such as listening to the patient's breath sounds, to more invasive procedures, such as the pelvic exam, while maintaining the privacy and dignity of the client. As previously stated, the use of a Wood's lamp to perform a cursory general inspection of the body may be performed at this time. As the forensic examiner completes each step of the exam, she should clearly, objectively, and thoroughly document all findings. Specific, detailed forms for physical examination documentation are often provided in the sex crimes kit, although this type of form should be used whether utilizing a sex crimes kit or not. These forms provide specific cues to the examiner in addition to diagrams of both the anterior and posterior body and both male and female genitalia to aid in documenting the client's condition and any injuries or other findings noted during the examination. When injuries are identified, complete documentation should include the locations, dimensions, and descriptions of those findings.

The examiner looks for all abnormal findings and may categorize most injuries according to the acronym **TEARS**—tears, ecchymosis, abrasions, redness, and swelling (Slaughter & Brown, 1992). Following this sequence to make observations and notations during the physical examination simplifies and standardizes documentation of injuries. It is critical that the examiner use a point of reference adjacent to the site of the injury to provide the appropriate perspective of size. This reference may be any appropriate scale, such as a tape marked with millimeters or centimeters on it. When making notations during the physical examination, the examiner should state clearly and objectively what was found and should avoid any attribution to the cause of an injury unless readily deduced from the actual observation of the injury. The SAFE should also use consistent terminology in any descriptions throughout the examination process. Careful examination of the oral cavity should be performed, especially if it is reported as a site of assault. Forensic and medical specimens may be obtained at this time.

Patterns of injuries may be determined through examination and description of injuries, such as a circular ecchymotic area, which could indicate a finger imprint or a bite mark pattern. These patterns are important to note because they may provide consistency with the client's history. Photographs of injuries are helpful as they provide a visual document of the injuries. Forensic cameras that have magnifying features are available so that nongenital injuries may be more easily visualized. It is advisable to obtain the client's written consent to use photographs as part of the documentation prior to doing so. Photographs generally remain with the client's medical record, and the number of photographs taken as well as what areas of the body are being photographed should be clearly documented in the record. Each photograph should also be individually identified, along with the client's name, date, time, and name of the examiner. No photograph should ever be discarded, even if not well developed. A system should be developed to maintain the integrity of the photograph, including appropriate storage. If photographs are handed over to law enforcement, a chain of evidence should be maintained. A more detailed discussion of this documentation process may be found in Appendix 4 of this text.

After all areas of the body have been examined, the forensic examiner should then conduct the pelvic and rectal examinations. Only water should be used to lubricate the speculum initially if one is used, so that forensic specimens may be obtained. Following the collection of forensic specimens, a lubricant may be used to conduct the rest of the exam. If available, a **colposcope** may be used for the pelvic exam. The client should be informed of the use of the colposcope as it is a large piece of equipment and may be intimidating to the client. Studies have shown that using the colposcope improves the detection of genital trauma in sexual assault cases, as opposed to a gross visual exam, because it allows magnification of the sites (Slaughter, 1991). A study by Slaughter and Brown (1992) reported that genital trauma or injury visualized with a colposcope was as high as 87%, as opposed to detecting 10–30% with unaided visual examination. If a colposcope is used, it should be noted in the documentation along with the degree of magnification. A stain, such as toluidine blue, can be applied to stain the mucosa, which may enhance the visibility of any injuries (Lenahan, Ernst, & Johnson, 1998). Some colposcopes are equipped to take photographs or videos of genital injuries. If this feature is used, the client should provide written consent. Chain of evidence should be maintained with colposcope photographs, as with other evidence.

A standardized and accepted method of describing the location of injuries in the female genital area is to mentally superimpose the face of a clock over the genital area, with 12:00

at the mons pubis and 6:00 at the perineum (Girardin et al., 2002). Any injuries visualized may then be described on the medical record by using the previously mentioned acronym *TEARS* along with measurements and location within the context of the clock (e.g., a 2-cm tear at 6:00 at the posterior fourchette). Multiple studies have shown the most common location of genital injury in the female client is the posterior fourchette. Slaughter (1997) determined that the most common sites of injury by penile penetration of the vagina included the posterior fourchette, labia minora, hymen, and navicular fossa. Once injuries have been identified, forensic and medical specimens may then be obtained.

The rectal area should also be inspected at this time, along with appropriate specimen collection. Depending upon assessment findings, it may be necessary for the examiner to use an anal scope for better visualization. Superimposing the face of the clock over the anal area can also be helpful in the description of the location of any identified injuries, again using the acronym *TEARS*.

Once the examiner has completed the physical assessment and has obtained appropriate specimens to medically treat the patient and forensic evidence for the sex crimes kit, the topics of **prophylaxis** of both pregnancy and STIs should be discussed. Adults should be allowed to make informed decisions surrounding these issues. The examiner should be aware of any drug allergies or other health issues that the client has at this time. The examiner should also be sensitive to the person's religious and other beliefs and provide factual information to the client. In fact, the religious orientation of the organization in which the client is being treated at times may be a factor in providing pregnancy prophylaxis. (The examiner should have addressed any potential conflicts in this area and developed acceptable protocols prior to providing care to any client.) Generally, pregnancy prophylaxis may be provided when the sexual assault occurred within 72 hours of the exam and the patient has tested negative for pregnancy. Testing can be done with serum or urine. There are a variety of prophylactic medications available, and more recent medications have very few side effects.

Untreated, STIs cause major health problems with far-reaching consequences, with treatment expenses as high as $8.4 billion annually (Reid, 1999). STIs may include gonorrhea, chlamydia, syphilis, human papillomavirus, herpes, trichomoniasis, and bacterial vaginosis, and HIV. The most frequently transmitted include gonorrhea, chlamydia, trichomoniasis, and bacterial vaginosis (Centers for Disease Control and Prevention, n.d.). Factors affecting the transmission of STIs include the type and nature of the assault, the extent of the injuries, number of assaults, multiple perpetrators, susceptibility of the client, and known STI status of the perpetrator(s). This information should be assessed and discussed with the client to determine prophylaxis and follow-up care. Baseline specimens for STIs may be taken during the exam; however, depending upon the timing of the assault, this testing may only provide information related to the client's condition prior to the assault. This fact should be discussed with the adult client.

STI testing is often carried out with children because assaults are generally repetitive and occur over a period of time; however, the type and nature of the assault(s) are taken into consideration, along with the child's presentation.

The decision to obtain specimens for STIs should be made prior to the exam so that the appropriate specimens may be collected at the same time as the forensic evidence collection. For many clients, it is advisable to provide STI prophylaxis at this time because many clients will not continue with follow-up appointments. Ideally, clients should be retested again in 2 weeks regardless of findings to assure that test results remain or become negative for sexually transmitted diseases. Also, testing for syphilis should be repeated 12 weeks after the assault. Many protocols provide for prophylaxis of gonorrhea, chlamydia, trichomoniasis, and bacterial vaginosis following Centers for Disease Control and Prevention guidelines.

Hepatitis B may also be transmitted from a sexual assault. Transmission depends on the nature and type of assault, extent of injuries, and the known hepatitis B infection state of the perpetrator. The clinician should determine whether the client has previously received the hepatitis B vaccination series. Often, administration of the hepatitis B vaccine provides sufficient prophylaxis; however, depending upon the nature of the assault or the infection state of the perpetrator, it may be advisable to administer hepatitis immunoglobulin vaccine. Clients should be referred for follow-up doses as needed.

One of the greatest fears of many clients is the contracting of HIV from a sexual assault. Some studies have indicated that there is generally a low risk of transmission from a single encounter (Giardino, Datner, & Asher, 2003). Like other STIs, however, transmission is dependent upon the type and frequency of the assault (oral, vaginal, or anal), the type of injuries sustained along with exposure to blood and secretions, the presence of other STIs, and if known, the serological and clinical status of the perpetrator (Gostin et al., 1994). Prophylaxis is based upon this risk assessment, and all information should be discussed with the client to provide reassurance and allow for consideration of risks and benefits of prophylactic treatment. It is often considered more appropriate to have a lengthier discussion surrounding baseline testing and/or HIV prophylaxis at a follow-up exam, allowing for more time to weigh the risks and benefits of treatment. Clients, however, should make informed decisions as to how to proceed. In some situations, the forensic examiner may consult with the infectious disease specialist in order to provide the client with specific data related to the nature of the assault and enhance decision making related to testing and prophylaxis. Additional testing may be required at 3 and 6 months postassault.

Following the examination, the patient may be provided a shower and change of clothing, along with something to eat and drink. Specific referrals should be made for medical follow-up, along with individualized needs such as counseling. It is critical that the client be provided with simple discharge instructions that include telephone numbers of identified resources such as the forensic examiner or the investigating officer. Additionally, the client should have an information sheet that describes exactly what was provided to the client at the time of the exam, and what to do next. The examiner should assist the client with discharge to a safe environment, and supportive family or friends to transport the client there. At times, the SACS counselor can assist with these arrangements.

Many states also have an office of victim services that can provide financial assistance for those clients who are victims of a crime and cannot afford ongoing medical or other related expenses. Generally, the only obligation of the client is to file a police report. The SACS counselor can assist the client with completing the forms to apply for reimbursement.

Care of the sexually assaulted client is both comprehensive and lengthy. Based upon the setting that the examiner will be working in, it is advisable to develop protocols in caring for clients that allow specific direction and guidance to simplify the care and direct the examiner as needed. Also, it is helpful to have other specialists available for consultation, such as the communicable disease specialist, to address more complex needs of the client.

Sexual Assault Response Teams

Many communities have started sexual assault response teams that provide a multidisciplinary approach to the client. One of the original sexual assault response team models was developed in California and involved a coordinated response to the needs of the client from the time the client reports the assault, through any services necessary to assist the victim, to the prosecution of the crime. Generally, team members include the SAFE or emergency department medical personnel, law enforcement, prosecutor, and counselor(s). A sexual assault response team may also include other types of professionals who are available as needed, based upon the location and needs of the community or individual client. In some locations, the actual team arrives and works together with the client to provide comprehensive care. Other models involve the team meeting at regular intervals to establish a better understanding of each other's roles, to utilize each other as resources and experts, and to share data to enhance the care provided to all clients.

Summary

The forensic examiner provides a highly skilled level of care from the onset of the client seeking care. He or she provides physical, emotional, forensic, and legal care that continues to benefit the client long after the client has left the examiner.

 QUESTIONS FOR DISCUSSSION

1. What is sexual assault?
2. Who is at risk for sexual assault?
3. What are the consequences of sexual assault?
4. What is the role of the sexual assault forensic examiner?
5. What does the forensic exam involve?

REFERENCES

Adams, J., Harper, K., Knudson, S., & Revilla, J. (1994). Examination findings in legally confirmed child sexual abuse: It's normal to be normal. *Pediatrics, 94*(3), 310–317.

Aiken, M. M. (1993). False allegation. *Journal of Psychosocial Nursing, 31*(11), 15–20.

American College of Emergency Physicians. (1999). Evaluation and management of the sexually assaulted or sexually abused patient. Washington, DC: U.S. Department of Health and Human Services, Health Resources and Services Administration, Maternal and Child Health Bureau, Contract No. 98-0347(P).

Burgess, A. W., & Holmstrom, L. L. (1974). Rape trauma syndrome. *American Journal of Psychiatry, 131*(9), 981–986.

Centers for Disease Control and Prevention. (n.d.). 2002 sexually transmitted disease treatment guidelines. *Morbidity & Mortality Weekly, Report,* 51 (RR06), 1–80.

Commission on the Standardization of the Collection of Evidence in Sexual Assault Investigations. (2010). *State of Connecticut Technical Guidelines for Health Care Response to Victims of Sexual Assault.* Hartford, CT.

The Commonwealth Fund Survey of the Health of Adolescent Girls: Highlights and Methodology. Annual report, 1998. (1999, October). *Juvenile Justice,* VI(I). Retrieved from http://www.ncijrs.gov/pdffiles1ojjdp/178254.pdf

ElSohly, S. J. S. (1999). Prevalence of drugs used in cases of alleged sexual assault. *Journal of Analytical Toxicology, 23,* 141–146.

Federal Bureau of Investigation. (2009). *Uniform crime reports, 2009.* Retrieved from www2.fbi.gov/ucr/cius2009/index.html

Fergusson, D., Horwood, J., & Lynskey, M. (1997). Childhood sexual abuse, adolescent sexual behaviors and sexual revictimization. *Child Abuse and Neglect, 21*(8), 790–803.

Fisher, B., Cullen, F. T., & Turner, M. G. (2000). *Research report: Sexual victimization of college women.* Washington, DC: National Institute of Justice.

Giardino, A., Datner, E., & Asher, J. (2003). *Sexual assault victimization across the life span* (pp. 331–332). St. Louis, MO: G.W. Medical.

Girardin, B., Faugno, D., Senski, P., Slaughter, L., & Whelan, M. (2002). Developing a sexual assault response team. Frankfort, KY: Kentucky Association of Sexual Assault Programs.

Gostin, L., Lazzanini, Z., Alexander, D., Brandt, A., Mayer, K., & Silverman, D. (1994). HIV testing, counseling, and prophylaxis after sexual assault. *Journal of American Medical Association, 271*(18), 1436–1444.

Haddix-Hill, K. (1997). The violence of rape. *Critical Care Nursing Clinics of North America, 9*(2), 167–174.

Hampton, H. (1995). Care of the woman who has been raped. *New England Journal of Medicine, 332*(4), 234–237.

International Association of Forensic Nurses. (1996). *Sexual assault nurse examiner standards of practice.* Silver Spring, MD: Author.

LeBeau, M. (1999). Toxicological investigations of drug-facilitated sexual assaults. *Forensic Science Communications, 1*(1). Retrieved from http://www2.fbi.gov/hq/lab/fsc/backissu/april1999/index.htm

Ledray, L. (1990). Counseling rape victims: The nursing challenge. *Perspectives in Psychiatric Care, 26*(2), 21–27.

Lenahan, L., Ernst, M., & Johnson, B. (1998). Colposcopy in evaluation of the adult sexual assault victim. *American Journal of Emergency Medicine, 16*(2), 183–184.

New Hampshire Sexual Assault Protocol Revision Committee. (1998). *Sexual assault: A hospital protocol for forensic and medical examination* (2nd ed.). Concord, NH: New Hampshire Office of the Attorney General.

Ramin, S. M., Satin, A.J., Stone, I. C., Jr., Wendel, G. D., Jr. (1992). Sexual assault in postmenopausal women. *Obstetrics and Gynecology, 80*(5), 860–864.

Reid, J. (1999). Sexually transmitted disease in the U.S. *ADVANCE for Nurse Practitioners, 7*(8), 45–50.

Riggs, N., Houry, D., Long, G., Markovchick, V., & Feldhaus, K. (2000). Analysis of 1,076 cases of sexual assault. *Annals of Emergency Medicine, 35*(4), 358–362.

Sievers, V., Murphy, S., & Miller, J. (2003). Sexual assault evidence collection more accurate when completed by sexual assault nurse examiners: Colorado's experience. *Journal of Emergency Nursing, 29*(6), 511–514.

Slaughter, L. (1991). Cervical findings in rape victims. *American Journal of Obstetrics and Gynecology, 164,* 528–529.

Slaughter, L. (1997). Patterns of genital injury in female sexual assault victims. *American Journal of Obstetrics and Gynecology, 176*(3), 609–616.

Slaughter, L., & Brown, C. (1992). Colposcopy to establish physical findings in rape victims. *American Journal of Obstetrics and Gynecology, 166*(1), 83–86.

State of Connecticut Supplemental Guidelines. (1998). *Child sexual abuse examination.* Hartford, CT: St. Francis Hospital and Medical Center.

U.S. Department of Justice, Bureau of Justice Statistics. (1994). The cost of crime to victims. *Crime Data Brief.* Washington, D.C.: U.S. Department of Justice.

U.S. Department of Justice, Office of Justice Programs, Bureau of Justice Statistics. (2010). *Criminal Victimization 2009 NCJ 231327.* Washington, D.C.: U.S. Department of Justice.

U.S. Department of Justice, Office of Violence Against Women. (2004). *National Protocol for Sexual Assault Medical Forensic Examinations.* Washington, D.C.: U.S. Department of Justice.

Welner, M. (2001). The perpetrators and their modus operandi. In M. LeBeau & A. Mozayani (Ed.), *Drug facilitated sexual assault* (p. 41). San Diego, CA: Academic Press.

SUGGESTED FURTHER READING

Campbell, R., & Wasco, S. (2005). Understanding rape and sexual assault: 20 years of progress & future direction. *Journal of Interpersonal Violence, 1,* 127–131.

Elis, C. (2002). Male rape: The silent victims. *Collegian: Journal of the Royal College of Nursing Australia, 9*(4), 34–39.

Hazelwood, R., & Burgess, S. (Eds.). (2009). *Practical aspects of rape investigation* (4th ed.). Boca Raton, FL: CRC Press.

Ledray, L. (2010). Expanding evidence collection time: Is it time to move beyond the 72-hour rule? How do we decide? *Journal of Forensic Nursing, 6*(1), 47–50.

Loger, T, Cole, J., & Capillo, A. (2003). Sexual assault nurse examiner program characteristics, barriers and lessons learned. *Journal of Forensic Nursing, 3*(1), 24–34.

Rosay, A., & Henry, T. (2008). *Alaska sexual assault nurse examiner study* (Report 2004-WG-BX-0003). Washington, DC: U.S. Department of Justice. Retrieved from http://www.ncjrs.gov/pdffiles1/nij/grants/224520.pdf

CHAPTER 19

Correctional Nursing

Anita G. Hufft

In a 1979 film from the American Medical Association, Out of Sight—Out of Mind, Dr. Alvin J. Thompson remarked, "Professionalism in medicine depends on our ability to provide quality care to the least of us" (Anno, 1991). If the care and treatment provided to the incarcerated is a reflection of the degree of professionalism attained in a healthcare field, it seems logical that advanced practice nurses working as correctional specialists provide leadership in the care of those in our jails and prisons, instituting best practices, supervision, and role modeling in secure settings.

CHAPTER FOCUS

- » Advanced Practice Correctional Nursing
- » Growth of Correctional Institutions as Healthcare Settings
- » Factors Affecting Health Care in Corrections
- » Major Healthcare Challenges
- » Prisoner Populations: Culture of Corrections

- » The Prison Subculture
- » Special Prison Populations
- » Advanced Practice Nursing in Correctional Settings
- » Professional Correctional Nursing Development

KEY TERMS

- » adjudication
- » deterrence
- » evidence-based practice
- » federal prisons
- » incapacitation
- » jail
- » lock-up

- » malingering
- » manipulation
- » maximum-security facilities
- » medium-security prisons
- » rehabilitation
- » restorative justice
- » subculture

Introduction

It has been said that to understand society, one only needs to look within its prison walls where one can see people affected by racism, poverty, and illiteracy. In 2008, over 7.2 million people were on probation, in jail or prison, or on parole, which accounts for 1 in every 32 adults (U.S. Bureau of Justice Statistics, 2009a). Observations of prison settings reveal the fact that a majority of prisoners are people of color and underrepresented minorities, and those from economically impoverished communities. African Americans and Hispanic Blacks make up 12.6% of the total U.S. population as of 2008, but comprise 39.4% of the prison population (U.S. Census Bureau, 2010; U.S. Bureau of Justice Statistics, 2009b). As a result, prisons comprise a microcosm of marginalized and oppressed populations normalized within a unique structural and cultural institution. The poor healthcare status observed in prisoners is not surprising given that poverty and race status are known factors affecting incidence and prevalence of communicable diseases and mental health problems. Within prison walls are individuals who have often lacked access to health care and who often received poor healthcare services prior to incarceration. Consequently, prison offenders present unique challenges to the nursing and healthcare staff charged with their care.

On January 27, 2003, United Press International released a news brief from its chief White House correspondent regarding a report on inmate medical care in the United States. This report revealed the results of a National Institute of Justice study, which found that many prisons and jails in the United States did not meet the established guidelines for the delivery of healthcare services, resulting, upon release from incarceration, in the eventual introduction into the community of many offenders with serious health problems such as HIV/AIDS, tuberculosis, hepatitis, and mental disorders (Potter & Tewksbury, 2005). Ironically, correctional facilities are mandated to provide health care at a level that exceeds the experience of many Americans, and therefore often provide the best, and sometimes the only, health care many offenders have ever received (Hofacre, 2003). Correctional health care, and the nursing care within it, represents part of the overall healthcare delivery system for the most vulnerable of society. Because corrections directly impacts the overall delivery of health care to a very high-risk population, correctional nursing is in a position to help improve the health of offenders and, in turn, to positively impact the general public health.

Advanced Practice Correctional Nursing

This chapter is not intended as a comprehensive reference on correctional nursing. The purpose of this chapter is to review the role of advanced practice nursing in correctional settings and propose strategies for the identification and implementation of advanced practice correctional nursing as a specialty of forensic nursing. Advanced practice correctional nursing involves the direct care of incarcerated persons in traditional as well as expanded roles within secure settings of jails and state or federal prisons. Advanced practice correctional nurses are nurse practitioners or clinical nurse specialists prepared at the graduate level. They use in-depth knowledge of healthcare policy, organizational behavior of secure settings, ethical and legal issues in correctional health care, role development in correctional nursing, diversity and cultural competency in corrections, and health promotion and disease prevention among correctional populations. Advanced practice correctional nurses implement highly autonomous and collaborative nursing roles primarily aimed at conducting comprehensive health assessments, diagnosing and treating complex responses to actual or potential health problems of individuals and groups within offender populations, and formulating clinical decisions to manage acute and chronic illness and promote wellness in prison and jail settings. The range and depth of competencies and knowledge of advanced practice correctional nurses result in a broader repertoire of effective strategies to meet the needs of inmate patients and correctional healthcare systems, and they are therefore suited to manage more complex, more uncertain, and resource-limited situations that characterize correctional settings (American Association of Critical Care Nurses, 2003).

Growth of Correctional Institutions as Healthcare Settings

Although incarceration rates in the United States have leveled off since the dramatic increases in the 1980s and 1990s, the number of adults and juveniles in correctional facilities has seen unprecedented growth. At the end of the 20th century, the United States put more people behind bars than at any other time; over 2 million people were housed in prisons or jails (Jamison, 2002). Unlike decades past, when rates of incarceration rose and fell with wars, depressions, and economic booms and busts, as well as with the rise and fall of crime rates, the current growth in incarceration has continued to increase. In 2009, 7.2 million people were on probation, in jail or prison, or on parole. Currently, 1 in every 32 adults is under the supervision of the criminal justice system (U.S. Bureau of Justice Statistics, 2009a). According to the U.S. Department of Justice (2003), the incarcerated population grew an average of 3.6% annually, with the largest growth occurring in federal prison (5.8%) and local jails (5.4%) between 1995 and 2002 (U.S. Department of Justice, 2003).

In the United States, the rights of offenders are based on interpretations of the Eighth Amendment to the United States Constitution, which prohibits cruel and unusual punishment. Both federal and state laws, along with professional standards of correctional health care, serve as guidelines for the administration of safe and ethical health care to offenders. The basic assumption upon which professional and ethical standards of care are developed in correctional settings, and for which advanced practice nurses are responsible for providing oversight, is that incarceration does not, by itself, deprive individuals of rights, although these rights must be administered within the scope of legitimate needs of penal authorities to preserve security, control, and rehabilitation (American Nurses Association [ANA], 1998b; American Psychiatric Association, 2000; ; National Commission on Correctional Health Care, 2002d). All correctional facilities are designated as providers of health care, either directly or indirectly through the establishment of contractual arrangements.

The introduction of professional nursing to prisons and jails has become common only within the last 20–30 years; it is therefore important for advanced practice correctional nurses to understand the evolution of jails and prisons as settings for societal sanctions available to the courts to deal with those who commit criminal offenses. The first prisons were created in the Middle Ages by the Christian church to house those who offended canon law. Debtors' prisons followed in the 1400s for the purpose of housing those who violated civil laws (Schmalleger, 1999). The prison or jail, as we know it, emerged out of the 16th century with the building of the prototype house of correction, the London Bridewell. Prior to Bridewell, prisons were used as detention settings for those awaiting punishments such as the ducking stool, the pillory, whipping, branding, or the stocks (Howard League, 2003). Evidence suggests that the prisons of this period were badly maintained and often controlled by negligent prison wardens. Many people died of diseases such as typhus. Houses of correction evolved out of the "Poor Law," and were intended to instill habits of industry through prison labor. Most of those held in detention were nonviolent offenders convicted of petty theft, being vagrants, or being disorderly local poor. During the 18th century, large numbers of British prisoners were transported to Australia and America for the purpose of imprisonment and hard labor. The first correctional institution in the United States, the Walnut Street Jail, opened in Philadelphia in 1790 and, unlike previous institutions, was established purely for the purpose of punishment (Wrobleski & Hess, 1997). Also referred to as the Philadelphia Penitentiary, the Walnut Street Jail housed offenders in solitary confinement so that they could address their inner evil, study the bible, and be reformed (Schmalleger).

The rehabilitation era of the Pennsylvania style prison gave way to the mass prison era of the 1800s in an attempt to lower costs and increase access to group workhouses (Schmalleger, 1999). Between 1876 and 1890, Alexander Maconochie and Sir Walter Crofton's efforts in Australia and Ireland to change prison conditions and focus influenced Gaylord Hubbell, warden of Sing Sing prison in New York, to create a reformatory based upon concepts of earned early release if the inmate reformed himself. Men and women of vision met at the first National Prison Association conference in 1870 to propose the ideal prison system, emphasizing rehabilitation of first-time offenders. The eventual failure of this system has been attributed to cultural orientation of prison staff that overemphasized confinement and institutional security rather than reformation. It is important to remember that the conflict between custody and reform remains with us today, and is highlighted in the recurring role conflict between custody and caring experienced by correctional nurses (Maeve, 1997; Peternelj-Taylor & Hufft, 1997; Peternelj-Taylor & Johnson, 1995).

Three basic types of facilities make up the correctional institutions found in the United States today: jails, state prisons, and federal prisons. **Jails** are locally operated correctional facilities that confine persons before or after **adjudication**. Offenders sentenced to jail usually have a sentence of 1 year or less, although this can vary from state to state. Jails also incarcerate persons in a variety of other categories, such as persons being held pending arraignment, trial, conviction, or sentencing; those who have been returned to custody following violation of the terms of their release on probation or parole; and persons being transferred to the custody of other criminal justice or correctional authorities. **Lock-ups**, commonly located in city halls or police stations, differ from jails in that they are temporary holding facilities authorized to hold individuals for a maximum of 48 hours. Either a state or the federal government operates prisons, and they confine only those individuals who have been sentenced to 1 year or more of incarceration. Generally, persons sentenced to prison have been convicted of a felony offense (National Institute of Corrections, 2003).

Organization and delivery of nursing and health services is in part determined by the physical and procedural limitations of the correctional facilities in which they are offered. Offenders in prisons and jails are classified by security levels designated to match physical and procedural restrictions with the prisoner's risk to the population in terms of violence or escape. **Maximum-security facilities** house the most dangerous of offenders and tend to locate cells and other inmate living facilities in the center of the institution and place a variety of barriers between the living area and the institution's outer perimeter. **Medium-security prisons** generally afford more freedom of movement and activity and are under less intense supervision than maximum-security facilities, particularly in relation to associations between offenders, movement in the prison yards, and use of facilities such as exercise rooms, libraries, showers, and bathrooms. Head count is an important security measure and is usually taken several times throughout the day. All activities, including health care, must conform to security routines in correctional facilities. The lower a facility's security level, generally the more comfortable the environment. There is generally more room for movement, more windows, more programming, and more opportunities for social interactions. These environmental concerns are important factors affecting psychosocial and biophysical health, and an in-depth knowledge of facilities and the rationale for those facilities is a critical component to assessment and planning for advanced practice correctional nurses.

The federal prison system was implemented in 1895 with the conversion of Leavenworth Prison from military confinement to civilians convicted of violating federal law. The Federal

Bureau of Prisons was established in 1930 to adequately oversee the 11 **federal prison** facilities existing at that time and to provide a professional framework for the development of prison standards. As of 2011, there are 100 institutions, 6 regional offices, a central headquarters, 3 staff training centers, and 28 community corrections offices. In addition, the Bureau of Prisons provides health care for most offenders within the correctional institutions. For those who need hospital care, there are 7 inpatient medical referral centers with about 2,000 inpatient and chronic care beds (U.S. Department of Justice, 2001).

Current trends in prisons and jails affecting nursing and health care include expanding populations of offenders and those ordered for evaluation prior to trial or sentencing, shortages of nursing staff, limitations in financial and physical resources, role ambiguity and role conflict as a consequence of caring and security goals, and the necessity of adapting to the values and transactions inherent in prison culture. A recent survey conducted by the National Institute of Corrections cited widespread deficiencies in medical staff in prisons or other units housing offenders with medical needs, particularly in women's care units and for mentally ill offenders (National Institute of Corrections, 2002). Advanced practice nurses with backgrounds in women's health care and psychiatric nursing are particularly needed in correctional settings.

Factors Affecting Health Care in Corrections

Both physical setup and procedural restrictions serve as mechanisms to preserve security and promote control in correctional settings. Restrictions in movement, interactions with staff and other offenders, and physical barriers introduced to prevent escape are common in correctional environments. Locked doors, high fences, and barred windows are part of the physical reality of prisons and jails. Rigid schedules for daily activities, required attendance at scheduled meals and work details, along with mandatory silence at lights out are a few of the temporal limitations of life in a correctional setting. Understanding the relationship between the physical and logistical demands of a correctional setting and the procedures used to implement health care is essential for developing optimal systems of care.

Before seeing a healthcare provider, offenders must usually complete a written request, indicating the nature of the health problem for which care is sought. Depending on the institution, the request for health services may be evaluated by individuals with little or no medical training, and in some instances, correctional officers, whose knowledge and assessment of the conditions warranting routine or emergency care may be limited or biased by security concerns. When healthcare triage decisions are unduly influenced by security concerns, delay or denial of healthcare requests can occur. In some settings, the disorganization or limitation of services delaying routine sick call requests results in unnecessary declarations of emergency by offenders.

Like the emergency room used for routine health care, the misuse of emergency declarations overtaxes healthcare systems in corrections and may result in sanctions or higher levels of eligibility before an offender can be seen. Advanced practice nurses in correctional settings are responsible for the review of policies and procedures related to access to health care. Recommendations for procedures that facilitate the availability of healthcare services to inmates, along with the development of documentation systems verifying appropriate screening, referral, and delivery of healthcare services by qualified healthcare staff, require negotiation with security staff and health authorities. Advanced practice nurses must be aware of threats to security and a variety of options for the delivery of healthcare services so that recommendations can be adapted to the specific needs of the institution.

Growing numbers of correctional institutions require inmates to pay a minimal, but unaffordable to some, co-pay for care. Long waiting periods, sometimes in very uncomfortable conditions outside, without cover, serve as another deterrent to those seeking care. Often inmates are restricted to sick call-out at only one time each day. Sick call may be as early as 6:00 a.m., with the request needing to be posted the day before. Any healthcare concern that is not an emergency that occurs after that time would need to be postponed until the next day. When attending clinics or sick call, inmates miss meals, work assignments, or special programming. In some instances, missed days of work add days to the sentence, a disincentive to those seeking medical care. Many times inmates will postpone medical care until an emergency exists, making their conditions more severe and more difficult to manage.

Inmates on medication face difficulties related to accessing their medications, maintaining privacy in terms of what medications they are taking, and timing of medications. Any activity related to security, such as head counts or lockdowns, interrupt any other activity taking place in the institution and may contribute to missed medication and medications dispensed without regard for food and beverage ingestion. When unable to take their medications with prescribed food or on an empty stomach, inmates may experience side effects, drug resistance, or exacerbation of a medical condition.

Perhaps the greatest barrier to inmates in accessing and using health care in correctional settings is the culture of the institution itself. Prison culture does not tolerate weakness, and those with medical problems can be viewed as outcasts and deviants by inmates and by correctional staff. Suspected of manipulation, inmates seeking health services, particularly those who complain of pain, are often marginalized and disrespected. Responding to the need for acceptance among their peers and out of a need for self-preservation, offenders may elect not to access healthcare services. *Noncompliance* is a common term used in corrections, because many offenders view medication refusal as a way of asserting their independence in a setting in which they have very little control. Understanding the organizational behavior exhibited within corrections, among both staff and offenders, is a critical element to the organization of healthcare services. The advanced practice nurse is in a position to not only influence policy directly, but also, through the education and development of correctional staff, increase the manpower available to deal with special needs populations such as the mentally disordered and chronically ill (Tahir, 2003).

The prison healthcare setting is, by its very nature, an environment unconducive to clinical productivity. Low productivity among healthcare staff results in underused healthcare resources and denial of access to facilities by inmates. Overcoming issues such as organization of efficient nursing staff to support medical and nursing interventions, management of laboratory reporting processes, and low administrative support of healthcare functions is a priority in all correctional settings (Anno & Dubler, 2002; Bachmeier, 2003; Paris, 2003). Advanced practice nurses must be able to implement productivity measures in order to develop staffing formulas appropriate for the setting. Warden's meetings, inmate transportation, inmate count or attendance, and reducing paperwork associated with documenting services are all points of activity for the management of effective and efficient correctional healthcare services.

Major Healthcare Challenges

Although offenders represent the larger communities from which they come, individuals in prison and jail settings reflect major categories of acute and chronic illnesses at greater rates than the public. Major responsibilities of the advanced practice nurse in corrections include knowledge of policy, institutional culture and organizational behavior, and standards of correctional nursing care to establish nursing systems for implementation of the nursing process and attainment of institutional health benchmarks.

Screening and Assessment

Critical to the successful management of health care in correctional settings is the development of effective screening procedures and accompanying policies and protocols to deliver appropriate healthcare interventions. An example of an opportunity for critical assessment of screening tools is the use of instrumentation to assess drug use among offenders. Current legislation requiring mandatory sentencing for drug-related crimes has resulted in significant numbers of offenders with substance abuse histories. Presented with growing numbers of drug-involved offenders and limited resources, it is essential for advanced practice correctional nurses to provide oversight and guidance to the development of protocols for nursing involvement in drug screening and treatment facilitation. Instrumentation for nursing assessments of substance abuse in correctional settings is implemented to help mental health staff identify candidates for levels of treatment designed for maximum impact and avoid spending time and money on intensive treatment of low-risk offenders. Any mandatory and routine assessments or screenings done by nursing staff should be subject to review by nurses, who are accountable for ensuring that the cost, length of time to administer, scope, and application of drug and alcohol treatment options are appropriate for the instruments being used (Peters et al., 2000; Wells, 2003).

Identification of Nursing Priorities

Identifying major nursing diagnoses for those offenders presenting for nursing care is helpful in the development of plans of care for groups of offenders. Major infectious diseases such as HIV/AIDS, tuberculosis, and hepatitis B and C occur at significant rates in correctional settings.

Prisoner Populations: Culture of Corrections

The goal of culturally competent care for clients in correctional settings is to encourage appropriate exchanges and collaborations among offenders, healthcare providers, and correctional staff. These collaborations should foster equitable health outcomes and result in the identification and provision of services that are responsive to issues of race, culture, gender, sexual orientation, and social and economic status. Being competent in cross-cultural functioning means learning new patterns of behavior and effectively applying them in appropriate settings.

The American Nurses Association has asserted that culturally competent nursing care goes beyond cultural sensitivity and awareness of different cultures to specific knowledge and skills that can help the nurse change situations of oppression and avoid stereotypical assumptions (ANA, 1998a). Based on the anthropological concept that all human communities develop through learned and shared information about what is acceptable and expected behavior, nursing has evolved as a scientific practice discipline rooted in our own cultural values of caring, compassion, and technical competencies. The prison or correctional setting represents a challenge to nursing as offenders represent a multitude of cultures within a unique culture of the prison itself. Culture is a distinctly human capacity for adapting to circumstances and transmitting this coping skill and knowledge to future generations. The prison culture has its own attributes, forming a sense of identity, a set of expected behaviors, and distinct goals for those who are incarcerated and for those who care for them. Prison becomes a setting in which persons from various cultures and criminal backgrounds come together in a contrived culture derived from values and dictates of the criminal justice system and the participants in the operations of the institution.

Prisons mirror those characteristics of any culture through expression of values and norms, beliefs and attitudes, relationships, communication and language, sense of self and space, appearance and dress, work habits and practices, and food and eating habits. Correctional nurses who are aware of the cultural backgrounds and characteristics of offenders are in a position to adapt healthcare practices to meet client needs and avoid imposing their own attitudes and approaches on others.

Historically, prisons have served five major purposes in American society—retribution, deterrence, incapacitation, rehabilitation, and restoration (Schmalleger, 1999). Retribution represents punishment for the sake of punishment—also referred to as revenge. Retribution focuses on the crime itself rather than on the offender's needs or the needs of the community. **Deterrence** relies on incarceration as a means to prevent future criminal actions and is more proactive and functional than retribution. **Incapacitation** refers to making it impossible for offenders to commit other crimes and has the goal of segregating offenders from the rest of society to protect them. **Rehabilitation** has the goal of correcting deviant behavior. In and out of favor in the criminal justice system and dependent upon funding, rehabilitation is the focus on medical and mental health treatment for many offenders whose offense is related to their pathology. Due to critical levels of funding and questions about the effectiveness of rehabilitation in light of high rates of recidivism among offenders, the prevailing approach of the criminal justice system in relation to corrections currently focuses on punishment or retribution. An evolving paradigm of justice, called **restorative justice**, focuses on problem solving and repair of social injuries incurred through criminal behavior (Wrobleski & Hess, 1997). Restorative justice acknowledges the relationship between the offender and the victim, the rights of the victim, and the need for society to be repaired through the offender making retribution for injuries perpetrated in criminal offenses. This approach recognizes the ability of the stigma of offense to be removed through repentance and forgiveness and, while implemented in probation sentencing, does not represent the current model of prison culture.

The prison culture values order and obedience, power over the weak or disenfranchised, and strict adherence to policies and procedures. Many prisons are characterized by a culture of fear (Ramsbotham, 1999) and underscored by actions by offenders and staff suggesting racism and sexism. Normative behavior often includes widespread use of drugs and physical and mental abuse among offenders. Prison culture is heavily oriented toward security, with offenders being kept powerless and forced to rely on correctional officers for the delivery of services, particularly health care (Blair, 2002).

In 2003, 31% of individuals incarcerated were convicted of drug offenses (Bewley-Taylor, Hallam, & Allen, 2009). The prison population in general is characterized by low levels of formal education, socially disadvantaged backgrounds, and a lack of significant vocational skills. Most adult offenders have served considerable time in juvenile correctional facilities and evidence acculturation to the prison.

Correctional nurses must be aware of the culture shock most offenders experience upon first entering a correctional setting. Culture shock is a psychological disorientation related to inaccurate interpretation of role expectations or cues from another culture (American Correctional Association, 2003). In addition to being cast into interactions with persons of diverse and often unknown cultural backgrounds, the prison itself presents an environment requiring adaptation. Offenders must adhere to sets of policies dictating every movement and event from when they eat and sleep to what they wear, when they can speak, and what work they will do each day. They are cut off from family and social support systems and subjected to lack of privacy, changes in stimulation and recreation, and limited access to physical and emotional stress management options. Offenders in prison must learn vocabulary and postures in order to fit in. They must quickly identify the power structures among the other offenders and among the staff in order to avoid becoming a victim of abuse or ridicule. Offenders with physical problems, developmental problems, or mental disorders are particularly vulnerable to segregation and victimization. All offenders share common deprivations of liberty, goods and services, heterosexual relationships, autonomy, and personal security. These are the common stressors that link the offenders in prison.

One approach to the study of prison culture is based on the work of Erving Goffman (1961). He described total institutions as places where the same people work, play, eat, sleep, and recreate together on a daily basis. Such places include prison, concentration camps, mental institutions, and seminaries. Total institutions are small societies cut off from the larger society either forcibly or willingly. They evolve their own distinctive values and styles of life.

The Prison Subculture

Two realities exist in prisons. One is the official structure of rules and procedures dictated by the state department of corrections or the federal government. The other is the more informal but more powerful inmate culture—the prison **subculture**.

Offenders have to learn all the rules and regulations set by the corrections administration, but they must also learn very quickly the unwritten rules dictated by the prison subculture incorporating inmate concerns, values, roles, and even language (Schmalleger, 1999). The inmate learns an unwritten code that dictates five common elements:

1. Do not interfere with the interests of other offenders. Never rat on a con.
2. Do not lose your head; play it cool and do your own time.
3. Do not exploit offenders. Do not steal. Do not break your word; be right.
4. Do not whine. Be a man.
5. Do not be a sucker. Do not trust the guards or the staff.

Prison subculture is constantly changing and probably represents the greater culture of criminals existing outside of prisons. Structural dimensions of prison subculture often determine how prison culture is described. These include the degree to which the staff and the offenders are alienated, the three general categories of offense types among the offenders, how work gangs and cell houses are organized, racial groups, the power of inmate leaders, the degree of sexual abnormality presented by an inmate, and personality differences existing among individuals (Schmalleger, 1999).

Special Prison Populations

Since the 1960s, a growing concern for the rights of ethnic minorities, women, the physically and mentally challenged, and many other groups has extended to the issue of unfair and inequitable treatment by the criminal justice system. A special population is identified as any group of individuals who present patterns that distinguish them from other individuals and whose patterns of behavior or physical characteristics affect their health or experience of health and health care. Within the prison culture there are specific groups needing nursing assessment and intervention. Major groups identified as special prison populations upon which one can focus culturally competent nursing intervention strategies include women, homosexuals, juveniles, gang members, ethnic and racial minorities, the elderly, and those with chronic illnesses.

Women

Although women represent only 10% of the country's correctional population, they are the fastest growing group in jails nationwide (Harrison & Beck, 2005). On average, female offenders are 2.5 years older than their male counterparts, are less likely to be convicted of a violent offense, and are more often than not victims of sexual or physical abuse, involved in drug use or drug trade, and have children (Greenfeld & Snell, 1999). Women live in prison within complex social systems based on close emotional relationships with other offenders. Women find prison life harder than men, crave affection, and are more vulnerable to homosexual relationships (Heidensohn, 1995).

Women are especially vulnerable to the stress of separation from family and children. Women's correctional facilities often suffer from a lack of resources as compared to men's, due to a lack of funding equity. Fewer women in prison results in numbers too low to justify many programs. In addition, women in prison are subject to sexual misconduct in the form of sexual contact between women offenders and staff, name calling, and inappropriate leering. The great imbalance of power between health or correctional staff and offenders makes the notion of consent impossible and the resulting vulnerability serves as a constant source of stress (Coolman, 2003).

Incarcerated women use healthcare services at a significantly higher rate than men due to the greater complexity of a woman's reproductive system, a high rate of sexually transmitted disease, and pregnancies. Women entering correctional settings report problems with alcohol abuse, headaches, fatigue, drug abuse, and sexually transmitted diseases (National Commission on Correctional Health Care, 2001; National Institute of Corrections, 2002).

Women in prison present unique healthcare challenges due to poor self-care, high levels of drug use and histories of abuse, high-risk pregnancy, and dysfunctional family histories. Diets high in fat and carbohydrates often lack nutrients considered essential in the prevention of heart disease and hypertension, loss of bone mass, and anemia.

Although women tend to resist prison subculture and are more likely to have more trusting relationships with staff, they are often viewed by the correctional staff as complainers and whiners. Their physical and emotional complaints are often viewed as malingering or manipulation. Women are typically underserved in correctional settings due to underprogramming, fragmentation of services, inconsistent treatment philosophies (especially in areas of mental health and comorbidity), and lack of gender-specific treatment alternatives (Dolan, Kolthoff, Schreck, Smilanich, & Todd, 2003).

Women tend to organize themselves into prison families, creating artificial relationships that mirror the outside world. These relationships produce three primary responses and distinct personality types; square, cool, and life (Pollock, 1998; van Wormer, 2001). The squares identify predominantly with conventional norms and values and have had little previous experience with the criminal justice system. Cools represent those women who isolate themselves and are career offenders. Lifers are full participants in the prison culture, usually taking leadership roles.

Lifers represent those women who have no meaningful relationships or identity outside prison and find prison culture their only source of self-concept and status. A new category of female offender, the "crack kid," exhibits a lack of respect for traditional prison values, for their elders, or even for their own peers. They are frequently involved in fights and their lack of even simple domestic skills estranges them from others.

It is important to note that women who deliver their babies while incarcerated are not allowed to keep their baby and often do not see the baby before he or she is in the custody of protective services. Grieving and bereavement services may not be available, thus these women are compromised once more. It is in this area that the correctional nurse must step in and provide not only postpartum care once the patient is discharged from the hospital but the opportunity to mourn over the loss of her baby. Although families are asked to step in, this may not be acceptable to the inmate who has little or no control over the decision. Postpartum depression is another reality for many of these women and the referral to behavioral health services is essential.

The risk of suicide in the general prison population is of concern, and screening for suicidal behavior is a high priority. However, the coping strategies for this population are limited, thus the vigilance of the nurse along with superior assessment skills may prevent an attempt or completion by the suicidal inmate.

Homosexuals

Homosexual activity in prisons is universally condemned and prohibited by formal prison policy and, at the same time, encouraged and promoted by the environmental and social structures supporting prison subculture. There are two major male types of homosexual activities in prison. One type of homosexual activity involves predatory behavior of heterosexual males reacting to the constraints of prison life that prohibit heterosexual liaisons. The other involves those men who participated in a homosexual lifestyle outside of prison. Homosexual activity among females is less aggressive than males and involves the need for attention and affection (Potter & Tewksbury, 2005).

Newly admitted offenders may be sought out by older offenders looking for a sexual union. They will ingratiate themselves by offering cigarettes, money, drugs, and other favors and then demand sexual favors in return. The inmate code calls for the payment of debt and the inmate is therefore obliged to perform sexual favors or be subject to inmate justice.

Rape among male offenders has been reported as high as 28% (Lockwood, 1978). Although most sexual aggressors do not consider themselves homosexuals and sexual release is not the primary motivation for sexual attack, many aggressors continue to participate in gang rape activity in order to avoid becoming a victim of rape. Twelve percent of all hate crimes in prison are perpetrated against males believed by their victimizers to be homosexuals (Schmalleger, 1999), and this aggression often continues into the correctional setting against homosexual offenders. In 2003, the Prison Rape Elimination Act was signed by then-President George W. Bush. The act includes the following measure:

> ... carry out, for each calendar year, a comprehensive statistical review and analysis of the incidence and effects of prison rape; include, but not be limited to the identification of the common characteristics of—(A) both victims and perpetrators of prison rape; and (B) prisons and prison systems with a high incidence of prison rape (Bureau of Justice Statistics, 2003).

The act also seeks to utilize "a random sample, or other scientifically appropriate sample, of not less than 10 percent of all Federal, State, and county prisons, and a representative sample of municipal prisons; use surveys and other statistical studies of current and former inmates; and provide "a listing of those institutions in the representative sample, separated into each category ... and ranked according to the incidence of prison rape in each institution" (Bureau of Justice Statistics, 2003, p. 117) and "a listing of any prisons in the representative sample that did not cooperate with the survey" (Bureau of Justice Statistics, 2003).

Juveniles

In the last decade of the 20th Century, juvenile drug use, gun use, and gang involvement increased, the presence of juveniles in correctional settings has increased by more than 300% during the 1990s. Mirroring the adult population, most juvenile offenders are male, and the female population is growing at an unprecedented rate (U.S. Department of Justice, 2002).

Taken as a broad category of the correctional population, juveniles are characterized as "rejecting middle class values of social duty and personal restraint" (Schmalleger, 1999, p. 578). Increasing experience with problems of drug and alcohol abuse, violence, gang membership, separation from family and home, and sexual and physical abuse affect the growth and development of the juveniles seen in the criminal justice system. The rates of self-destructive behavior such as self-mutilation and attempted and completed suicide are on the rise among juveniles in the correctional population at higher rates than in the general population (American Academy of Pediatrics, 2001).

Ethnic and racial diversity among juveniles is a complicating factor influencing diagnosis and implementation of responsive and appropriate healthcare strategies, particularly in mental health (Canino & Spurlock, 2000). Inability to focus on the subtleties of cultural variance in symptoms of illness can delay onset of treatment or selection of appropriate treatment. This has been a factor in the persistent lack of resources and adequate health care for youths in detention and correctional facilities.

Routine childhood and adolescent developmental issues must be integrated into any plan of care for juveniles in corrections. A complete assessment includes immunization updates, the need for crisis intervention and suicide prevention, and risk factors such as domestic violence, drug use, and assaultive behavior. In addition, specific policies related to parental notification and consent for treatment must be instituted. Unlike adult populations, the impact of healthcare services may be *greater among juveniles. If juvenile* offenders receive intensive intervention while incarcerated, during their transition to the community, and while they are under community supervision, they will benefit from improved family and peer relations, education, job skills, substance abuse levels, mental health, and recidivism levels (Bradley & Kalfs, 2003).

Gang Members

Prisons began to have noticeable increases in gang activity when states enacted tougher laws for gang-related crimes in the 1980s. Documented as an inner-city phenomenon in the United States since the 1920s, gangs have experienced a growth in numbers and power inside prisons. Many individuals who had previously never associated with gangs become gang members during incarceration (Egley, 2005; Egley & Arjunan, 2002; Schmalleger, 1999; Thornberry, Huizinga, & Loeber, 2004). Correctional facilities bring members of gangs together in a setting without natural boundaries, creating tensions over turf and opportunities for competition for space, power, and membership. Male gang members tend to adopt a defensive worldview evidenced by a feeling of vulnerability and suspicion, a general mistrust of others, the need to maintain social distance, a proclivity toward violence as a problem-solving mechanism, and an attraction to others who are defensive. Gang members tend to come from dysfunctional families and are less likely than nongang members to complete high school. They are known as predators, taking advantage of and exploiting other juveniles and adults. Extreme risk takers, gang members are frequently involved in accidents as well as altercations, making them frequent visitors to the infirmary (Esbensen, 2000; Howell, 2000; Howell & Lynch, 2000).

Gangs can be extremely well organized, many hold regular meetings with a rigid set of rules and even requiring regular payment of dues. Violence is often used as a rite of passage, and up to 40% of gang members report rape of females and other violent crimes, especially on rival gang members (Schmalleger, 1999). Most gangs are ethnically diverse (70%), but few allow female membership or female leadership roles. Exclusively female gangs are increasing in number, particularly among the Hispanic population. The one thing that most gang members have in common is a tendency to violence and delinquency before joining a gang (Esbensen, 2000). However, most gang members claim that, if given a second chance, they would not have joined a gang. The correctional environment, however, with its emphasis on sustaining tightly controlled reference groups, does not promote the success of programs designed to discourage gang affiliation.

Ethnic and Racial Minorities

The recognition of hate crimes—offenses in which aggression is based on actual or perceived race, color, religion, national origin, ethnicity, gender, or sexual orientation— emphasizes the segregated and heterogeneous nature of American society. White supremacist and separatist groups adhering to an identity theology further marginalize and segregate ethnic and racial groups (Marable, 2000; Schmalleger, 1999). Racial and ethnic minorities such as African Americans, Native Americans, and Hispanics are overrepresented in U.S. prisons and jails. Factors contributing to this minority overrepresentation in our correctional systems include biases and deficiencies in our justice system, socioeconomic conditions, educational systems, and trends in family structures and instability (Devine, Coolbaugh, & Jenkins, 1998). Although African American males are so visible in our prisons, they are more likely to be a victim of violent crime than any other segment of our population. In contrast, the correctional staff and healthcare professionals caring for correctional populations are predominantly white.

African Americans account for over 50% of the correctional population, and Hispanics represent 15% of those incarcerated, far exceeding their numbers across the nation. In predominantly Hispanic or African American communities, these statistics are even higher (Harrison & Beck, 2005). Correctional communities solidify segregation of racial and ethnic minorities, increasing opportunities for friction and suspicion based on racial and ethnic identity and differences.

Growing numbers of non-English-speaking offenders from ethnically isolated Asian or Middle Eastern communities present special needs. Restricted financing for prisons and jails and difficulty recruiting a diverse workforce in corrections limits the ability to provide multilingual services.

The Elderly

The elderly (those 55 years of age and older) represent a growing population in correctional settings. Growing numbers of elderly in prisons are the result of (1) increasing crime among those over 50; (2) the gradual aging of society from which the offenders come; (3) a trend toward longer sentences, especially for violent offenders with previous offenses; and (4) the gradual accumulation of older habitual offenders in prison. Similar to over-representation in other prison age groups, elderly offenders serving life sentences or long sentences tend to be African American (Harrison & Beck, 2005; Neeley, Addison, & Craig-Moreland, 1997).

Common characteristics among elderly offenders include physical impairments and chronic illnesses, a lack of sustained contact with family or regular visitation, and a lack of interest in rehabilitation programs. Elderly offenders may have chronic, pervasive stress levels that are subsumed under a stoic or tough outward appearance and behavior, particularly if they have been institutionalized for a long period of time. Dealing with the threat or experience of violence present in correctional settings can be especially difficult for this population (Parrish, 2003; Smyer, Gragert, & LaMere, 1997; Yates & Gillespie, 2000).

The Chronically Ill

The growth of HIV and AIDS among prison offenders is a serious healthcare problem facing the United States. Positive HIV seroprevalence rates vary from region to region, from 2.1% to 7.6% of all men and between 2.5% and 14.7% of women (Day, 2004; Seiter & Kadela, 2003). HIV appears to be spreading in prison through homosexual activity, intravenous drug use, and the sharing of tainted tattoo and hypodermic needles. Most offenders report high-risk behaviors before entering prison, especially intravenous drug use. Most reports indicate that HIV transmission within prisons is minimal (Macalino et al., 2004). Often offenders who are HIV positive do not have their confidentiality protected. Knowledge of their status results in avoidance by staff and offenders, and denial of certain jobs, home furloughs, and visitation.

Other special populations can include those with terminal illnesses, those living on death row, and political offenders, who, by nature of their unique circumstances and backgrounds, each provide distinct cultural characteristics and considerations. They are often grouped together, segregated by the nature of their offenses, and therefore bonded by collective notions of victimization or unjust treatment. Many offenders with chronic illnesses will eventually be reintegrated into society after incarceration. The period of incarceration provides an opportunity for effective treatment and illness management.

The moral and social philosophies associated with the definition of crime and the associated appropriate and proportionate justice response are integral to the understanding of individual and collective healthcare response to patient needs among offenders (National Commission on Correctional Health Care, 2002b).

There is a trend toward providing hospice care to the terminally ill inmate—other inmates are trained to provide this care under the guidance of the nurse. Hospice care was put in place as part of the care given to HIV/AIDS patients in New York state prisons, which saw a dramatic decrease in the number of deaths due to HIV/AIDS from 26.3 per 10,000 in 1996 to 6.1 per 10,000 in 1998 (CDC, 2001).

Culturally Competent Nursing in Correctional Settings

Nurses working in corrections must adapt to the culture and mandates of the setting. Healthcare priorities are subsumed into the larger mandate for confinement and punishment, and resources for rehabilitation are often diverted to structures and staff focusing on security. Nursing efforts must be highly focused and clearly substantiated through accurate and reliable assessments of patient needs that incorporate advanced health assessment skills. The use of master assessments of physical, psychosocial, and cultural indicators is essential for efficient and effective care. The preservation of ethnic identity and personal self-concept is a right that must be sustained within the confines and restrictions of correctional environments that demand close inspection of and impose restrictions on verbal and nonverbal communication. Acceptance of authority, particularly from female correctional officers or healthcare staff; ways in which stigma or shame are dealt with; and the struggle to maintain individual identity, particularly in the area of healthcare choice, need to be included in any health promotion plan of care (DuPont & Halasz, 1998).

Specific strategies for the implementation of culturally competent care include the assessment of the cultural groups present in the correctional facility and an inventory of practices, beliefs, and needs affecting health behavior that distinguish those groups. Advanced practice correctional nurses are expected to provide leadership in this endeavor and provide education to healthcare personnel. An understanding and respect for differences, although critical to cultural competency, is difficult to promote in an environment that emphasizes conformity. Advanced assessment skills are essential to quality health care for offenders in correctional settings and must be grounded in awareness of population characteristics, differentiating them from myths about inmates. Biases toward prisoners greatly impact the care they receive while in correctional settings and revolve around several myths. Many people believe that all prisoners are dangerous and need constant surveillance and restraints, despite the fact that most prisoners have not committed violent crimes. Additionally, a myth exists that all offenders are drug seekers, noncompliant with medications, not interested in health, malingerers, and manipulative. Although it is true that some inmates exhibit these characteristics, it is not the case with all, and designation of such should be on the basis of assessment and evidence, not myth. It is essential that advanced practice correctional nurses understand these labels and reserve them for appropriate circumstances, based on evidence collected in health history and assessment.

Drug-seeking behavior is a common phenomenon in correctional settings. Requests for narcotics or psychotropic medications are accompanied by common complaints of back pain, headache, extremity pain, and dental pain. Without a thorough history and assessment, the nurse will not be able to confirm the frequency of those requests and physical complaints not supported by physical assessment findings. The challenge to the advanced practice correctional nurse will be to accurately assess the need for medication and appropriately avoid rewarding drug-seeking behavior, while avoiding using the label *drug seeking* without sufficient cause. Many inmates will present physical or psychological symptoms in an effort to avoid work details or other undesirable assignments, to escape exploitation by other inmates, to defy or control the system and its authority figures, or to self-manage undiagnosed psychological disorders or substance abuse withdrawal.

Manipulation is a way of life and a primary means of goal-oriented behavior and satisfaction for those with whom many advanced practice correctional nurses work. A behavior common in personality-disordered individuals in secure settings, manipulation has primary aims of securing privileges to which individuals are not eligible, escaping boredom, establishing or maintaining a sense of power, and sustaining inappropriate boundaries for self-image and self-esteem. Mastering techniques for recognizing manipulation and dealing positively with this behavior is essential in forensic nursing. It is important for the nurse not to take manipulation personally, because one of the most powerful outcomes of manipulation is to make someone in authority angry, self-conscious, or fearful.

Although manipulation cannot be totally eradicated among the incarcerated, it can be managed. Systematic, thorough assessment based on fact and observation, along with consistency in the application of policies and procedures, is crucial to limiting the impact of manipulation among inmates. The use of a matter-of-fact, nonjudgmental approach to interactions with inmates strengthens interventions aimed at understanding what the inmate hopes to achieve and how he or she understands his or her acts of manipulation. Underlying effective nursing responses to manipulation is the ability to communicate the absence of power, the need, or the interest in assisting the inmate to achieve the goals of manipulation.

Malingering is the fabrication or exaggeration of psychiatric symptoms occurring in association with a clearly identifiable secondary gain (American Psychiatric Association, 1994). Malingering is characterized by significant exaggeration or faking of psychiatric symptoms for a conscious gain or purpose; the malingerer is fully conscious of the intended purpose of personal gain or advantage. Malingering is prevalent in correctional populations, estimated to occur in 8–37% of individuals referred for pretrial evaluations and up to 46% of inmates claiming psychological impairment (Norris & May, 1998). Motivation to malinger is similar to that of manipulation and includes benefits such as avoidance of responsibility or punishment, better living quarters, medications, declaration of incompetence to stand trial or to use the insanity defense, or obtaining medical benefits after release from prison. Screening measures specific for malingering are being used with some success in correctional settings and are more successful in identifying malingerers than a structured clinical interview, distinguishing most malingerers in correctional settings as less educated and younger than nonmalingerers (Hall, 2000; Hall & Pritchard, 1996; Norris & May, 1998; Reid, 2000). This finding may imply that malingering is an adaptation tool for those less capable of sophisticated decision-making and those who are more impulsive. Often malingerers begin malingering before they are incarcerated, subsequently obtaining a psychiatric diagnosis that is assumed to be a preexisting condition upon admission to the correctional facility. Familiarity with current specialized screening and assessment tools is an essential skill of advanced practice correctional nurses in order to determine the correlation between inmate patterns of behavior and complaints of psychiatric illness.

Factitious disorders are similar to malingering in that the offender presents physical or psychological symptoms in order to assume the sick role and associated benefits. Unlike the malingerer, who is conscious and aware of the intended benefit to be derived from their feigned illness, the person experiencing a factitious disorder is not aware of the drive underlying the intent to mislead (American Psychiatric Association, 1994). Although the act of malingering can sometimes be adaptive, as in the case of hostages, the absence of external incentives for the presenting symptoms in factitious disorders always signifies psychopathology. It is important to understand that, in the correctional setting, the object or goal, whether conscious or not, often is placement in the healthcare unit and the adoption of the sick role as a means to receive caring that is not present in other correctional settings. Although there is no known cause for factitious disorder, some theories suggest a history of abuse or neglect as a child or a history of frequent illnesses that required hospitalization may be factors in the development of the disorder. Advanced practice correctional nurses have the responsibility to ensure that health history forms and data collection include nursing assessment of history of abuse in order to affirm or add to the findings of other healthcare providers. Significant numbers of female offenders express their disorder as Munchausen syndrome by proxy, an extreme form of the disorder manifested by the creation of symptoms in their children, particularly infants, in order to present to healthcare providers as a heroic and tragic parent figure. Held in particular disdain by other offenders and staff, these patients present challenges for the advanced practice correctional nurse in terms of effective management of staff and inmate behavior as well as establishment of therapeutic care (Eminson & Atkin, 2000; Maden, 1996).

Nurses must work with correctional staff and administration to identify appropriate opportunities for individualization of healthcare interventions and link these to an overall plan for health promotion for offenders and staff within the institution. Acknowledging the importance of staff health and concerns is an important first step to gaining the cooperation needed to implement individualized care for offenders. Opportunities to substantiate outcomes of nursing intervention with scientific or data-based information can be a powerful tool in enlisting support. The nurse who links the provision of privacy during medication administration and teaching offenders about their treatments and medications with decreased problems of noncompliance and/or disruptive behavior during pill call will be very successful in getting the administration's attention. Nurses must recognize the importance of their roles as *continuous* change agents.

Having served their time, over 80% of all offenders will return to their previous communities. There has been steady growth in the offender populations with special needs such as the mentally ill, women, and the elderly. Responsibilities of the advanced practice correctional nurse include the discharge planning and case management of offenders, particularly those with chronic physical and mental health illnesses. Among successful approaches used to promote health in community-based offenders is the Girls Assets Program, a combination of therapy and mentoring used to decrease recidivism among at-risk youthful offenders (Eels, 2003; Evans, 2003). The nurse must build documentation of assets and resources for the offender within the correctional setting and in the community into which the offender will go upon release. Assets can be grouped into two categories: external and internal. External assets include positive resources such as social support systems, activities and goals for empowerment, setting boundaries, and assistance for time and resource management. Internal assets include those values and skills the offender has acquired in order to promote his or her health and to maintain medical compliance.

The experience offenders take with them, including the type and nature of health care provided to them, can be a determinant of whether or not they reoffend. Culturally competent nursing care in corrections is dependent on the incorporation of fundamental principles such as inclusiveness, reflecting the diversity of the community served, valuing cultural differences, employment equity, service equity, and involving everyone in the setting.

The first obligation of the culturally competent correctional nurse is to become exposed to information about and opportunities to be involved with the cultures represented in the correctional setting. Accepting the value of differences is a personal decision necessary to cultural competency and precedes all other professional development. The culturally competent nurse recognizes the personal responsibility and accountability for continuous professional development through formal educational opportunities or informal lectures and events. The nurse must organize information about cultural groups for whom care is provided and document standards of care incorporating interventions that have meaning specific to individual cultural considerations. Hiring practices and the recruiting of new staff should be guided by a commitment to inform and educate potential staff regarding the cultural groups represented in the institution (DuPont & Halasz, 1998).

Language, customs, and practices should be maintained as much as possible, within the security restrictions of the setting. Healthcare staff must work with correctional staff to identify maladaptive or dysfunctional cultural behavioral patterns, such as tattooing or gang raping as an initiation to a gang, and target them for extinction through therapeutic as well as policy mechanisms.

Core symbols of culture need to be examined within each cultural group to verify how they are acted out in the correctional setting. Issues of collectivism, individuality, positivism, genuineness, assertiveness, orientation to time, and secrecy are common themes distinguishing cultural groups that are modified in correctional settings. Nonviolent posturing as a form of emotional expressiveness among African Americans must be distinguished from intent to act. Understanding that Hispanic male youths often act out aggressively rather than withdraw when they are depressed is essential to assessment of emotional and psychiatric state. Additionally, understanding that among Muslims, Islam is always the determining factor in decision-making processes and there is no distinction between secular and religious life is critical to explaining why even small concessions to dietary or dress rituals demanded in correctional settings is intolerable and is a source for violent response (American Correctional Association, 1993).

Nurses must break down barriers to culturally competent care from within their own ranks, learning how to recognize and confront prejudice, stereotyping, and discrimination. We need to think about ways we apply profiling to groups of offenders or clients, whether it be assuming all victims of rape should be willing to report the assault, or assuming that nurses who work with drug addicts must themselves be in recovery. Nurses must identify sources of friendly fire in the form of biased language, grouping people as having a characteristic simply because of where they come from, mislabeling groups, addressing persons in a familiar way when is it not warranted, and using inappropriate titles and terms. Nurses must learn to apply principles of physical and psychosocial assessment in a culturally competent way, particularly in corrections where eye contact may be discouraged not only as part of cultural heritage, but also as learned behavior initiated by expectations of punitive correctional staff. Recognizing when behavior is consistent with the correctional culture and when it is a product of another cultural context is a difficult and ongoing process that correctional nurses must master. Even nursing goals for patient behavior may be inconsistent with expectations of the prison culture, such as promoting trust and openness during psychiatric encounters, when this behavior may actually be life threatening in the correctional setting.

Finally, nurses must take an environmental inventory of the ecological factors affecting and predominating in the correctional setting. Nurses need to take the lead in asking the questions that raise awareness of and appreciation for the need for cultural competency.

Professional Correctional Nursing Development

The development of programs for discipline-specific training and continuing education for correctional nursing staff is a major responsibility for advanced practice correctional nurses. Topics for continuing professional development should be based on a needs assessment specifically identifying competencies and interests directly associated with nursing productivity, positive nursing intervention outcomes, nursing work satisfaction, and the expectations of those interfacing with nursing. Among topics common for development are physical and mental healthcare issues of offenders, especially special populations, and the role of the professional forensic nurse working in correctional facilities. Issues such as ethical/legal implications of practice in correctional settings, acute and chronic disease management, and special vulnerabilities in the areas of communicable diseases, suicide and self-destructive behavior prevention, and assaultive behavior management are high priorities in correctional settings. More training is needed in mental health issues related to offenders and the relationship of race and ethnicity to mental health assessments, which are important education areas. The mastery of boundaries of practice and relationships with correctional staff and the offender are recurrent dilemmas for correctional nurses. Primary learning needs are centered on the correctional culture and how nurses reconcile the demands of the correctional setting with their professional code (Hufft & Peternelj-Taylor, 2000). In addition, there is a need for strong leadership in correctional nursing, reflected in the feelings among nurses that they are undervalued and neglected in major decision making related to nursing services. Advancing the skill sets in areas of leadership, management, and administration are essential to advancing the correctional nursing role.

Expectations for professional performance emphasize **evidence-based practice** and individual and departmental accountability in corrections. Major cultural changes for the nursing staff are outcomes of professional role modeling, including the following:

1. Policies and procedures are revised to conform to national standards, rather than focusing on specific institutional correctional preferences.
2. Nursing roles are defined in terms of the healthcare agency rather than correctional confinement or control goals.
3. Relationships with correctional officers are redefined from subservient to collaborative.
4. Institutional policies are not an excuse for lack of professional accountability.
5. Success is defined in terms of healthcare outcomes of offenders, rather than in terms of logistical expediency or security goals.

These changes are a necessary foundation for the transition to better health care for the offenders and part of the overall change in values that are the responsibility of advanced practice nurses in corrections. Although security and confinement will always be very important factors affecting the healthcare delivery system, the roles of correctional officers and nursing staff must be clarified, freeing nurses to care for and be responsive to the needs of the people in their care.

Summary

Advanced practice correctional nurses must intervene sensitively, creatively, and responsibly on the basis of scientific and evidence-based knowledge, and must also extend their roles to include that of personal advocate for competent care for offenders in correctional facilities. Their roles include development and implementation of correctional healthcare policy, development of organizational culture to promote collaborative models of healthcare delivery, advancement of ethical and legal nursing practice, development of professional nursing roles within correctional facilities, and facilitation of diversity and culturally competent health promotion and disease prevention. Increasing inmate satisfaction and the effectiveness of health care received in correctional facilities may provide a basis for offenders trusting and participating in healthcare strategies and self-care health promotion during their incarceration and after their release.

Advanced practice correctional nurses are in a unique position to provide leadership in the efficient and effective implementation of nursing and healthcare standards in correctional settings. New standards for health services in prisons and jails were published by the National Commission on Correctional Health Care (NCCHC c,d) in 2002, which distinguished between prisons and jail settings and emphasized educational material enabling facilities to assess their compliance with the standards using the same indicators used by NCCHC accreditation surveyors. Advanced practice correctional nurses are well prepared to serve as surveyors for the NCCHC.

Internal classification systems, those used to determine appropriate custody, housing, and programming within a facility, use policies and procedures for screening and evaluating prisoners who are management problems and those who have special needs. In particular, these criteria and procedures are used to assign offenders to administrative segregation, disciplinary segregation, and protective custody. Mental healthcare units and medical healthcare units must be part of the system. Advanced practice correctional nurses involved in the assessment of offenders for classification not only will provide expert administration of reliable and valid instruments, but also will advise and collaborate in decisions regarding options for using the results of such assessments in determining appropriate designation of offenders, ensuring involvement of the inmate in the process. The nurse should ensure that the inmate is informed and has a copy of the classification assessment. In addition, the nurse should ensure periodic review of any nursing assessments and be involved in the design and implementation of the classification process as it involves nursing and health assessments (Schneider, 2002).

Managing risk in a correctional healthcare setting is an especially important priority for advanced practice nurses due to the increased threats to security and the unique nature of the offenders, including the health risks they present. Significantly higher proportions of inmate populations, as compared to nonprison populations, are exposed to HIV and tuberculosis, experience substance abuse and physical trauma, and have mental disorders. Suicide rates in jails have been reported as high as 40% (Goss, Peterson, Smith, Kalb, & Brodey, 2002; Robertson, 2004). The advanced practice role includes surveillance, infection control, and risk management roles and the implementation of a systematic approach to problem identification and analysis of adverse events related to correctional health care (Valente, 2002). Suicide, exacerbations of psychiatric conditions, undetected or delayed diagnoses of medical conditions, and detection of active tuberculosis represent major foci of risk management programs in correctional settings. The advanced practice correctional nurse uses the public health model to construct nursing policies and procedures to document critical health events occurring in inmate and staff populations.

Advanced practice correctional nursing roles include that of mentor. Designed to improve the professional lives of correctional healthcare staff, mentoring focuses on the support, counsel, friendship, reinforcement, and constructive feedback necessary for successful professional practice. The Academy of Correctional Health Professionals has established a formal mentoring program and provides training at national meetings (National Commission on Correctional Health Care, 2002b). Nurses in advanced practice are expected to possess skills in listening and demonstrating caring for coworkers. Bringing new generations of correctional nurses into professional and social maturity occurs best through close and nurturing relationships with experienced expert nurses who not only provide practical information related to the policies and procedures of secure settings, but also provide guidance and modeling of evidence-based approaches to analytical problem solving and culture building. Building trusting relationships with correctional officers and establishing meaningful boundaries with staff and offenders is essential to successful professional practice. A correctional nursing mentor focuses on his or her career and institutional goals while maintaining professional standards of practice and upholding ethical and intellectual principles supporting nursing.

Privacy provisions established by the Health Insurance Portability and Accountability Act of 1996 (HIPAA) represent a unique challenge for correctional healthcare settings (Orr & Hellerstein, 2002). Impacting primarily the operations and finances of healthcare providers and payers, HIPAA privacy requirements regarding general consent and the privacy practice notification specifically exclude offenders. Translating these protections into best practices reflecting appropriate policies for correctional healthcare settings requires analysis and input from advanced practice nurses.

Establishing a therapeutic relationship with any patient can be a challenge, particularly if that individual has a mental disorder or is otherwise suspicious or paranoid. When the patient is an inmate, challenges to the therapeutic alliance include suspiciousness associated with prison culture and inmate socialization and conditions imposed on professional and personal boundaries related to security. Advanced practice nurses are prepared to present nursing models of care that incorporate strategies for adapting and caring for unique interpersonal relationships represented in the correctional population.

In extraordinary circumstances, patients are informed specifically not to engage in treatment, as in the case of sex offenders, because information revealed to counselors or nurses can be used to confine them in a postrelease treatment facility. Since 1999, the U.S. Supreme Court has allowed sex offenders to be confined in treatment facilities after their release from prison, if it is determined they are at risk for reoffense. There is no current data on how many sex offenders in correctional facilities refuse treatment or reasons why those refusing treatment do so. Advanced practice nurses are positioned and educated to collaborate with other healthcare providers to deliver therapeutic programs for special populations such as sex offenders.

Correctional health care provides a means to advance the public health agenda by caring for those who are among society's most vulnerable. Advanced practice correctional nurses are positioned to create and manage a closed healthcare system in which they can identify and treat high-risk patients, monitor their care, and support lifestyle changes. Advanced-practice correctional nurses have the skills and knowledge needed to advance nursing care as the most powerful change agent in correctional settings (Vitucci, 2001). Ultimately, the health care of the community is positively impacted.

 QUESTIONS FOR DISCUSSSION

1. What does the dress code adopted in a correctional setting, for staff as well as offenders, say about us?
2. How do the furnishings and layout of the physical setting affect emotions, perceptions, stress, and functional ability to carry out daily routines?
3. What does the vocabulary we use in the correctional setting say about our attitudes, beliefs, and philosophy of nursing care? Does it matter whether we use the terms *inmate, patient, client, youth, felon,* and *perp*?
4. What does the history of the institution tell you about how we nurse those in our care? What roles have nurses taken? What part of the budget has been given to nursing? At what meetings or activities have nurses regularly been included? Where and when are nurses mentioned in official documents? How often and in what context do nurses interact with administration?

REFERENCES

American Academy of Pediatrics. (2001). Health care for children and adolescents in the juvenile correction care system policy statement (RE0021). *Pediatrics, 107*(4), 799–803.

American Association of Critical Care Nurses. (2003). *What is an advanced practice nurse?* Retrieved from http://www.aacn.org/AACN/Advanced.nsf

American Correctional Association. (2003). *Understanding cultural diversity.* Lanham, MD: Author.

American Nurses Association. (1998a). *Culturally competent assessment for family violence.* Washington, DC: Author.

American Nurses Association. (1998b). *Legal aspects of standards and guidelines for clinical nursing practice.* Washington, DC: Author.

American Psychiatric Association. (1994). *Diagnostic and statistical manual of mental disorders* (4th ed.). Washington, DC: Author.

American Psychiatric Association. (2000). *Psychiatric services in jails and prisons* (2nd ed.). Washington, DC: Author.

Anno, B. J. (1991). *Prison health care: Guidelines for the management of an adequate delivery system.* Chicago, IL: National Commission on Correctional Health Care.

Anno, B. J., & Dubler, N. N. (2002). Confidentiality in corrections: Examining the ethical issues. *CorrectCare, 16*(4), 12.

Bachmeier, K. (2003). Addressing quality health care in the correctional setting. *Corrections Today, 65*(6), 76–77.

Bewley-Taylor, D., Hallam, C., & Allen, R. (2009). The Incarceration of Drug Users: An Overview. The Beckley Foundation Drug Policy Programme. Report 16. Retrieved from: http://www.idpc .net/sites/default/files/library/Beckley_Report_16_2_FINAL_EN.pdf

Blair, P. (2002). Correctional nursing: What's wrong with this picture? *CorrectCare, 16*(4), 8.

Bradley, J., & Kalfs, E.M. (2003). Identification and management of chronic medical problems in juveniles. *Corrections Today, 65*(6), 86–89.

Bureau of Justice Statistics (BJS). (n.d.). *Prison Rape Elimination Act (sexual violence in correctional facilities).* Updated August 9, 2010. Retrieved from http://bjs.ojp.usdoj.gov/index .cfm?ty=tp&tid=20

Canino, I. A., & Spurlock, J. (2000). *Culturally diverse children and adolescents: Assessment, diagnosis and treatment.* Amherst, MA: BOSC Books.

Centers for Disease Control and Prevention. (2001). *Providing services to inmates living with HIV.* Retrieved from http://www.cdc.gov/idu/facts/cj-hiv.pdf

Centers for Disease Control and Prevention. (2003). *Routine HIV testing of inmates in correctional facilities.* Retrieved from http://www.cdc.gov/hiv/partners/Interim/routinetest.htm

Coolman, A. (2003). Sexual misconduct in women's facilities: The current climate. *Corrections Today, 65*(6), 118–120.

Day, R. F. (2004). HIV/AIDS in prison: Crisis of the confined. *Body Positive.* Retrieved from http://www.thebody.com/bp/oct04/prison.html

Devine, P., Coolbaugh, K., & Jenkins, S. (1998). Disproportionate minority confinement: Lessons learned from five states. *Juvenile Justice Bulletin (NCJ 173420).* Washington, DC: Office of Juvenile Justice and Delinquency Prevention, Office of Justice Programs, U.S. Department of Justice.

Dolan, L., Kolthoff, K., Schreck, M., Smilanich, P., & Todd, R. (2003). Gender-specific treatment for clients with co-occurring disorders. *Corrections Today, 65*(6), 100–107.

DuPont, K., & Halasz, I. M. (1998). *Diversity: Communicating effectively; Professionalism in corrections.* Lanham, MD: American Correctional Association.

Eels, S. (2003). Providing therapeutic mentoring. *Corrections Today, 65*(6), 20–22.

Egley, A., Jr. (2005). *Highlights of the 2002–2003 national youth gang surveys.* OJJDP fact sheet. Washington, DC: U.S. Department of Justice.

Egley, A., Jr., & Arjunan, M. (2002). *Highlights of the 2000 national youth gang survey.* OJJDP fact sheet No. 4. Washington, DC: Office of Juvenile Justice and Delinquency Programs.

Eminson, D. M., & Atkin, B. L. (2000). The dangerousness of parents who have abnormal illness behavior. *Child Abuse Review, 9*(1), 68–73.

Esbensen, F. (2000). *Preventing adolescent gang involvement bulletin. Youth Gang series.* Washington, DC: U.S. Department of Justice. Office of Justice Programs, Office of Juvenile Justice and Prevention Programs.

Evans, D. G. (2003). New AAPA president faces today's challenges. *Corrections Today, 65*(6), 24–27.

Goffman, E. (1961). On the characteristics of total institutions. In D. R. Cressey (Ed.). *The Prison.* New York, NY: Holt, Rinehart & Winston.

Goss, R. J., Peterson, K., Smith, L. W., Kalb, K., & Brodey, B. B. (2002). Characteristics of suicide attempts in a large urban jail system with an established suicide prevention program. *Psychiatric Services, 53*(5), 574–579.

Greenfield, L. A., & Snell, T. L. (1999). *Bureau of Justice Statistics: Women offenders.* Washington, DC: U.S. Department of Justice.

Hall, H. V. (2000). *Detecting malingering and deception: Forensic distortion analysis* (2nd ed.). Los Angeles, CA: CRC Press.

Hall, H. V., & Pritchard, D. A. (1996). *Detecting malingering and deception: Forensic distortion analysis (FDA).* Delray Beach, FL: St. Lucie Press.

Harrison, P. M., & Beck, A. J. (2005). *Prison and jail inmates at midyear 2004.* Washington, DC: Bureau of Justice Statistics, Office of Justice Programs, U.S. Department of Justice.

Heidensohn, F. (1995). *Women and crime* (2nd ed.). New York: New York University Press.

Hofacre, R. (2003). The correctional health care debate. *Corrections Today, 65*(6), 8.

Howard League. (2003). *A short history of prison.* London, England: The Howard League for Penal Reform Publications.

Howell, J. C. (2000). *Young gang programs and strategies.* Summary. Washington, DC: U.S. Department of Justice, Office of Justice Programs, Office of Juvenile Justice and Delinquency Prevention.

Howell, J. C., & Lynch, J. P. (2000). Youth gangs in schools. *Young Gang Series Bulletin.* Washington, DC: U.S. Department of Justice, Office of Justice Programs, Office of Juvenile Justice and Delinquency Prevention.

Hufft, A., & Peternelj-Taylor, C. (2000). Forensic nursing. In J. T. Catalano (Ed.), *Contemporary Professional Nursing* (2nd ed.). Philadelphia, PA: Davis.

Jamison, R. (2002). The punishing decade: Prison and jail estimates at the millennium. Retrieved from http://www.cjcj.org/pubs/punishing/punishing.html

Lockwood, D. (1978). *Sexual aggression among male prisoners.* Ann Arbor, MI: University Microfilms International.

Macalino, G. E., Vlahov, D., Sanford-Colby, S., Patel, S., Sabin, K., Salas, C., & Rich, J. D. (2004). Prevalence and incidence of HIV, hepatitis B virus, and hepatitis C virus infections among males in Rhode Island prisons. *American Journal Public Health, 94*(7), 1218–1223.

Maden, T. (1996). *Women, prisons, and psychiatry: Mental disorder behind bars. Jordan Hill.* Oxford UK: Butterworth-Heinemann.

Maeve, M. K. (1997). Nursing practice with incarcerated women: Caring within mandated alienation. *Issues in Mental Health Nursing, 18*(5), 495–510.

Marable, M. (2000). Racism, prisons, and the future of black America. Along the color line. Retrieved from http://www.peaceworkmagazine.org/pwork/1200/122k05.htm

National Commission on Correctional Health Care. (2001). *Women's health care in correctional settings position statement.* Chicago, IL: NCCHC.

National Commission on Correctional Health Care. (2002a). *The health status of soon-to-be-released inmates: A report to Congress.* Retrieved from http://www.ncchc.org/pubs_stbr.html

National Commission on Correctional Health Care. (2002b, October). Mentoring: A great way to give back to your profession. *CorrectCare,* p. 4.

National Commission on Correctional Health Care. (2002c). *Standards for health services in jails.* Chicago, IL: NCCHC.

National Commission on Correctional Health Care. (2002d). *Standards for health services in prisons.* Chicago, IL: NCCHC.

National Institute of Corrections. (2002). Staffing analysis in women's prisons and special prison populations. *Special Issues in Corrections.* Retrieved from www.nicic.org/pubs/2002/018602.pdf

National Institute of Corrections. (2003). Frequently asked questions. Retrieved from http://www.nicic.org.FAQ.aspx

Neeley, C., Addison, L., & Craig-Moreland, D. (1997). Elderly offenders: the forgotten minority. *Corrections Today, 44,* 14–16.

Norris, M. P., & May, M. C. (1998). Screening for malingering in a correctional setting. *Law and Human Behavior, 22*(3), 315–323.

Orr, D., & Hellerstein, D. (2002). Controversy, confusion herald HIPAA. *CorrectCare, 16*(4), 1, 22.

Paris, J. E. (2003). Overcoming barriers to correctional physician productivity. *Corrections Today, 65*(6), 72–75.

Parrish, A. (2003). Reaching behind the bars. *Nursing Older People, 15*(3), 10–13.

Peternelj-Taylor, C. A., & Hufft, A. G. (1997). Forensic psychiatric nursing. In B. S. Johnson (Ed.), *Psychiatric-mental health nursing: Adaptation and growth* (4th ed., pp. 771–785). Philadelphia, PA: Lippincott-Raven.

Peternelj-Taylor, C. A., & Johnson, R. L. (1995). Serving time: Psychiatric mental health nursing in corrections. *Journal of Psychosocial Nursing and Mental Health Services, 33*(8), 12–19.

Peters, R. H., Greenbaum, P. E., Greenbaum, M. I., Steinberg, M. L, Carter, C. R., Ortiz, M. M., ... Valle, S. K. (2000). Effectiveness of screening instruments in detecting use disorders among prisoners. *Journal of Substance Abuse Treatment, 18*(4), 349–358.

Pollock, J. M. (1998). *Counseling women in prison.* Thousand Oaks, CA: Sage.

Potter, R. H., & Tewksbury, R. (2005). Sex and prisoners: Criminal justice contributions to a public health issue. *Journal of Correctional Health Care, 11*(2), 171–190.

Ramsbotham, D. (1999). Report on a full announced inspection of HMP Exeter. Retrieved from http://www.homeoffice.gov.uk/docs/exetcpe.html

Reid, W. H. (2000). Malingering. *Law and Psychiatry, 6*(4), 226–229.

Robertson, J. E. (2004, Summer). Inmate suicide litigation redux. *Jail Suicide/Mental Health Update, 13*(special issue 1), 1–20.

Schmalleger, F. (1999). *Criminal justice today: An introductory text for the twenty-first century* (5th ed.). Upper Saddle River, NJ: Prentice Hall.

Schneider, J. W. (2002). Managing inmate populations. *Correctional News, 8*(6), 20–21.

Seiter, R. P., & Kadela, K. R. (2003). Prisoner reentry: What works, what does not, and what is promising. *Crime and Delinquency, 49*(3), 1–7.

Smyer, T., Gragert, M. D., & LaMere, S. (1997). Stay safe! Stay healthy! Surviving old age in prison. *Journal of Psychosocial Nursing & Mental Health Services,* 35(9), 10–17.

Tahir, L. (2003). Supervision of special needs inmates by custody staff. *Corrections Today, 65*(6), 110–111.

Thornberry, T. P., Huizinga, D., & Loeber, R. (2004). The causes and correlates studies: Findings and policy implications. *Juvenile Justice, 9*(1), 3–19.

U.S. Census Bureau. (2010). Overview of race and Hispanic origin. Retrieved from: http://www.census.gov/prod/cen2010/briefs/c2010br-02.pdf

U.S. Bureau of Justice Statistics (2009a). Total Correctional Population. Retrieved from: http://bjs.ojp.usdoj.gov/index.cfm?ty=tp&tid=11

U.S. Bureau of Justice Statistics. (2009b). Prison inmates at midyear 2009-statistical tables. Retrieved from http://bjs.ojp.usdoj.gov/index.cfm?ty=pbdetail&iid=2200

U.S. Department of Justice. (2001). *About the Federal Bureau of Prisons.* Lompoc, CA: Federal Bureau of Prison Industries.

U.S. Department of Justice. (2001). Criminal offenders statistics. Retrieved from http://www.ojp.usdoj.gov/bjs/crimoff.htm

U.S. Department of Justice. (2002). *Bureau of Justice Statistics: Demographic trends in jail populations.* Retrieved from http://www.ojp.usdoj.gov/bjs/glance/tables/jailagtab

U.S. Department of Justice. (2003). *Nation's prison and jail population 2002.* Retrieved from http://www.ojp.usdoj.gov/bjs/pub/press/pjim02pr.htm

Valente, S. (2002). Overcoming barriers to suicide risk management, *Journal of Psychosocial Nursing and Mental Health Services, 40*(7), 22–33.

van Wormer, K. (2001). *Counseling female offenders and victims: A strengths restorative approach.* New York, NY: Springer.

Vitucci, N. (2001). Innovation leads to DC jail transformation. *CorrectCare, 15*(1), 1, 12.

Wells, D. (2003). Drug-assessment instruments: Making wise choices. *Corrections Today, 65*(6), 28–30.

Wrobleski, H. M., & Hess, K. M. (1997). *Introduction to law enforcement and criminal justice* (5th ed.). Minneapolis, MN: West.

Yates, J., & Gillespie, W. (2000). The elderly and prison policy. *Journal of Aging and Social Policy, 11*(2–3), 167–175.

SUGGESTED FURTHER READING/RESOURCES

Ackerman, J. (Director). *Trapped: Mental illness in America's prisons* [film].

American Nurses Association. (2007). *Corrections nursing: Scope and standards of practice.* Silver Spring, MD: American Nurses Association.

American Nurses Association. (2010). Scope and standards of nursing practice in correctional facilities. Washington, DC: National Commission on Correctional Health Care. Retrieved from http://www.ncchc.org

Anno, B. J. (2001). *Correctional health care: Guidelines for the management of an adequate delivery system.* Chicago, IL: National Commission on Correctional Health Care.

Cohen, F. (2008). *The mentally disordered inmate and the law.* Kingston, NJ: Civic Research Institute.

Greifinger, R. B., Brick, J. A., & Goldenson, J. (2007). *Public health behind bars from prisons to communities.* New York, NY: Springer.

National Hospice and Palliative Care Organization. (2009). Quality guidelines for hospice and end-of-life care in correctional settings. Retrieved from http://www.nhpco.org/files/public/access/corrections/CorrectionsQualityGuidelines.pdf

Ray, M. A. (2010). *Transcultural caring dynamics in nursing and health care.* Philadelphia, PA: F.A. Davis.

CHAPTER 20

The Forensic Nurse Witness in the American Justice System

Elaine M. Pagliaro and Bonnie R. Bentley Cewe

By its very nature, forensic nursing requires regular interaction with some aspect of the American justice system. A clear understanding of the various courts, their jurisdictions, and the stages of proceedings is vital. This chapter provides an overview of the trial process and the requirements for admissibility of evidence. This chapter also seeks to highlight the conduct of witnesses and the importance of expert testimony. The standards for expert witness testimony are also addressed. It also illuminates some of the negative fallout that may result from the provision of such testimony.

CHAPTER FOCUS

- » Overview of the Federal and State Court Systems
- » Case Procedure
- » Evidence Standards
- » Overview of Criminal Procedure
- » History and Standards of Expert Testimony
- » Expert Testimony
- » Preparing the Case

KEY TERMS

- » admissibility
- » civil action
- » competence
- » *Daubert*
- » evidence
- » expert witness
- » *Frye*
- » jurisdiction
- » relevance
- » reliability
- » *voire dire*

Forensic nurses likely will, at some point during their careers, be called upon to testify in a court of law and, thus, should possess at least a basic understanding of the American system of justice and court structure. Insight into the processing of cases and the application of the information presented in this chapter will undoubtedly aid the forensic nurse by providing the legal context within which forensic nursing is practiced. The forensic nurse's credibility within the legal system, with other practicing professionals, and with a judge or jury might seriously be diminished by an unfortunate display of lack of awareness of the details of the legal system.

Space constraints limit this discussion to a basic overview of the justice system. Ideally, a more specific understanding of the legal system and a rudimentary appreciation for the laws of a particular **jurisdiction** in which the forensic nurse will practice should be sought. The most effective way to become familiar with the workings of the legal system is to spend some time observing the proceedings in criminal and civil courtrooms during daily court activities and especially during trials. The roles of the forensic nurse as consultant and expert witness require a thorough understanding of the proceedings and procedures of the court, as well as the statutory requirements that must be met for a case to go forward in either criminal or civil court.

CASE STUDY 20-1

A "Battered Woman"

A victim of interpersonal violence recounted the following story to the hospital workers and later to the police:

... about 3 a.m. We went to bed and he began to accuse me of cheating on him. He took a pillow and put it over my face. I couldn't breathe. I gasped for air. He let me go and took a rope and tied my hands and feet together behind my back. It hurt. He kept putting the knife on my mouth and chest while he sat on my chest and put his knees on my arms. He said he was going to kill me. He cut the top of my lip and the bottom of my lip.. He kept saying he was going to kill me and my family, my two daughters and two sons. He had a lit cigarette which he threw on the bed. It landed next to me. I thought the bed sheets would catch on fire. He then said, "I missed you," picked up the cigarette and put it on my chest. . .

The victim subsequently recanted her statement. Emergency department personnel who treated this woman noted various injuries and bruises and included her statements in the treatment notes. When the medical personnel later provided testimony, they met with the prosecutor for about 10 minutes and then were sequestered until their testimony. In addition to questions about the physical injuries, the nurse was asked questions about the cause of the injuries and about battered woman syndrome. Several objections were made; the jury was dismissed from the courtroom several times and the nurse was required to provide testimony outside the hearing of the jury so the judge could make her ruling. What this medical expert believed was going to be a short, primarily fact-based testimony turned into an extensive and sometimes confusing courtroom experience. Complete pretrial preparation with the attorney would have made this experience more helpful to the trier of fact and more positive for the nurse.

The American System of Justice

The system of justice in the United States is an adversarial system; that is, there exist two sides in a case, each of which presents its own point of view. *Black's Law Dictionary* defines an adversarial system as "characterized by opposing parties who contend against each other for a result favorable to themselves" (*Black's*, 1999, p. 446). Consequently, each side of a dispute must present **evidence** in support of his or her side of the case. Simultaneously, each side strives to challenge, limit, or object to the evidence presented by the other side. Courtroom and evidence rules and procedures help to keep the proceedings fair and to prevent questionable facts from being presented to the jury. The case is carried out in front of a neutral judge whose job is to ensure that such rules and procedures are followed. When all the facts have been presented, it is up to the trier of fact, usually a jury, to weigh the facts and reach a conclusion about the case. The American justice system, which is also an accusatorial system, assumes the defendant is innocent unless and until guilt is proven. In an accusatorial system, the defendant is identified as having caused a harm, either civil or criminal, but the burden of proof rests on the accuser to prove guilt.

In a criminal trial, the justice system has developed a series of steps that must be followed according to specific rules so the rights of the parties are upheld while society attempts to prove the case against the defendant. As everyone who watches television knows, the standard of proof for a criminal trial is beyond a reasonable doubt. That proof must be in the form of evidence that is obtained in an appropriate manner without violating the rights of the accused. Also, the constitutional right against self-incrimination means that the defendant has an absolute right to remain silent concerning criminal charges. It cannot be stressed enough that a defendant's silence cannot be interpreted negatively. The state also has the burden of persuasion in most instances in a criminal trial because of the defendant's fundamental rights.

Civil trials proceed differently than criminal trials, as will be discussed briefly in this chapter. Because there is no criminal wrongdoing at question and the state is not bringing the charges, many of the individual protections of the Bill of Rights do not apply. In addition, the burden of proof in a civil case is more likely than not. Thus, because the accusation must be proved only by a predominance of the evidence, a person could be found liable in civil court using evidence that would not meet the burden of proof in a criminal case. One of the most prominent examples of this potential disparity in trial outcome is the O.J. Simpson cases. O.J. Simpson was tried for the murders of his ex-wife, Nicole Brown, and an acquaintance. After months of highly publicized testimony, Simpson was acquitted of all criminal charges related to their deaths. Several months later, a civil case was held, charging Simpson with the two untimely deaths. A jury found Simpson civilly liable for the two deaths and awarded the families $30 million (*Louis H. Brown, Estate of Nicole Brown Simpson v. Orenthal James Simpson*, 1995).

Sources of Law

The U.S. Constitution

The U.S. Constitution enumerates rights to which the citizens of this nation are entitled, including certain rights applicable in any federal or state court of law. The U.S. Constitution was drafted in response to actions by the government upon the citizenry. The federal system was designed to limit such governmental intrusion by dividing sovereign power between a central (federal) government, which would coordinate issues of interest to all the states, and state governments, recognized as representing local interests and opinions. Although the U.S. Constitution clearly identifies and guarantees certain rights of the people under the federal sovereign, when the Bill of Rights was written, it applied only to the actions of the federal government; initially, states were not required to guarantee these enumerated rights. Subsequent amendment of the Constitution required that states act in accordance with maintaining those basic, individual rights. In addition to the U.S. Constitution, the constitutions of individual states set forth the rights of persons in each state. Many state constitutions currently provide greater rights and protections to individuals *residing in those states* than the U.S. Constitution. These constitutional protections form the standard against which all statutes, regulations, rules, and procedures must be measured.

Common Law

Common law, or judge-made law, as it also is known, was developed over centuries. Numerous cases, involving different factual situations, came before judges for decision. Eventually judgments became more uniform, reflecting legal principles that were derived from the usages and customs of the people, affirmed and enforced by the courts. Common law consists of legal principles created and developed by the courts independent of legislative enactments. The common law developed and applied by American courts has its roots in the English common law. In England, such law came to be known as common law because it applied generally throughout medieval England and, thus, replaced a less uniform system of customary law dispensed in local or regional courts and in the private courts of feudal lords.

Although the courts in each state are free to develop the common law of that state in a manner that reflects local policies, to a surprising degree, federal courts and courts in different states share common views on general principles of law. This consistency is due in part to the fact that the decisions of the court are "inspired by natural reason and an innate sense of justice" (Mosk, 1988, p. 35) and in large part from the doctrine of *stare decisis*. *Stare decisis* is grounded in the belief that "security and certainty require that accepted and established legal principles ... be recognized and followed" (*Otter Tail Power Co. v. Von Bank*, 1942, p. 607). Accordingly, once a court has established a principle of law that is applicable to a certain set of facts, future courts should adhere to that principle and apply it in similar future cases unless the court subsequently finds that justice requires otherwise.

Legislation

The third source of law in the United States is the legislatures. Consistent with their role as the primary policy-making body, federal and state legislatures enact laws, known as statutes, to address problems that they have concluded were not adequately addressed by the common law. Because the legislature is the paramount law-making authority, a legislative enactment supersedes common law if a discrepancy exists between the sources of law. Today, the causes of action in civil cases and criminal charges are primarily outlined in state statutes. Over time, legislatures have created comprehensive bodies of legislation known as codes. A code, as distinguished from a statute, contains a systematic compilation of related enactments. As of 2011, federal and state legislation have so proliferated that most American jurisdictions are code jurisdictions. For example, every forensic nurse is likely familiar with the codes that establish licensing and professional standards within each state.

As discussed in Chapter 22, the forensic nurse may be called upon to act as an advocate to the legislature during the development of its laws and regulations. For example, testimony by nurses at a hearing committee before a final vote has had significant impact on legislation in areas such as victims' rights, domestic violence and partner abuse, the standardization of sexual assault examinations, and the statute of limitations elimination for cases involving DNA.

Overview of the Federal and State Court Systems

Two separate but interrelated court systems coexist in the United States. Article III of the U.S. Constitution establishes the federal courts and the areas of law that can be tried in those courts. The federal system includes the United States Supreme Court, established by the U.S. Constitution, and the federal district courts, courts of appeal, and several specialized courts of limited jurisdiction, allowed for in the U.S. Constitution and established by Congress. State courts, created by the states, hold the residuum of jurisdiction. State court structure and jurisdiction is the sole responsibility of the states. State decisions cannot be overturned by the federal court unless the state has based its decision on an erroneous interpretation of the U.S. Constitution.

Most court systems in the United States function as a hierarchy; that is, there are supreme courts that make final decisions in appeals of disputes brought to lower courts. Most states and the federal system also have an intermediate court to which a party can appeal if there are questions about the verdict in a case. Cases are first heard at the entry level. In the federal system, these are the district courts. In states, lawsuits or prosecutions are brought in courts of limited jurisdiction or general jurisdiction. Limited jurisdiction includes minor courts that hear a wide range of cases, such as police courts, small claims courts, and magistrate's courts. General jurisdiction courts hear most of the criminal cases in the states. All trial courts, whether federal or state, are courts of record. This means that a verbatim record is kept of each proceeding.

The United States Supreme Court

As the only court in the federal court system to be specifically established by the U.S. Constitution, the U.S. Supreme Court sits atop the federal court hierarchy. Although certain cases may be filed directly in the Supreme Court, such as cases in which one state is suing another state, most cases brought to the Supreme Court seek review of the judgments of lower courts. Most of these cases are appeals from the judgments of either federal courts of appeals or of state courts of last resort that dealt with questions of federal law. In a few types of cases, which are becoming increasingly rare, the Supreme Court hears an appeal from a district court without any intermediate appeal to the circuit court. The Supreme Court has the discretion to refuse to hear cases in which review is sought. Most cases that are appealed to the Supreme Court are refused a hearing. Each case is heard in the Supreme Court by the nine Supreme Court justices. On rare occasions, a case may be heard by fewer justices, but the quorum is never fewer than six. The U.S. Supreme Court is the final arbiter of federal law and federal constitutional issues.

State Court Jurisdiction

State courts are courts of general jurisdiction and are governed by state law. They are subject only to specific limitations set forth in the U.S. Constitution or by acts of Congress. Most states have a trilevel court structure that is similar to the federal court system—trial-level courts that possess general jurisdiction; intermediate appellate-level courts that hear appeals taken from trial-level cases; and a high appellate court, often called the state supreme court, or court of last resort. Some states have only a high appellate court, with no intermediate appellate courts.

Like the federal court system, state court systems also typically have several courts of limited jurisdiction called inferior courts, which hear only specified matters. These courts typically are less formal than superior courts and often are not courts of record; that is, detailed transcripts of court proceedings are not regularly kept. Examples of inferior courts are probate courts, traffic courts, administrative courts, and small claims courts. Jurisdictional divisions among inferior courts vary widely. In some instances, appeals can be taken from an inferior court to be heard in a superior court.

State Appellate Courts

Each state has its own system of appellate courts. As previously mentioned, some states have an intermediate appellate level and a high appellate court, whereas some have only a high appellate court. Some states, especially those with an intermediate-level appellate court, provide for an appeal as a matter of right from a trial court decision. Other states provide for appeals only in certain circumstances. State high appellate courts generally select from among the applications those cases that it considers appropriate for consideration. An appellate court may decide to hear a case because it presents an important issue, perhaps of constitutional magnitude, or perhaps poses an important question that requires a rule binding on all lesser courts within that state in order to ensure judicial consistency.

State High Appellate (Supreme) Courts

Every state has a high appellate court that serves as the ultimate authority of issues of state law within that state. Generally, in states with intermediate appellate courts, high appellate courts consider appeals only from those intermediate courts. Appeals from intermediate appellate courts to high appellate courts typically require some type of application process, sometimes called certification or *certiorari*. In states without intermediate courts, appeals to high appellate courts are taken directly from trial court decisions. High appellate courts also can exercise their authority to take appeals directly from trial courts whenever the high court considers the case to be one of special interest to the court.

The Case Procedure

All legal disputes or cases arise out of some type of event. In a criminal case, the event is the commission or omission of an act that constitutes a crime. The flow of a case in a criminal proceeding is shown in **Figure 20-1**. In a civil case, it might be the commission of a negligent or intentional act that causes harm to an aggrieved party, the breach of a contract between parties, or even the dissolution of a marriage. The type of event matters with regard to whether the result is a criminal action or a civil action. Ultimately, in either type of action, the case must be proven by the presentation of evidence pertaining to the event.

The Role of Evidence

Evidence is defined as any physical, circumstantial, or direct information that is offered in a proceeding to prove or disprove an issue in dispute. Evidence may include all statements, perceptions, physical evidence, and knowledge presented that pertains to the elements of a case. The adversarial system allows each side to present evidence that is most favorable to its side, while allowing challenges to the evidence of the other side. Generally, unless the opposing side successfully objects to its admission, proffered evidence will be available for

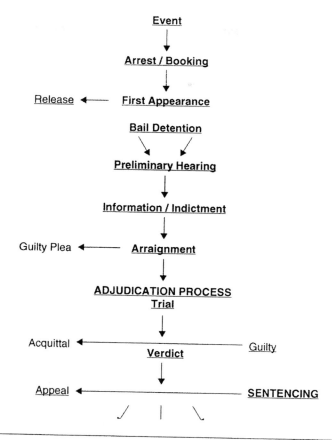

Figure 20-1   The criminal justice process.

the trier of fact (judge or jury) to consider in its deliberations. Once evidence is admitted at trial, the jury has sole discretion and responsibility to decide what weight to accord each item of evidence and to determine what evidence is credible.

After centuries of looking to the common law rules of evidence, the federal government determined that a more uniform set of evidence rules was necessary. In 1975, Congress enacted the Federal Rules of Evidence (FRE), which were standardized versions of the existing common law rules. In order to create workable rules that allowed for the flexibility necessary to address the myriad evidentiary questions facing judges every day, the FRE were drafted using general language that allows judges a great deal of discretion. Hence, judges must still rely on the vast body of the common law for application of the FRE in specific circumstances. In addition, the FRE did not address certain evidentiary issues, such as spousal privileges. Like the rules of procedure, the FRE are dynamic. For example, the FRE were revised to reflect the change in the federal admissibility standards for scientific evidence outlined in *Daubert v. Merrell Dow Pharmaceuticals* (1993).

In general, evidence can be divided into the following four categories: (1) witness testimony; (2) real, or physical, evidence; (3) documents or writings; and (4) demonstrative evidence (i.e., visual or audio materials presented to assist the jury). Such broad categories inevitably allow for evidence in many formats to be presented during a trial. Although the actual form and origin of the evidence may influence the judge's decision about whether it can be used in a particular proceeding, three basic requirements must be considered by the court: relevance, reliability, and competence. Evidence that is not relevant, reliable, and competent cannot be effectively tested by the opposing side and, therefore, is not an appropriate part of a fair trial process.

Relevant Evidence

According to common law and FRE 401, relevant evidence is any evidence that has "any tendency to make the existence of any fact . . . more probable or less probable than it would be without the evidence" (FRE, 2003). For evidence to be relevant it must pertain to the case at hand in such a way that the trier of fact could find this information useful during deliberations. Relevancy is essentially a logical evaluation of the evidence. Usually if there is a logical relationship between the evidence and the case the judge will allow its presentation. Admitting relevant and excluding irrelevant evidence is a practical rule, as well. The relevancy rule limits the scope of the topics that can be addressed during trial. Thus, the need for relevancy saves time during both case preparation and the actual court proceedings. Relevancy also helps to prevent the admission of evidence that may be misleading or confusing to the fact finder. Some experts have suggested that the relevancy rule also improves society's perception of a trial by requiring that the proceedings actually have something to do with the charge (Best, 2000).

Relevancy functions as the initial filter of evidence, based on the particular case scenario. For example, if J.J. is charged with forging checks, and during the investigation it is found that he has been carrying out a business in a residential zone, that evidence would likely be found inadmissible because it is irrelevant. Although some may consider J.J.'s acts as proof of his willingness to disregard the zoning law, this fact is not relevant because it is not of consequence to the determination of whether J.J. forged checks. On the other hand, if J.J. has a broken hand at the time of his arrest, the court may allow medical testimony from a nurse or physician to establish whether J.J. had a broken hand at the time the checks were forged. An example of an evidence rule based on the concept of relevancy that is of significance to the forensic nurse is the rape shield rule. (This rule has been codified by Congress and most state legislatures.) Generally, evidence of a sexual assault victim's prior sexual history is considered not relevant to the determination of whether she or he was sexually assaulted by the accused. This rule protects the privacy of the victim and prevents prejudice and confusion among jurors as to the significance of any prior sexual activity. However, in some instances, such as when the prosecution presents evidence that semen was found during a forensic examination of the victim, the court may allow the defendant to present scientific evidence that the recovered semen came from someone with whom the victim had consensual relations.

Reliable Evidence

Evidence must also be reliable to be admissible. **Reliability** of evidence may be established in several ways, depending on the nature of the evidence presented. Witnesses generally may testify to what they directly saw or did. The opposing party has the right to challenge those actions or perceptions through cross-examination. The freedom of a witness to testify regarding what she or he heard, however, is significantly more limited due to concerns about the reliability of such evidence. Although testimony that a witness heard a loud noise outside her window would be admissible (if relevant), *her testimony that another witness told her that the defendant did not commit the crime* would be barred by what is commonly known as the hearsay rule.

Hearsay is defined as "a statement, other than one made by the declarant (witness) while testifying at the trial or hearing, offered in evidence to prove the truth of the matter asserted" [FRE, 2003 § 801(c)]. This rule essentially prevents the admission of evidence that relies on the truthfulness of someone who is not present in court and whose veracity and perceptions cannot be challenged, which is guaranteed by the 6th Amendment of the U.S. Constitution. Although many out-of-court statements are generally deemed unreliable, and therefore rendered inadmissible, certain categories of out-of-court statements are made under circumstances that imbue them with a presumption of reliability. Those categories form numerous exceptions to the hearsay rule.

One hearsay exception known as the diagnosis and treatment exception is of importance to forensic nurses because the rule may permit the practitioner to testify to the statements of another made during a medical examination. The reliability of such statements is based on the premise that a person seeking medical assistance would speak truthfully to a medical provider in order to obtain appropriate care. Some attorneys have questioned whether the medical diagnosis exception will continue unchallenged in light of the Supreme Court decision in *Melendez-Diaz v. Massachusetts* (2009). As of the publication of this book, however, there have been no effective challenges to medical personnel including statements made by victims of interpersonal violence or sexual assault during examination and treatment.

Certain types of evidence, such as documents, photographs, and physical evidence, must be authenticated prior to presentation in order to establish their reliability. Some items may be considered as self-authenticating, such as certified public documents, but in general, authentication is done by a witness who can attest to the reliability of the item. If the item of evidence is a photograph, for example, the witness will be asked whether the image depicted is a fair and accurate representation of what was viewed by that witness. If physical evidence is collected from a scene, the witness will be asked about the chain of evidence to show its reliability. Discussion of physical evidence collection and how to maintain the proper chain of custody can be found in Chapter 14.

Scientific, medical, and other pieces of evidence presented by an expert witness are established as reliable when certain requirements for admissibility, as outlined in Supreme Court and state court decisions and rules of evidence, are met. According to FRE 702 "if the scientific . . . knowledge will assist the trier of fact to understand the evidence or to determine a fact in issue, a witness qualified as an expert . . . may testify thereto" (FRE, 2003 § 702). The current common standards for scientific and other expert evidence are described in the Supreme Court's decisions of *Frye v. United States* (1923) and *Daubert v. Merrell Dow Pharmaceuticals* (1993). These cases make it clear that the judge must act as a gatekeeper, determining if evidence is reliable and relevant prior to the evidence being presented to the jury. Thus, it is the court that first rules whether any witness is qualified as an expert and may testify on a particular subject. Then, even if the court finds that a witness qualifies as an expert, the judge may determine that a particular subject of the testimony is *not* admissible because it does not meet the criteria for scientific or medical evidence laid out in *Daubert* and FRE 702.

Admissibility of Scientific, Medical, or Technical Evidence

A forensic nurse may be called upon to testify as an expert witness concerning some aspect of technical, scientific, or medical evidence. Forensic testimony may pertain to subjects such as protocols, interpretations of data or medical records, or the administration of tests or treatments. Such testimony falls under the rules of expert witness testimony. Thus, a brief discussion of the development and requirements of the rules regarding expert testimony follows.

The *Frye* Standard. In 1923, the Federal Court of Appeals established the standard for the **admissibility** of scientific evidence that became the predominant rule for 70 years and still remains in effect in several states. In refusing to admit a polygraph result, the court stated that to be admitted into evidence, a scientific procedure must have gained general acceptance in the relevant scientific community (*Frye*, 1923). Critics of the ***Frye*** standard claimed that this test did not guarantee that evidence was reliable or even that it was the result of good science; *Frye*, they claimed, only required that a significant number of people recognize or use the test and any subsequent results. Questions also were raised about who constituted the relevant scientific community in which there was general acceptance. As technology boomed in the 1980s, the question of what actually makes a technical, scientific, or medical result reliable was revisited.

The Relevance Standard. Some states use what they call a **relevance** standard for admissibility of medical or technical evidence. Under this standard, scientific evidence may be admitted if the evidence has more than a minimum of probative value and the method used is supported by accumulated experience and court precedent.

The *Frye*-Plus Standard. As more complex and varied testing became available in the 1970s and 1980s, some states, particularly California and New York, adopted what is sometimes called the *Frye-Plus* or *Super-Frye* standard (*People v. Kelly*, 1976). Under this expanded test, the party offering the evidence is still required to show that the scientific method or standard applied to the evidence is generally accepted in the relevant scientific community. *Frye-Plus* also requires that the party offering the evidence show that those procedures were appropriately followed and that the results are reliable. This standard has been applied primarily for new technologies, such as DNA testing.

The *Daubert* Standard. *Daubert v. Merrell Dow Pharmaceuticals, Inc.* (1993) revolutionized the way courts look at scientific and medical evidence. In ***Daubert,*** the Supreme Court overturned a lower court ruling that excluded research evidence because it failed to meet the *Frye* general acceptance test. The Court held that, although general acceptance in the scientific community was an important factor, other factors should also be considered when determining whether such evidence is reliable. Emphasizing Federal Rule 702 and the judge's role as gatekeeper, the Court presented several factors to weigh in deciding whether to admit scientific evidence:

1. Is the method generally accepted within the relevant scientific community (the *Frye* test)?
2. Has the technique or theory been tested and validated?
3. Have the procedures or technique been reviewed by other scientists in the field or published in a peer-reviewed journal?
4. What is the error rate of the technique or the theory?
5. Are there standards applicable to the theory or techniques applied?

The Supreme Court clearly stated that no one factor is more important than any other, and that all factors do not have to be satisfied for the court to admit the evidence. On the other hand, even if all these factors are met, a judge may still exclude evidence if other issues raise questions about the reliability of the evidence. Some courts have held, for example, that although a procedure may generally be accepted, the specific application in a particular case is not. (Other courts have ruled that the application of procedures to a specific piece of evidence is a matter of weight and not admissibility.) In 1999, the Supreme Court held that the *Daubert* standard applied to all types of technical expert witness testimony, not just the traditional sciences and medicine (*Kumho Tire Co. v. Carmichael,* 1999).

Since the *Daubert* decision, most states have revisited the issue of expert witness testimony and the admission of scientific/medical evidence. Most states have adopted the *Daubert* standard or some modification of that standard for the admissibility of scientific evidence. Some state courts have added factors for consideration by the court in determining relevance and reliability of scientific evidence. Those factors include considerations such as the reputation of the expert and the extent to which a protocol previously has been accepted in the courts.

Competent Evidence

In some situations, even if evidence is determined by the judge to be relevant and reliable, the judge will not allow its use during a legal proceeding. Most relevant and reliable evidence will be found competent and admissible; however, there are certain situations, defined by the courts and rules of evidence, in which otherwise admissible evidence may be barred. If a witness is deemed unable to appreciate the duty to testify truthfully or is incapable of perceiving, remembering, or describing the incident in question correctly, that witness will be found incompetent. In some situations the testimony of a proposed witness, although relevant and reliable, may be protected by a legally recognized privilege of the defendant. For example, the defendant in an assault case may have told his doctor that he received his injuries during an ambush of the assaulted party. If this statement were made to the accused's neighbor it would likely be admitted by the judge as an admission by the defendant; however, because the statement was made to his physician as part of his medical treatment, most likely the doctor–patient privilege would apply and the doctor would be barred from testifying about the defendant's statement. Spousal privilege may prevent testimony of a spouse in certain circumstances. Another common situation in which evidence is not competent is when the exclusionary rule is applied by the court. The exclusionary rule is applied as a sanction in criminal cases when otherwise relevant evidence was obtained in violation of the accused's constitutional rights. For example, the exclusionary rule will be applied when evidence has been obtained in violation of the search and seizure protections of the defendant guaranteed by the U.S. Constitution (*Black's,* 1999). This is why it is important for the forensic nurse to ensure proper written consent or a search warrant has been obtained before the collection of reference biological samples from a suspect brought to the medical facility by investigators.

Other Evidence Considerations

In addition to the three basic requirements for the admissibility of evidence, the court will consider several other factors to ensure the fairness of a trial. In all cases the court must determine whether the probative value of relevant, reliable, and competent evidence is "substantially outweighed by the danger of unfair prejudice, confusion of the issues, or misleading the jury" (FRE, 2003 § 403). In other words, the judge must determine whether the impact of the evidence may be so great that it will affect the fact finder in a way that limits his or her ability to reach a reasonable, fair verdict. The court must weigh the probable effect of the evidence against the tendency of that evidence to prove or disprove a fact that is important to a case. If the court determines that the prejudicial impact outweighs the value of the evidence, it will bar that evidence. Not all prejudicial evidence will be excluded. It is axiomatic that evidence presented at trial against a defendant, whether by the prosecutor or plaintiff, will be prejudicial to some extent. Generally, *excludable* prejudicial evidence falls into two categories: evidence that will likely create prejudice in the juror's mind that is unrelated to the case, and evidence that has the risk of having undue impact on a juror and, thus, will be given extra weight during deliberations. The latter situation is sometimes described as evidence that will inflame the passions of a juror, which would prevent a cool-headed deliberation of the case against the defendant.

Evidence may also be excluded if it is cumulative, that is, if the court finds that the evidence is offered as proof of a fact that has already been supported by sufficient evidence. Such repetitious evidence may be barred because it can waste time, may confuse the jury, or may lead to a juror placing too much weight on a particular fact. The judge also has the discretion to exclude evidence that comes as a surprise to an opponent. The court excludes such surprise evidence to ensure a fair trial, especially when the surprise is the result of less than full compliance with applicable discovery rules. Several other areas of relevant testimony that are specifically excluded on the basis of a fair and efficient trial system can be found in the FRE and common law.

The court will consider the reliability, relevance, and **competence** of evidence as it applies to the admissibility of the testimony of the expert witness.

The Legal Nurse Consultant

The role of the legal nurse consultant is to evaluate, analyze, and render informed opinions on the delivery of health care and the resulting outcomes (American Association of Legal Nurse Consultants, 1995). In reviewing a case for possible medical malpractice or personal injury, for example, individuals involved in these cases typically have suffered some type of injury and that injury may have been caused by one or more individuals. Although this may not be a case that reaches the level of criminality, it may end up in the civil court system. Whether the injury occurred at a nursing home, hospital, clinic, physician's office, stand-alone surgical center, rehabilitation center, or any other place a patient received medical care, the medical records are the starting point in an investigation. Upon receiving the complete medical file, the legal nurse consultant uses both nursing assessment skills and the skills obtained through forensic training to review these materials. She evaluates the records and policies of the healthcare facility objectively and determines if the record indicates that the appropriate standard of care was applied in the case. The legal nurse consultant will also make determinations as to what other medical and forensic expertise is necessary to evaluate the case fully and appropriately. Legal nurse consultants may also be involved in the investigation of insurance fraud, Medicare abuse, OSHA violations, or other administrative case investigation.

Role of the Expert Witness

An expert is unique within the legal system. Only the expert can offer an opinion in court; that opinion may be based on personal study, educational background, experience, or review of the work of other individuals. An expert witness, by definition, possesses specialized knowledge that is beyond the experience of most persons and is called to testify to explain or elaborate on a particular issue in question. The role of the expert is to help the trier of fact understand a particular specialty or issue. People who are familiar with the judicial

TABLE 20-1   Guidelines for the Expert Witness

- Discuss parameters of the case prior to case acceptance.
- Set fees and expectations in a written agreement.
- Establish limits of expertise early in case discussions.
- Review all available, pertinent case materials.
- Offer both strengths and weaknesses of the case during evaluation and discussion with client or attorney.
- Testify only after pretrial conference.
- Maintain a dispassionate, professional demeanor.
- Let the truth of your testimony speak for itself.
- Answer all appropriate questions without argument.
- Learn from each experience as an expert witness.
- Seek advice if ethical issues arise.

system only through watching television or movies or by reading crime novels believe that the most important work conducted by an expert witness is in the courtroom. At that time the expert can provide the smoking gun—the information that the attorney can use to find the real criminal or to nail a conglomerate who is flouting the law that resulted in harm to an unsuspecting community, as in the movie, *Erin Brokovich*. However, most of the work of a good expert is accomplished outside of the courtroom. Through a disciplined, scientific approach to his or her area of expertise and the case facts provided, an expert witness assists the legal team in many ways. For example, the forensic nurse consultant may provide important insight into improper procedures that led to injury of a patient in the emergency room. In addition, he or she may point out that all guidelines were properly adhered to, saving the attorney much time and energy in pursuing what would ultimately be an unsuccessful challenge in a medical malpractice case. In fact, the attorney will depend on the forensic nurse to act as a true professional, pointing out both strengths and weaknesses in a particular argument. The forensic nurse must have the knowledge necessary to support his or her viewpoint with theory and practical examples. She or he must also provide an overview of contrary opinions that may be offered in a case and the strength of those arguments. In addition, the forensic nurse must be aware of the limitations of his or her expertise. Although the expert may have sufficient knowledge to review a case, other experts with detailed scientific knowledge may be required to effectively assist the client or attorney.

How an expert witness proceeds from the first contact at the beginning of a case through testimony and any subsequent contacts about his or her involvement will ultimately determine his or her success. **Table 20-1** provides a list of guidelines for the expert witness during this process. Although not exhaustive, these guidelines should provide a road map for the successful and ethical expert witness. The following discussion will expand on some of those points, although space does not permit a thorough treatment. Several very good references and many articles are on the market today to help the beginner become an effective and ethical witness.

The Expert Witness

As stated previously, whether someone can testify in a court of law or at a legal proceeding as an **expert witness** is ultimately determined by the judge. Acting as gatekeeper, it is up to the judge to determine who is an expert and the area of expertise about which that person may testify. Through a process called **voire dire**, the judge and/or attorneys will ask a series of questions designed to demonstrate the education, training, and experience of the proffered expert. The judge will then determine if the witness is indeed qualified to testify as an expert and the area of expertise.

However, many experts never go to court, but provide information and services to attorneys, managers, and others responsible for handling investigations, trials, and hearings. This is a very common aspect of the expert witness experience, so it is important to consider how user groups determine who is a suitable expert for a case. It is equally important for experts to consider whether a case is suited for their particular skills and temperament.

Many expert witnesses, even when hired as full-time employees, list their general qualifications and areas of expertise in an expert witness registry or advertise in legal and bar association publications. This is an efficient and cost-effective method of reaching those people most likely to need the expert's services. Once an expert is well established in his or her field, advertising is often not necessary, and the expert has more work than can be accepted. However, even the well-seasoned expert may find it necessary or desirable to expand his or her pool of potential clients. Because only a small amount of information, and perhaps a curriculum vitae, can be provided prior to involvement in a case, it is extremely important that the expert witness discuss his or her areas of expertise and limitations prior to accepting any case.

One of the biggest mistakes some expert witnesses make is to go beyond their specializations. For example, one forensic odontologist was reported as testifying to tool marks made by a knife at the crime scene, even though he had no specific training in that area (Saviers, 2002). In *Porter v. Whitehall Laboratories, Inc.* (1993), the opinions of three medical professionals as to the cause of renal damage from postsurgical medication were excluded because they had neither appropriate specialized experience nor studies on which they based their medical conclusions. Unfortunately, offering opinions beyond one's expertise can happen even to people who frequently act as experts if the boundaries are not carefully watched. This problem can be avoided from the beginning, however, if experts clearly delineate the knowledge, skills, and abilities they have to offer. Once the parameters have been established, it is easier for the expert to maintain those boundaries. Many attorneys are not aware of the different backgrounds and training necessary for some specialties, or they may misunderstand scientific and medical information. It is therefore up to the expert witness to explain any unique aspects of forensic nursing that are applicable in a case. For those who are employed full-time by a firm or institution, although sometimes difficult, it is still important for the expert to review the facts and to determine if it is appropriate to take on a case without assistance.

When providing testimony, the forensic nurse must be careful to remain within the purview of the medical expert. In *Velazquez v. Commonwealth of Virginia* (2002), the Virginia supreme court held that, while the sexual assault nurse examiner correctly testified to medical causation of injuries, her testimony improperly invaded the province of the jury when she stated that the injuries were not only inconsistent with consensual intercourse but added that they were the result of nonconsensual intercourse. The determination of the ultimate question—whether sexual assault occurred—can only be decided by the trier of fact. The forensic nurse will go through several steps in the process of serving as an expert, as explained in the following sections.

Initial Consultation

The initial consultation is a critical step for the expert witness. This initial discussion need not take a long time, but should provide the expert with sufficient information to gauge the situation and to decide if he or she is suited for the case. Because people seeking an expert often have little time and do not want to waste resources, they may provide little unsolicited information. One approach is to develop a series of questions to ask someone seeking your professional assistance. Questions such as, "How do you think I can help you?" or "What are the basic facts in dispute?" may quickly get to the heart of the matter. During an initial contact in a legal case, for example, an attorney should provide a short outline of the case, the specific expertise that is being sought, and a time estimate for the expert's work review/report and testimony, if necessary.

Often attorneys will ask colleagues for expert witness names, especially those experts who have been successful supporters and advocates for their side. Some who require specialized expertise will go expert shopping, seeking a witness who will support their view of a situation no matter what the facts may indicate. All experts should be wary of this possibility. You should make it clear during the initial contact that an unbiased, scientific approach to data evaluation and only appropriate testimony will be provided. For example, although the forensic nurse may be an advocate for victims of domestic violence, the attorney should not assume that this will ensure her testimony that interpersonal violence caused a documented injury.

If the expert cannot meet the expertise required or the time restraints presented in the initial inquiry, it is important to state that fact up front. If the time factor is critical to the case, then the expert may provide the names of people who may be more appropriate for the case needs. It is ethical behavior and proof of your professionalism to do so. Many experts get into trouble because they have case overloads and cannot complete work in a timely fashion. No matter how important an issue appears or intriguing a case may sound, if you cannot fulfill your professional obligations, that information will soon become general knowledge.

If an expert is unsure about a case or whether he or she has time for a particular case, it is usually a good idea to request further information for review and consideration prior to committing to the project. Usually the expert can be provided with materials with the understanding that those materials are confidential, even if he or she decides not to act as the expert after case evaluation. If this review does occur, however, the expert should be aware that it would be unethical to serve subsequently as an expert for opposing counsel.

After the basic outline of the problem has been provided, the expert should also make a clear statement about his or her fees, including any requirements if he or she needs to testify. It is difficult for some people to discuss fees, especially if they are accustomed to doing the same work for someone else at a salary or as government employees. Fees are necessary and an expected part of dealing with an expert witness. All fees should be reasonable and customary. For example, if you normally charge $200/hour for your expert services, this would likely be considered reasonable to review case materials and consult with the attorney about your findings. However, if in a similar case involving a well-known celebrity you charged $800/hour for the same type of work, there may be some question about the ethics of your agreement. Inevitably a question concerning fees will be asked during the testimony of a private expert witness, but most jurors understand that seeking payment for one's special skills is reasonable and necessary. It is important to realize that you, as an expert, are not paid for your opinion, but for your time used to apply your specialized knowledge. Usually, only when the fees appear to be unreasonable or to be influencing (buying) the expert's testimony will the jury consider those funds a factor in the credibility of the expert witness. Once you have agreed to participate as an expert witness, the terms should be written in a letter of agreement from you, the other party, or both.

Case Review and Evaluation

The expert witness provides appropriate assistance in a case only when all relevant materials are provided from the client. Some clients will not always pass along all information in a case because they do not realize what is relevant or are in the habit of passing along only minimal information. Attorneys like to control the direction of their cases and may, in the mistaken belief that they are doing the best for their clients, limit the materials released to experts. Every expert witness should ask for *all* documents, interviews, photographs, depositions, and other significant material pertaining to the case or fact at issue. The expert should make a list of information not provided that might clarify points and should note all questions that arise during the case evaluation. Rules of evidence recognize that many opinions of experts rely on data other than that presented in court to reach their conclusions.

It is obviously common practice to interview a party when physical or psychological status is at issue in a case, such as with an insanity or syndrome defense (e.g., battered spouse syndrome, rape trauma syndrome). Several approaches exist for carrying out these interviews. No matter the approach, the effectiveness of an expert will depend on the thoroughness of his or her preparation for that interview. Appropriate documentation and notes must be maintained during this process. Some experts are afraid that notes may be subpoenaed. However, without such notes there may be little factual information that the expert can provide in a trial or hearing that takes place years after the evaluation. In addition, notes and other documentation provide material to refresh the recollection of the expert prior to testimony. It should be understood that notes of the expert may be covered by the confidentiality of work produced at the request of the attorney and may not be available for review in certain circumstances.

If an expert has been objective, professional, and thorough in his or her evaluation, she or he should not be afraid to have an expert from the other side review that documentation. Often, when the forensic nurse acts as an expert, the situation provides opportunities for interaction with the client or patient. Although this relationship may provide added insight for the expert and the opportunity to assist the client in many ways, the expert must be careful to maintain an unbiased approach to the case. Even if the witness is personally committed to the client, emotional separation is necessary in the courtroom to best serve the client's interests. Although some experts may find this professional separation difficult to maintain, the forensic nurse has training and experience that is especially useful in situations that require such professionalism.

Preparation of a Report of Findings

After thorough evaluation, interviews, and study of supporting materials, the expert witness will usually prepare a report of his or her findings. This report should answer the overall question and provide the necessary data to support his or her conclusions. This report will be the basis of the expert's subsequent testimony in most cases. With the final report, both parties in the case will be able to see those factors the expert considers significant and the logic applied when analyzing the case. Theories of outstanding experts in the field that substantiate conclusions are important to point out. In addition, when appropriate, the expert witness should point out opposing theories, especially if they may have an impact on the case if presented by opposing counsel's expert. Reconstructions of probable actions that led to an injury, for example, may require reference to facts that support this as the most likely scenario, while indicating that other interpretations may be possible. This approach to case evaluation and report writing is an extension of the scientific objectivity that the expert must maintain throughout the case.

Expert Witness Testimony

Most cases in which an expert is involved never come to trial. The information that the expert provides in her written report may be used by the attorney to negotiate a settlement in a civil case or plea bargain before a criminal trial. As important and common as that process is, the expert should always be prepared to testify to her findings and support her conclusions on the witness stand or in sworn deposition. During oral testimony the expert has the opportunity to explain to the trier of fact opinions and interpretations of the data obtained. Prior to testifying, the expert witness should always have a pretrial conference with the attorney. Even if there have been several previous conversations concerning her report, no expert should get on the witness stand without such a meeting. Campbell et al. (2007) found that 58% of sexual assault nurses who provided testimony experienced difficulties in court. Many of the examples they discuss could be eliminated or reduced if the forensic nurse prepares thoroughly and meets with counsel before testimony. The purpose of the pretrial meeting is twofold. First, the expert will have a final opportunity to review her or his position and highlight significant points with the attorney. The attorney should review with the expert the questions he or she will ask and make sure of the likely answer. Second, if any additional issues have arisen during the trial, the pretestimony meeting is the only way that the expert can be aware of any changes in strategy or possible unanticipated questions that opposing counsel may raise. There is nothing more frightening to the conscientious expert than an attorney who will spend little time with her before testimony; when the attorney says, "Don't worry, I know what I'm doing," or "I'll leave it up to you, you're the expert," the expert witness may be justified in beginning to worry!

Prior to being qualified as an expert witness by the judge, the expert will be asked a series of questions designed to outline his or her educational background, training, and experience. Questions about membership in professional organizations, publications, and faculty appointments will also be put forth. The expert should be careful not to inflate his or her qualifications in an effort to impress the court or the jury. Even small overstatements, such as claiming association with illustrious leaders in forensic nursing when having taken only a course from that expert, can be fatal to one's career. In one case, when the expert presented himself as having been on the faculty of a university, this statement was effectively challenged by the defense attorney who knew that the expert only worked under an on-site, grant-funded project. Once the facts came to light, the judge barred any further testimony and warned of possible perjury charges (*State of North Carolina v. Peterson,* 2003). In another instance, the state's expert in a murder trial testified that he had a master's degree; in fact, he had completed the coursework, but not his thesis for this graduate-level degree. Ultimately he was found guilty of instances of this perjury in several cases, and his professional career was ruined (Maier & Quittner, 1987).

Oral testimony is a somewhat unique situation. Although testimony provides an opportunity to educate the trier of fact to the issues and the expert's opinion, it is unlike a typical educational setting. Generally, direct testimony is most like a classroom and provides a setting in which the expert can present clearly, in his or her own way, significant data and opinions. Even on direct examination, however, the attorney controls the flow of the discussion and decides which questions will be asked in what order. With appropriate preparation and a pretrial meeting with the attorney, the expert should be able to lay out her opinion in a clear and concise manner with few interruptions.

The expert witness is usually asked to give her opinion according to reasonable scientific or medical certainty. This terminology is sometimes difficult for the expert witness to deal with, because experts often deal with possibilities and likelihood and not certainty. When an attorney asks about reasonable scientific or medical certainty, this does not mean that there is no uncertainty associated with the opinion. As explained by Fields (1999), this term is usually thought of as a likelihood of more than 90%, "derived from the statistical data on the sources of measurement" (Fields, p. 53) and not taken as an absolute. However, this certainty must be based on information gathered using practices acceptable to the relevant medical community.

Witness Demeanor

Rightly or wrongly, the expert's demeanor during testimony plays a large part in his or her effectiveness. The expert does not have to maintain a solemn expression, but there are few opportunities in court to make jokes during testimony. This does not mean that the expert should be wooden or expressionless. On the contrary, the animated expert usually retains the attention of the jury. An expert's presentation style may go a long way in getting a jury to listen carefully to the expert's opinion. Usually it is more difficult for the expert who appears condescending or pompous to testify effectively. Unfortunately, the expert witness may not be aware of her or his pomposity. Using medical terminology without defining it to the members of the jury may confuse them; explaining procedures and opinions in a condescending manner has reportedly caused juries to ignore a witness. An expert witness should seldom lose his or her temper, even when being pressured in a continuous attack by a ruthless attorney. In fact, that is usually the questioner's purpose. In such a situation, the expert actually wins high points with the jury for remaining cool under fire. Some experts who are even-tempered during direct questioning have been known to become argumentative on cross-examination. Behaving in this manner will give the impression that the witness is biased or has something to hide from the court. Remember that it is the attorney's job to represent his or her client vigorously. The witness should not take personally any attempts of the attorney to do so.

Nurses have a great advantage when serving as expert witnesses. They are used to dealing with members of the public in a straightforward manner, explaining difficult concepts to patients and family members with compassion. Their experience working with people gives most nurses an ability to provide knowledge without appearing condescending. National polls have shown that nursing is the most trusted profession when honesty and ethical standards are considered (ANA, 2009). This general belief by the public goes a great way to giving the nurse expert great credibility, even before he or she opens his or her mouth!

An expert witness should have an open, natural manner and look often into the eyes of the jury. This personal contact instills a feeling of trust and maintains the interest of the jury during testimony. Of course, the most important aspect of the expert's testimony is a strict adherence to an ethical code that requires scientific objectivity.

Bias

The expert testifies ostensibly because her opinion will support the side calling her to court. The expert will explain clearly her conclusions and support these with studies and facts from other experts, where appropriate. Espousing a particular viewpoint, however, does not remove the responsibility to acknowledge other possible interpretations of the same data. When asked about other theories that could be in opposition to the expert's testimony, the witness should be prepared to explain why his or her explanation or application is more reasonable under the specific case circumstances. A forensic nurse must be aware of any limitations of the tests performed or interpretations of data and the error rate associated with any statistical analyses. Objectivity is important if a forensic nurse is going to be an effective expert. Canaff (2009) purports that, in fact, all roles of the SANE are improved by maintaining a neutral stance. He stresses that the credibility of the witness is enhanced when the scientific neutrality is reflected in testimony. The expert should be careful not to allow any previous role as an advocate to color testimony. In *Hussen v. Commonwealth of Virginia* (1999), the sexual assault nurse examiner testified that, in her opinion, injuries noted during her medical examination of the victim were the result of rape. When pressed further, she stated that consensual sex was out of the question because injuries such as those observed did not occur when the sexual response was triggered. Objections were raised by the defense about the bias inherent in such a conclusion. Although the Virginia Supreme Court ultimately upheld the SANE as an expert in the examination and medical evaluation of sexual assault, some of the defense community are still disturbed by her testimony. Few still argue that the judge erred when he recognized the years of experience in the emergency room and the training as a SANE that gave the forensic nurse an appropriate background as an expert. However, some defense attorneys believe that the SANE's refusal to consider any other modalities, even when the victim had not had intercourse previously, pointed to a biased and unscientific medical evaluation. Supporters of the forensic nurse argue that as an expert she gave her opinion based on direct observation of the injury and her expertise, and the SANE role as an advocate for the victim did not color her testimony. Similar controversies will no doubt occur in the future, especially in areas in which the forensic nurse combines her medical training and advocacy role.

Follow-Up After Testimony

After an expert has testified, he or she should directly leave the court or hearing room in a professional manner. The effective expert will *never* stop to shake hands with the attorney or client, which can communicate a bias to the jury. When the trial is finished, the expert may want to contact the attorney and analyze the testimony or discuss the more effective testimonial techniques. In addition, the expert witness should seek feedback from *both* attorneys, if possible, to improve her testimony skills. Some experts refuse to seek the opinions of opposing counsel, especially after criminal trials. However, since the opposing counsel did not invest much time or money in the other side's witness, comments from that attorney may prove most helpful, especially to the novice.

 ## QUESTIONS FOR DISCUSSION

1. Describe the desirable characteristics for an effective expert witness.
2. How are the credentials of an expert witness assessed?
3. Discuss the potential pitfalls that await the expert witness during trial testimony. What are some steps that can be taken to minimize or avoid them?
4. In what ways can a team of attorneys use an expert witness besides direct trial testimony?
5. Discuss some strategies for managing the potential conflict between the role of the nurse as advocate and the role of the expert witness in cases such as intimate partner abuse.

REFERENCES

American Association of Legal Nurse Consultants. (1995). *Standards of legal nurse consulting practice and professional performance.* Glenview, IL: Author.

American Nurses Association. (2009, December 11). Gallup poll votes nurses most trusted profession. *Medical News Today.* Retrieved from http://www.Medicalnewstoday.com/articles/173627.php

Best, A. (2000). *Evidence* (4th ed.). New York, NY: Aspen.

Black's Law Dictionary (7th ed.). (1999). St. Paul, MN: West.

Bosk, S. (1988). The common law and the judicial decision-making process. *Harvard Journal of Law and Public Policy 1*(11), 35–41.

Campbell, R., Long, S., Townsend, S., Kinnison, K., Pulley, E., Adames, S., & Waco, S. (2007). *Journal of Forensic Nursing, 3*(1), 7–14.

Canaff, R. (2009). Nobility in objectivity: A prosecutor's case for neutrality in forensic nursing. *Journal of Forensic Nursing, 5*(2), 89–96.

Daubert v. Merrell Dow Pharmaceuticals, Inc., 509 U.S. 579 (1993).

Federal Rules of Evidence, Public Law 93-595, revised December 1, 2003.

Fields, R. (1999). The science of expert opinions. In M. Shiffman (Ed.), *Ethics in forensic science and medicine* (pp. 50–63). Springfield, IL: Charles C. Thomas.

Frye v. United States, 293 F. 1013 at 1014 (D.C. Cir. 1923).

Hussen v. Commonwealth, 414 S.E. 2d. 597, 243 Va. 262 (1999).

Kumho Tire Co. v. Carmichael, 119 S. Ct. 1167 (1999).

Louis H. Brown, Estate of Nicole Brown Simpson v. Orenthal James Simpson, No. SC036876, Superior Court, State of California, County of Los Angeles (1995).

Maier, T., & Quittner, J. (1987, April 15). Crime 'expert' admits lying on credentials: felony conviction endangered. *Newsday.* Retrieved from www.corpus-delicti.com/dubey_041587.html

Melendez-Diaz v. Massachusetts, 129 S.Ct. 2527 (US 2009).

Otter Tail Power Company v. Von Bank, 8 N.W. 2d 599 (1942).

People v. Kelly, 17 Cal 3d 24 (1976).

Porter v. Whitehall Laboratories, Inc. 9 F. 3d 607, Court of Appeals 7th Cir. (1993).

Saviers, K. D. (2002). Ethics in forensic science: A review of the literature on expert testimony. *Journal of Forensic Identification, 52*(4), 449–462.

State of North Carolina v. Peterson, 652 S.E. 2d 216 (2003).

Velazquez v. Commonwealth of Virginia, 557 S.E. 2d 213, 263 Va 95, Va Supreme Ct. (2002).

SUGGESTED FURTHER READING

Bond, C., Solon, M., Harper, P., & Davies, G. (2007). *The expert witness: A practical guide* (3rd ed.). Kent, England: Shaw & Sons.

Cashman, D., & Beerrak, L. (2008). Preparing staff for testimony in sexual assault cases. *Journal of Forensic Nursing, 3*(1), 47–49.

Golan, T. (2004). *Laws of man and laws of nature: The history of scientific expert testimony in England and America.* Cambridge, MA: Harvard University Press.

Kohler, S. (2009). Types and roles of a witness. *Journal of Forensic Nursing, 5*(3), 180–182.

Matson, J. (2004). *Effective expert witnessing: Practices for the 21st century.* Boca Raton, FL: CRC Press.

CHAPTER 21

Disaster and Emergency Management

David Duff and Deborah Smith

The term disaster has been described throughout history as any event, natural or man made, that happens with or without warning, negatively affecting the life and safety of those within a community. This event further requires the coordinated use of services and organizations from multiple agencies to mitigate the effect and limit the damaging consequences of the event. The attacks of September 11, 2001 and subsequent anthrax attacks brought the attention of the U.S. government to establish policies to strengthen its preparedness activities to prevent and respond to threatened or actual domestic terrorist attacks, major disasters, and other emergencies. Nursing plays a unique role in this country's preparedness and response activities as nurses have the ability to utilize their critical thinking and problem-solving skills to improvise and adapt their care practices to effectively deliver care after a disaster. Those in forensic nursing, by virtue of their specialized training, have the opportunity to bring the distinctive skills of their practice to mitigate the effects of a disaster by their education in medical response, in postmortem response, and in the medical-legal implications in the postdisaster environment.

CHAPTER FOCUS

» Definitions of Disasters
» Principles of Emergency Management
» Incident Command Systems
» Terrorism and Weapons of Mass Destruction

» Psychosocial Issues
» Personal Preparedness Activities

KEY TERMS

» disaster
» emergency management
» hazard vulnerability
» incident command system (ICS)
» man-made disaster
» mitigation
» natural disaster

» planning
» preparedness
» recovery
» response
» terrorism
» weapons of mass destruction

Introduction

The term *disaster management* conjures up the images of the terrorist attacks of September 11, 2001, and the subsequent response. This large-scale **disaster** served as a wake-up call, alerting the Western world that nontraditional warfare has become the preferred weapon for use by terrorists and/or religious zealots to advance their causes. The Western world, specifically the United States, realized it was no longer immune to the actions of organizations based in many second- or third-world countries, as the members of these organizations are willing to attack the countries perceived as supporting their enemies. This nontraditional, limited warfare, also known as **terrorism**, is an ideal weapons platform for a less technologically advanced country or organization to confront a stronger opponent. One must query the purpose of the terrorist organization and its intended gains by performing such horrific actions against a civilian population. The goal is often as simple as wishing to disrupt the lives of the targeted country, using fear to alter how that country's inhabitants attend to their daily activities or to force a change in how governmental policy is created or enacted. This disruption is most evident today in the United States, Great Britain, Australia, France, Germany, and other Western republics/democracies. Such societies must now reconfigure their prevention and response apparatus to confront new threats. This has resulted in the construction of new government entities, with a tremendous channeling of fiscal and manpower resources toward the concept of strengthened homeland security. The creation of the Department of Homeland Security within the United States, with the concomitant commitment of resources, is intended to prevent or at least limit the impact of new disasters perpetrated by terrorist groups. As a study in the social sciences, this would generate endless perspectives to consider in the debate of what is terrorism vs. an act of war. However, as this chapter is designed to serve as a basic primer in disaster management, we will not delve further into the motivations of such actions. Rather, we will examine some of the steps that are taken to prepare for such actions and to reduce the impact of these activities.

Although terrorism preparedness and response is the overwhelming issue presented in media discourse, it is not the only concern of the emergency manager. Many disasters frequently impact the population. These disasters range from intense forest/brush fires (Australia, western United States, and several of the European nations) to floods, hurricanes, blackouts, and earthquakes that may cause loss of life and property. The disaster/emergency manager must be prepared for a rapid response to both natural events and terrorist actions. The forensic nurse specialist may play an important role in responding to either type of crisis as well as assisting in the evaluation of the causative action/agent.

The Definition of Disaster

A disaster is an occurrence or event that exceeds the capabilities of the available resources of a business or governmental jurisdiction (Federal Emergency Management Agency, 2005). The term *disaster management* not only includes the immediate response by a person, group, or agency to a traumatic event, but it also encompasses a greater scope of management. Although a large, powerful storm might wreak havoc through a region, it might not be defined as a disaster if the local government meets the needs of the citizenry with the available resources. If the ability to respond to the event exceeds the available resources of the jurisdiction, then the event will be classified as a disaster. In the United States, all disasters begin as local events. Local governments are responsible for responding to the needs of their particular jurisdiction. Once the local government's resource needs exceed its current capabilities, then assistance is sought from the next level of government. This process continues up the chain of governance until the disaster exceeds the capabilities of the state or group of states to adequately assist in the response. The governor of the affected state must request a declaration from the president of the United States for a situation to be deemed a federal disaster.

Another basic concept to understand is how the Federal Emergency Management Agency (FEMA) defines a disaster. Currently, FEMA categorizes disasters into two types, natural and technological (Federal Emergency Management Agency, 2010a). The term **natural disaster** includes events such as tidal waves, earthquakes, floods, forest fires ignited by lightning, blizzards, and heat waves. The term **man-made disaster** (or *technological disaster*) refers to those disasters that are caused by man, including terrorist acts (chemical, biological, radiological, explosive, and incendiary), blackouts, computer system failures, failure of telecommunication systems, arson, computer viruses, and accidents that may involve hazardous material spills, oil spills, and shipping.

Principles of Emergency Management

In order to understand the role of nursing in disasters, it is first important to understand the principles of **emergency management**. In the post–September 11, 2001 and post–Hurricane Katrina world, all levels of government understand the need to protect against, respond to, and recover from a wide array of manmade and natural disasters. To address this need, the president of the United States signed a series of Homeland Security Presidential Directives (HSPDs) in order to provide an integrated approach to disaster preparedness and response activities. These included:

» **HSPD-5, Management of Domestic Incidents.** HSPD-5 identifies steps for improved coordination in response to incidents. It requires the Department of Homeland Security to coordinate with other federal departments and agencies and state, local, and tribal governments to establish a national response plan and a national incident management system.[1]

» **HSPD-8, National Preparedness.** HSPD-8 describes the way federal departments and agencies will prepare. It requires the Department of Homeland Security to coordinate with other federal departments and agencies—and with state, local, and tribal governments to develop a national preparedness goal.

» **HSPD-18, Pubic Health and Medical Preparedness.** HSPD-18 describes the need for preparation against an attack by terrorist forces using a weapon of mass destruction. It acknowledges that having sufficient resources on hand at all times and at all places is not a realistic possibility. The policy set forth in the HSPD is a two-tiered approach for development and acquisition of medical countermeasures.

» **HSPD-21, Pubic Health and Medical Preparedness.** HSPD-21 describes the principles set forth in *Biodefense for the 21st Century* (April 2004) to transform the country's approach to protecting the health of the American people against all disasters. This approach included biosurveillance, epidemiologic surveillance, and ensuring public health and medical preparedness activities including the concept of *surge* to allow response to an event that threatens a large number of lives.

---

[1] In January 2008, Department of Homeland Security issued the National Response Framework (NRF) that supersedes the national response plan.

In March 2007, a group of emergency management practitioners from the Emergency Management Institute gathered to come to a consensus of principles that would guide the development of a doctrine of emergency management. The principles outlined by the group would be described as comprehensive, progressive, risk driven, integrated, collaborative, coordinated, flexible, and professional.

The process by which emergency management is based to effectively integrate all directives and principles to effectively prepare for, respond to, and recover from all disasters are considered the phases of emergency management or the emergency management cycle. The emergency management cycle stretches across all aspects of the disaster and includes:

» **Mitigation,** the process of proactively reducing the potential impact that disasters may have on the community over the long term. Mitigation is the opportunity to save lives and reduce the future costs associated with responding to a disaster.
» **Preparedness,** the process of **planning,** organizing, supplying, training, exercising, and evaluating activities to ensure effective capabilities to respond to any natural or man-made disaster or act of terrorism.
» **Response,** the ability to mobilize the necessary assets and first responders to effectively respond to a disaster area.
» **Recovery,** the process to restore an affected organization or community to predisaster status (Kaiser Foundation Health Plan, Inc., 2001).

Hazard Vulnerability Analysis

Disasters are by definition events that are often accompanied by significant destruction and loss. However, as was previously discussed, the mitigation phase of the disaster cycle allows an organization to minimize the amount of potential losses that may be incurred. To proceed with the mitigation phase in an organized fashion, organizations perform a **hazard vulnerability** analysis. The hazard vulnerability analysis may be presented in several forms, including a written analysis or a matrix format. The written analysis is normally the most complete form of threat analysis performed, but it may be difficult to decipher by those unfamiliar with the business or jurisdiction. The matrix format is a simple method that assigns a score to each potential disaster. The higher the score, the more likely the threat would cause damage or disruption in services. The matrix is the most common form used, at least within the healthcare community.

The first step to perform is to identify which hazards may confront the particular organization. The items in this list of potential hazards are normally categorized as technological threats or natural threats.

Once the list of hazards is developed, the next step is to evaluate the likelihood of the event occurring within or to the organization. Using the matrix format, the hazard is assigned a number from zero (unlikely to occur) to three (highly likely to occur during the period covered by the hazard vulnerability analysis). In attempting to determine the probability of an event occurrence, it is important to consider historical occurrences, known threats, and any intelligence provided by the law enforcement community.

The hazard is then evaluated for the risk that organization faces for each identified disaster. Risk is a category that evaluates the potential for harm or loss from each specified disaster. Risk may include posing an immediate threat to life or health, the disruption of services (including information technology services), damage to critical infrastructure,

Hazard And Vulnerability Assessment Tool Naturally Occurring Events — KAISER PERMANENTE.

Event	Probability	Severity = (Magnitude - Mitigation)						Risk
		Human Impact	Property Impact	Business Impact	Preparedness	Internal response	External response	
	Likelihood this will occur	Possibility of death of injury	Physical losses and damages	Interuption of services	Preplanning	Time, effectivness, resouses	Community mutual aid state and supplies	Relative threat*
Score	0 = N/A 1 = Low 2 = Moderate 3 = High	0 = N/A 1 = Low 2 = Moderate 3 = High	0 = N/A 1 = Low 2 = Moderate 3 = High	0 = N/A 1 = Low 2 = Moderate 3 = High	0 = N/A 1 = High 2 = Moderate 3 = Low or none	0 = N/A 1 = High 2 = Moderate 3 = Low or none	0 = N/A 1 = High 2 = Moderate 3 = Low or none	0 - 100%
Hurricane								
Tomado								0%
Severe thunderstorm								0%
Snow fall								0%
Blizzard								0%
Ice storm								0%
Earthquake								0%
Tidal wave								0%
Temperature extremes								0%
Drought								0%
Flood, External								0%
Wild fire								0%
Landside								0%
Dam inundation								0%
Volcano								0%
Epidemic								0%
Average score	0.00	0.00	0.00	0.00	0.00	0.00	0.00	0%

* Threat increases with percentage.

Risk = Probability + Severity
0.00   0.00   0.00

Figure 21-1   Hazard vulnerability analysis.
Source: Powers & Daily, 2010.

the loss of goodwill or trust, financial impact, or legal impact on the organization. Risk is scored on a scale of one (the lowest risk) to five (the highest level of risk to life and property).

The final component of the matrix is the evaluation of the organization's level of preparedness to respond effectively to each specific hazard. This is often done using a scale of one to three. The lower the score assigned, the better the preparation of the organization in meeting the potential threat. In considering preparedness, the organization should include such issues as insurance, availability of resources, readiness of response plans, and most importantly the training status of the responders and supervisors in the implementation of the plan. By identifying the greatest vulnerabilities, the emergency manager may address the most significant in the mitigation process. **Figure 21-1** shows a sample hospital hazard vulnerability analysis chart.

Nursing and the Phases of Emergency Management

Successful disaster planning, response, and recovery require an integrated, collaborative approach to address the varieties of hazards produced by the disasters themselves. Each phase of emergency management is a distinct component of a total process that is required to provide an effective response to a disaster event. Nurses, utilizing their knowledge, critical thinking, and assessment skills have the opportunity to guide process development for effective healthcare response during a disaster. Nursing expertise may guide planning by effectively assessing medical needs, determining staffing requirements, determining triage, surge management needs and care patterns, and evaluating alternate care resources (Federal Emergency Management Agency, 2010b).

Incident Command System

Given the large number of events that may be termed *disasters*, the forensic nurse specialist should have a basic knowledge of the incident management system used by most jurisdictions as well as many private institutions to manage disaster response activities. The **incident command system (ICS)** is a standard, on-scene, all-hazard management concept that represents best practices and has been adopted as the standard to incident management across the country. Incident command is a flexible management structure that may be used to coordinate both large and small events. ICS was originally developed by those involved in wildland fire management in the mid-1970s. It is designed to provide an effective coordinated response that may span over multiple jurisdictions (National Wildfire Coordinating Group, 1994). Since its inception, the ICS structure has been integrated into hospitals and other healthcare organizations and has become a requirement for all Joint Commission–accredited healthcare organizations. ICS provides consistency, with a clear chain of command, common language among responding agencies, and is flexible and scalable to all types of disasters (Hogan & Burstein, 2002).

The incident command system is divided into five management functions (see **Figure 21-2**) that provide the foundation for all response activities. These primary management functions may expand or contract to meet the needs of the incident. They include:

1. *Incident Command.* This position is responsible for the overall management of the response, setting the objectives and priorities that the team will attempt to accomplish.
2. *Operations.* This section conducts the tactical operations to achieve the objectives set by the incident commander. The operations section chief develops tactical objectives, is responsible for organizational development, and directs assigned resources.
3. *Planning.* This section is tasked with the development of the strategic objectives and the operations plan, as well as monitoring the long-term availability and deployment of resources.

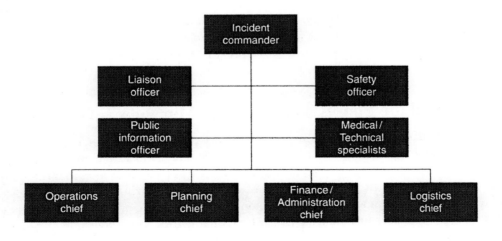

Figure 21-2 Incident command structure.

4. *Logistics.* This section provides and maintains the available resources and necessary supplies as well as supporting services to all staff (food, transportation, medical care, etc.).

5. *Finance/Administration.* This section monitors costs related to the incident, provides for accounting, establishes procurement contracts, monitors worker's compensation issues, provides time recording, and handles cost analysis.

The ICS structure is designed to coordinate activities and provide an organized approach necessary to establish and sustain the necessary level of capability during a disaster. This organized approach includes:

» *Defined primary functions.* These functions provide a structural matrix upon which additional activities may be added and defined as the incident grows and evolves.

» *Chain of command.* ICS provides for an orderly ranking of management positions. A clearly defined hierarchical structure provides for a clear line of supervision and stability in the implementation of the emergency operations response guidelines.

» *Organizational flexibility.* Although a position is listed, there is no mandate that it must be filled. The functions required to accomplish the mission determine the necessity of positions.

» *Common terminology.* Common vocabulary is important when working with multiple agencies and jurisdictions. Common terminology is applied to organizational elements, position titles, resources, and facilities.

» *Span of control.* This is a critical ICS issue. Span of control describes how many people or units may safely and effectively serve under each position. This management concept includes up to seven people or units serving under each position, with five being the ideal number. When additional resources or units are required, the incident commander, using the organizational flexibility of ICS, may add an additional management position in order to maintain a safe operational response.

» *Planning by operational period.* The concept of developing a written incident action plan for each operational period is novel to many responders. This plan is developed by the planning section in coordination with the operations section and supervised by the incident commander.

Terrorism

Terrorism is defined as the unlawful use of force or violence against persons or property to intimidate or coerce a government, the civilian population, or any segment thereof, in furtherance of political or social objectives. Since 1986, terrorism has become a common occurrence across the world. From 1969 through 1983, there were approximately 220 terrorist bombings, killing 463 persons and injuring 2,894 others. From 1984 through 1994, attempted or actual terrorist bombings increased by 400% (Hogan & Burstein, 2002). Since that time, the world has seen the 1995 Oklahoma City bombing, the attacks on the World Trade Center and the Pentagon on September 11, 2001, the 2002 Bali nightclub bombing, the 2004 Madrid train bombings, the 2005 London train bombings, and the 2008 Mumbai attacks which, combined, killed approximately 4,000 people and injured thousands more. As terrorism grows around the world, so does the need to understand the consequences of such attacks so as to more successfully prepare for an effective response.

Terrorist attacks may come in many different forms. Most commonly, terrorists will employ the use of explosive devices, as they are high profile, cause many casualties, and disrupt the local infrastructure. However, the potential for use of **weapons of mass destruction**—specifically chemical, biological, or radiological devices—continue to remain a significant risk.

In the event of a deliberate terrorist attack within the United States, the key governmental directive of concern to the forensic healthcare provider is Presidential Decision Directive 39 (Hogan & Burstein, 2002). Presidential Decision Directive 39 (1995) clearly defines roles and responsibilities of federal agencies in the event of such an attack. The Federal Bureau of Investigation is designated as the primary law enforcement agency responsible for preventing attacks and also for handling the postevent investigation. Although this appears to contradict the previous adage that all events are local, one must remember the potential scope that this investigation may entail. If a weapon of mass destruction is used, it would be considered an act of war if the action was sanctioned by a nation-state or an act of aggression if committed by saboteurs/illegal combatants and/or terrorists. Weapons of mass destruction use by terrorists may represent a cause with a multinational operational profile, like the group al-Qaeda. A multinational profile impedes tracking and the identification of the terrorists; thus the Federal Bureau of Investigation, in coordination with all of the available federal resources, becomes the ideal entity to deal with threat prevention and the capture of the fugitives postevent.

It is important for the forensic nurse specialist to understand the role that the Federal Bureau of Investigation plays in responding to potential acts of terrorism. The forensic specialist may be required to assist in the collection or examination of evidence, such as bodies, clothing, visual imagery, and documented observations of survivors. If a weapon of mass destruction is used, there will be casualties of the attack and potentially many more people affected by the psychological impact associated with the use of chemical, biological, or radiological devices. Early in the response to an event, these victims will require medical and crisis interventions. The response to such an event necessitates a combination of medical and legal knowledge, so the forensic nurse specialist appears the ideal candidate to assist the community, given the definition of forensic nursing provided by Lynch (Lynch, 1991). Lynch describes forensic nursing as the combined application of forensic science and clinical nursing in the scientific investigation and treatment of trauma, death, violence, and criminal activity.

This collaboration of medical care and forensic science seen in forensic nursing gains greater significance as institutions focus on initiating a proactive response to a terrorist attack. If a terrorist attack contains a chemical, biological, or radiological material and people are believed to be contaminated, one of the first responses is to remove all the clothing and perform thorough decontamination upon the person or patient presenting. Due to the nature of the event and the emergency department's primary goal of saving the patient, regard to the preservation of evidence will not be the primary focus of attention. Lynch emphasizes that appropriate forensic nursing techniques are vital in the emergency department, as the nurse is frequently the first to see the patient, to handle patient property, and to handle lab specimens. The emergency nurse must recognize that any patient with potentially liability-related injuries, whether victim or victimizer, living or dead, is a clinical forensic patient (Lynch, 1995). This last phrase from Lynch highlights an important detail to consider when dealing with patients from a weapons of mass destruction incident—that some of the patients may have perpetrated the incident. Therefore, the application of appropriate forensic technique, even amidst the mayhem of the response, is critical. The development of this protocol should be a joint effort among forensic specialists, law enforcement, and healthcare institutions.

The most important aspect for a forensic nurse specialist to consider before being called to such an event is the early development of a positive working relationship with local and federal law enforcement agencies. One of the basic tenets within emergency management is that the first contact between responders or agencies should occur over coffee before an event, not during the event. The development of such a rapport is critical to all aspects of emergency management and will improve the interactions of the forensic nurse with those with whom he or she may be working.

Weapons of Mass Destruction
Chemical Weapons

By definition, chemical weapons are any chemical agent used with intent to kill or injure or incapacitate an enemy. The term *chemical agent* may include weapons primarily found within the military, as well as industrial chemicals that are used to cause harm through intentional exposure (Encyclopedia Britannica, n.d.).

Humans have used chemical weapons for thousands of years, dating back to the Roman Empire and beyond. Military use of chemical weapons began in World War I with use of gas warfare resulting in more than 1 million casualties. In the ensuing years, chemical weapons have been employed numerous times, most recently in the Iran–Iraq War (1980–1988). Throughout recent history, countries around the world have stockpiled enormous amounts of chemical weapons; however, with the end of the Cold War (1945–1991), international agreements have been reached to ban chemical weapons developed since World War I. Despite international bans on chemical weapons, the threat of use by terrorists' entities remains real. As a point of fact, terrorists used sarin, a nerve agent, in an attack in Japan in 1995.

The threat of chemical weapons for use by terrorists may be significant for several reasons: the relative ease of acquiring the chemical intermediates required for the manufacture of the poison, the creation of immediate casualties and fear in the target population, the relative stability of the substance over a long period of time, and the use of modern devices to assist in the dispersal of the agent. However, there are also negative aspects for the terrorist to consider. A chemical attack is geographically limited in the extent to which it may effectively cause injuries to the intended target population. Another drawback is that a chemical exposure is unlikely to create additional patients from person-to-person contact. This lack of transmission is not only due to the agent's volatility, but also because responders have become aware of signs and symptoms that result from chemical agents and are more likely to take precautionary steps in dealing with consequences of such attacks. The last drawback to consider is that it is possible for the terrorist to be overcome by the agent, becoming a casualty along with the targets. As was mentioned previously, this is an important consideration for the forensic nurse specialist—any patient with injuries related to a man-made disaster is a clinical forensic patient. The actions of the forensic nurse specialist may assist in the retention of vital evidence that may be used to further the investigation into the terrorist act and also within the courtroom if the perpetrators are apprehended.

Chemical agents are classified by primary site of effect: blood agents (cyanide), nerve agents (tabun, sarin, VX), pulmonary/choking agents (phosgene or chlorine), blister agents (mustard types, lewisite), and incapacitating/riot agents (tear gas–type agents). In this section we will briefly review the pulmonary agents and the nerve agents.

The fact that many of the pulmonary agents are also common chemical precursors within modern industry means that there is a relatively abundant supply of these substances throughout the country. A terrorist who can effectively identify an opportune situation might decide to use one of these agents in an area that could affect thousands of people. The well-prepared emergency manager will understand the risks within the jurisdiction and develop a mitigation plan to reduce the continued threat that exists from this chemical type, whether it is an accidental release or an intended one aimed at creating terror, injuries, death, and financial impact.

Nerve agents were accidentally discovered in the mid-1930s by German scientists performing research to develop improved insecticides. The research into these agents, commonly known German gas A (GA, a.k.a. tabun), German gas B (GB, a.k.a. sarin), German gas C (GC, a.k.a. soman), and German gas F (GF, a.k.a. cyclosarin), was discontinued due to their extreme toxicity. Another nerve agent that is frequently mentioned is VX. VX, where the *V* stands for venomous, was originally developed in the 1950s in the United Kingdom. It is considered much more toxic than sarin and is considerably less volatile; therefore it may be more persistent in the environment.

Nerve agents are chemicals that act on the nervous system of victims, overstimulating the nerve receptors. Nerve agents bind acetylcholinesterase, preventing the enzymatic degradation of acetylcholine at the nerve receptors. The binding of the acetylcholinesterase leads to the overstimulation of muscles and glands. The acronym *SLUDGE* (salivation, lacrimation, urination, defecation, gastrointestinal distress, and emesis) may help people remember the effects of nerve agents on the human body. To counter these effects, atropine and pralidoxime chloride (2-PAM Cl) are provided to the victims via either intramuscular injection or intravenous access.

As was mentioned previously, the overwhelming amount of casualties requiring medical attention is an important consideration for the forensic nurse specialist. Any patient with injuries related to a chemical attack would be considered a clinical forensic patient warranting procedures necessary for evidence collection. The actions of the forensic nurse specialist will be paramount in the retention of vital evidence that may be used to further the investigation into the terrorist act and also within the courtroom if the perpetrators are apprehended.

Biological Weapons

Biological weapons are disease-producing agents, bacteria, virus, or toxins, with the ability to infect and spread through a population with the intent to be used as weapons against people, plants, or animals. Humans have used biological weapons throughout history. The first known uses took place in the 6th century BC, when the Assyrians used rye ergot to poison the wells of their enemies. Recent history includes use during World War I where German agents inoculated horses and cattle with glanders in the United States before the animals were shipped to France. In addition, the United States researched the use of biological weapons up until 1969, when President Nixon ordered that all offensive biological and toxin weapon research to end. As with chemical weapons, the potential use of biological weapons has not been swayed as a result of national and international agreements

(History of Bioterrorism, n.d.). Incidents including use of ricin as an assassination weapon in London in 1978 and the 2001 anthrax attack of members of the U.S. Congress and media outlets resulting in five deaths continue to demonstrate the use of biological weapons remains an undeniable threat.

The Centers for Disease Control and Prevention have designated several biological organisms or their toxins as potential weapons when used in a manner not conforming to legitimate research. These biological agents are divided into specific categories based upon those agents that are considered readily weaponized, and (1) are stable for storage and transportation, (2) are known to produce stable aerosols, (3) can be produced in large quantities, (4) are known to be highly infectious with high mortality, and (5) may be spread person-to-person with persons having little or no immunity. In addition, these biological agents have a strong potential to eventually be refined into weapons-grade material. The agents listed in this highest risk category (Category A diseases) are:

- » Anthrax (*Bacillus anthracis*)
- » Smallpox (variola virus)
- » Plague (*Yersinia pestis*)
- » Tularemia (*Francisella tularensis*)
- » Botulism (botulinum toxin)
- » Viral hemorrhagic fever

This section on biological weapons is intended only as a quick summary of the potential effects of biological agents that may be used as weapons. It is not intended to provide the medical practitioner with care or treatment guidelines. Guidelines for the recognition, care, and treatment of patients who may have been exposed to these biological agents can be obtained from the Centers for Disease Control and Prevention (CDC) website, www.bt.cdc.gov.

Although most known agents are not considered transmissible between humans, there are some notable exceptions. Smallpox (variola virus), which was eradicated through a worldwide vaccination program, is considered to be highly contagious between humans (WHO, 2001). The last remaining known caches of the virus are held by the Russian and United States governments. There is considerable supposition that additional countries may have retained their virus stocks or may have stock that was surreptitiously obtained. Smallpox has proven itself as an efficient weapon, assisting the Europeans in their conquest of the indigenous people located in both of the American continents. The fear that it may be reintroduced has led to a dramatic policy change and the re-creation of a vaccine to limit its spread. Again, note that fear of man-mediated events drives security, political, and fiscal policy decisions of the government.

For centuries, the plague (*Yersinia pestis*), otherwise known as Black Death, has remained a problem for man. The plague in 14th-century Europe is estimated to have led to the deaths of one third of the population. Plague is still endemic in many regions of the world. This historical success makes the plague and smallpox potentially lethal choices as weapons. Like smallpox, the plague has the potential for human-to-human transmission (Decameron, 2004).

The use of biological agents as weapons provides an unusual set of challenges for the healthcare professional. First, it would be unlikely that a biological attack would produce a large influx of patients requiring immediate medical care as biological agents require varying incubation periods. In addition, the ability to recognize a biological attack is extremely difficult as initial presenting signs and symptoms mimic that of common influenza. Recognizing that the differential diagnosis for influenza includes some of these diseases is vital to the containment of the outbreak. In addition, time is of the essence, not just for patient care, but also for evidence collection. In the time it takes to draw the distinction between a simple flu outbreak and the suspected use of a biological agent, damages may escalate from minimal fatalities to hundreds or thousands dead. Additionally, due to the current mobility of the population, containment of a biological attack may no longer be feasible. An excellent example of how a disease can rapidly spread before it is recognized is the outbreak of severe acute respiratory syndrome in the fall of 2002 to the summer of 2003. This disease spread from a rural Chinese province to many developed countries of the world in under a year. This inadvertent spread had a disastrous impact on many populations. An engineered bioweapon containing a transmissible agent may have a far greater impact on the world.

The use of quarantine is a much debated topic in emergency management and public health circles. Quarantine was used with some mixed results during the initial severe acute respiratory syndrome pandemic. Because of the varied results, albeit in very different cultural settings, the efficacy of both voluntary and involuntary quarantine measures is not fully understood. In addition to this issue, there are still questions on how the implementation of mass quarantine would be accomplished within the United States, as this would depend on the potential scale of the disease outbreak. The political jurisdiction might be able to effectively limit the movements or isolate several individuals, but as the numbers of individuals affected by the epidemic increases, there may be increasing difficulty in implementing quarantine orders. This decrease in the ability to effectively implement quarantine orders may be linked to several issues, including lack of political will to order the implementation of quarantine, overworked public health employees, the need to cohort patients in specific healthcare facilities, media broadcasts fanning the anxiety of the populace, and civil resistance. The ability to quarantine may also be limited by the lack of empowering legislation or by potential backlash from individuals claiming that the quarantine order violates their civil rights.

In a biological attack, the challenge to both the healthcare and law enforcement fields is in recognizing that an outbreak is indeed an intentional act and in the identification of the source of that act. The forensic nurse specialist may plan an important role as the conduit between healthcare personnel and law enforcement, with the CDC and the Department of Homeland Security providing their expertise by interpreting epidemiologic surveillance and assistance with evidence collection that may be used for further investigation to determine the source of the biological attack.

Radiological Weapons

A radiological weapon is a device used to spread radioactive contamination, either to cause panic, injury, or death to a population. Radiological weapons do not generally have practical military applications. American generals first studied the possibilities of using radiological devices as weapons during World War II. Their conclusion determined that mortality may not occur for days or weeks and their use would contaminate the target area. However, since World War II, radiological devices have remained a small but lasting threat. The threat of use by terrorist organizations remains real due to their ease of construction once the terrorists have acquired the appropriate materials. This section will discuss the properties of radiological devices in order to understand their use during a terrorist attack.

Radiological dispersion devices, also known as dirty bombs, are simple radiological devices combined with a conventional explosive device. A conventional explosive is used and mixed with a radioactive material. The actual radioactive material used may come from a variety of sources. Many abandoned medical facilities contain equipment that used radioactive materials for diagnosis and treatment. Academic research facilities and industrial equipment sterilizing companies often contain sources of radioactive material. Terrorists may break in to these facilities and retract the radioactive material, thereby "orphaning" it. While a radiological dispersion device detonation will most likely expose those in the immediate area to radioactive material, the actual exposure levels will likely be low, and cases of significant exposure including acute radiation syndrome will be minimal. While the consequences of radiation exposure will be nominal, fear of radiation exposure may cause panic and will easily overwhelm the local healthcare system.

In contrast to a radiological dispersion device, a radiation emission device is a nonexplosive device that emits radiation and has no explosive component. A radiation emission device is designed to be placed in a busy or populous location and has the ability to emit radiation, thus irradiating anyone who passes by. In contrast to a radiological dispersion device, a radiation emission device has the potential to lethally contaminate those in its proximity.

The priority of care of victims of radiological weapons varies from other hazardous materials exposure and contamination. In contrast to chemical contamination, the first priority for medical staff after a radiological attack is to treat patients with life-threatening traumatic injuries prior to decontamination. Since these patients remain contaminated during lifesaving treatment, staff caring for these patients will require additional personal protection, which includes respiratory protection from the inhalation or ingestion of particulate radioactive matter, skin protection, and monitoring of radiation exposure.

The use of these types of radiological weapons will produce an overwhelming amount of casualties, including those requiring medical attention and those who believe they have been radioactively contaminated (the worried well). Since the use of a radiological dispersion device or a radiation emission device will be considered a terrorist act, all patients may be classified as clinical forensic patients, thus warranting procedures necessary for evidence collection. Again, the forensic nurse specialist will have an integral role in retention of vital evidence and collaborating and coordinating with local and federal law enforcement agencies during the incident investigation.

Psychosocial Issues of Terrorism and Weapons of Mass Destruction

Earlier in this chapter, the discussion of terrorism suggested that terrorists are attempting to make political changes or statements, to force policy changes within the targeted nation-state's foreign affairs, or to disrupt the economy and lifestyle of the targeted population. The essence of terrorism is to force expanded expenditures, to make life uncomfortable for the citizens of the targeted nation, and to force them to change how they live and thereby demand their government to change its policies. In the end, terrorism is more of a psychological weapon aimed at making socioeconomic and political changes than a weapon to destroy people.

Given that a terrorist group is interested in creating fear, the mere threat of using a weapon of mass destruction is often sufficient to achieve its goals. In their text, Maniscalco and Christen (2002) use the nomenclature of *weapon of mass effect* as a new way of viewing the potential use of weapons of mass destruction materials, as the terrorist seeks to disrupt society by creating fear and preventing normal operations. The threat of such weaponry may encourage a society to change its operations. Excellent examples of these adjustments can be seen with the CDC's efforts to restart the smallpox vaccination process, the creation of a new large governmental organization (Department of Homeland Security), and the reallocation of scarce monetary resources into counterterrorism activities. We have dramatically changed our priorities in the United States as a result of persistent threats.

Beyond just terrorism, any disaster, whether natural or man-made, causes a disruption of societal norms. The physical damage may be great, but often the population's psychological response to a disaster may be much greater. The citizenry involved in a disaster or terrorist attack may respond in many ways. Each type of response will require different event and postevent recovery assistance. Psychosocial assistance is not meant to pathologize the response of the participants; on the contrary, the psychosocial response is meant to provide those affected with the tools required to cope with the immediate time period during and after the disaster. Psychosocial response recognizes that many people are by nature resilient to the effects associated with a traumatic event. This type of intervention is intended to enable disaster victims to retain at least minimal function. The psychosocial intervention is also meant to identify individuals who may require additional mental health assistance beyond the scope of the psychosocial assistance; these individuals would be immediately referred to psychiatric specialists for more intensive interventions.

The event may continue to significantly affect some individuals weeks, months, or years after the traumatic experience. These individuals may require extended medical care and mental health assistance. Posttraumatic stress disorder treatment is an example of one intervention that is performed by licensed professionals over a lengthy period of time to assist with the coping of those involved in traumatic events. A more thorough discussion of posttraumatic stress disorder can be found in Chapter 12 of this book.

Personal/Family Preparedness Issues

Disaster readiness is an issue not only for governments or businesses, but also for you and your family. If you are expected to respond to and provide assistance in a disaster, then the development of your own personal preparedness plan is imperative. To assist in personal preparedness planning, many resources, including the CDC and FEMA (http://www.ready.gov) have been developed to provide a framework for plan development. While the actual content of personal preparedness activities vary from organization to organization, the basic principles remain the same. Personal planning principles include the following:

» Gather emergency supplies (see www.bt.cdc.gov/preparedness). If a disaster strikes your community, essentials such as electricity, food, and water may not be initially available. Create an emergency supply stockpile in your home to include:
  ■ Bottled water
  ■ Medications
  ■ Food that does not require refrigeration for the family as well as the pets
  ■ Flashlights with replacement bulbs
  ■ Battery-operated radio
  ■ Batteries

- Prepare a "go bag" for each person that, at a minimum, contains:
  - Clothing (socks, underwear, shirts, pants, and sweatshirts for 3–5 days)
  - Shoes
  - Personal care supplies (shaving kit, toothbrush, toothpaste, soap, shampoo, and other personal hygiene materials)
  - Medications (30-day supply of prescriptions and photocopies of prescriptions)
  - Cash
  - Books, playing cards, or some other form of entertainment/diversion that does not require power or batteries
- Create a family emergency plan (see www.ready.gov for complete details).
  - Identify an out-of-town contact. It may be easier to make a long-distance phone call than to call across town.
  - Be sure every member of your family knows the phone number and has the ability to call the emergency contact (via cell phone or prepaid phone card).
  - Teach family members how to use text messaging (also known as SMS or short message service). Text messages can often get around network disruptions when a phone call might not be able to get through.
  - Subscribe to alert services. Many communities now have systems that will send instant text alerts or e-mails to let you know about bad weather, road closings, local emergencies, etc.
  - Prearranged evacuation route and reunification location for family.
  - Make arrangements for child care and pick-up from school.
  - Arrangements for pet care.

Summary

The knowledge base of the forensic nurse specialist continues to expand, as does the variety of potential disasters. Basic concepts of emergency management have become one of many new tools for the forensic nurse. Though many may think of emergency management as the response and recovery from an act by a terrorist, it is actually based on developing a program to address the needs presented by all hazards. This all-hazards approach to emergency management contends that the emergency management cycle needs to equally address the many potential threats presented by the modern world. Even though terrorism is the hot topic of emergency management, it is essentially just a disaster that is mediated by man to increase either the probability for an event to occur or the degree of impact of the event upon the community. Because of the use of an all-hazards approach to planning, the prepared emergency manager should have, at a minimum, a basic response model for each event. A chemical terror attack is similar to a chemical release from a factory or transport vehicle, whereas a biological attack is an epidemic that is intentionally released on the target population.

Emergency management emphasizes mitigation as the best way to reduce the impact that disasters may have on a jurisdiction. By increasing training and readiness as well as improvements to the physical environment protected by the emergency manager, the potential impact that an event may have on the region is lessened. As responders, it is important that forensic nurse specialists, as well as their families, be prepared to respond to an event. Personal and family preparedness will allow for a quicker response time as well as less time devoted to concern over the well-being of one's family. Having made adequate preparations, the responder should have fewer worries concerning the safety of his or her family and therefore be better able to concentrate on his or her performance.

The evolving field of emergency management depends on many different governmental agencies, businesses, nongovernmental organizations (American Red Cross, United Way, Doctors Without Borders, etc.), and individuals prepared to enact their response plans in the event of a calamity. A forensic nurse specialist has the potential to play an essential role, utilizing his or her experience in coordination, delegation, and care management coupled with expertise in forensic science in all phases of disaster preparedness, response, and recovery. It will be up to the forensic nurse specialist to engage in the process, providing input and ensuring the highest level of care to all patients he or she might serve.

QUESTIONS FOR DISCUSSION

1. What are the steps in the disaster cycle?
2. What are some strategies for an organization to be prepared for and deal effectively with a disaster?
3. What governmental response units are available to respond to a disaster? What is the role of each unit, and how do these interact with each other and with local management teams?
4. What difficulties are inherent in dealing with terrorist-type disasters?

REFERENCES

Decameron Web. (n.d.) *The coming of the plague to Italy.* Retrieved from http://www.brown.edu/Departments/Italian_Studies/dweb/plague/origins/spread.php

Encyclopedia Britannica. (n.d.). Chemical weapon. Retrieved from http://www.britannica.com/EBchecked/topic/108951/chemical-weapon

Federal Emergency Management Agency; Emergency Management Institute. (2005, July). *The ICS/EOC interface.* Emmitsburg, MD: The Department of Homeland Security.

Federal Emergency Management Agency; Emergency Management Institute. (2010a, August). *Fundamentals of emergency management.* Retrieved from http://training.fema.gov/EMIWeb/IS/is230a.asp

Federal Emergency Management Agency; Emergency Management Institute. (2010b, August). *Introduction to the incident command system for healthcare/hospitals.* Retrieved from http://training.fema.gov/EMIWeb/IS/is100HClst.asp

History of bioterrorism: A chronological history of bioterrorism and biowarfare throughout the ages. (n.d.). Retrieved from http://www.bio-terry.com/HistoryBioTerr.html

Hogan, D. E., & Burstein, J. L. (2002). *Disaster medicine.* Philadelphia, PA: Lippincott Williams & Wilkins.

Homeland Security Presidential Directive. (2004).Biodefense in the 21st Century. Office of the Press Secretary. The White House. Retrieved from: http://www.fas.org/irp/offdocs/nspd/hspd-10.html

Kaiser Foundation Health Plan, Inc. (2001). *Kaiser Permanente HVA.* Retrieved from http://www.njha.com/ep/pdf/627200834041PM.pdf

Lynch, V. A. (1991). Forensic nursing in the emergency department: A new role for the 1990s. *Critical Care Nursing Quarterly, 4*(3), 69–86.

Lynch, V. A. (1995). Clinical forensic nursing: A new perspective in the management of crime victims from trauma to trial. *Critical Care Nursing Clinics of North America, 1*(3), 489–507.

Maniscalco, P. M., & Christen, H. T. (2002). *Understanding terrorism and managing the consequences.* Upper Saddle River, NJ: Prentice Hall.

National Wildfire Coordinating Group (1994). Incident command system: National training curriculum. History of ICS. Retrieved from http://www.nwcg.gov/pms/forms/compan/history.pdf

Powers, R., & Daily, E. (2010). *International disaster nursing.* Cambridge, UK: Cambridge University Press.

World Health Organization. (2001). *Smallpox, historical significance.* Retrieved from http://www.who.int/mediacentre/factsheets/smallpox/en

SUGGESTED FURTHER READING/RESOURCES

Agency for Healthcare Research and Quality. (2007). *Nursing homes in public health emergencies: Special needs and potential roles.* Rockville, MD: U.S. Dept. of Health and Human Services.

Beach, M. (2010). Disaster preparedness and management. Philadelphia, PA: F. A. Davis.

Holloway, A. (1990). *Disaster reduction: What it means for nurses.* Emmitsburg, MD: National Emergency Training Center.

Powers, R., & Daily, E. (Eds.). (2010). (2010). *International disaster nursing.* Cambridge, UK: Cambridge University Press. Available at http://www.cambridge.org/aus/catalogue/catalogue.asp?isbn=9780521168007

Sundnes, O. K., & Birnbaum, M. L. (2003). *Health disaster management: Guidelines for evaluation and research in the Utstein Style.* [United States]: Prehospital and disaster medicine.Vol 17 Supplement 3. Retrieved from: http://www.wadem.org/guidelines/intro.pdf

Veenema, T. G. (2003). *Disaster nursing and emergency preparedness for chemical, biological, and radiological terrorism and other hazards.* New York, NY: Springer.

World Association for Disaster and Emergency Medicine website. Available at http://www.wadem.org

CHAPTER 22

Forensic Nursing in the Community: Public Policy and Public Relations

Michael E. Moynihan, Tracy A. Swan, and Anne Klein

Forensic nurses often find themselves involved in key interactions with the public. These roles range from influencing public policy to interacting with the public and the media to promote these policies or during medical interventions. This chapter will review, define, and describe public policy and the ways in which policy decisions influence nursing practice. The various roles of the forensic nurse sometimes lead to interactions with the public in nontraditional ways. Because the forensic nurse may be involved in high-profile cases or serve as an advocate or spokesperson, knowledge of how the media function and the best way to work with the media to achieve success for both parties is critical. This chapter will enhance current knowledge and assist in developing new knowledge that can be applied to addressing the development of forensic nursing practice in the 21st century.

CHAPTER FOCUS

- » Definition of Public Policy
- » Categories of Public Policy
- » Types of Public Policy
- » Public Policy-making Process/Cycle
- » Administrative Agencies
- » Policy Makers
- » Policy Influencers
- » Specific Policy Areas of Interest to Forensic Nurses

- » Advocacy Role of Forensic Nurses and Associations
- » Understanding the Media
- » Monitoring the Media
- » Developing a Strategy to Work with the Media
- » Developing a Proactive Plan to Manage a Crisis
- » Understanding Media Terminology

KEY TERMS

- » administrative agencies
- » advocacy
- » agenda
- » authoritative technique
- » broadcast media
- » capacity technique
- » distributive policy
- » executive department
- » follow-up questions

- » for background only
- » hortatory technique
- » incentive technique
- » independent agency
- » interest groups
- » key message
- » legislature
- » not for attribution
- » off the record

KEY TERMS

- » on the record
- » outreach
- » policy adoption/decision making
- » policy formulation
- » policy implementation/administration
- » print media
- » problem recognition
- » professional associations
- » programs

- » public policy
- » redistributive policy
- » regulations
- » regulatory commission
- » regulatory policy
- » rule making
- » spokesperson
- » talking point

Introduction

A bill creating a program for sexual assault nurse examiners was passed in 2008 in the state of Connecticut. This bill was the culmination of years of work by many who knew of the successes in other states toward providing consistent care for victims. While the state was in the forefront of creating a multidisciplinary team to standardize evidence collection and provide training to emergency personnel, the next step of creating a sexual assault nurse examiner program was elusive. A collaborative effort involving the state's commission for the standardization of sexual assault evidence, the Connecticut chapter of the International Association of Forensic Nurses, state medical societies and associations, sexual assault counseling services, (the state victim's **advocacy** organization), state's attorneys, scientists, and many others eventually brought about this monumental event. This bill was one of many, including the elimination of the statute of limitations on sexual assault, that was possible through the public policy efforts of nurses joining with other groups. The coalition that formed typified the effectiveness of nurses joining forces to affect public policy in a positive way.

Nurses historically have not been very involved in either developing policies or lobbying for or against policies that impact nursing practice. With significant forensic nursing issues often in the forefront of today's healthcare legislation and on the front page of newspapers, forensic nurses must step out of the traditional roles and develop skills that will help them work effectively with politicians, public agencies, nonprofit groups, and the media. The International Association of Forensic Nurses maintains a government affairs committee and actively encourages forensic practitioners to become active voices for important legislation. "With respect to forensic health care policy, there is very likely no one who can speak better to the issues at hand than a forensic nurse" (International Association of Forensic Nurses, 2006, para. 1). Some specific issues that may be of interest to those in the field of forensic nursing are DNA analysis; sexual assault forensic examiner, forensic nurse examiner, and sexual assault nurse examiner certification; prevention of violence and abuse; specifically sex-based crimes; prisoner rights; healthcare services in prisons; bioterrorism; forensic examination protocol; patient education programs for at-risk populations; web-based crimes; and, of course, the adequate funding and support to address these issues. Forensic nurses can have great influence in the current debates about statutes of limitations related to sexual assault, child abuse, and other crimes, status of the death penalty and its implementation, and treatment of offenders who are minors.

One of the very first proactive conversations you should have is with reporters to educate them about forensic nursing—what it is, why it is a cutting-edge profession, and what you, as a forensic nurse, do. When television shows or movies focus on forensics for solving crimes, many assume this to be your principal role. This is where being credible is essential. You will want to point out the differences between entertainment and real life, then take this excellent opportunity to explain the various specialties (in particular your specialty) within forensic nursing practices. As a forensic nursing professional, you must know how and when to work with the news media to achieve policy goals. You also need to know what your role is in other professional situations where the media may be involved. You need to know what you can say without compromising a case you are working on or jeopardizing the security, safety, or health of the people with whom you are working, while protecting your own credibility.

Well-honed communication skills can often help bridge the gaps among the healthcare system, the justice system, legislation, and the public. A thorough knowledge of public policy and creative, effective communication methods can help achieve the goals of forensic nursing in the 21st century.

What Is Public Policy?

Public policy is a relatively stable, purposeful course of action followed by a government in addressing some problem or matter of concern that is shared by a substantial number of individuals, corporations, or organizations (Anderson, 2003, p. 2). Public policies are government policies based on law and are authoritative and binding (O'Connor & Sabato, 2002, p. 430). There are several categories of public policies: substantive, procedural, material, symbolic, distributive, regulatory, self-regulatory, redistributive, and those policies involving public or private goods. The types of public policies that affect the field of forensic nursing and that would be of most interest are distributive, regulatory, and redistributive. These kinds of policies differ from other types by their effect on society and the relationship among those involved in the formation of the policy (Anderson, p. 7).

Distributive policies involve allocation of services or benefits to particular segments of the population—individuals, groups, corporations, or communities. Some distributive policies may provide benefits to just one or a few beneficiaries, whereas other distributive policies, like health aid for the elderly, tax deductions for home mortgage interest payments, free public school education, and job training programs, provide benefits to a vast number of individuals. Distributive policies typically involve using public funds—taxes—to assist particular groups, communities, or industries (Anderson, 2003, p. 7).

Redistributive policies involve deliberate acts by the government to shift the allocation of wealth, income, property, or rights among a broader class in society or to specific groups, like from the wealthy to the poor. This type of policy is usually heatedly debated in the media, among elected officials, and between political parties because redistributive policies transfer some power, rights, or money from one group to another. Examples of some successful redistributive policies are the graduated income tax, Medicare and Medicaid, the Voting Rights Act, and the Civil Rights Act (Anderson, 2003, p. 10).

Regulatory policies impose restrictions or limitations on the behavior of individuals, groups, and industries. This type of policy reduces the freedom or discretion to act of those regulated, whether they are bankers, utility companies, liquor stores, physicians, or engineers. The most extensive variety of regulatory policies deals with criminal behavior against individuals and property. The formulation of regulatory policies usually occurs because of conflict between two groups or coalitions of groups, with one side seeking to impose some sort of control on the other side. Typically, the other side views the proposed control as unnecessary or inappropriate for the desired result and, thus, opposes the regulation.

Regulatory policies take several forms. Some set general rules of behavior, directing that certain actions be taken or not taken. Others set standards for quality—quality of goods, services, or information—as with the Food and Drug Act, Consumer Credit Protection Act, or the hundreds of professions that require licensing in order to practice (Anderson, 2003, pp. 8–9).

When Does a Problem Come to the Attention of the Public?

The extent to which an issue is perceived to be a problem and is shared by many is the catalyst for generating interest in addressing/solving the issue. Four factors can influence the perception of an issue as a problem that must be addressed:

1. *Image of the problem:* Is the problem one that is truly shared by many and worthy of being addressed? Can the problem be solved or impacted in a meaningful way?
2. *Influence and number of constituents affected by the issue or interested in the issue:* The greater the number of individuals affected by the issue and the greater their political clout—voting power or financial influence—the more likely the issue will be considered.
3. *Political acceptability of the issue:* Can policies be developed that would have an impact on the issue? Do voters care about this issue?
4. *The issue's point in history:* Must the issue be dealt with now? Can it be put off until later?

Some problems will never rise to the level of public concern because they are accepted as trivial, appropriate, inevitable, or beyond the control of government (O'Connor & Sabato, 2002, p. 432). **Figure 22-1** depicts the relationship between the political environment and the policy-making process.

Public policies are created out of a need, which can be social or economic, as already discussed. The need usually requires some kind of change, such as greater access to health care for the retired, more employment opportunities for those on welfare, lower interest rates in order to spur buying and borrowing, or stronger restrictions on pollution in order to enjoy cleaner air and water. When the government steps in to create a policy, regardless of whether the proposed policy is social or economic, it is usually to promote efficiency in situations where the market (our economy—the exchange of goods and services) is believed to have failed or to foster a more desirable distribution of goods, services, and rewards among individuals in society (Starling, 2002, p. 31).

The Environment

Markets fail in four distinct ways:

1. They organize themselves such that there is little or no competition, which can cause prices to skyrocket (e.g., a monopoly).
2. They release a byproduct that is harmful to the public/environment, such as pollution, when manufacturing their goods.
3. They tend not to produce or underproduce a needed/wanted public good (e.g., public roads, parks, defense, judicial system) because they find it difficult to make a profit selling the public good.

The Environment

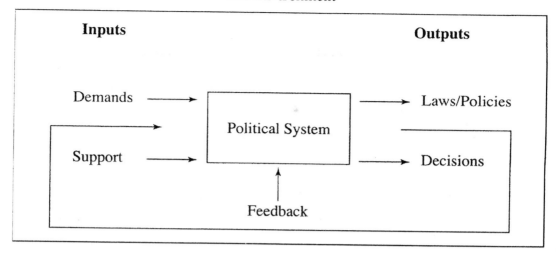

Figure 22-1   A model of the political environment where policy is created.
Source: Anderson (2003), p. 15.

4. They withhold vital consumer information such as drug side effects or qualifications of professionals, like physicians, that could lead to consumer harm.

Besides market failures, some other situations in which private issues can rise to the level of public concern and warrant attention as part of the public agenda include:

» Breakdowns of systems, such as family relationships
» Low living standards that result from well-functioning markets that do not reward individuals very generously if they lack marketable assets and skills
» Discrimination against racial and other minorities
» Areas where government is expected to function effectively, but in fact is not, such as providing excellent public education (Bardach, 2000, pp. 3–4).

Leadership and Policy Initiatives in Forensic Nursing

According to Beatty, Glendon, and Williams (2006), the future of forensic nursing is directly related to the need to develop well-prepared nurse leaders who can assume positions of power and influence. In these positions, forensic nurses can affect decision-making bodies throughout the nursing profession and make policy at the local, state, national, and international levels. To reach this goal, forensic nursing must foster articulate leaders through education and assessment. The assessment tool was developed by Goldwater and Zusy (1990) and proposed for use by Beatty et al. This tool can be used to evaluate nurses' political acumen and raise awareness of the steps each nurse can take to affect policy.

The Policy Process/Cycle

Political scientists and other social scientists have developed many theories and models to explain the public policy process. Presented here is a widely used model that outlines the process as a sequence of stages or functional activities. As you review the model presented in this chapter (see **Figure 22-2**), please keep in mind that sometimes in the policy process some of the stages may merge, such as the policy formulation and adoption stages, or the adoption and budgeting stages. Also, it is important to recognize that what happens at one stage in the policy-making process affects action(s) at later stages, and sometimes such action is done deliberately with these effects in mind. For instance, how does the content of legislation (policy formulation) ease or complicate its implementation? Or, how does implementation affect its impact (evaluation)? Also, the policy cycle is flexible and open to change and refinement as the policy progresses through the stages. The cycle also highlights the relationships, or interactions, among the participants in the policy-making process. Political parties, interest groups, legislative procedures, presidential commitments, public opinion, and the media can be tied together as they drive and explain the formulation of the policy (Anderson, 2003, p. 30).

Problem Recognition and Definition

In the **problem recognition** and definition stage, a problem is identified as some condition or situation that causes distress or dissatisfaction or generates needs for which some kind of relief or corrective action is sought—often from the government (national, state, or local) (O'Connor & Sabato, 2002, p. 432). Often there is not a single agreed-on definition of the problem. This can lead to political struggle because how the problem is defined helps determine what sort of action is appropriate to adopt.

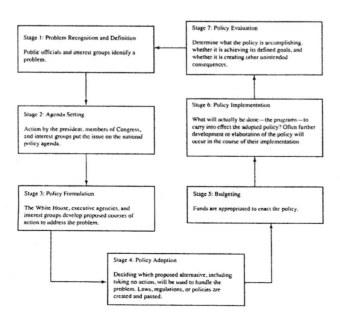

Figure 22-2 Stages of the policy-making process.
Source: O'Connor & Sabato (2002), p. 431.

Agenda Setting

Once a problem is recognized and defined, it must be brought to the attention of public officials and it must secure a place on the government's **agenda**—a set of problems to which policy makers believe they should be attentive (O'Connor & Sabato, 2002, p. 433). Not all the problems that attract the attention of public officials have been widely discussed by the general public; also, not all the problems widely discussed by the general public attract the attention of public officials. The two most pressing factors for a shared problem to receive attention from public officials are the influence and number of constituents affected by or interested in the problem and the political acceptability of the problem and its solution.

Policy Formulation

The **policy formulation** stage involves the crafting of appropriate and acceptable proposed courses of action, or policy alternatives, to ameliorate or resolve the public problem. Policy formulation may be undertaken by various players in the political environment—from the president and his aides to agency officials, from appointed task forces and commissions to interest groups, from think tanks to legislators and their staffs. In developing the policy alternatives, often a preliminary analysis of their success, which includes costs and practicability for implementation and political acceptability, occurs.

Many different methods for analysis can be used here or as part of the next stage. The most commonly used method is a cost–benefit analysis. This method compares the costs of creating and implementing each policy alternative (usually in terms of expense, but also political feasibility) against that alternative's benefits. The analysts need to determine if the benefits outweigh the costs, or if the benefits justify the costs regardless of how high they are.

To evaluate an alternative's political feasibility, an analyst looks at whether elected officials would vote for the proposal and make it law *and* whether appointed officials will support the law and implement the policy in a way that makes its success possible (Munger, 2000, p. 15). There is only one way to ensure that politicians and bureaucrats will be likely to support a policy, or at least not to oppose it: get them involved from the beginning of the cycle. The two most important stages in which to get these officials involved are in the problem recognition and definition stage and in the policy formulation stage. Because politicians and bureaucrats have different kinds of veto power over many policies, it is especially important to get their views on each policy alternative before you move on to the next stage in the policy-making cycle (Munger, p. 15).

Policy Adoption

In the **policy adoption** stage, also referred to as **decision making**, the different policy alternatives are compared to determine which alternative is the most appropriate and usually the most cost-effective to address the defined problem. The adoption of one alternative must be approved by the people with the requisite authority to do so, such as the **legislature** or chief executive. This approval gives the policy legal force. Successful policy adoption requires the building of majority coalitions like interest groups, labor organizations, political parties, or general citizenry. Policy adoption is political in that it usually includes conflict, negotiation, the exercise of power, bargaining and compromise, and sometimes even deception and bribery (Anderson, 2003, p. 29). *It is crucial that the policy* adopters correctly state in specific language what the policy is to accomplish, and by whose authority, so as to adequately guide the implementation of the policy and to prevent distortion of legislative intent (O'Connor & Sabato, 2002, p. 434).

Not all policy adoption requires the formation of majority coalitions. Presidential decision making, such as on foreign affairs and military actions, is often unilateral. Although inundated with information and advice from many aides and advisors, the final decision rests with the president. Also, the president also has the power to veto a bill—a piece of legislation that would address a public, shared problem—passed by the legislature.

Budgeting

As with most things, a crucial stage in the policy-making cycle is funding. Most public policies require financial support in order to be carried out successfully. Many of the distributive and redistributive types of policies involve the transfer of money from taxpayers to the government and back to those individuals whom the policy was created to benefit. Whether a policy is well funded or not has a significant effect on its scope, impact, and effectiveness. An absence of funding or a refusal to fund can virtually nullify a policy. Also, other plans or **programs** developed to meet the objectives of the policy can suffer from inadequate funding, such as the No Child Left Behind Act (O'Connor & Sabato, 2002, p. 435).

The budgetary stage also gives the president and Congress an opportunity to review the hundreds of government policies and programs, to inquire into their administration, to appraise their value and effectiveness, and to exercise some influence on their conduct (O'Connor & Sabato, 2002, p. 435).

Policy Implementation

The **policy implementation** stage (also referred to as **administration**) defines *how* policies are carried out. Most public policies are implemented primarily by **administrative agencies**. These administrative agencies are given a mandate by Congress to create the necessary programs that will meet the objectives of the policy passed by the legislature. While creating the programs, administrative agencies often engage in elaboration of the policy and even creation of policy through enactment of the programs' rules and standards. **Figure 22-3** shows how a public policy is implemented through agency plans, which are administered through various programs that reflect policy goals.

Administrative agencies may be enabled to use a number of techniques to implement policies in their jurisdictions. These techniques can be categorized as authority, incentive, capacity, and hortatory techniques.

Authoritative techniques are based on the assumption that people's actions must be directed or restrained by government in order to prevent or eliminate activities or products that are unsafe, unfair, evil, or immoral. Examples of these actions are driving while intoxicated, manufacturing unsafe consumer products like poorly designed baby cribs, or broadcasting obscenities over the radio. Agencies enforce policies by issuing rules and standards that individuals and corporations must follow. Compliance with these rules and standards is determined through inspections and monitoring. Penalties may be imposed if individuals or corporations are in violation of the rules and standards that are set forth in a particular policy.

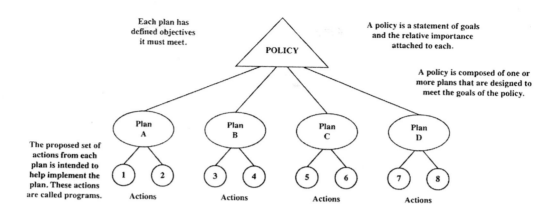

The proposed set of
actions from each
plan is intended to
help implement the
plan. These actions
are called programs.

Each plan has
defined objectives
it must meet.

A policy is a statement of goals
and the relative importance
attached to each.

A policy is composed of one or
more plans that are designed to
meet the goals of the policy.

Figure 22-3 The structure of a public policy.
Source: Starling (2002), p. 187.

Incentive techniques are based on the assumption that individuals are maximizers of goods and services and act in their own best interest, and thus must be provided with pay-offs or financial inducements to get them to comply with the policy. Examples of financial inducements to create certain desired behaviors are tax deductions for charitable dona-tions or grants awarded to companies for installing pollution control equipment. Also, sanctions such as high taxes imposed on luxury goods (such as furs and diamonds) and sin goods (such as gasoline, tobacco, and liquor) are intended to discourage consumption of these products.

Capacity techniques are based on the assumption that society has the incentive or the desire to do what is right but lacks the capacity to act accordingly. This technique provides individuals with information, education, training, and resources that will enable them to undertake the desired activities. Examples of this are job training for the unemployed and accurate information about interest rates for consumers.

Hortatory techniques are based on the assumption that people decide to act on the basis of their personal beliefs and values, such as equality, justice, and what is right and wrong. These techniques encourage individuals to comply with a policy by appealing to their better instincts, such as the "Only you can prevent forest fires," "Don't be a litterbug," and "Just say no" publicity campaigns (Anderson, 2003, pp. 220–221). The effectiveness of public poli-cies depends largely on the ability of the agencies to promote understanding and consent, thereby reducing violations and minimizing the use of sanctions (Anderson, p. 236).

Policy Evaluation

The policy evaluation stage determines whether the course of action—the program—is achieving its intended goals and objectives. Policy evaluation may be conducted by a variety of players from congressional committees to presidential committees, from admin-istrative agencies to university researchers, and from private research organizations or think tanks to the General Accounting Office of the federal government. Evaluations may lead to amendments that would hopefully correct problems or shortcomings in the policy.

Who Creates Policy?

Official policy makers are those who have the legal authority to engage in the formation of public policies. These policy makers include legislators (federal, state, and local), executives (president, governor, county executive, and mayor), administrative agencies, and judges. They each perform somewhat functionally different policy-making tasks from one another (Anderson, 2003, p. 46).

Policy makers can be broken up into two distinct categories: primary and supplementary. *Primary policy makers* have direct constitutional authority/power to create policy. These include legislators and executives. The main function of our legislature is to engage in the central political tasks of lawmaking and policy formation in our political system (Anderson, 2003, p. 47). Our president's authority to exercise legislative leadership is clearly established by the U.S. Constitution and legislation and is an accepted practical function and political necessity of the executive branch. Presidents are generally more interested in policy initiation and adoption than in policy administration (Anderson, p. 52).

Supplementary policy makers, such as administrative agencies and judges, operate from the power granted to them by primary policy makers. Due to our increasingly complex society and its social, technical, and economic needs, as well as a lack of time for legislators to become experts in the vast number of policy areas, our political system created administrative agencies for the specific purpose of adequate control of public policies. This creation caused the delegation of much discretionary authority, which often includes extensive rule-making power, from legislatures to administrative agencies. Consequently, administrative agencies make many decisions and issue many rules that have far-reaching political and policy consequences (Anderson, 2003, p. 53).

Rule making by administrative agencies is the creation of agency statements of general applicability and future effect that concern the rights of private parties. These guidelines have the force and effect of law. Under the requirements of the federal Administrative Procedures Act, general notice of a proposed rule must be published in the *Federal Register* so interested parties can have the opportunity to present their opinions on it through a presentation of written data. The *Federal Register*, published five days a week, also lists the latest presidential orders and rules adopted by agencies and a great variety of other official notices (Starling, 2002, p. 58). In addition to adopting new policies, rule making also involves modifying existing policies.

As administrative agencies implement policy, conflicts can and do arise between the agencies and individual citizens. *Adjudication* is a quasijudicial process conducted by agencies to determine if their decision on some matter involving an individual or corporation was within their scope of jurisdiction (for example, denial of a permit).

The courts, specifically the national and state appellate courts, have often greatly affected the nature and content of public policies through their powers of judicial review and statutory interpretation. Judicial review is the power of courts to determine the constitutionality of actions by the legislative and executive branches of our government. Courts can declare actions null and void if they find them in conflict with the U.S. Constitution. Courts also interpret and decide the meaning of statutory provisions that are ambiguous or unclearly stated and open to conflicting interpretations. When the court accepts one interpretation over another, it in effect gives preference to the winning party's explanation of the policy (Anderson, 2003, pp. 54–55).

Who Influences Policy?

In addition to the primary and supplementary policy makers, several other entities influence policies through their opinions, specialization and expertise, and ability to influence others. Some of these entities are individual citizens, labor unions, professional organizations, research organizations, media, nonprofit groups, public corporations, lobbyists, political parties, legislative staff, and interest groups.

A pictorial representation of these influences on the policy-making process is shown in **Figure 22-4.**

Individual citizens—constituents—can influence policy in three distinct ways: voting, party affiliation, and political activism. Some policies are taken to the public for a vote (for example, referendums and propositions), whereas other policies are actually proposed by the people—initiatives. Also, constituents who are unhappy with elected officials and the officials' policy decisions and adoptions can always exercise their right to vote against them in the next election. Individuals can also influence policy by their support of certain policies or elected officials through volunteerism, contributing financial resources, and advocating in the political environment for or against a public policy, such as staging protests.

Legislators are targets of a wide variety of lobbying activities from both *professional lobbyists* and **interest groups.** These activities consist of congressional testimony from experts in policy areas, letters of interest from group members, campaign contributions, and sometimes even the outright payment of money for votes (O'Connor & Sabato, 2002, p. 371). Interest groups try to work closely with agency administrators in an effort to

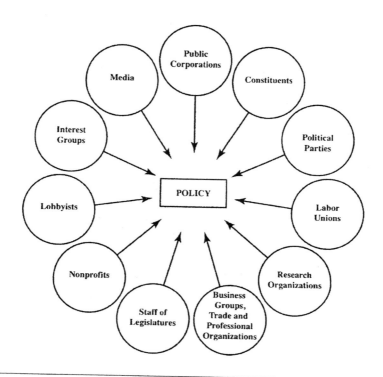

Figure 22-4 Influences on policy making.

influence policy formulation and, more importantly, policy implementation. Lobbyists and interest groups are often seen as experts on a particular issue (for example, the environment, the elderly, or gun control), and thus are consulted by policy makers. Interest groups are especially poised to help policy makers form coalitions in order to successfully adopt a particular policy alternative.

Political parties greatly influence policy through their endorsements of specific candidates and domination of elected seats in government. Parties endorse candidates by raising and donating money for their campaigns and recruit and organize volunteers for campaign efforts and other group efforts like get-out-the-vote campaigns. Also, by creating a new political party, like the Green Party, a candidate can help to spotlight an issue of concern.

Keep in mind that the president appoints most high-level positions in the administrative area of our government (**executive departments**, **regulatory commissions**, and **independent agencies**), with approval from the Senate. Also, elected officials' staffs are hand picked by the elected official. It stands to reason that the president, and thus the president's political party, will appoint leaders who share the same political views and ideals as they do. In general terms, the Republican Party tends to be more conservative on issues and the Democratic Party tends to be more liberal. Whichever party controls the presidency and the majority in Congress tends to advance more of its own views on public issues during its term.

Research organizations are composed of policy analysts and researchers. They exist to provide policy makers with information and data on policy alternatives and even on proposals for new policy alternatives. Also, they provide the public with their opinions on the effectiveness of public policies. These organizations usually have a policy bias and distinct ideological leanings—conservative or liberal.

Other entities that may lobby policy makers or contribute financially to elected officials' campaigns in exchange for favorable votes on policies are corporations, labor unions, nonprofit organizations, business groups, and trade and **professional associations**.

One of the most influential entities regarding policy, at least on the evaluation of public policies, is the media. Again, different media outlets usually have political biases and specific ideologies that affect their evaluations of elected officials and their policies.

Key Techniques for Influencing Policy

There are several techniques forensic nurses can employ to influence policies that are of interest and impact their occupations:

» *Join a professional organization* such as the American Nurses Association, the International Association of Forensic Nurses, or the regional forensic nurses association.

» *Determine the specific public and health issues of interest* that impact the field of forensic nursing.

» *Become informed* about the public policies and health policies currently under consideration at the federal level of government.

» *Study the federal rule-making process* and learn how to present one's opinions for consideration by an administrative agency.

» *Become familiar and comfortable with the* Federal Register. It will publish directions on where to send comments and the deadline for the public comment period.

» *Offer one's expertise* to the state's nurses association in assisting with the development of new **regulations** or modifying existing regulations. Also, offer one's expertise to help the association prepare comments on proposed regulations (American Nurses Association, n.d.).

» *Interact effectively with the media* to influence policy and reorient any media outlet that has misconceptions concerning the policy and the role of the forensic nurse. Effective interaction with the media is discussed in detail in the following sections of this chapter.

» *Create a social networking group site* to gain supporters for the policy, for comments, and to make the issues known to a large portion of the public.

The Media, Public Policy, and the Forensic Nurse

As a forensic nurse, you might be called upon someday to be an official **spokesperson** to the news media, especially if you are actively involved in the policy process. You may think that it is unlikely, but in today's era of all news, all the time, chances are that sooner or later you will be contacted or confronted by at least one reporter seeking factual information or just wanting your comments when something major occurs or as an advocate for a particular cause or group. Forensic nurses may be asked to comment on the latest health-related issues as a representative of the forensic community. Competition requires that reporters go to anybody they can find to give them responses to whatever questions they have. Because forensic nurses help bridge the gap between the healthcare system and the legislative and the justice processes, the range of possible instances where reporters might seek you out for information or opinion, even when you are not an official spokesperson, is enormous. This is why it is so important that, as a forensic nursing professional, you know how and when to work with the news media.

The following sections will provide an overview of the news media and some basic coping skills when working with reporters and other news professionals. Topics that will be examined include:

» the different types of news media and how their roles and needs differ.
» the differences between proactive and reactive media relations.
» what you can and cannot say to the media—and when and how to say it.
» how to develop key messages and how to stay focused on them.
» how to prepare responses well in advance of actually being asked questions.
» how to answer questions you don't really want to answer, without having to say, "No comment."

You will learn how to work with the media so that both their needs and yours are satisfied without violating your professional code of ethics.

Understanding the Media

All news media generally want the same information:

Who (Who was involved?)
What (What happened?)
When (When did it happen?)
Where (Where did it happen?)
Why (Why did it happen?)
How (How did it happen?)

But all media are not necessarily looking for identical answers. That is because each medium operates differently, with different time and space constraints, and with different audience needs. Consequently, what you say must be tailored to the needs of each specific medium.

Traditionally, news media have fallen into two broad categories—print and broadcast/cable. In recent years the Internet, which combines print and broadcast/cable with immediacy and instant availability, has been growing as a major source of news information.

Print Media

Print media include newspapers, magazines, and national news (also known as wire) services such as The Associated Press (AP), Dow Jones, and Reuters. Print media reporters often have more time than their broadcast brethren in which to research and write their stories. This often gives them the time and the ability to do in-depth research. It also enables them to look for more relevant material and different angles from what the **broadcast media** will have reported because of their earlier and more-or-less instant deadlines.

This difference can be especially beneficial when you need to explain complex material. Because print reporters generally have the time to delve into details, it gives you the opportunity to cover material that may have been ignored or played down by broadcast media in their rush to be first with the news. There is also a very good chance that more of what you have to say will be quoted in print. In turn, this enables you to be able to give perspective to your story for people who may have only gotten a quick summary from the broadcast coverage.

However, this opportunity can also pose a danger if you are not careful. Because so much more of what you say can and, most likely, will be reported, you need to be careful not to ramble on and on. The more you keep talking, the more there is a danger you may say something you shouldn't. If this *faux pas* appears in print, the likely result will be embarrassment for you and your organization.

There is also the danger that the reporter may go off in a wrong direction. If the reporter does not completely understand the subject, he or she can do a lot of harm. Therefore, when working with print media, use the opportunity to tell your story in depth, but make certain the reporter is properly focused and understands what you are saying at all times. Consider the interview an opportunity to educate the reporter. If the reporter is confused when he or she begins to write the story, the result can be a professional disaster.

Broadcast/Cable Media

In contrast to print media, broadcast media—that is, radio and television—and cable TV news channels are not usually interested in extended, in-depth reports. In most instances, stories prepared by broadcast reporters run anywhere from about 30 seconds to a couple of minutes. If you are lucky and have given the reporter a good, concise interview, you may have a chance to be quoted in your own voice as part of that news report. The problem is that you will usually have perhaps only 15 to 20 seconds in which to state your case. This means that the message you want to convey to the public about key issues has to be well organized and framed clearly in one or more concise sound bites. If your answers are too lengthy, only a portion of one of your responses will be used to highlight a particular point that the reporter wants to make during the broadcast. Unfortunately, because the reporter is choosing the portion of the interview to air, unless you have chosen your words carefully, the report may not have the impact you intended.

There are significant differences among the various broadcast media. Because radio conveys sound only, you want to try to frame your comments for the listening audience in a way that will help listeners form mental pictures. Radio can be an important news medium for your organization as long as you remember to speak your message clearly and concisely. When you do that you can be reasonably certain that what you have to say will be reported fairly and accurately on radio.

Television reporters, on the other hand, want more than just your voice. They are equally concerned about getting pictures to show along with their reports, so you may want to give thought beforehand to any picture possibilities to go along with your comments. It is not unusual for TV reporters to use the spokesperson's voice (but not his or her face) while relevant pictures are being shown. That is referred to in TV parlance as a *voice-over*. When dealing with TV, it is important to try to frame what you say to go along with particular images you may have in mind. The use of demonstrative props while speaking or requesting the interview be filmed in a setting that conveys part of your message are two examples of framing your message. For example, an interview about forensic nursing education might be best in an interactive educational setting.

Another problem often encountered when dealing with TV is its use of live pictures as events are unfolding. Frequently, the anchorperson back in the studio who is trying to describe the pictures that are going out over the air has only scant information about what is happening, so he or she will keep repeating what has been previously said. This can be advantageous to you if you can get your quote on the air early. If studio news anchors keep repeating the forensic nurse's perspective of an incident or issue, it can help assure that your message is getting out to the public.

When the TV or radio industry devotes extended time to a news story, reporters often have to fill a lot of air time with relatively few facts to report. That often leads to on-the-air speculation. In such situations, it becomes especially important that you not join in the speculation or allow yourself to be goaded into voicing your own speculative thoughts. We have all seen forensic professionals asked to speculate about the types of evidence or other factors influencing high-profile cases. Too often they provide on-the-spot commentary that later comes back to haunt them or they comment on apparent facts that are later shown to be rumor. Remember, when you are addressing the news media officially or unofficially, professionalism demands that you speak only from a strictly informed and factual perspective; otherwise, you risk your personal and professional credibility.

The Internet

The Internet is quickly becoming an important third major news medium. The Internet has the unique ability to combine print, sound, photos, and moving images and present them on demand, thereby combining the best features of newspapers, radio, and TV, along with the major news services. Recent studies have shown that an ever-increasing number of people are turning to the Internet as their first source of information about breaking news. Real-time transmission of information often requires Internet sites to seek out various sources of information that will keep the viewer returning to the site.

Today, nearly every major news outlet, from national to local newspapers and magazines and from national broadcasters to local broadcasters, has a website where people can turn for the latest news. Working with reporters for Internet news feeds is not any different than working with regular print or broadcast reporters; they are usually the same people, and that means we can expect their news reports will be professional, fair, balanced, and accurate.

Unfortunately, not all information on the Internet meets professional journalistic standards. Chat rooms, rogue websites, and bloggers who maintain online journals and diaries answer to no professional authority and often dispense disinformation, rumor, and innuendo. Monitoring such sites is extremely difficult, if not downright impossible. Therefore, it becomes even more important to maintain good relations with the professional mainstream media to ensure that your story is being properly told.

The Internet can also prove a valuable tool in promoting policy or generating public interest in a forensic nursing concern. Local and international professional websites can provide basic information about key issues, links to educational sites, and video feed. Social networking outlets are quickly becoming a source of information and discussion for many in today's society. The more than 722 million members of Facebook can befriend a group formed in support of a particular issue or promoting policy, make comments, and provide feedback for the forensic nurse involved in policy making (Boyd, 2008).

All these tools can counter misinformation or speculation found at other Internet sites.

Develop a Proactive Plan for Working With the Media

Can you imagine any forensic nurse proceeding with a patient examination without any advance preparation or planning? Of course not. Not if the nurse wants to maximize success and minimize risk. The same is true when it comes to working with the media. The more prepared you are, the greater the chance of achieving your goals. The best way to work with the media is proactively. The more you work with the media before a serious situation arises, the more effective you will be working with the media when public policy issues or high-profile incidents do occur.

Media Outreach

To start, build a list of reporters, editors, and broadcast news producers and directors at all of the local media outlets that might cover your organization, healthcare issues, and the justice system. Call them to introduce yourself and, in the process, explain to them how forensic nursing is the bridge between the healthcare system and other processes or agencies. Then meet in person and get to know them. The idea of this **outreach** is to let them get acquainted with you before the need ever arises for them to have to seek you out.

Getting better acquainted means learning what kinds of stories interest them. It means learning what their deadlines are and honoring those deadlines. It means being open and friendly and willing to help the reporter or editor as much as you can. It means being prompt in returning phone calls or e-mails and offering them help on stories on which they are working that may not even be related to your organization. It means holding seminars on purely technical subjects for no purpose other than to provide background information even when you are not looking for publicity or a credit line. It means introducing reporters who cover crime, healthcare, or legal issues to your key executives and other individuals in your organization who can provide information when needed. It means developing credibility in their eyes long before you may ever need it in reaction to a crisis situation.

As a forensic nurse, you are a professional with a specific area of expertise. Reporters seek experts as they write their stories. If you are called by a reporter, remember these guidelines and you will have a good experience:

1. **Treat reporters as professionals** and recognize they have a job to do.
2. **Confine your responses to your area of expertise.**
3. **Know in advance what you want to say, and stick to it.** Write it down and keep your notes with key message points handy.
4. **When you are a spokesperson, ask to be briefed by the public relations staff prior to a media interview,** especially if the reporter has provided questions in advance. Anticipate other questions the reporter may ask.
5. **Take time to formulate your answers before responding,** especially for more difficult questions. If you need more time to prepare your answer, ask the reporter to repeat the question. Don't digress. Stick to the main facts.
6. **Never lie to a reporter. Be as honest, open, and helpful as you can** when answering a reporter's questions. Remember, a reporter's job is not to serve as an advocate or foe of a particular organization or individual. Reporters want a good story. You can put your best foot forward and help them by following this open honesty rule.
7. **Cooperate with a reporter** because he or she will get the story whether you help or not. If you don't give reporters the facts, they will find someone who will, including people who don't know the answers but will talk anyway. If you don't cooperate, you can't complain if the story that gets published or broadcast is based on hearsay and conjecture.
8. **Convey medical and technical information in lay terms** whenever possible. Be patient if reporters seem to have difficulty understanding the information you are conveying. Try using a second approach to explaining the material. If you can, give reasonable analogies that the public can relate to. You want the reporter to get the information right.
9. **Repeat information or review what could be considered confusing details.** This is particularly important during a crisis situation, when information must be accurate to avoid confusion of the facts.
10. **Provide plenty of background information** about your organization and your job. Use any background information you have available, especially about forensic nursing and your role as a responder.
11. **Do not answer a question if you don't have the facts and do not give out any unconfirmed facts.** Say, "I don't know, but I will get that information for you." Then, get back to the reporter as soon as possible.
12. **Stop talking after you have answered a reporter's question.** Don't ramble on. This is when many comments are made that were not meant to be made. Reporters will sometimes use awkward silences to their advantage. If there is a long pause after you have given an answer, ask, "Do you have another question?"
13. **Always ask what a reporter's deadline is and honor it** when you must get back to him or her with information. If you cannot honor it, say so.
14. **Keep your word.** If you promise to arrange an interview or to get more information for an answer, be certain you follow through, even if it is only to let the reporter know you are still working on it.
15. **Never play favorites when it comes to providing newsworthy information.** If you do offer a reporter an exclusive feature or background story, then it should remain exclusive until both you and the reporter agree it is not.

16. **Do not *ever* respond to a question with "No comment."** It is *never* an acceptable answer. If you cannot comment, explain why.

17. ***Never* talk off the record.** An excellent rule to remember is, "Never say anything you do not want to see in print or hear on the air." Assume the microphone is on whenever a reporter is present. Unless you have a long-established relationship with a reporter, **off the record** entails considerable risk.

18. **Never ask to see a story or news report before it is printed or aired.** Reporters and editors do not look kindly on this practice. They regard it as an intrusion on the tradition of a free press and an attempt on your part to censor their coverage.

19. **Be alert to inaccuracies in a printed or aired story.** If there are major inaccuracies in a printed or aired story, call the reporter, explain the error, and ask him or her to correct the file or database. Do not demand a retraction or correction unless absolutely necessary. You do not want to prolong the story.

20. **Do not offer the reporter gifts.** Good intentions can be misconstrued.

21. **Build relationships.** Get to know reporters you might be working with and what types of stories they like to work on. If you have a story idea for them or information to help them do their jobs better, call them.

22. **Provide telephone numbers** where you can be reached in an emergency.

23. **Avoid an initial overreaction during a crisis.** You are a professional. Try to remain calm and speak to the reporter in a conversational tone. When you get angry, you lose control of the situation and lessen the chances for ensuring that your information is reported properly and correctly. Do your best to be helpful. Don't guarantee how quickly you can provide answers.

24. **Notify the media before they contact you** if having the media first learn about a situation from someone else would damage you or your organization's image or credibility.

Build Goodwill

Build on your media contacts in positive ways. For example, you might develop a series of news releases or feature articles introducing reporters to forensic nursing and covering the differences between fictional drama and reality. You could provide information on ways the public can protect itself should an environmental hazard occur. You can provide key information related to upcoming healthcare legislation, particularly those issues of forensic nursing interest. Or you might discuss the implications of school bullying and other antisocial behavior. Or, as still another example, you might identify risk factors and cues for violence in healthcare and workplace settings. These are only a few of the many informational news stories you could offer the news media that would not only help explain what it is you do, but also build a working relationship and establish credibility with the news people who cover your field.

The more goodwill you develop with the members of the news media, the more residual goodwill you will have when a crisis or disaster strikes and you are forced to go into reactive mode. Remember that the reporters who will most likely cover your organization when trouble strikes will be the same ones you will have been working with proactively. If you have already established your credibility with them and earned their trust, they will be far more likely to be receptive to what you have to say, and they will likely be more cooperative.

Identify Potential Scenarios

Start by identifying every potential situation or scenario you might have to face that could require interfacing with the media. Ask yourself such questions as: What are the key policy issues that will be raised? What opposition to this public policy might be encountered? Where are the greatest risks in our organization? What specifically might happen? How likely is it? How severe could the impact be? What groups would be affected? What is our organization's position if this type of incident occurs? What is our organization's philosophy on how to respond to this situation? What is my role?

Some potential situations and scenarios that readily come to mind include:

» Child, elder, and spousal abuse
» Sexual assault
» Environmental hazards
» Internet crime
» Pornography, especially if it involves children
» Bullying in schools
» Issues of competence
» Treatment of prisoners in custody
» Treatment of crime victims
» Criminally induced trauma
» Maladaptive social behavior
» Assessment of inmates in a psychiatric facility
» Preservation of evidence
» Investigations of death and violence

You might encounter other situations in your work. They, too, should be considered, because if you do not know how you will respond to that very first reporter's call, it is almost a foregone conclusion that the first story written or broadcast will be negative or, at best, simply incorrect. Unless you handle the call properly, your credibility, your competence, or both, will be questioned.

Identify Spokespersons

Once you have identified the potential policy and crisis scenarios you might face, then determine who within your forensic nursing organization or sphere of work will be the official spokesperson. Will it be someone from the public relations or public affairs department? Someone from legal? Someone from management? You?

Where and when do you fit into the picture? Regardless of your assigned or unassigned role, it is still a safe bet that sooner or later you will be approached by someone from the news media, so it is best to be prepared. This is especially true if you have taken the time to develop a relationship with the media in your area. You will be their go-to person, whether or not you are the official spokesperson or even directly involved in the crisis situation.

Develop Key Messages

Once all the potential policies, situations, and scenarios have been identified, the next step is to determine how you or other designated spokespersons will respond to the media.

That means developing **key messages** and talking points for each potential incident. You cannot respond adequately to an inquiry unless you have prepared in advance.

Key messages are simply short, concise statements (sound bites) that help you explain the main points you want to make. **Talking points** are additional statements that expand, explain, or support your key messages. In working with the media, your key messages will help them understand who you are, what you do, and how well you do it; for example: "I am a forensic nurse. This is what I do. . . . These are the steps or protocols involved in a situation such as this. . . ." Your talking points then become the facts you use to describe how you do your job.

It is essential that you give your key message up front before discussing or addressing other issues. In a fast-paced environment, you never know when you will be interrupted. Unless you are focused on your messages, it is easy to be led off the topic to other subjects by reporters. When that happens, you never get to talk about what *you* want to talk about. In more extreme cases, you may need to consider how to respond to a hostile reporter; points to consider in this situation are outlined in Figure 22-3.

Your key messages should be the three or four most important sound bites that you want the reporter to use. They should not be rambling sentences. A good guideline to remember is that you should be able to complete a response in the time it takes for a three-or-four-floor elevator ride.

Prepare for Follow-up Questions

After you have determined your key messages, you are not yet finished. Reporters always ask **follow-up questions**. Anticipate media questions in advance. Remember that reporters always want the answers to questions that start with the words who, what, where, when, why, and how. Knowing what questions to expect makes preparing answers in advance that much easier. But unless you have carefully thought about the many scenarios related to a proposed policy or forensic crisis, you won't know what to say to the media. You will hesitate or perhaps say the wrong thing and make matters worse. Your responses, especially to the question, "What are you going to do about it?" should be a reflection of your ethics and those of the healthcare or forensic nursing organization. Most importantly, your responses should reflect your professionalism and competence in doing your work.

Know Your Job

In many instances, your best response to reporters' questions about forensic nursing and policies may simply be to describe for them what protocols you follow in the performance of your duties in response to a specific incident or issue. It might be a statement that begins, "I am a forensic nurse. In a situation such as this, involving (fill in the incident: child abuse, sexual assault, autopsy assistance, etc.), these are the protocols I normally follow." When related to developing or endorsing certain public policy, that statement can be expanded to include "This is what the (fill in the desired legislation) will do to help me be more effective in my job as a forensic nurse," and then begin to describe for the reporter or reporters the specific effects on how you perform your duties in this matter. The advantage of this type of response is that it grounds your answer in fact, not speculation, and you don't need to worry about having given an answer that may violate professional ethics. This is an especially effective way to respond to questions from the media when an *ongoing criminal* investigation prevents any discussion of the particulars of the specific case, evidence, or your involvement. Answering in this fashion also educates the reporter about your professional role and relieves you of having to say, "No comment."

The most important thing to remember when you are working with the media is that you can control what you say. You have the ability to give out as much or as little information as you choose. Never forget that!

Understanding Media Terminology

Members of the news media operate under an unwritten code of ethics that spells out what they may and may not print or air based on agreements they make with news makers. But if you expect reporters to adhere to these agreements, it is important that both you and the reporter have the same understanding about what you have agreed to. This is why it is critical that you learn the meaning of some basic media terms. Otherwise you may think that what you are telling a reporter in an attempt to be helpful will not be printed or used on the air and then be shocked or horrified when it becomes public.

1. **On the Record:** This means exactly what it sounds like. Everything you say can be used or reported at the reporter's discretion. If you say it, its use is fair game. You can't take back anything you said—even if you didn't mean to say it.

2. **Off the Record:** This is the opposite of on the record. It means that anything you say "off the record" may not be reported. But it is not that simple. There are protocols to be followed; otherwise, despite what you think, you may still be on the record, not off.

    First of all, if you want something to be off the record, you must say so in advance, not after you have spoken it. Once the cat is out of the bag, you cannot change your mind and declare the previous remarks to be off the record. It just doesn't work that way.

    The reason for telling reporters that what you are about to say is off the record is to give any of them a chance to say, no, they do not wish to go along with an off-the-record presentation. Sometimes reporters don't want to accept off-the-record information because they want to be free to report it. Agreeing to accept off-the-record information in effect commits the reporter to secrecy (until you put it on the record) and blocks him or her from reporting that information.

    In other words, just saying something is off the record is no guarantee it will not be reported. But you can minimize the risk by asking reporters to agree in advance before you tell them what they can't report.

3. **Not for Attribution:** This is pretty much what it seems. It means reporters can use the information you gave them, but they cannot identify you as the source. As with off the record, not-for-attribution remarks must be prefaced in advance and agreed to by those present. The purpose of not-for-attribution remarks is to help reporters round out their stories with more facts or details than they otherwise could if it would appear the information came from you. When, for instance, you read a news story that attributes the source as "a high-ranking government official," it sometimes may even be the president or vice president of the United States. But by speaking not for attribution, they can say things or reveal information they otherwise could not say formally on the record.

4. **For Background Only:** This is also sometimes known as for deep background only. Either way the meaning is the same. As with not for attribution, the information given out is intended to put developments into perspective or context for reporters so they can write a more accurate and meaningful story for their audiences. For example, background information may explain how or why something came about, or it may make reference to similar situations or incidents, or developments that reporters would not otherwise know about that would better help explain their stories.

The important point to remember in talking with the news media is that you can control what you say so that you and your organization gain the maximum benefit. Knowing how and when to go on or off the record, on background, or not for attribution maximizes that control. But still that control is not absolute. It is the reporter, not you, who ultimately controls what gets reported. That's why the *best* policy is simply to forget about off the record, not for attribution, and background. You will never get burned if you follow this simple advice: Never say *anything* that you wouldn't want to see on the front page of the newspaper or on the evening TV news.

Summary

Governmental policy, whether federal, state, or local in origin, develops through the many stages discussed in this chapter. These stages provide numerous opportunities for the forensic nurse to help shape policy and its implementation in programs that will serve clients in diverse populations. Much of that shaping and influence involves working with the media to get your message across. The forensic nurse often has little experience with governmental agencies or policy administration. In addition, their interactions with the media are also very limited. Without appropriate planning and preparation, the processes involved in developing policy and taking that message to legislators and the public may not be totally effective. Therefore, forensic nurses should familiarize themselves with the policy-making process by taking advantage of opportunities to participate at the local and state levels in grassroots organizations, to raise local awareness of issues of interest, and to network with individuals from other professions who have similar interests and concerns. They should learn to have a good working relationship with the media to provide educational opportunity regarding forensic nursing interests while allowing the media to do their job.

One way to network with groups and forensic nurses in other jurisdictions is through the use of the Internet. Most national, international, or advisory groups have websites that are readily accessed. Forensic nurses can use the information provided by these groups to supplement their own experiences and understanding of an issue as they work to shape public policy. In addition, the forensic nurse should access all appropriate federal executive and legislative branch websites. This will help when evaluating local and national trends in policy making. These same websites are used by administrators and legislators themselves to research policies and programs and to develop ideas for legislation. Thus, one can anticipate statutory trends and responses by legislators by studying the same materials they rely on. The forensic practitioner can develop the skills necessary to further public policy in areas of interest by utilizing all available resources and working with legislators and administrators to respond to clients' needs.

QUESTIONS FOR DISCUSSION

1. What is public policy?
2. When does a problem rise to the attention of the public?
3. What are the steps in the policy-making process?
4. Who creates policy?
5. Who influences policy?
6. What strategies might the forensic nurse employ to influence policy and assist in its implementation?
7. Identify the common public media with which the forensic nurse often interacts. In what ways do these media differ? What different skills might be required with each?
8. In what ways can the forensic nurse work with the media to develop goodwill and to highlight areas of forensic interest for both parties?
9. A critical incident has occurred in a local healthcare facility that may involve intentional harm to patients caused by one of the staff. What special concerns might arise when addressing such a case with the media?

REFERENCES

American Nurses Association, Government Affairs—"ANA in Action" (n.d.). Retrieved from www .ana.org/gova

Anderson, J. E. (2003). *Public policymaking* (5th ed.). Boston, MA: Houghton Mifflin.

Bardach, E. (2000). *A practical guide for policy analysis.* New York, NY: Seven Bridges.

Beatty, E. R., Glendon, M., & Williams, M. J. M. (2006). Leadership in forensic nursing. In R. Hammer, B. Moynihan, & E. Pagliaro (Eds.), *Forensic nursing: A handbook for practice* (pp. 130–156), Sudbury, MA: Jones and Bartlett.

Boyd, D., & Ellison, N. (2008). Social network sites: Definitions, history and scholarship. *Journal of Computer-Mediated Communication, 13*(1), 210–230.

Goldwater, M., & Zusy, M. J. (1990). Prescription for nurses: Effective political action. St. Louis, MO: Mosby.

International Association of Forensic Nurses. (2006). *Government affairs.* Retrieved from www.iafn .org/governmentaffairs

Munger, M. C. (2000). *Analyzing policy.* New York, NY: Norton.

O'Connor, K., & Sabato, L. J. (2002). *Essentials of American government: Continuity and change.* New York, NY: Addison Wesley Longman.

Starling, G. (2002). *Managing the public sector* (6th ed.). Belmont, CA: Wadsworth/Thomson Learning.

SUGGESTED FURTHER READING

Attrobus, S., & Kitson, A. (1999). Nursing leadership: Influencing and shaping health policy and nursing practice. *Journal of Advanced Nursing, 29*(3), 746–753.

Faford, P. (2008). *Evidence and healthy public policy: Insights from health and political sciences.* National Collaborating Centre for Healthy Public Policy. Available at www.nccnpp.ca/docs/ fafardEvidence08June.pdf

Farnan, J., Paro, J., Higa, J., Edelson, H., & Arora, V. (2008). The YouTube generation: Implications for medical professionals. *Perspectives in Biology and Medicine, 51*(4), 517–524.

Ollerhead, S. (2010). *Establishing acceptable "rules of engagement" to encourage young fathers to access services at Sure Start Children's Centres through social networking.* Available at http:// chesterrep.openrepository.com/cdr/handle/10034/108997

CHAPTER 23

Forensic Nursing Education: Developments, Theoretical Conceptualizations, and Practical Applications for Curriculum

Arlene Kent-Wilkinson

Forensic nursing's time has come. Events covered in the media have contributed to public awareness of how the applied sciences are used to help solve crimes, to determine psychiatric assessment of those accused, and to educate professionals in the identification, treatment, and prevention of trauma and catastrophic injuries. Now students from all over the world are inquiring about how they can become forensic nurses and where and how they can take forensic nursing courses. To meet these requests, forensic nursing education programs are rapidly becoming part of the curricula of leading colleges and universities. This chapter provides practical applications for developing forensic nursing and multidisciplinary curriculums using classroom, distance, and online delivery modalities. Images detailing many facets of course development are included, showing frameworks for content structure and content concepts, as well as teaching and learning strategies for forensic interactivities. Visual learning objects include the use of animation, Macromedia Shockwave, and Internet resources in combination with an international perspective to the fascinating forensic field.

 ## CHAPTER FOCUS

- » Systems and Services Where Forensic Nurses Work
- » How Do I Become a Forensic Nurse?
- » Educational Levels of Forensic Nursing Courses
- » Policies and Standards Guiding Forensic Nursing Education
- » Responsibilities of Forensic Nurse Educators
- » Methods (Modes) of Course Delivery (On site/Online)
- » Forensic Nursing Curriculum Content
- » Effective Teaching and Learning Strategies
- » Research in Online Forensic Nursing Courses
- » The Future of Forensic Nursing Education
- » Forensic Nursing Programs Globally

KEY TERMS

- » Courseware Blackboard
- » international perspective
- » learning objects
- » WebCT

Introduction

How can I become a forensic nurse? What education do I need? Students all over the world are inquiring about where they can take forensic nursing courses and where to find jobs that employ forensic nurses.

Although forensic nursing courses have been rapidly appearing in curriculums of many leading colleges and universities, forensic nurse educators themselves also have questions, including, "How do we best organize and disseminate this unique body of knowledge?" and "What content should be included in each course or program of study?" Perhaps the most important questions educators have is this: "Are we conceptualizing forensic nursing consistently with other programs locally, nationally, and internationally?"

The different on-site and online choices in delivery modalities will be described with content outlines that have been used in specific forensic nursing programs. Samples of **learning objects** for student interactivities will be included. Finally, to answer the universally asked question, "Where are the programs?"

Systems and Services Where Forensic Nurses Work

Forensic nurses practice not only in the complex organization of hospitals within the healthcare system, but also in facilities of many interfacing systems: the criminal justice system, the mental healthcare system, the medical examiner/coroner system, the child welfare system, and in government-approved facilities. Forensic nurses have adapted to practices within many systems and with many disciplines on interdisciplinary teams, but their practice remains within the scope of nursing.

How Do I Become a Forensic Nurse?

The generic undergraduate baccalaureate degree in nursing is first required, as forensic nursing is a specialty that requires additional skills and knowledge in a specific area. Several graduate programs are available in forensic nursing, and more are in the planning stages. However, it is possible to attain additional skills in particular areas of forensic nursing, such as sexual assault nurse examiner (SANE) or legal nurse consultant through programs of continuing education rather than through formal graduate study. Students enrolled in undergraduate nursing programs who have an interest in forensic nursing could inquire into the possibilities of forensic placements for a clinical practicum and could focus written assignments on a forensic nursing role, or a forensic health issue.

Because forensic nursing education is relatively new, the programs of study are in the early development stages at colleges and universities scattered around the world. The courses for the most part have been and are being written by forensic nurse clinicians and nurse educators with a passionate interest in the area. Because educational programs were not previously available, nurse educators developing the programs are drawing from their own forensic clinical experiences and/or from what has been published in the forensic nursing literature.

Many nurses identified themselves as forensic nurses and practiced with forensic populations long before education was available in this specific field. This is similar historically to many nursing specialty areas, including emergency, critical care, and nurse midwifery.

Educational Levels of Forensic Nursing Courses

By the end of the 20th century, it was evident that an exciting movement toward forensic nursing was taking place internationally in every method of educational delivery possible: traditional classroom, distance, and Internet delivery with varying levels of certificate, diploma, baccalaureate, and graduate credit. With many different levels of forensic nursing courses and programs becoming available, it is difficult for student nurses and anyone interested in the forensic area to sort out what level of program is best to take for their individual situation. The following sections discuss the main levels of nursing education in general, and specify whether programs or courses of study exist in forensic nursing at that level.

Certification

Certification is an examination process that verifies whether a professional has a sufficient amount of current knowledge in a selected specialty area. Usually the professional organization in the field of study determines the criteria for certification and the length of time for which the certification is valid. Certification is separate and different from a formal academic diploma or degree, neither of which guarantees qualifying for employment in the area of practice. In some countries, and for some specialties of nursing, students are expected to achieve advanced practice certification appropriate to their specialty after graduation with a diploma or baccalaureate degree in nursing. For example, in the United States, the American Nursing Credentialing Center offers certification exams for some nursing specialty areas; in Canada, the Canadian Nurses Association offers certification exams for some nursing specialties, such as mental health nursing.

With regards to forensic nursing, certification already exists for some of its subspecialties: correctional nursing has certification examinations offered by the National Commission on Correctional Healthcare; the American Association of Legal Nurse Consultants provides legal nurse consultants with certification examinations; and the International Association of Forensic Nurses (IAFN) began offering SANE certification in 2001. Only some areas of nursing practice require certification to obtain employment; thus far it is not a requirement for most areas of forensic nursing. However, New Jersey has made SANE programs mandatory in its counties in an effort to improve the care and treatment of sexual assault survivors (Naught, 2002).

Certification examinations are often developed by a professional interest group or association, which determines whether the level of certification is at the advanced practice graduate level or at the diploma/baccalaureate level. Although certification for the subspecialties of forensic nursing (correctional nursing, legal nurse consulting, and SANE) is at the diploma/baccalaureate level, those who wish to sit for the certification examination for forensic nursing in general, when it is available, will be required to have a graduate degree in nursing.

Certificate Program

A certificate program is a series of courses in a selected specialty of professional practice (e.g., mental health, emergency, critical care, neonatology, gerontology). After completion, the student has a certificate in a specific area of practice. A certification program is required in some areas of practice to obtain employment. A certificate forensic nursing program is a series of courses in the specialty of forensic nursing (e.g., forensic heath studies certificate). After completion, the nurse has a certificate in specific areas of forensic nursing.

Graduate Degree Nursing Programs

A master's of nursing degree requires advanced practice nursing studies, which are beyond a baccalaureate degree in nursing and include graduate nursing courses.

> Advanced practice nurses (APNs) are taking their place in the forefront of the rapidly changing health care system, developing a myriad of roles in organizations that aim to provide cost-effective, quality care . . . APNs were traditionally educated to provide advanced nursing care in a specific system or setting such as a hospital unit or clinic, it is now fairly common for APNs to work across system boundaries to follow their patients in a multifaceted care delivery arena. (Jansen & Zwygart-Stauffacher, 2010, p. 3)

When studying for a master's degree in nursing, students may choose to focus on the specialty area of forensic nursing or forensic healthcare issues for their articles or thesis. A graduate degree forensic nursing program provides a master's degree in the specialized area of forensic nursing study.

Doctoral Degree Nursing Program

A PhD nursing program of study (which culminates in a doctoral degree in nursing) requires studies beyond a graduate degree in nursing. When pursuing a doctoral degree in nursing, students may want to focus on the specialty area of forensic nursing or forensic healthcare issues for their research or dissertation. A forensic nursing PhD program requires studies beyond a graduate degree in nursing where the special focus of the program is advanced practice forensic nursing at the doctoral level.

None of the previously mentioned levels of education guarantees obtaining employment in the area of forensic nursing practice. Currently, certification in forensic nursing is not required in most forensic nursing subspecialties to obtain employment, but due to the laws of supply and demand, as with many other nursing specialties, certification may be required in the future. Nurses, like most other healthcare professionals, may choose to take educational programs outside of their discipline. Many forensic nursing courses could easily be designed or already are designed for multidisciplinary study, and most are recognized within other disciplines.

Policies and Standards Guiding Forensic Nursing Education

Nurses, as the largest group of healthcare professionals, have advantages when marketing, developing, and delivering programs for forensic nursing and multidisciplinary educational programs at all levels. The discipline of nursing has a strong and clear metaparadigm with a professional scope as well as standards of practice, a code of ethics, and ideologies that provide a framework for the development of forensic nursing educational programs.

IAFN Educational Policies and Standards of Practice

Clearly delineated standards of nursing practice inform professional nursing care and provide a framework for responsibility and accountability. The IAFN has begun to make a significant contribution to global policies for forensic nursing education. The *Sexual Assault Nurse Examiner Standards of Practice* (IAFN, 1996) and the *Forensic Nursing Standards and Scope of Practice* were both developed by the IAFN membership (ANA, 1997). Forensic nursing certification became available in 2001 for the subspecialty of sexual assault nurses. On October 1, 2001, an IAFN resolution on terrorism called for worldwide support of nursing education that includes mass disaster preparedness (IAFN, 2001a). At the same time, an IAFN resolution on forensic nursing education called for the development and implementation of comprehensive forensic nursing content at all levels of formal nursing education (IAFN, 2001b).

The IAFN policies encourage forensic nurses to acquire and maintain current knowledge in forensic practice (ANA, 1997). The forensic nurse may seek additional knowledge and skills appropriate to the practice setting by participating in educational programs and activities, conferences, workshops, interdisciplinary professional meetings, and self-directed learning, thereby embracing a lifelong learning policy. The IAFN has taken a leadership role in the health policy arena to champion positions on national and international issues. IAFN nursing leaders have had the opportunity to participate in meetings about national policy regarding sexual assault victims and interpersonal violence.

Responsibilities of Forensic Nurse Educators

Although it is a privilege for forensic nurse educators to develop some of the first forensic nursing and forensic multidisciplinary academic programs, it is also a responsibility. The media, through magazines, movies, and television, have played a role in enhancing awareness of the forensic area, but forensic nurse leaders in the field are responsible for communicating their unique knowledge of the specialty. These forensic nurse specialists have to take responsibility for making both themselves and their specialty understood. Articulating the specialization in any discipline is serious, rigorous, and demanding. It requires the members of each area of specialization, beginning with the leaders and scholars in each field, to take on the hard work of defining what they do. To date, forensic nurses globally have authored an impressive body of knowledge. Discourse is alive in the important debates of the specialty in forensic nursing's current years of early development.

Forensic nurse educators also have a responsibility to mentor and advise those interested in a forensic nursing career. Forensic nurse educators need to be knowledgeable and up front that some areas of forensic nursing, particularly in certain locations, have very few available jobs. Advising newcomers to the forensic specialty as to where forensic nurses have pioneered their own jobs and how they made these inroads provides insight as to current and future career opportunities within the forensic arena. Forensic areas can exist anywhere healthcare professionals deal with victims or perpetrators of catastrophic accidents, physical or emotional trauma, violence, and crime.

Nursing professional bodies in North America and around the world have mandated that nurses become more culturally aware and sensitive to the diversity of their patients. Cultural components are required to be included in nursing educational curriculums and registration examinations (ANA, 1991, 2007; CNA, 2000, 2004). Students learn to under-stand and appreciate diverse perspectives through a dialogue with their peers, facilitated by a dialogue with the instructor, who helps students learn the unique knowledge content of forensic nursing. Many subspecialties of forensic nursing are exposed to the dilemma of crime or culture when caring for culturally diverse groups. Health-related issues of female genital mutilation raise many ethical concerns for nurses who care for these female clients. Nurses must interact in a culturally sensitive manner and know when and to whom to voice their concerns about cultural practices.

Methods (Modes) of Course Delivery (On Site and Online)

Whenever a new teaching method comes along in education, educators and students debate which teaching and learning modalities (i.e., classroom, distance, and most recently online distance education) are the most efficient and effective models. Arguments about the role of technology in education go back at least 2,500 years. For the ancient Greeks, oratory was the means by which people learned and passed on learning (Bates & Poole, 2003). Oratory was soon challenged by the advent of reading and writing, and the debate then turned to a concern for which of the two was more effective for learning.

Today, one of the prominent educational debates concerns the efficacy of on-site educa-tion versus online or distance education. We are beginning to realize that virtual or online education is not necessarily better or worse than face-to-face education. The old distinc-tion between on-site and distance technology blurs rapidly as the increasing availability of network resources and collaborative software stimulates a convergence of the two.

The Classroom/On-Site Experiences/Lecture Method

For hundreds of years, the lecture format was traditional for classroom delivery. The word *lecture* stems from the Latin word for *reading* because it was mainly based on readings in Latin from ancient handwritten manuscripts. The philosophical position that informs this teaching method is scholasticism, which trains students to consider a text according to certain preestablished, officially approved criteria, which are painstakingly and pain-fully drilled into them (Bates & Poole, 2003). The traditional classroom teaching method has evolved to include numerous delivery methods for the exchange of information. The lecture, the seminar, group discussion methods, and elaborate multimedia technology enhancements make this an effective and more enjoyable learning mode than the original lecture format.

Classroom forensic nursing courses can be multidisciplinary in nature, overviewing the emerging forensic specialty. During a classroom forensic nursing course, experts in the unique forensic practice areas can be brought in as guest lecturers. Complementing the classroom instruction are field trips or clinical practicums organized to include local forensic facilities, such as secured facilities (jails or penitentiaries), young offender cen-ters, forensic psychiatric units, homeless shelters, courts of law, women's shelters, or the medical examiner's or coroner's offices. These on-site experiences introduce students to the actual clinical settings where roles for forensic health professionals are clearly visible in practice. Classroom forensic courses, including a variety of teaching approaches, can be duplicated in any educational institution teaching forensic nursing.

Distance Education

Distance education is learning that takes place when the instructor and student are not in the same room but are separated by physical distance. It is therefore a solution for those who require a creative and flexible way to learn. Many associate distance learning with correspondence learning, the original form of distance learning. Distance education has gone through four or five generations of technology throughout its history. These generations are print, audio/video teleconferencing, computer-aided instruction, e-learning/online learning, and computer broadcasting/webcasting, etc. (Taylor, 2003).

When first introduced, distance education was considered a prepackaged text or audio-visual course, with little or no interaction between the student and the instructor. Today's evolving interactive communication technology allows learning experiences to occur at any time between instructor and student, student and student, and student and expert. When developing a course online, many elements of the classroom can be incorporated (**Figure 23-1**). Hybrid courses that combine the traditional classroom with online methods are commonly being used, and evaluations suggest that this combination provides for more resources and more efficient communication.

Forensic Nursing Curriculum Content

The most difficult aspect of course development for nurse educators is how to best organize and structure the forensic course content. This task is magnified for forensic nursing content because there are many subspecialties of forensic nursing; many concepts are similar among all the specialties, but some content is unique to each subspecialty. In addition, the courses are often written for a multidisciplinary audience with an **international perspective** to the forensic issues. Forensic nursing content can be organized and disseminated in many

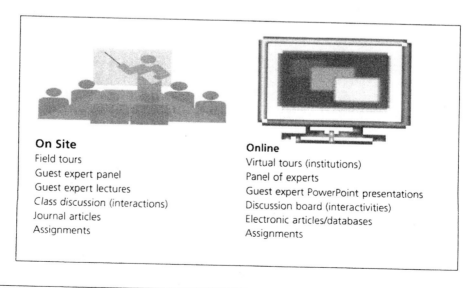

On Site
Field tours
Guest expert panel
Guest expert lectures
Class discussion (interactions)
Journal articles
Assignments

Online
Virtual tours (institutions)
Panel of experts
Guest expert PowerPoint presentations
Discussion board (interactivities)
Electronic articles/databases
Assignments

Figure 23-1 On-site and online parallels of course content.
Source: Kent-Wilkinson (2001).

different ways. The challenge of turning the content of a successful classroom-delivered forensic nursing course into content delivered online is an onerous undertaking.

An introductory course on all subspecialties of forensic nursing is perhaps the most difficult course to develop. Deciding what to include and what to leave out from a massive amount of theoretical and clinical concepts is overwhelming. The job at hand is to include only an overview of the key roles and concepts.

Often an undergraduate course on forensic nursing may be only a single course within a nursing baccalaureate degree or postregistration program. When this is the case, there is not a continuous series of courses, each focusing on a different subspecialty. Therefore, the challenge is to organize a single course that provides a student with the best overview possible of this umbrella specialty.

When the concepts to include have been decided, then decisions must be made as to how to organize the content. The author has included a navigation framework unit or module outline that she developed (**Figure 23-2**). This framework serves equally as well for forensic nursing courses as, for example, a cultural diversity and Aboriginal health course. The content of many different courses can be inserted into the categories of this framework.

Although forensic nursing course content may be structured or organized into many different overall sections/units, one of the challenging points to sort out is the hierarchical structure of the terms for the course—index, topics, sections, units, and modules. Terms differ when developing courses with different instructional design teams, at different universities, and in different countries. The term *topics* in Australia seems to correspond to the term *sections* in North America, and within these are units and modules.

Course Management Systems and Templates

There are also many different ways in which a course can be delivered. The choice of model will depend on the scale and complexity of the course and the centrality of the use of technology (Bates & Poole, 2003). Since the late 1990s, the two most popular course management systems for online course templates have been **WebCT** and **Courseware Blackboard**. Within the online educational community, there is a debate: Is the software

Forensic history/laws

Forensic theories/philosophy

Forensic specialties/roles

Forensic systems/services

Forensic practice/prevention

Forensic populations (at risk)

Forensic concepts

Forensic issues

Forensic education

Forensic research

Forensic career opportunities

Figure 23-2   Section/unit outline for forensic nursing content.
Source: Kent-Wilkinson 1997; 1999; 2002.

version of Blackboard better than WebCT? Both support excellence in online teaching and learning with course tool software, resources, and academic expertise.

The Future of Forensic Nursing Education

Significant changes are occurring in nursing education around the world as institutions restructure to address financial constraints and the changing needs of the profession. Many universities are implementing specialized forensic programs and developing an educational niche for themselves driven by the passion of forensic nurse experts, many of whom have pioneered forensic nursing roles in their clinical practice and/or published early works on forensic nursing concepts. Specialization in forensic nursing is a popular focus area that many universities are embracing. In addition, forensic areas of research with regard to prevention and marginalized populations are gaining attention as important areas of funding.

Not only is there a need for more forensic nursing programs, but there is also a need for a forensic nursing educational framework to promote standardization and program structure. This framework should emphasize international concepts within the forensic nursing curriculum.

Summary

Forensic nursing has and is an essential area of nursing practice. In order for nursing assessment to be accurate and comprehensive, a best practices model is essential. This model requires a multidisciplinary, evidence-based approach (Lippincott Williams & Wilkins, 2007). Forensic nursing utilizes a multi-disciplinary, collaborative patient care model in order to achieve the best patient care outcome. We have collaborated with experts in various disciplines in revising and updating this text with the goal of forensic nursing practice being a model for best practices.

Acknowledgment

The author acknowledges the international experts, the instructional designer teams, and the computer technicians who participated in the panels and interactivities, globally, for their clerical and administrative support that make the content of forensic nursing courses a virtual reality: Mount Royal College and University in Calgary, Alberta and the University of Saskatchewan in Saskatoon, Canada. Also, a special thank you to Lydia Lanxner for her contributions.

QUESTIONS FOR DISCUSSION

1. Where can I work as a forensic nurse?
2. How are on-site and online forensic nursing courses similar and different?
3. What content can I expect in forensic nursing courses?
4. What teaching and learning strategies have been effective in forensic nursing courses?
5. Where can I take forensic nursing courses?

REFERENCES

American Nurses Association. (1991). *Ethics and human rights position statements: Cultural diversity in nursing practice.* Washington, DC: Author. Retrieved from http://www.nursingworld.org/MainMenuCategories/EthicsStandards/Ethics-Position-Statements/prtetcldv14444.aspx

American Nurses Association. (2007). Nursing's legislative and regulatory initiatives for the 110th congress: Nursing shortage. Silver Spring, MD: Author.

Bates, A.W. & Gary Poole. (2003). *Effective teaching with technology in higher education: Foundation for success.* Indianapolis: IN: Jossey-Bass.

Canadian Nurses Association. (2000, February). Cultural diversity: Changes and challenges. *Nursing Now — Issues and Trends in Canadian Nursing, 7.* Retrieved from http://www.cnanurses.ca/_frames/search/searchframe.htm

Canadian Nurses Association. (2004). *Promoting culturally competent care* [position statement]. Retrieved from http://www.cna-nurses.ca/CNA/documents/pdf/publications/PS73_Promoting_Culturally_Competent_Care_March_2004_e.pdf

International Association of Forensic Nurses. (1996). *Sexual assault nurse examiner standards of practice.* Thorofare, NJ: Slack.

International Association of Forensic Nurses. (2001a, October 1). *Resolution I: Terror on September 11.* IAFN 9th Annual Scientific Assembly, Orlando, FL: Author.

International Association of Forensic Nurses. (2001b, October 1). *Resolution II: Forensic nursing education.* IAFN 9th Annual Scientific Assembly, Orlando, FL: Author.

Jansen, M. P., Zwygart-Stauffacher, M. (2010). *Advanced practice nursing: Core concepts for professional role development* (4th ed.). New York, NY: Springer.

Kent-Wilkinson, A. (1997). *FORE 4401 - Forensic history, risk population and issues. Forensic Studies.* Calgary, AB, Canada: Mount Royal College. Retrieved from http://mtroyal.ca/ProgramsCourses/FacultiesSchoolsCentres/HealthCommunityStudies/Programs/ForensicStudiesCertificate/CurriculumCourses/fore5501.htm

Kent-Wilkinson, A. (1999). *FORE 4403 — Forensic history, risk population and issues.* Forensic Studies. Calgary, AB, Canada: Mount Royal College.

Kent-Wilkinson, A. (2001, October 17). *Forensic nursing: International educational technologies.* [Invited plenary address]. Psychiatric Nurses Association (FPNA), Blackpool, England, UK.

Kent-Wilkinson, A. (2002). *NURS.503.08. Focus on forensic: Forensic nursing and health care in forensic populations* [Course content index]. Post Registration BN Program, Calgary, AB, Canada: University of Calgary. Retrieved from http://www.forensiceducation.com/forensic_edu/uofc.htm

Lippincott Williams & Wilkins. (2007). *Best practices: Evidence-based nursing procedures.* Philadelphia, PA: Lippincott Williams & Wilkins.

Naught, P. (2002). Compassionate care: Flight nurse heads program to assist sexual assault victims. *Forensic Nurse Magazine.* Retrieved from http://www.forensicnursemag.com/articles/281feat2.html

Taylor, J. C. (2003, June). The fifth generation of distance education. Translation in the *Chinese Journal of Open Education Research, 3,* 25–27.

SUGGESTED FURTHER READING

Lewin, R. (2009). *The handbook of practice and research in study abroad: Higher education and the quest for global citizenship.* New York, NY: Routledge.

Mashaba, T. G., & Brink, H. (1994). *Nursing education: An international perspective.* Kenwyn: Juta.

APPENDIX 1

Internet Resources

American Bar Association
  http://www.abanet.org

American Medical Association (AMA)
  www.ama-assn.org

American Nurses Association (ANA)
  http://nursingworld.org

American Psychological Association
  http://www.apa.org

Ana Definition Of Advanced Practice Nursing
  http://www.nursingworld.org/readroom/fsadvprc.htm

Anthrax And Smallpox—Being Prepared For Bioterrorism
  http://www.immunization.org

Bioterrorism And Disaster Planning
  http://nursingworld.org/news/disaster/bioprep.htm

Brookings Institution (Public Policy)
  http://www.brookings.org

Centers For Disease Control And Prevention (CDC)
  http://www.bt.cdc.gov

Children, Bioterrorism, And Disasters
  http://www.aap.org/advocacy/releases/cad.htm

Competencies For Mass Casualty Response
  http://www.aacn.org/AACN/pubpolcy.nsf/vwdoc/Sept11

Credentialing
  http://nursingworld.org/ancc

Department of Homeland Security
  http://www.dhs.gov/dhspublic

Department of Justice
  http://www.usdoj.gov

Elements Of Effective Bioterrorism Preparedness—A Planning Primer For Local Public
  Health Agencies
  http://www.naccho.org/files/documents/Final_Effective_Bioterrism.pdf

Federal Bureau Of Investigation
  http://www.fbi.gov

Food and Drug Administration
  http://www.fda.gov

Group Violence
http://www.heal-reconcile-rwanda.org

An Introduction to Firearms Identification
http://www.firearmsid.com

Johns Hopkins University Center For Gun Policy and Research
http://www.jhsph.edu/gunpolicy

Managing Radiation Emergencies: Guidance For Hospital Medical Management
http://www.orau.gov/reacts/care.htm

Men Stopping Violence
www.menstoppingviolence.org

National Academies Press Terrorism and Security Collection
http://www.nap.edu/terror

National Association of Clinical Nurse Specialists
http://www.nacns.org

National Center on Elder Abuse
http://www.elderabusecenter.org

National Center For Policy Analysis (NCPA)
http://www.ncpa.org

National Committee To Prevent Child Abuse
http://www.childabuse.org

National Criminal Justice Reference Service
http://www.ncjrs.org

National Institutes of Health
http://www.nih.gov

National League For Nursing
http://www.nln.org

Nurse Advocate: Nurses and Workplace Violence
http://www.nurseadvocate.org

Nursing Network on Violence Against Women, International
http://www.nnvawi.org

Nursing's Agenda for the Future
http://www.nursingworld.org/naf

Physicians For Social Responsibility (PSR)
http://www.psr.org

Physicians For A Violence-Free Society
http://www.pvs.org

Public Health—American Public Health Association (APHA)
http://www.apha.org

Public Health Foundation (PHF)
http://www.phf.org

Regional Healthy People 2010 Events And Priorities
http://www.phf.org/HPtools/regions.htm

Sexual Assault Nurse Examiner-Sexual Assault Response Team
http://www.sane-sart.com

Smallpox, Big Problem?
http://www.nature.com/nsu/011213/011213-15.html

Thomas
http://thomas.loc.org

U.S. Agency For Healthcare Research And Quality (AHRQ)
http://www.ahrq.gov

U.S. Census Bureau
http://www.census.gov

U.S. Institute of Peace
http://www.usip.org

Workplace Violence
http://nursingworld.org/dlwa/osh/violence.htm

APPENDIX 2

Legal Issues in Forensic Nursing: Search and Seizure of Evidence

Mary M. Galvin

Forensic nurses by definition are required to navigate the areas where law and medicine intersect. Some of these areas include sexual assault examinations where medical treatment is administered and evidence is collected for use in court; medical examiner autopsies and investigations; child sexual abuse interviews and examinations; treatment for physical assaults and domestic violence; and forensic mental health assessments and examinations.

This appendix is intended to provide an overview of certain areas of the law that will frequently arise in the forensic context. Forensic nurses should be aware of the basics of search and seizure law, the requirements for chain of custody of evidence, the admissibility of statements made by defendants and others, and legal foundations for expert opinion testimony.

Fourth Amendment

The Fourth Amendment to the U. S. Constitution commands that:

> The right of the people to be secure in their persons, houses, papers, and effects, against unreasonable searches and seizures shall not be violated, and no warrants shall issue, but upon probable cause, supported by oath or affirmation, and particularly describing the place to be searched, and the persons or things to be seized. (U.S. Const. amend. IV)

The U.S. Supreme Court has ruled that the Fourth Amendment protects any person who has a "reasonable expectation of privacy" (*Katz v. U.S.,389 U.S. 347, 356,* 1967). This means that if police search a person or his or her property for which there is a reasonable expectation of privacy, then either the officer must have a search warrant issued by a judge or there must be an exception to this warrant requirement. When a defendant in a criminal case claims that the Fourth Amendment has been violated, he does so by moving to suppress the evidence. The court's suppression of improperly seized evidence is done pursuant to what is called the exclusionary rule. In addition, a defendant must have standing to claim a violation of Fourth Amendment rights. The doctrine of standing requires that the police must have violated the *defendant's* individual right to privacy, not someone else's. In other words, the defendant cannot use the exclusionary rule to exclude evidence based on a violation of a victim's or third party's Fourth Amendment rights. The defendant can only use this right to claim a violation of his or her *own* privacy rights. As a result, a motion to suppress evidence from the medical examination of the victim based on a claim of an improper search or seizure would not be available to a defendant in a criminal case.

The forensic nurse should recognize that the use of a criminal search warrant is one proper way that the police comply with the U.S. Constitution. There are also exceptions to the warrant requirement, and these also comply with the U.S. Constitution. It is perfectly proper for the police to use one of the following exceptions to seize evidence:

» Plain view
» Exigency
» Consent
» Inventory
» Caretaker
» Stop and frisk
» The car doctrine
» Search incident to a lawful custodial arrest

Some of these will be explained in this section. There are also three areas where it has been held that the Fourth Amendment does not apply and does not provide its protection:

1. Open fields
2. Private party searches
3. Abandonment

Of these various warrantless searches, a forensic nurse is most likely to encounter the exceptions of exigency, plain view, consent, caretaker, or search incident to a lawful custodial arrest. The other exceptions to the warrant requirement are usually found in contexts that do not involve a forensic nurse.

The exigency exception applies to situations in which the police must act hastily to enter a location in order to prevent the loss of evidence, to alleviate danger to life, or to prevent the escape of a wanted felon. Furthermore, when police come upon the scene of a homicide or serious assault, they may perform certain legitimate emergency activities without a warrant. At such a scene, the police may make a search for other victims or for suspects and may seize any evidence that they find in plain view during these legitimate emergency activities (*Mincey v. Arizona*, 1978).

The plain view doctrine allows law enforcement officers who are in a place where they have a legal right to be to seize any item that they have probable cause to believe is evidence of a crime.

A properly executed consent to search constitutes another exception to the warrant requirement of the Fourth Amendment. A valid consent to search must be freely and voluntarily given by a person who is capable of giving that consent. A reviewing court will examine various factors including age, education, intelligence, and physical condition to decide if the person is capable of giving a valid consent. As a result, police may inquire of a nurse as to whether an individual is competent to give consent. Police officers often will prefer a written consent because it is usually easier to establish in court than a verbal consent. Although the person giving consent is not required to have direct physical control over the item that is the object of the consent, that person must have mutual authority over the property or must have joint use of the item if it is shared property. Sometimes this means that a parent may legally consent to a search of his or her child's belongings.

Caretaker searches occur when law enforcement officials seize property as part of their caretaking function. The courts rarely utilize this exception; some of the few situations in which it has come up involve the seizure of clothing cut off of a patient by a nurse or EMT. Such removal of clothing has been held to constitute abandonment of neither the clothing nor any possessions contained within the clothing. Nevertheless, the seizure of such property may be upheld under the caretaker exception, because the items were taken into custody to protect them and take care of them. In some jurisdictions, a warrant or consent will be required before any further examination or testing can be performed on items seized under the caretaker exception.

When an arrestee is taken into lawful custody, the police may seize his or her clothing as an incident of that arrest. This is often referred to as a station house seizure of clothing, and it is done to preserve the clothing for evidence and for forensic examination and testing. An arrestee's clothing can be a valuable source of evidence, including bodily fluids, hair, and trace evidence. "Stop and frisk" and the car doctrine are two additional exceptions associated with law enforcement activities when there is no arrest.

In conclusion, the Fourth Amendment protects citizens from unreasonable searches and seizures. These rights are individual and must be asserted by the person whose privacy interests have been impacted. Therefore, when a victim is examined, and evidence is seized from the victim, the offender cannot claim a Fourth Amendment violation because the offender's reasonable expectation of privacy is not involved. Only the victim's expectation of privacy is involved in such an examination. A defendant's Fourth Amendment rights are personal and must arise from his or her own reasonable expectation of privacy.

Chain of Custody

When clothing or evidence is seized from a victim of a crime, some common legal challenges to the admission of that evidence are based upon improper chain of custody, contamination of the evidence, or spoliation of the evidence.

The law requires that a proper chain of custody be kept on seized evidence to the extent necessary to provide a reasonable assurance to the court that the evidence to be introduced is the same evidence that was seized by the police and that its condition is substantially unchanged. Therefore, unique or individualized items will generally require a less strict chain of custody than generic or fungible items. When evidence is seized during a medical examination of a victim, it is very important to properly document who has obtained the evidence, who packaged the evidence, and the police officer to whom any evidence was given. All of these steps are necessary to ensure a proper chain of custody. Claims that evidence was contaminated can involve situations where samples are mixed or improperly packaged. Spoliation of evidence can occur when an item is not properly preserved, when it is discarded, or when relevant evidence is not seized and is therefore lost.

Expert Opinion

Pursuant to Rule 702 of the Federal Rules of Evidence (2003), an expert may render opinion testimony:

If scientific, technical, or other specialized knowledge will assist the trier of fact to understand the evidence or to determine a fact in issue, a witness qualified as an expert by knowledge, skill, experience, training, or education, may testify thereto in the form of an opinion or otherwise, if

1. the testimony is based upon sufficient facts or data.
2. the testimony is the product of reliable principles and methods.
3. the witness has applied the principles and methods reliably to the facts of the case.

Before allowing such expert testimony, the court may examine the expert's credentials and qualifications to make sure that the witness is qualified to render an expert opinion. Nurses have been qualified to render relevant opinions in courts in the United States. The specific science that an expert like a nurse is testifying about may also be reviewed by the court and must be found to be reliable. The case of *Daubert v. Merrill Dow Pharmaceuticals* (1993) controls the admission of expert testimony and requires that before an expert is allowed to testify, his or her science must pass through the following gatekeeper test for expert testimony:

1. The scientific theory or technique can be and has been tested.
2. The theory or technique has been subjected to peer review and publication.
3. The scientific technique has a known or potential rate of error or follows set standards.
4. The theory or technique has general acceptance in the relevant scientific community.

Essentially, the *Daubert* gatekeeper test guarantees that any expert testimony given by a nurse be about a scientific theory or technique that has been established as valid and reliable. The thrust of the *Daubert* case was to make sure that courts don't admit junk science or untested theories.

Statements

Questions frequently arise about the admissibility of statements that are obtained in a hospital. Such statements may be obtained from defendants who are receiving treatment and are being questioned by the police. Sometimes statements from victims or other witnesses are given while seeking treatment and become part of the hospital record. The law makes provisions concerning the admissibility or inadmissibility of these various statements.

When a defendant makes a statement in a hospital or in the presence of a nurse, that statement may be admissible as evidence against the offender at trial. Some important legal requirements must be met before the defendant's statement will be admitted into evidence. If the defendant was in police custody at the time of questioning, then he must be advised of his rights pursuant to *Miranda v. Arizona* (384 U.S. 436, 86 S.Ct. 1602 [1966]) before questioning begins. The defendant must waive these rights and agree to talk to the police. Another constitutional requirement that must be met in order for an offender's confession to be admitted is voluntariness. In order for a statement by a defendant to be admitted in court, the statement must have been "the product of his free and rational choice" (*Mincey v. Arizona,p. 398,* 1978). If the defendant's physical condition is impaired to the degree that she cannot exercise her free and rational choice, then her statement will not be admitted in court. As a result of this rule, police will frequently check with the nurse or head nurse in a hospital before questioning a suspect. The fact of hospitalization does not preclude a finding of voluntariness of a confession. The court will review each situation on a case-by-case basis to assess whether a defendant was capable of giving a voluntary statement. It is not uncommon for police to request the presence of medical personnel when they take a statement or confession from a hospitalized person. This is done to ensure that the police officer will not be accused of overriding the suspect's free will and so that medical personnel will be available to testify accurately concerning the suspect's condition and ability to speak with the police.

Although many out-of-court statements are excluded from evidence by the hearsay rule, the statement of a victim or witness made for the purpose of medical diagnosis or treatment is admissible under an exception to the hearsay rule. The following reflect Rule 803 (4) of the Federal Rules of Evidence concerning hearsay exceptions:

> Statements made for purposes of medical diagnosis or treatment and describing medical history, or past or present symptoms, pain, or sensations, or the inception or general character of the cause or external source thereof in so far as reasonably pertinent to diagnosis or treatment. (Federal Rules of Evidence, Rule 803[4], 2003)

This hearsay exception is carved out to specifically address the situation of an individual presenting himself to a hospital for diagnosis or treatment. Statements made to a doctor or nurse can fall under this exception to the hearsay rule, and if so, will be admissible into evidence. This exception is relevant when a sexual assault victim presents at the hospital, and it allows such hearsay statements to be presented in court. Therefore, the importance of accurately recording statements made by victims and witnesses in the medical record is obvious for both medical and legal purposes.

In addition, some states have a doctrine called constancy of accusation, wherein certain statements made by rape victims within a short time after the crime are admissible as evidence. It is not unusual for a nurse to be a constancy of accusation witness, specifically in the context of a prompt report and presentation for treatment by the victim. Again, the laws of each state apply, and there is wide variation in the existence and application of this hearsay doctrine.

Victims' Rights

All states have some form of assistance for victims of crime, and every state has passed some type of statute to provide assistance to victims. In fact, some states have enacted constitutional amendments to their state constitutions that can afford substantial rights to victims of crime. Some of the statutory provisions that have been passed to assist victims include notification requirements, compensation for various types of economic loss, rape shield laws, protection of personal information, and the right to be heard in court. Because significant differences exist among the states on the rights that are afforded to victims, it is necessary to review each state's statutes in order to ascertain which rights are provided to a victim in a specific state.

Potential victims also have a right to be notified of certain dangers. If a person seeing a therapist, which can include a psychiatric nurse, gives reasonable cause to believe the patient is dangerous to a third person, then the therapist has a duty to warn that potential victim (*Tarasoff v. The Regents of the University of California*, 1976).

Individual states may afford their citizens, including victims and wrongdoers, greater rights than the U.S. Constitution provides (in other areas of constitutional and statutory law that are discussed in this appendix). In other words, the U.S. Constitution sets the minimal level of constitutional rights that must be afforded to every citizen. The states may give their citizens greater, but never less, protection than the federal constitution.

TABLE A1-1 Other Relevant Legal Citations

Exclusionary rule	*Mapp v. Ohio,* 367 U.S. 643, 81 S.Ct. 1684 (1961).
Standing	*Rawlings v. Kentucky,* 448 U.S. 98, 100 S.Ct. 2565 (1980).
Plain view	*Horton v. California,* 496 U.S. 128, 110 S.Ct. 2301 (1990).
Consent	*Schneckloth v. Bustamonte,* 412 U.S. 218, 193 S.Ct. 2041 (1973).
Third-party consent	*United States v. Matlock,* 415 U.S. 164, 94 S.Ct. 988 (1974).
Caretaker	*Cady v. Dombrowski,* 413 U.S. 433, 93 S.Ct. 2523 (1973); *State v. Joyce,* 229 Conn. 10 (1994).
Search incident	*United States v. Edwards,* 415 U.S. 800, 94 S.Ct. 1234 (1974).
Accusation constancy/consistency	*State v. Roldan,* 257 Conn. 156 (2001).

Summary

Forensic nurses practice at the crossroads of law and medicine. They are in a field where knowledge of both medicine and law is essential. Although their emphasis is on the science of nursing, to be forensic, they must also learn the law. The rulings in **Table A1-1** outline several other relevant court decisions on evidence search and seizure.

REFERENCES

Daubert v. Merrill Dow Pharmaceuticals, 509 U.S. 579, 113 S.Ct. 2786 (1993).
Federal Rules of Evidence (2003) Public Law 93-595.
Katz v. U.S., 389 U.S. 347, 88 S.Ct. 507 (1967).
Mincey v. Arizona, 437 U.S. 385, 98 S.Ct. 2408 (1978).
Tarasoff v. The Regents of the University of California, 17 Cal. 3d. 425; 551 P.2d 334 (Ca.1976).
U.S. Const. amend. IV.

APPENDIX 3

Photography in Forensic Nursing

Kenneth B. Zercie and Paul Penders

> ## CASE A2.1
>
> *A child was brought to the emergency department of a city hospital with what was reported by her parents as an animal bite. Suspicions were aroused for various reasons and hospital personnel were concerned that the child was a victim of abuse. The nurse on duty in the emergency department was trained in forensic photographic documentation. The bite marks on the child's legs were photographed with and without a scale, using a digital camera. The bite mark images were retained in the patient's records according to hospital protocols. Swabs were also taken of the bite mark areas, but no DNA profiles were developed from this evidence. After a brief investigation, the parents were arrested and charged with child abuse. They were subsequently found guilty and the father was sentenced to several years' incarceration.*
>
> *The photographs of the bite marks taken by the nurse were obtained by the appellate attorney and submitted to a forensic dentist for examination. The expert was able to use the scaled photographs to demonstrate that the appearance and dimensions of the bite marks were not consistent with a human bite. This photographic evidence was sufficient to secure additional tests of the swabs, which revealed DNA from a canine. Because of the accurate and appropriate photographic documentation of the child's injuries, justice was obtained for an innocent man.*

Introduction

The forensic nurse is faced with the same challenges that any investigator has with respect to photography. He or she must understand the importance of being able to create good quality images of any observations, knowing that those pictures may be used in a court of law as documentation that an injury or event took place. The ability to capture an image using instant imaging, film, video, or digital media is critical for the patient, client, investigator, and judicial system. Proper photographic documentation lets all concerned parties see at a later time and place the forensic nurse's firsthand observations. The use of only verbal descriptions can leave out much detail. Written notes allow for interpretation, even if testimony is given as to what the forensic nurse is trying to communicate. Images that present a true and accurate rendering will facilitate the understanding of others when they supplement written notes and sketches. Images also provide for the possibility that an independent evaluation may be necessary as part of a case or incident. The forensic nurse recording an image does not have to be an expert in the field of photography but should possess the technical skill and basic knowledge necessary to perform the function well and defend his or her choices in a court of law, if required to do so.

Photographic Equipment

This appendix will deal with the traditional camera, lens, film, procedures, techniques, image composition, and exposure. Most of these items and principles apply to both film and digital photography. Digital imaging has recently become very popular, and a section on digital photography is included. The application of digital imaging differs from traditional film mostly by the methodology of capture.

The Camera, Lens, and Film

The camera is the basic component of the photographer's equipment.

Most 35-mm single lens reflex cameras function in a similar fashion (i.e., image viewing is done through the lens). Several controls are present on the camera, including the shutter button, film advance and rewind cranks, shutter speed, film speed, and exposure. A light meter is also used to determine proper shutter speed and aperture settings, which allow one to properly expose an image onto a piece of film. Manual cameras allow photographers to adjust all of these settings as they see fit for each situation. Many modern cameras have internal computers that will automatically set the camera to take an average exposure of a scene. In most cases these automatic settings will provide acceptable images for basic documentation purposes. The automatic modes are: program, aperture priority, and shutter speed priority.

The camera is designed to allow various types of lenses to be attached to the camera body. The camera lens is essentially a series of lenses that collect light and focus it on the film plane. The aperture (f-stop) of the lens controls the amount of light passing through the lens to the film plane. The aperture works much like the iris of the eye, decreasing in diameter in bright light and opening wider in low light. A focusing ring allows the photographer to bring items into clear view in the viewfinder and thus into focus on the film plane. Another important indicator on most lenses is the depth of field indicator. Pairings of aperture numbers appear on the barrel of the lens. Once the image is in focus the photographer can look at the measurement on the distance scale and determine the area of the object (composition) that is in sharp, acceptable focus.

Basic Photography

The following factors are necessary to produce a good, clear, sharp image:

» The proper amount of light must reach the film.
» The focus must be accurate.
» The equipment must be steady and free of movement.

The Amount of Light

The amount of light entering the camera is controlled by the size of the aperture opening, the speed of the shutter, and the speed of the film if traditional film medium is used, identified by its ASA/ISO numbers. The aperture or lens opening controls the amount of light entering the camera. The aperture openings are designed with a mathematical progression, where each succeeding lens opening (f-stop) allows either one half or twice the amount of light to strike the film than the preceding f-stop. In this context, f stands for the focal length of the lens when focused at infinity. The f-stops commonly found on most cameras are f-1.4, f-2.0, f-2.8, f-4, f-5.6, f-8, f-11, f-16, f-22, and f-32. The lower the number of the f-stop, the larger the iris opening is. For example, f-8 (1/8) allows one half the light of f-5.6 (1/5.6) to fall on the film plane; f-11 (1/11) allows twice as much light as f-16 (1/16), the next highest f-stop.

The shutter speed is the second method used to control the amount of light entering the camera. This control, much like the aperture openings, is designed in a mathematical progression and will either cut in half or double the amount of time the shutter will remain open, allowing light to pass through the aperture to the film. Common shutter speeds of a camera range from several seconds to one thousandth of a second. The letter B on the shutter dial indicates *bulb*. When the shutter is set at B, it stays open as long as the shutter button remains depressed. This setting is used for taking timed exposures or when using a technique called painting with light.

When traditional film medium is used, the third method that controls film exposure is the film speed. The film speed rating indicates the film's capacity to absorb light. The number ratings are known as ASA (American Standards Association) or ISO (International Organization for Standardization) and are the same throughout the film manufacturing industry. A low ASA number, such as 25 or 64, indicates a low-speed film; that is, the capacity of the film to absorb light is low. This type of film would be ideal for photographing fixed objects, laboratory imaging, or copy work when fine detail is needed. Slower film has the ability to record in greater detail. Medium-speed film would have an ASA rating of 100 or 200. This type of film is ideal for general daylight photography and recording of scenes and evidence. When used with an electronic flash, medium-speed film may also be used in limited-distance, low-light situations. High-speed films would have an ASA of 400 or higher, and will allow you to use a faster shutter speed to stop action.

The forensic nurse should be aware that all film is not balanced for daylight photography (sunlight or electronic flash). If such is not the lighting situation, the nurse may need to employ color correction filters. For all general photography and overall documentation, daylight type film can usually be used successfully.

There may be occasions when taking photographs that are critical to an investigation present circumstances that will fool the meter. For example, subjects dressed in all white or all black will fool the meter, resulting in either too much or too little exposure. To avoid this situation, the photographer should bracket exposures by altering the f-stops.

Supplemental Lighting

Many images will require the use of electronic flash to supplement or replace the lack of light. Experience has shown that the full-time use of an electronic flash can aid the photographer in establishing repeatable exposures, removing shadows, and balancing the light when artificial lighting is present. Cameras have connectors to mount an electronic flash in a holder called the hot shoe. Some manual cameras still require a wire connection to the camera's X sync. Failure to properly seat the unit in the hot shoe or attach the sync cord to the correct terminal will result in an improper exposure. The recommended shutter speed and any speed slower will allow the flash to expose the film. However, at slow shutter speeds movement becomes a consideration. A common technique for indoor photography with a flash is to bounce the light off the ceiling. Generally this will give more even illumination for the subject and avoid harsh bright areas. Avoiding bright spots is important for the proper documentation of wounds and similar evidence. If the ceiling is of normal height and white in color, the flash can be bounced at the ceiling instead of the subject. When taking photographs of objects very close to the camera and flash unit, the forensic nurse should consider removing the flash and angling the light toward the object of interest. A clean handkerchief, Kimwipe® disposable wipe, or neutral density filter may also be used to reduce the intensity of the light being produced.

Focus

You can focus your camera on the subject in several ways. Many manual cameras have manual lenses that require the photographer to rotate a focusing ring on the lens until the subject is in sharp focus in the viewfinder or until the split image finder shows a vertical line in the viewfinder and the images come together.

Modern cameras have many advantages over the manual variety. With the advent of features such as auto-focus, auto-aperture, auto-shutter speed, auto-advance and rewind of film, program modes, and auto-flash synchronization, most of the guesswork is gone from traditional photography.

A photographer adjusts for factors that may affect photographic quality by using the various controls on the camera, choosing the proper light environment or flash, and selecting the appropriate film. Ultimately, the skill of the photographer can compensate for some limitations in any of these areas. By planning ahead, the forensic nurse can provide for the various types of photographs that he or she may be required to take for examination, documentation, and presentation in court.

Location and Subject Matter

Each of the following areas presents its own set of requirements, equipment, and specialized techniques. As the responsibility to document an item, scene, or individual changes, the conditions under which the images must be taken will also change. For these reasons, the forensic nurse photographer must have knowledge of the legal requirements, capability of the equipment, and how best to get the desired results for eventual presentation. Photographs are also used as evidence in court when presented as a true and accurate rendering of what is depicted. This true and accurate requirement means you must use photographic techniques appropriate for the situation. Although not all possible environments and their effect on the forensic nurse photographer can be addressed at this time, the following are some common situations that may affect documentation.

Crime and Death Scene Documentation

The scene of an incident creates the most challenging set of problems for the photographer. The photographer has no control over location, time of day, position of evidence, hazards that may be present, weather conditions, or other environmental factors that will affect how you complete your tasks. For example, a nurse death investigator may be required to document an outdoor scene in the middle of winter at the base of a mountain. The primary consideration is to know your responsibility at the scene. This includes how you interface with other investigative groups, such as the police, medical examiners, fire department and other emergency services personnel, and forensic scientists. It is important to remember that you are at the scene as part of a team. As with all teams, there are specific lines of authority and responsibility that should be clear to all involved. Knowledge of these factors will make documentation at the scene faster and easier and will likely facilitate efforts by the forensic nurse to learn supplemental information as part of his or her investigation.

The purpose of scene documentation is to record the location of evidence in its original position and condition before any alterations have taken place. Another use is as a reference for further investigation, deposition, courtroom presentation (both civil and criminal), and to refresh the memory. Photographs should be taken of the entire area of involvement showing spatial relationships of items, perspectives of witnesses, and views as noted by other involved parties at the scene. This initial documentation provides the forensic nurse and others with a firsthand representation of observations. An accurate depiction allows anyone to observe at a remote time and place what was seen and the conditions that existed at the moment you took the photograph. As noted previously, photographs do not stand alone as the only form of documentation; notes, video recordings, and sketches all complement each other and are essential supplements used to record the scene. When these documentation methods are combined during courtroom testimony, the trier of fact will have a clearer understanding of relevant observations. Proper photographic documentation will also help to establish the credibility of the forensic nurse as part of the investigative team.

There is no specific number of photographs to take at any given crime scene. Once an item or person has been moved from the scene or patterns have been cleaned up, the forensic investigator can never recover those images. Therefore, it is necessary to document all aspects of the scene as completely as possible.

Stepwise Approach to Incident and Scene Photography

The investigator often needs to photograph a scene quickly and accurately. Good planning before an incident will provide the forensic nurse with a basic set of procedures that can be modified, as necessary, to meet the specific needs of an individual case. The following are guidelines to follow when conducting photographic documentation at a scene.

1. Arrive at the incident scene as soon as possible. Check in with the individual in charge.
2. Check your equipment to ensure that it is operational.
3. Upon arrival, consult with the first responders and determine if the emergency is ongoing. Also, identify if anything has been disturbed.
4. If the others are still dealing with the emergency, begin to document the surrounding area and people at the scene, if practical.
5. Once the emergency is under control, determine the scope of the scene and walk through it with the initial responders. Caution should always be taken so as to not destroy evidence (e.g., footprints, tire tracks, etc.). (Polaroid and digital imaging may be useful at this time.)
6. Begin to document your way into the scene. Consideration should be given to using a point of entry not used by any suspects.
7. First photograph items that are perishable or will be lost if not immediately seized.

8. If working at a death scene, photograph the decedent in place before disturbing the body. Photograph both sides of the decedent when moved and the area underneath the body.

9. Photographs should follow a general three-shot sequence of overall, medium and close-up shots of each item of significance. This is often called the "rule of three."

   a. Photograph a minimum of four overviews (one from each corner perspective) of each room and specific areas of involvement and patterns.

   b. Take medium close-ups of each item of significant evidence as it relates to its immediate surroundings.

   c. Take close-ups of specific items of evidence as found or processed (e.g., pill bottles, footprints).

10. Photograph all hallways, stairways, entrances, and exits.

11. Rulers, surveys tapes, and other measuring devices may be necessary to document blood spatter patterns. Number stands or attention devices may be used to supplement the initial images; photograph both with and without the device, if used.

12. Photograph the scene using only existing light as well as with electronic flash.

13. Maintain a comprehensive record of the images taken.

14. Have the film processed and printed or print digital images as soon as possible; review and mark the photographs as required. Preserve the film because it can be considered evidence.

A well-designed photographic system configuration is shown in **Figure A2-1**. Such a configuration will help to ensure repeatable quality once the photographer is familiar with and has tested the equipment in controlled conditions. As a general rule, color negative film is recommended for crime scene use. If using traditional format, film having an ASA of 100, 200, or 400 should give sufficient sensitivity to light, good color rendering, and, when used with electronic flash, is adequate for most outdoor and nighttime photography.

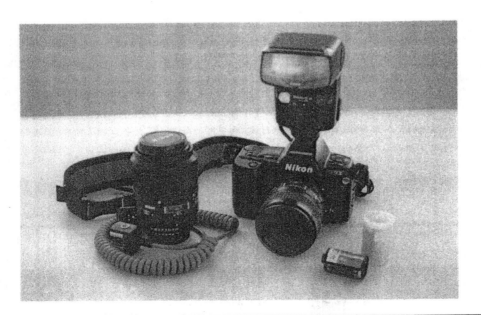

Figure A2-1 A well-designed photographic system includes a standard 35-mm camera, macro and zoom lenses, remote extension cord, electronic flash, and film.

Hospital Situations

The forensic nurse will be familiar with many of the situations in which the hospital is a setting for photographic documentation. Although the protocols of each institution may differ, written permission from the client is usually recommended prior to taking any photographs. Healthcare facilities do not always have clear protocols for the retention of photographs. Prior to taking any images, the forensic nurse should have established a procedure for proper storage of this type of documentation. Certainly client privacy and regulations such as HIPAA are considerations. In addition, improper storage of photographic records proffered for use as evidence could result in that evidence being barred from admission during trial. Before documenting injuries, the forensic nurse should always explain to the client why each photograph is being taken. It is important to exhibit great sensitivity to the client's physical comfort, emotional state, and need for privacy during this process. These concerns are best addressed if there are no interruptions during the photographic process and if the forensic nurse is familiar with the photographic equipment. The patient should be photographed in a position that creates the least amount of discomfort while still demonstrating the characteristics of the injury. In addition, it may be a good idea for the client to participate in the process, whenever possible. For example, the client can assist in draping and other acts to protect privacy and limit contact to achieve the correct photographic position. Often images taken in this setting are of a patient being treated for child abuse, domestic violence, sexual assault, physical assault, blunt trauma injuries, stab wounds, gunshot injuries, and surgical wounds.

Images of injuries, wounds, and scars should be taken both before and after treatment whenever practical, with the understanding that vital care for the patient always comes first. If images are to be taken after emergency procedures and while the patient is still in the hospital, then arrangements should be made with the treating physician and charge nurse if additional photographs are necessary to document injuries. For example, schedule time for the session during bandage changes to make the patient more comfortable. An overall photograph that shows the injury and the victim must be taken. In this way, the specific contusions, lacerations, and so on can be directly connected to the victim, because the close-up photograph of an injury must be linked to the victim in question. The use of a mirror may facilitate photographing the victim's face along with the injury itself. After documenting their locations, injuries must be photographed close up, with and without a scale. This documentation may be used for subsequent criminal and/or civil purposes. It is therefore important to consider the specific people who may use and access any photographs. To prevent an implication of bias or melodramatic court proceedings, the client should never be posed in an unnatural manner or to accentuate the injury for other than a scientific purpose.

The three-shot sequence described above and in Chapter 14 should be followed by a shot that gives the viewer the perspective of actually seeing the injury as observed at the time of treatment. An additional image is also required: a photograph of the injury or medical procedure using a scale of contrasting color. The American Board of Forensic Odontology standard scale is recommended since it will indicate any angles or contours in the wound area. Examples of various types of scales are shown in **Figure A2-2**. This scale is critical for pattern interpretation and the comparison with various edged or impact weapons to the injury. Including a scale allows better reproduction of the size and color. A scale also provides the necessary reference so that a life-size (1-to-1 ratio) image can be printed. Whenever possible, a color standard, such as a Macbeth

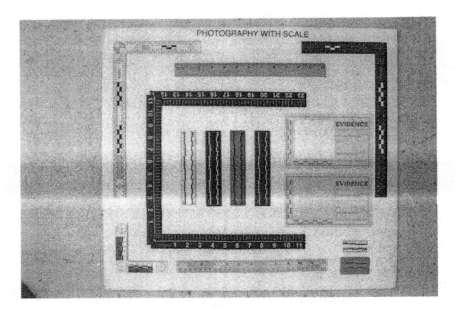

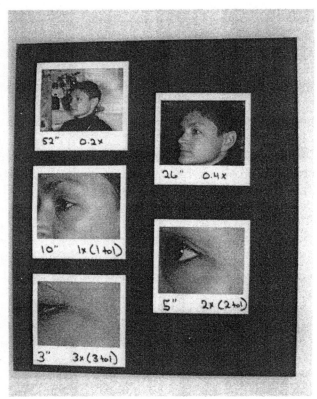

Figure A2-2 a/b Various types of scales available for photographic documentation are shown in the top photograph. The lower photograph shows how the use of scale and contrast facilitates subsequent examinations with enlargement to *life-size proportions for direct comparison.*

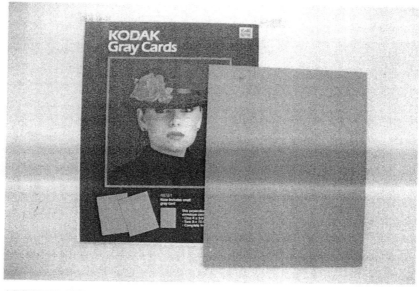

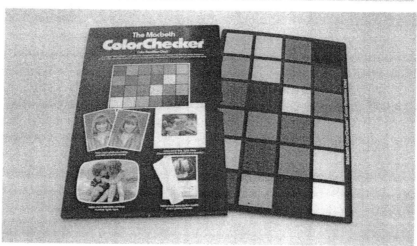

Figure A2-3 a/b Gray (upper photograph) and color (lower photograph) scales provide standards of color and exposure when images are printed. Use of scales is especially important to provide a true and accurate rendering when documenting injuries.

ColorChecker, or the Kodak Gray Card should be photographed under the same conditions as the area of interest (see **Figure A2-3**). Use of a color standard leads to more accurate reproduction and a truer rendering in the print. Although it is axiomatic that injuries must be documented before they heal, some injuries, such as bruises and bite marks, will become more apparent with the passage of time. Adequate images for scar evaluation may be difficult to produce with the flat lighting delivered by flash units built into a camera. Taking the time to use proper photographic procedures will give some creditability to the interpretation of bruises and wounds based on the color in the photographs, such as when aging bite marks.

Autopsy

The autopsy room presents several restrictions when documenting a deceased individual. The protocols of the agency and the needs and concerns of the pathologist must be considered. Whenever possible, the images of a deceased should not show background equipment such as tables or tools. A background of an 18% gray tone (standard color for all exposure balancing) provides a suitable backdrop in most instances. Photographs of the decedent should proceed in a logical sequence and should be taken from all angles. Close-up photographs of the face, injuries, clothing, footwear, and any other items of evidence or patterns of interest need to be taken prior to the removal of any garments. As layers of garments are removed, the documentation process should be repeated until the body is completely exposed. Additional images of the decedent should be taken after any blood or debris is removed or cleaned. These photographs will more clearly reveal the extent of injuries and damage.

Depending on the cause of death (homicide, suicide, accidental, natural, or undetermined), it may be advisable to document the body and evidence using an alternate light source. Available alternate light includes not only the commonly used ultraviolet lamp (Wood's lamp), but also a laser or variable-wavelength forensic light sources. Alternate light sources are particularly useful in identifying body fluid deposits and may provide better examination of the details of an injury pattern. This may be done when the decedent is received, as well as before and after clothing and areas of stain are removed. Alternate light may also enhance patterns and injury. Items that fluoresce must be documented before collection to show their location and relationship to the body. Photographs taken using alternate light sources follow the same metering and exposure guidelines as previously discussed. The program mode on automatic cameras is recommended, as is the use of a tripod to stabilize the image during long exposures. A barrier filter the same color as the viewing goggles must be used in front of the lens. **Table A2-1** identifies the recommended films, filters, and corresponding wavelengths to be used when photographing fluorescence or luminescence.

TABLE A2-1   Photographic Filters, Films, and Wavelengths

Color	Wavelength	Viewing/Camera Filter or Equivalent	Film Type
Ultraviolet	360–400 nm	Kodak Wratten	B&W, Color
Yellow	400–450 nm	Nos. 2A, 2B, 12 Absorption Kodak Wratten	B&W, Color
		No. 8 Yellow	
Blue-Green	450–540 nm	Kodak Wratten	B&W, Color
Blue	540–700 nm	No. 21, 22 Orange Kodak Wratten	B&W, Color
		No. 25 Red	
Infrared	700–1100 nm	Kodak Filters Nos. 15, 25, 29, 70, 87, 88A, and 87C	B&W high speed IR ektachrome Infrared

Evidence Documentation

Any item of interest in an investigation should be considered as evidence. Chapter 14 discusses in detail the proper recognition, documentation, and collection of physical evidence. The following discussion provides a general guideline for only the photographic documentation of evidence of interest. All evidence must first be documented in the place where it was found. These photographs show the condition of the evidence and its relationship with other items of interest. Evidence pictures generally follow the three-shot sequence described in the "Crime and Death Scene Documentation" section of this appendix. (See **Figure A2-4**) One additional image is usually necessary when specific items are documented—the fourth picture in this series is the specific item of interest with a scale. These additional images with a scale may be taken at the scene or under controlled circumstances, such as a laboratory, office, examination room, or studio. The use of a copy stand may be helpful for this detailed documentation at a later time, especially if an alternate light source is used. These additional photographs are critical because they are also used for comparison and analysis by other forensic examiners.

If evidence is to be processed, enhanced, or altered in any way, images should be taken at each step to document the process. Most processing methodologies alter, destroy, or change the evidence from its original condition. Capturing images at each step will preserve the item or pattern so that any following alternations will not interfere with the value that may have preceded the next examination. Once you destroy the patterns or remove the evidence it can never be put back to its original condition.

Flash Usage at the Scene

The photographer can take advantage of light-colored walls and ceilings to provide soft, even illumination when documenting an area. This procedure is called the bounce flash technique. When the flash is aimed at these surfaces, the flash will reflect off of them (bounce back), giving an indirect lighting effect. Using a bounce effect will eliminate intensity differences in the lighting and fall off that can produce sharp and distracting shadows. This type of lighting is useful when trying to show the orientation of several objects at various distances from the camera lens. The bounce flash technique also may provide additional details and eliminate misleading shadows.

Digital Photography in Forensic Nursing

The use of digital imaging or digital photography is the most common methodology used today. Some of the principal benefits of digital capture are:

» The photographer is independent of other photographic processing labs, and images can be processed and printed by a computer.
» The photographer can reasonably (but not critically) proof the image directly on the camera screen. In other words, the anxiety of whether the images came out can be relieved by proofing it on the spot before altering or releasing the subject. Because the victim may be covered with dressings obscuring the injury or other important details, photographing the body area to be covered beforehand may be important.

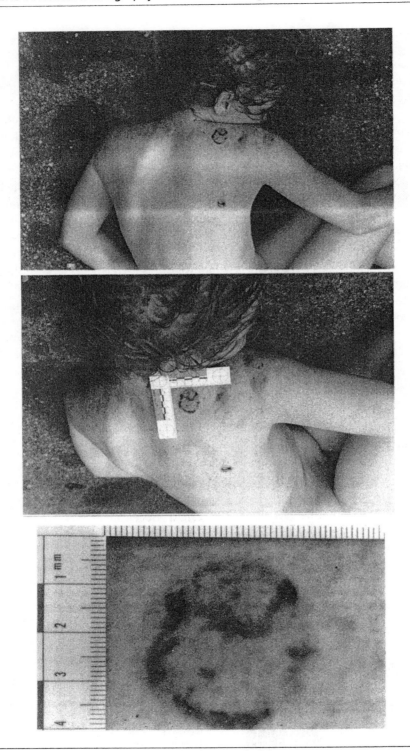

Figure A2-4 a/b/c Documentation at a homicide scene by a death investigator using the three-step photographic process. The top picture depicts an overall view of the decedent as she was found at the scene; the middle photograph is a closer view of her upper torso showing an area of injury; the last picture is a close-up view of the bite mark on the decedent's shoulder. (Note a scale has been placed in the area for size reference.)

» Viewing and critically evaluating the image on a monitor is the preferred method, because the image delivered to the camera's built-in display is quite small and of low resolution or quality.
» A digital file is capable of being exactly reproduced any number of times. The 20th copy is of the same quality as the original.

It is these characteristics of digital photography that have made it the method of choice for quick documentation and storage of multiple images. The choice of camera and the type of storage medium that the camera uses are critical considerations for the forensic nurse. As shown in **Figure A2-5**, digital cameras can range from expensive, professional style to affordable consumer models. The forensic nurse can view the subject on a screen as soon as the photograph is taken. Thus, the photographer can decide immediately if it is necessary to rephotograph the subject. If additional photographs are necessary, this can be done with minimal change in the environment or discomfort to the subject. When choosing a camera or other digital capture device, image quality is of great importance. Image quality is usually stated in megapixels. Image sizes typically used in e-mail attachments and for Internet display (72 dots per inch) are unsuitable for evidentiary documentation and/or analysis. A camera used for documentation should be toward the higher end of the scale in image quality. The final output will be only as good as the captured images.

Digital cameras also come with enhancements. For example, there should be a white balance capability as well as the ability to set your capture device to the light source (fluorescent, incandescent, daylight, electronic flash, etc.). Most digital systems also provide some close-up photographic capability. The extent to which the photographer can zoom in on the subject to capture close details is of particular importance when imaging contusions, lacerations, damage to clothing, and similar alterations. After photographs are taken, the forensic nurse must consider additional, practical parameters:

» How will the images be output? Will they be printed, transmitted via a network, or burned to a CD/DVD?
» Which software will you use for organization, display, access, and archiving of your images? Will it be the software included with the camera or something more specialized such as iPhoto, Adobe Album, or ImageAXS Pro?

The cost of a professional or advanced amateur digital camera system is in excess of $400. Although a serviceable, consumer-oriented capture device may be purchased for less, not all cameras are suitable for proper evidentiary documentation. Most cameras produced today are geared toward typical amateur snapshot usage such as birthday parties, graduations, sports events, and vacation scenes. At the very least, any digital camera used by the forensic nurse should be capable of producing quality close-up photographs.

Because many images taken by the forensic nurse may need to be accessed years from the date of capture, he or she must make every attempt to use a system that will allow this access. Thus, it is a real concern whether the software that created the files will soon be obsolete and whether the storage media will still be widely used, or at least readable, when the photographs are required. Also, forensic nurses' working environment may be unsafe for some digital image capture devices. Electromagnetic radiation, such as microwaves, can adversely affect or erase images on digital storage media, while liquid crystal displays on any camera can be damaged when brought in proximity to magnetic resonance imaging devices.

Digital image capture is well suited for low-volume output; that is, for images that will be stored and displayed or viewed electronically on a monitor or printed in very small

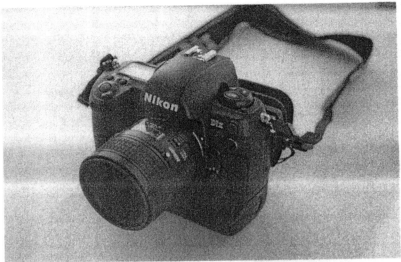

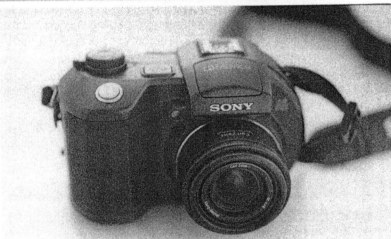

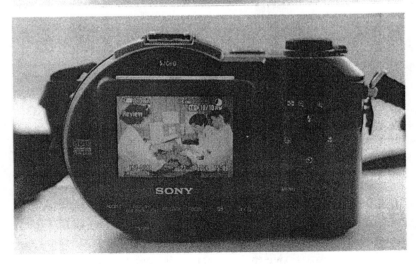

Figure A2-5 a/b/c A professional-style digital camera is shown in the top photograph. A front view and the viewing screen of a consumer-style digital camera are shown in the lower figures.

quantities. When the images are printed on paper, quality paper and inks must be used to produce quality photographs that show the detail required in court. In addition, characteristics of images printed on a desktop printer are typically poor because they tend to shift color. Color may play a key issue in a true and accurate representation of evidence that is of concern to the forensic nurse. Printer images also fade rapidly, especially when displayed. The cost of storage media for archiving digital images is also a concern. Additional media must be purchased and redundancy is often urged by experts in digital imaging. Clearly, photographs produced for criminal, civil, and death investigations must be handled and preserved to address legal admissibility and authenticity issues. The forensic nurse must be prepared to respond to questions concerning the potential for alteration or loss of digital images.

Photography in the Courtroom

Photographs are usually offered by the forensic nurse as demonstrative evidence (i.e., to show the existence of fact as depicted in the photograph). Although a more detailed discussion of evidence admissibility can be found in Chapter 20, this section addresses several issues specifically related to the use of photographs in the courtroom. The first area of concern relates to the training and experience of the photographer; the second set of issues concerns the photograph itself.

In most circumstances the forensic nurse has had some training in proper photographic documentation techniques. Some forensic nurses may enroll in courses on advanced scene techniques and procedures in specific environments, such as in the emergency room. However, few forensic nurses have extensive training and experience in photography that includes technical issues using various cameras, film, and lighting techniques. However, the fact that photography is not the primary function of the forensic nurse is not necessarily a problem. As a trained forensic observer, the forensic nurse must be able to state conclusively that the photograph accurately depicts the object or location recorded on film. If the photographs are used as part of the documentation record, information related to what was photographed and any special lighting or other techniques must be noted. The forensic nurse must know the effects of these procedures and the equipment used on the image in the photograph. It is important that the nurse photographer take many test shots under various conditions using the available equipment prior to use in an actual case. This experience will provide the forensic nurse with the background necessary to take photographs confidently. Some attorneys may attempt to draw the forensic nurse into a discussion of the fine points of photographic theory and camera operation. A witness should not hesitate to say, "I don't know" when asked a technical question concerning the photographic process. In most cases such knowledge will have little relevance to the accuracy and reliability of the photograph. If the forensic nurse follows the guidelines for thorough and appropriate photographic documentation, most images will be useful for future study or admission during testimony.

As stated previously, the primary purpose for photographic documentation by the forensic nurse is to provide a clear and accurate record of what was seen at the time of the incident. As such, a person (the photographer or someone else present) testifies in court to the accuracy of the depiction. It is this testimony—the authentication of the image—that is most significant. The photograph is used to convey to the trier of fact the appearance of the scene, evidence, or injury. In essence, the witness testifies to the condition observed, using the photograph as a means to demonstrate those observations. Although some differences between photographs and other demonstrative evidence have been noted by the courts, the witness is usually required to provide an explanation of the circumstances surrounding the production of an image. The opposing attorney will make every attempt, when appropriate, to point out discrepancies or variations between the witness's oral description or other witnesses' observations and the photographic depiction. Similarly, problems with the photographic technique may result in purported misrepresentations that can keep a photograph from the jury's inspection. Ultimately, the court will make every effort to see that a complete and accurate representation is shown in an image. For example, if only a close-up photograph of an injury is shown, the jury may misinterpret the size and extent of an injury. When the court allows all of the photographs taken in step-wise documentation, it ensures an accurate record for the jury to consider. Similarly, the court may limit the number of photographs admitted when a scene or injury is particularly gruesome. By limiting the exposure of the jury to such potentially shocking depictions, the court limits the potentially unfair bias that may be created in some of the jury as a result of the natural, human response to such evidence. If the forensic nurse is familiar with documentation guidelines and the abilities and limitations of available equipment, he or she can readily satisfy the basic requirements for use of photographs in court.

The practice of forensic nursing involves numerous areas of specialization. Key to good practice in all of these areas is proper and complete documentation. Whenever documentation of physical characteristics, a pattern, or other physical evidence is required, some form of photography should always be used to supplement and enhance other forms of documentation. As discussed in this chapter, the forensic nurse has several options when choosing what photographic equipment to use in his or her practice. Whatever equipment and techniques are employed, the forensic practitioner should be facile enough with these to produce quality images that will satisfy any legal and scientific requirements for the use of the photographs.

SUGGESTED FURTHER READING

Blaker, A. A. (1989). *Handbook of scientific photography* (2nd ed.). Stoneham, MA: Butterworth.

Davies, A., & Fennessy, P. (1998). *Digital imaging for photographers* (3rd ed.). Woburn, MA: Focal Press.

Davis, P. (1995). *Photography* (7th ed.). Stoneham, MA: Butterworth.

Hedgecoe, J. (1982). *The photographer's handbook* (2nd ed.). New York, NY: Random House.

Ledray, L. (2008). Consent to photograph: How far should disclosure go? *Journal of Forensic Nursing, 4*(4), 188–189.

McDonald, J. A. (1992a). *Close-up & macro photography* (2nd ed.). Arlington Heights, IL: PhotoText Books.

McDonald, J. A. (1992b). *The police photographer's guide.* Arlington Heights, IL: PhotoText Books.

Miller, L. S. (1998). *Police photography.* Cincinnati, OH: Anderson.

Pasqualone, G. (1995). The importance of forensic photography in the emergency department. *Journal of Emergency Nursing, 21*(6), 566–567.

Redsicker, D. R. (2001). *The practical methodology of forensic photography.* Boca Raton, FL: CRC Press.

Russ, J. C. (2001). *Forensic uses of digital imaging.* Boca Raton, FL: CRC Press.

Scott, C. C. (1969). *Photographic evidence* (Vols. 1–3). St. Paul, MN: West.

Vogley, E., Pierce, M., & Berbecci, G. (2002). Experience with wood lamp illumination and digital photography in the documentation of bruises on human skin. *Archieves of Pediatrics and Adolescent Medicine, 156*(3), 265–268.

APPENDIX 4

Selected Assessment Tools

The assessment tools included in this appendix may be useful in the evaluation of the forensic client. Forensic nursing practice involves treating or interfacing with clients from various age groups, ethnic groups, and socioeconomic levels and in a variety of settings. The reason for the client/nurse interaction may vary, ranging from treatment to risk assessment to preparation for trial. In order to provide the most effective intervention as well as establish needs and predictors for further interventions, various assessment tools have been created. It is essential that these tools be utilized by those who have the skills to administer, interpret, and draw conclusions from the data obtained. In order to develop a level of comfort and self-confidence in administering these tools, the nurse should review the action to be undertaken once the assessment has been completed. We have included selected international guidelines as well. Each chapter includes tools/guidelines specific to the content in that chapter. The practice of Forensic nursing continues to address previously unrecognized and/or unidentified populations; thus, the development of assessment tools is an ongoing challenge as we broaden the scope of practice in the 21st century.

Nurses must consider HIPAA and ethical guidelines and have informed consent prior to undertaking any assessment procedures. We have listed only a sample of the many varied assessment tools available to the forensic nurse—the large number of possibilities exceeds the scope of this appendix. The resources identified in this appendix represent a sampling of guidelines currently available, and at times represent "works in progress" to be further developed by those practicing in the field. The forensic nurse should research the various assessment tools available for specific purposes. The Internet is an invaluable source of information, as are peer review, networking, and the exchange of information among colleagues. Any screening tool or scale must be culturally sensitive and age appropriate, and utilize language that the client can understand. Assessment tools may not exist for certain forensic client populations. The role of the forensic nurse as researcher and collaborator becomes even more important in those situations.

Assessment Tools

Children & Adolescents

Dienemann, J., Campbell, J., Landenborrer, K., & Curry, M. A. (March 2002). The domestic violence survivor assessment: A tool for counseling women in intimate partner violence relationships. Patient Education and Counseling, 46, 221–228.

Otto, R. K., Douglas, K. S., (Eds.) (2009). Handbook of Violence Risk Assessment. International Perspective of Forensic Mental Health. New York, NY: Taylor & Francis Group.

Sherdan, D. J. (1988). The Harassment Instrument. Available from Dshen.dan@son.jhml.edu.

Council on Scientific Affairs. (1992). Violence against women relevance for medical practitioners. Journal of the American Medical Association, 267(23), 3184–3189.

Balaban, R., Stanger, V., Haruvi, R., Zur, S., & Ausarten, A. (2002) Suspected child abuse and neglect: Assessment in a hospital setting. Israel Medical Association Journal, 4, 617–623.

Elder Abuse

Wolf, R. (2003). Risk assessment instruments. Available from http://www.ncea.aoa.gov/ncearoot/
main_site/library/Statistics_Research/Research_Reviews/risk_assessment.aspx
Reis, M., & Nahmiash, D. (1998). Indicators of abuse screen. *The Gerontologist, 38*(4), 471–480.
Fulmer, T., Guadango, L., Bitondo, C., & Connolly, M. (2004). Progess in Elder Abuse Screening
and Assessment Instruments. *The American Geriatric Society.* Retrieved from: http://www.chcr.
brown.edu/PDFS/FULMER_ELDER_ABUSE_TOOL_2004.PDF

Post-traumatic Stress Disorder

National Center for Post-Traumatic Stress Disorder (2011): http://www.ptsd.va.gov/
This resource provides clinicians and researchers with descriptive, reference, and contact information
about child and adult measures of trauma exposure and response. This is a very valuable site
for the forensic nurse; however, there are strict ethical guidelines related to administration of
assessment tools.
American Psychiatric Association. (2000). Diagnostic and statistical manual IV-TR. Washington,
DC: Author.

Teen/Adolescence

Center for Disease Control and Prevention Youth Risk Behavior Surveillance System. Washington,
DC: Department of Health and Human Services. Retrieved from http://www.cdc.gov/
HealthyYouth/yrbs/index.htm
Merell, K. W. (2003). (2nd ed.). Behavioral, social, and emotional assessment of children and
adolescents. Mahwah, NJ: Lawrence Erlbaum Associates.

Domestic Violence/Intimate Partner Abuse

Centers for Disease Control and Prevention: Division of Violence Prevention (2011). http://www.
cdc.gov/ViolencePrevention/index.html
Chalk, R. (2000). Assessing family violence interventions: Linking programs to research based
strategies. *Journal of Aggression Maltreatment and Trauma, 4*(1), 29–53.
Knopp, P., Hart, S., Webster, C., & Evans, D. (1995). Manual for the spousal risk assessment guide.
Vancouver, Canada: British Columbia Institute on Family Violence.
McFarlane, J., & Parker, B. (1994). Abuse during pregnancy—A protocol for prevention and
intervention. New York, NY: National March of Dimes, Birth Defects Foundation.
McFarlane, J., Hughes, R. B., Nosek, M. A., Groff, J. Y., Swedland, N., & Mullen, P. D. (2001).
Measuring frequency, type and perpetrator of abuse toward women with physical difficulties.
Journal of Women's Health and Gender-Based Medicine, 10(9), 861–866.
McFarlane, J., Parker, B., Soeken, K., & Bullock, L. (1992). Assessing for abuse during pregnancy.
Journal of the American Medical Association, 267(3), 3176–3178.
The Effect of Domestic Violence on Pregnancy and Labour. The College of Family Physicians
of Canada. Discussion paper January 28, 2000. Commissioned by the CFPC's Maternity and
Newborn Care Committee. Prepared by Lent B., Morris P. and Rechner, S.
National Domestic Violence Hotline 1-800-799-SAFE (7233)1-800-787-3224 (TTY)
Rape, Abuse & Incest National Network/New Haven Sexual Assault Hotline1-800-656-HOPE
1-800-656-4673 www.rainn.org

Civil Rights

American Civil Liberties Union. 125 Broad Street, 18th Floor, New York, NY 10004. 212-549-2500.
National Association for the Advancement of Colored People. http://www.naacp.org/content/main
The Leadership Conference. http://www.civilrights.org

Collective Violence

Centre for the Study of Violence and Reconciliation www.csvr.org.za
Internal Displacement Monitoring Centre www.internal-displacement.org

Elder Abuse

Action on Elder Abuse www.elderabuse.org.uk
International Network for the Prevention of Elder Abuse www.inpea.net
National Center on Elder Abuse www.ncea.aoa.gov/ncearoot/Main_Site/index.aspx
National Committee for the Prevention of Elder Abuse www.preventelderabuse.org
World Health Organization. Mental Health http://www.who.int/mental_health/en
Substance Abuse and Mental Health Services Administration. (SAMHSA). http://www.samhsa.gov

Mental Health

National Alliance for the Mentally Ill (NAMI) www.nami.org
National Institute of Mental Health (NIMH) www.nimh.nih.gov
Prevention Institute www.preventioninstitute.org/mental.html
Mental Health America (MHA) http://www.nmha.org

Migrant Workers

Association of Occupational and Environmental Clinics www.aoec.org
Migrant Clinicians Network www.migrantclinician.org
National Alliance for Hispanic Health www.hispanichealth.org
National Center for Farmworkers Health www.ncfh.org

Suicide

American Association of Suicidology www.suicidology.org
Suicide Prevention Advocacy network http://www.spanusa.org
Center for Disease Control and Prevention: Suicide Prevention. www.cdc.gov/ViolencePrevention/
    suicide
Violence Against Women
Global Alliance Against Traffic in Women www.gaatw.org
National Sexual Violence Resource Center www.nsvrc.org
Office of Violence vs. Women www.ovw.usdoj.gov
Research, Action and Information Network for the Bodily Integrity of Women www.rainbo.org
Women Against Violence Europe www.wave-network.org

Youth Violence

Center for the Prevention of School Violence www.juvjus.state.nc.us/cpsv
National Center for Injury Prevention and Control www.cdc.gov/injury
National Criminal Justice Reference Service www.ncjrs.org/intlwww.html

Organizations

Amnesty International www.amnesty.org
Centers for Disease Control and Prevention: National Center for Injury Prevention and Control
    http://www.cdc.gov/injury
Centro Latino-Americano de Estudos sobre Violencia e Saude www.ensp.fiocruz.br/portal-ensp/
    departamento/claves

Human Rights Watch www.hrw.org

Inter-American Coalition for the Prevention of Violence www.who.int/violenceprevention/about/participants/iacpv/en/index.html International Center for the Prevention of Crime www.crime-prevention-intl.org

Trauma.org www.trauma.org

United Nations Research Institute for Social Development www.unrisd.org

World Health Organization http://www.who.int/violence_injury_prevention/publications/surveillance/surveillance_guidelines/en/index.html (injury surveillance guidelines)

Index

Figures and tables are indicated by *f* and *t* following the page numbers.